Neuroanesthesiology Case Companion

Neuroanesthesiology Case Companion

Shailendra Joshi
MBBS MD (Anesthesiology) FFARCS (I)
Diplomate of the American Board of Anesthesiology
Associate Professor
Department of Anesthesiology
Columbia University
New York City, New York, USA

Foreword
William L Lanier

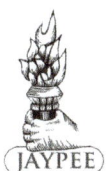

JAYPEE BROTHERS MEDICAL PUBLISHERS
The Health Sciences Publisher
New Delhi | London

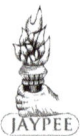 Jaypee Brothers Medical Publishers (P) Ltd

Headquarters
Jaypee Brothers Medical Publishers (P) Ltd
EMCA House, 23/23-B, Ansari Road, Daryaganj
New Delhi 110 002, India
Landline: +91-11-23272143, +91-11-23272703
+91-11-23282021, +91-11-23245672
Email: jaypee@jaypeebrothers.com

Corporate Office
Jaypee Brothers Medical Publishers (P) Ltd
4838/24, Ansari Road, Daryaganj
New Delhi 110 002, India
Phone: +91-11-43574357
Fax: +91-11-43574314
Email: jaypee@jaypeebrothers.com

Overseas Office
JP Medical Ltd
83 Victoria Street, London
SW1H 0HW (UK)
Phone: +44 20 3170 8910
Email: info@jpmedpub.com

EU GPSR Authorised Representative
Logos Europe, 9 rue Nicolas Poussin
17000, La Rochelle, France
Phone: +33 (0) 6 67 93 73 78
E-mail: Contact@logoseurope.eu

Website: www.jaypeebrothers.com
Website: www.jaypeedigital.com

© 2024, Jaypee Brothers Medical Publishers

The views and opinions expressed in this book are solely those of the original contributor(s)/author(s) and do not necessarily represent those of editor(s) or publisher of the book.

All rights reserved. No part of this publication may be reproduced, stored or transmitted in any form or by any means, electronic, mechanical, photocopying, recording or otherwise, without the prior permission in writing of the publishers.

All brand names and product names used in this book are trade names, service marks, trademarks or registered trademarks of their respective owners. The publisher is not associated with any product or vendor mentioned in this book.

Medical knowledge and practice change constantly. This book is designed to provide accurate, authoritative information about the subject matter in question. However, readers are advised to check the most current information available on procedures included and check information from the manufacturer of each product to be administered, to verify the recommended dose, formula, method and duration of administration, adverse effects and contraindications. It is the responsibility of the practitioner to take all appropriate safety precautions. Neither the publisher nor the author(s)/editor(s) assume any liability for any injury and/or damage to persons or property arising from or related to use of material in this book.

This book is sold on the understanding that the publisher is not engaged in providing professional medical services. If such advice or services are required, the services of a competent medical professional should be sought.

Every effort has been made where necessary to contact holders of copyright to obtain permission to reproduce copyright material. If any have been inadvertently overlooked, the publisher will be pleased to make the necessary arrangements at the first opportunity.

Inquiries for bulk sales may be solicited at: jaypee@jaypeebrothers.com

Neuroanesthesiology Case Companion

First Edition: 2024

ISBN: 978-93-90595-77-8

Dedicated to

The Residents and Fellows
Department of Anesthesiology, Columbia University
With the hope that they never forget that at the other end
of the needle is a person who is ailing, afraid, and anxious.
That they will always act with compassion, competence, and confidence.

Foreword

It is my pleasure to introduce readers to *Neuroanesthesiology Case Companion*, a book on clinical neuroanesthesiology written by my friend and fellow neuroanesthesiologist, Shailendra Joshi MBBS MD (Anesthesiology) FFARCS (I). The book represents yet another progressive step in the storied history of the neuroanesthesiology subspecialty.[1] Although the book will appeal to readers at all stages of anesthesiology training and practice, it is primarily targeted to those engaged in residency- or subspecialty education programs.

With this in mind, Dr Joshi envisioned that an anesthesiology resident physician will dedicate 2 or more months to neuroanesthesiology training. Accordingly, he organized the book into 62 chapters, each on a different topic, with the goal of having the trainee read one chapter per day in a single sitting. The chapters cover the breadth of neuroanesthesiology practice, have supporting reference materials, are thoughtfully organized, and provide space in the margins for the reader to add personal notes.

Dr Joshi is amply prepared to write such a book. He is currently an Associate Professor at one of the United States' premier medical centers and anesthesiology residency training programs: Columbia University's Irving Medical Center and Department of Anesthesiology, New York City, New York, USA. There, he engages in clinical care, teaching, and biomedical research. His research has focused on neuroanesthesiology topics and, more recently, the arterial delivery of drugs to treat malignant brain tumors. His research has resulted in unique discoveries in humans and laboratory animals, and the research has been funded in part by the United States National Institutes of Health. In another domain, Dr Joshi was for many years an editorial board member for the *Journal of Neurosurgical Anesthesiology* and, for a decade, was its Section Editor for Laboratory Reports.

Dr Joshi's academic path has had an interesting geographic and intellectual course. A native of India, Dr Joshi did his anesthesia residency at the All India Institute of Medical Sciences in New Delhi, India. He also trained in England before completing his neuroanesthesiology training under the mentorship of the renowned neuroanesthesiologist and researcher Professor William L Young at Columbia University. Since joining the Columbia University faculty, Dr Joshi has continued to travel between the United States and his Indian homeland to teach anesthesiology and participate in research activities.

Dr Shailendra Joshi's medical education and training in both India and the United States, and his direct contributions to the medical communities of both nations (and indirectly to the world) reflect the same type of activities by his venerated granduncle, Nielamber C Joshi MBBS. The elder Dr Joshi, after graduating from the Medical College of Lahore, Punjab University, initially practiced medicine in government hospitals. From records housed in Mayo Clinic's W Bruce Fye Center for the History of Medicine, we know that in 1917, Dr Nielamber Joshi traveled to the United States and my home institution, Mayo Clinic, in Rochester, Minnesota. There, he began a surgery residency in August 1917, under the direct tutelage of the two brothers, Drs William J Mayo and Charles H Mayo, responsible for the beginning and growth of

Mayo Clinic. In 1915, the Mayo Brothers organized Mayo Clinic's combined clinical and academic activities under the Mayo Foundation for Medical Education and Research. From these humble beginnings, Mayo Clinic ultimately became the largest site of graduate medical education in the world.[2] From its inception, the Foundation trained resident physicians from the United States and abroad, with Dr Nielamber Joshi being one of the first international trainees and the first to represent India. During his training at Mayo Clinic, Dr Nielamber Joshi was instilled with the values (now represented in the Institution's logo: the Triple Shield), that advances in medicine are predicated on simultaneous innovations in clinical practice, enlightened medical education, and progressive biomedical research. Dr Nielamber Joshi clearly embraced these values for the remainder of his professional life. After completing his Mayo Clinic surgical training in the fall of 1920, he returned to India to practice medicine and surgery and, a decade later, established India's first private surgical center. For many years, he corresponded with the Mayo Brothers, presumably to discuss applying their progressive approaches to clinical care, research, and education, to clinical and academic medical centers. With time, Dr Nielamber Joshi achieved greatness as a practitioner and leader in medicine.

It is clear that the intergenerational transfer of these values — from Dr Nielamber Joshi to Dr Shailendra Joshi— has informed the planning and writing of the current book *Neuroanesthesiology Case Companion*. Here, Dr Shailendra Joshi creates a method by which readers can use the interface of clinical innovations, education, and research to improve their own practices and the lives of the patients they treat.

As is true of all successful teachers, Dr Shailendra Joshi, in the pages of *Neuroanesthesiology Case Companion,* teaches learners not just what to think but additionally how to think about complex neuroanesthesiology issues. Hence, the reader is expected to acquire not only new knowledge but also acquire new attitudes about continuous learning throughout a career for the benefit of patients.

William L Lanier MD
Emeritus Professor of Anesthesiology
Mayo Clinic
Rochester, Minnesota, USA

1. Lanier WL. The history of neuroanesthesiology: The people, pursuits, and practices. J Neurosurg Anesthesiol. 2012;24:281-99.
2. Boes CJ, Long TR, Rose SH, Fye WB. The founding of the Mayo School of Graduate Medical Education. Mayo Clin Proc. 2015;90:252-63.

Preface

Books provide information, but most do not focus on recall. Information without recall and recall without application is relatively meaningless. It is not what the author provides but what the reader recalls that matters. I believe that the principal foundation of impactful higher education is the interest generated by the subject. The second most crucial component is the ease of learning and retention of information. True knowledge is an endless cycle of interest, learning, testing, and refining what one knows. Such a vision of adult education guided the preparation of this book, "Neuroanesthesiology Case Companion".

This book provides a broad clinical perspective needed for neurosurgical perioperative care. The information is structured as bulleted texts, tables, and simple figures. The layout provides margins for annotation and upgrading of the text. At the end of the clinical chapters are summaries of interesting neurosurgical cases culled from literature to encourage discussion and test application. Throughout the book are neuroscience vignettes meant to entice the reader.

On the operational side, the chapters are written with the following objectives:
- The 62 chapters amount to a chapter a day, the average days in neuroanesthesia rotations.
- The chapters are meant to be read in 30–45 minutes. A few topics are divided into two or more chapters at the cost of some repetition.
- The contents provide a practical plan for handling cases in the operating room.
- The emphasis is on clinical and operational information rather than academic discussions.
- The text is bulleted and follows a consistent layout.
- Numerical values are rounded, memory aids are included, and simple line figures and tables with text emphasis are provided to help with retention.

This book has four sections: *Section 1:* Applied Anatomy and Physiology; *Section 2:* Neuropathology for Anesthesiologists. Both these sections are similar to what one would have found in the erstwhile Foundation of Medicine series. These sections elaborate on the underlying concepts that are usually not a part of clinical discussions or need additional focus. *Section 3* is the primary clinical portion of the book. Each chapter begins with an introduction, then lists and elaborates on the neuroanesthetic concerns. At the end of each chapter, there are 3–5 case reports for further discussion. *Section 4* contains the Appendices, which contain essential information needed for clinical practice.

The target readers for this book are the anesthesia residents. This book will also benefit the neurosurgery, neurology, and critical care residents and fellows. Anesthesiologists in general practice can rapidly review neurosurgical topics. The vignettes will encourage medical students to seek a career in clinical neurosciences, specifically neuroanesthesiology.

Shailendra Joshi

Acknowledgments

It is an enormous undertaking to write an entire textbook on a subject. This one took over a decade. This textbook would not have been possible without the help of the Residents and Fellows in the Department of Anesthesiology, Columbia Presbyterian Medical Center, New York City, New York, USA. Many residents, during their neuroanesthesia rotation, have reviewed these chapters. Amongst those that stood out are: Anthony Auricchio, Brian Chang, Chung-Jen Chen, Stephanie Chen, James Colman, Julia Couto, Elizabeth Day, Caroline Eden, Christopher Folgueras, Justin Gengiano, Andrew Knapp, Laura McClung, Crystal Rui and Jamie Sack.

I am also grateful to Dr Pramod Bithal, Former Head of Neurosurgical Anesthesiology at the All India Institute of Medical Sciences, New Delhi, India. As my Senior Resident and despite three intervening decades, Dr Bithal did not abdicate from his responsibility of reviewing his junior's work and made invaluable suggestions and corrections to the final text.

Finally, I am indebted to Vidur Joshi, a Biomedical Engineering student at Stevens Institute of Technology, who helped edit the earlier drafts.

Contents

SECTION 1: Applied Anatomy and Physiology

1. Cell Biology of the Nervous System 3
2. Blood–Brain Barrier 11
3. Applied Anatomy of the Central Nervous System 16
4. Spinal Cord Anatomy 22
5. Visual Pathway 40
6. Auditory Pathway 44
7. Cerebral Circulation: Anatomy 49
8. Cerebral Blood Flow Regulation 55
9. Brain Metabolism and Flow Metabolism Coupling 64
10. Cerebrospinal Fluid Formation and Circulation 72
11. Hypothalamus—Pituitary Axis 83
12. Electrophysiological Monitoring 92
13. Neurological Monitoring and Imaging 106
14. Positioning during Neurosurgery 120
15. Anesthetic Neuroprotection and Neurotoxicity 127

SECTION 2: Neuropathology for Anesthesiologists

16. Raised Intracranial Pressure and CSF Drainage Procedures 137
17. Hydrocephalus in Children 146
18. Atherosclerotic Cerebrovascular Disease 151
19. Brain Tumor Pathology 159
20. Brain Edema and Herniation 166
21. Cerebral Aneurysms 173
22. Subarachnoid Hemorrhage and Cerebral Vasospasm 178
23. Pathophysiology of Arteriovenous Malformations 186

24. Surgical Treatment of Chronic Pain 193
25. Developmental Abnormalities of Spine and Scoliosis..201
26. Pathophysiology of Spinal Cord Injury..209
27. Movement Disorders..215
28. Seizure Types and Treatment...221
29. Venous Air Embolism 226
30. Traumatic Brain Injury..234
31. Targeted Temperature Management 240
32. Peripheral Neuropathies 246
33. Brain Death 250

SECTION 3: Neuroanesthesia Case Management

34. Preoperative Assessment of Neurosurgical Case..257
35. Routine Craniotomy under General Anesthesia 272
36. Awake Craniotomy for Seizure Disorders...291
37. Carotid Endarterectomy 301
38. Carotid Artery Stenting..317
39. Cerebral Arteriovenous Malformation Resection 331
40. Clipping of Cerebral Aneurysms 342
41. Treatment of Cerebral Vasospasm..357
42. Deep Hypothermic Circulatory Arrest 368
43. Management of Traumatic Brain Injury..376
44. Brain Herniation 389
45. Decompressive Craniectomy 401
46. Cerebrospinal Fluid Leak...411
47. Cervical Decompression 419
48. Acute Spinal Injury 428
49. Intraoperative Evoked Potential Changes 439
50. Posterior Fossa Surgery 446

51. Transsphenoid Hypophysectomy 458
52. Endoscopic Third Ventriculostomy and Shunt Procedures........................469
53. Anesthesia for Electroconvulsive Therapy 477
54. Pregnant Patient for Neurosurgery 486
55. Pediatric Neurosurgery Patient 495
56. Biopsy for Creutzfeldt–Jakob Disease..505
57. Postoperative Vision Loss..512
58. Robot-assisted Surgery and Laser Interstitial Thermal Therapy 520
59. Patient with Ventricular Assist Device 531
60. Post-craniotomy Pain Management...542
61. Massive Blood Transfusion 549
62. Brain Death and Organ Harvest 568

SECTION 4: Appendices

Appendix 1...579
Appendix 2...580
Appendix 3...581
Appendix 4...583
Appendix 5...584
Appendix 6...585
Appendix 7...587
Appendix 8...591
Appendix 9...594
Appendix 10 595
Appendix 11 597
Appendix 12 602
Appendix 13 606
Appendix 14 608
Appendix 15 609

Appendix 16 611

Appendix 17 613

Appendix 18 620

Appendix 19 623

Appendix 20 625

In Memoriam 627

On Teaching and Learning 628

Index 629

Section 1

Applied Anatomy and Physiology

- Cell Biology of the Nervous System
- Blood-Brain Barrier
- Applied Anatomy of the Central Nervous System
- Spinal Cord Anatomy
- Visual Pathway
- Auditory Pathway
- Cerebral Circulation: Anatomy
- Cerebral Blood Flow Regulation
- Brain Metabolism and Flow Metabolism Coupling
- Cerebrospinal Fluid Formation and Circulation
- Hypothalamus—Pituitary Axis
- Electrophysiological Monitoring
- Neurological Monitoring and Imaging
- Positioning during Neurosurgery
- Anesthetic Neuroprotection and Neurotoxicity

Chapter 1

Cell Biology of the Nervous System

INTRODUCTION

Cells of the nervous system are structurally diverse and complex **(Fig. 1)**. They have very specialized functions. Neurons, the primary cells of the system, generate, receive, store, and transmit information. Despite excessive metabolism, these cells lack substrate reserves. Hence, they are vulnerable to ischemic injury. When injured, the damage sustained is rapid, often catastrophic, and usually permanent. Cell biology provides us an insight into the functioning of the nervous system. It helps to understand the mechanism of injury at cell and tissue levels. It explains the uptake of drugs. Many drugs are excluded from the central nervous system by endothelial cells that form the blood-brain barrier (BBB), which poses treatment challenges.

KEY CELLS OF THE NERVOUS SYSTEM

- *Neurons:* Neurons can be: (1) *Projection* neurons that usually extend from the neuronal bodies to distant regions of the nervous system to

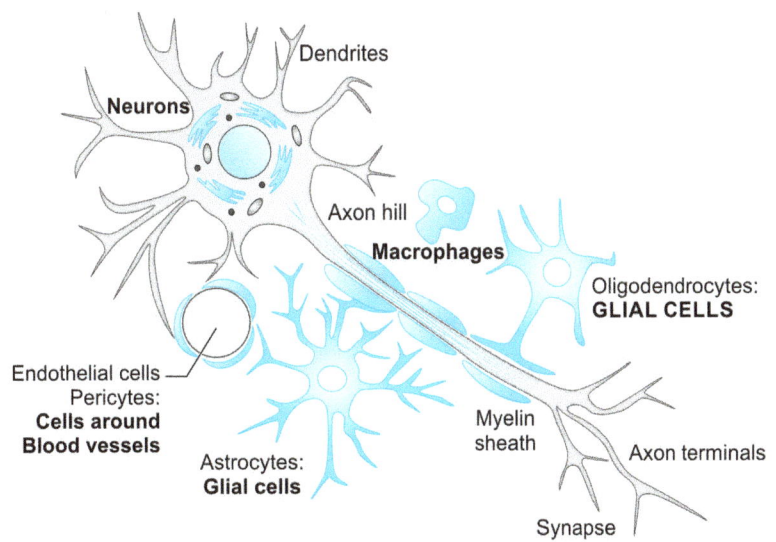

Fig. 1: Cell diversity of the nervous system.

transmit information. These can be *anaxonic* (amacrine cells of the retina), *unipolar* (absent in adult vertebrates), *bipolar* (retinal and olfactory neurons), or *pseudounipolar (dorsal root ganglia of the spinal cord)*. The latter are sensory neurons lacking dendrites but with naked or modified sensory nerve endings. (2) *Multipolar* neurons are the *commonest* type of neurons. Their dendrites densely communicate with each other and help to integrate information. Examples of multipolar neurons are motor neurons, pyramidal and Purkinje cells (**Fig. 2**). The process of creation of neurons is called neurogenesis.

- *Glial cells:* These are the non-impulse transmitting cells. They physically support the neurons, insulate them, supply nutrients, maintain homeostasis, and remove pathogens and dead cells. Types:
    - *Oligodendrocytes:* Cover the axons for faster impulse conduction.
    - *Microglial cells:* These are macrophages that remove cell debris.
    - *Astrocytes:* A component of the BBB, play a role in homeostasis, neurotransmitter recycling and are a source of growth factors.
- *Ependymal cells:* Line the ventricles and play a key role in cerebrospinal fluid (CSF) formation and resorption.
- *Endothelial cells:* Line blood vessels and are the major component of the BBB.
- *Pericytes:* Cells located in the vessel wall. They arise from the neural crest or the mesenchyme and play a key role in regulating the BBB.

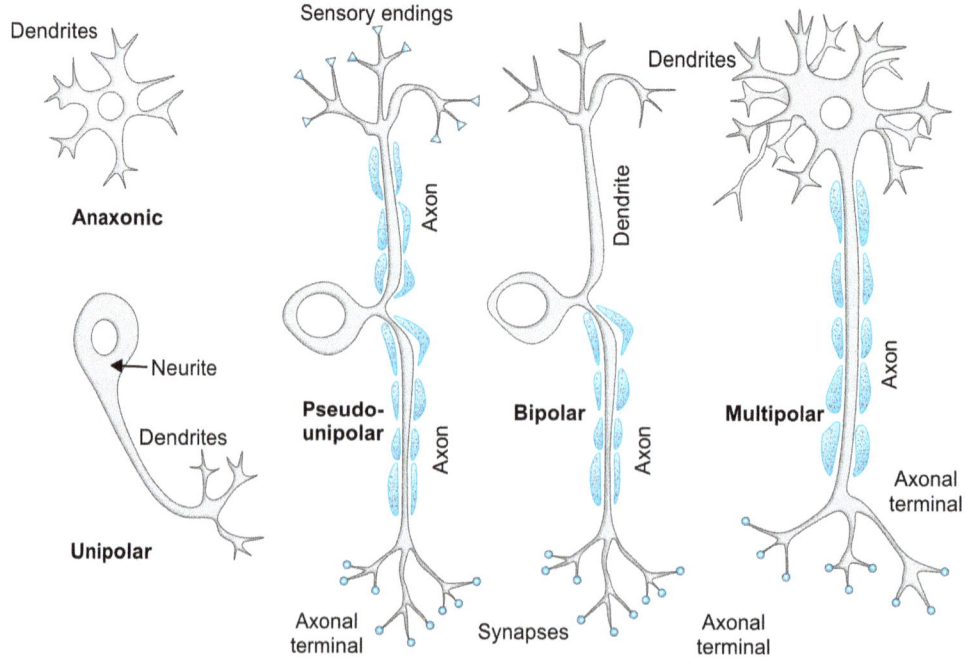

Fig. 2: Adult human neuron types.

- *Neural stem cells:* Dormant multipotent stem cells are found in several locations, such as the hippocampus, olfactory bulb, striatum, and septum. They have the potential to treat stroke and spinal injuries.

MEMBRANE POTENTIAL

Intracellular pumps create an ionic gradient across the cell membrane. The imbalance of the charge results in *transmembrane potential*. Nernst's equation describes the potential as a function of the ion concentrations as:

$$\text{Nernst equations (E)} = \frac{RT}{nF} \ln \frac{[\text{Ion out}]}{[\text{Ion in}]}$$

Where E is the equilibrium potential for a given ion, R is the universal gas constant, T is the absolute temperature, Ion out and Ion in are ion concentrations outside and inside the cell, respectively, and n is the valance. F is the Faraday constant or the charge per mole of electrons. Using this equation, the net charge on the neuronal membrane is -70 mV, which is closer to equilibrium potential due to K^+ (-90 mV) than Na^+ ($+45$ mV) ions.

Action Potential

The action potential is the sudden change in polarity of the axonal cell membrane, which enables the transmission of nerve impulses. In contrast, the action potentials in the neuronal cell body are more complex and nuanced and help store information. Action potentials are triggered when the threshold depolarization is reached. When the threshold is reached, there is a rapid increase in the voltage-gated Na^+ conductance followed by a slower sustained increase in the voltage-gated K^+ conductance. The cell membrane depolarizes due to a transmembrane shift in Na^+ ions. The restoration and hyperpolarization of the transmembrane potential occur due to the migration of K^+ ions. The action potential lasts about 1 ms and is followed by hyperpolarization. Axonal depolarization also impedes repetitive impulse transmission. The refractoriness to impulse transmission is "absolute" during the depolarization phase. While it is "relative" during the hyperpolarization phase, as shown in **Figure 3** as "*AB*" and "*REL*", respectively.

Compound Action Potential

Stimulation of the mixed nerves results in a complex depolarization pattern due to different types of fibers. This complexity is due to differences in conducting velocities and the refractory state of individual nerve fibers (**Fig. 2**). The curve's shape depends on the fibers a nerve contains and the recording site and can be used to assess nerve function and fiber loss.

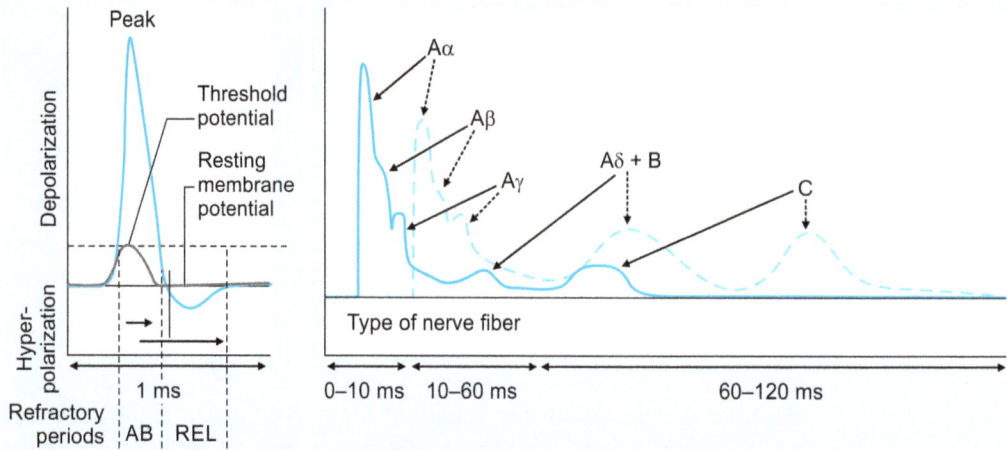

Fig. 3: Action potential recorded from a cell membrane versus compound action potential recorded from a mixed nerve proximally (solid line) and distally (dashed line). The shape of compound action potential changes due to interference between individual action potentials of different types of nerve fibers. (AB: absolute refractory period; REL: relative refractory period.)

SYNAPTIC TRANSMISSION

- Synaptic transmission involves the depolarization of the presynaptic terminal, increasing presynaptic Ca^{++} concentrations. Ca^{++} enables the binding of the neurotransmitter vesicles to the presynaptic membrane and their release into the synaptic cleft.
- The neurotransmitters **(Table 1)** diffuse across the synaptic cleft. They bind to postsynaptic receptors to depolarize the postsynaptic membrane.
- The postsynaptic membrane, such as in the neuromuscular junction, can be folded to increase the density of postsynaptic receptors. Increased postsynaptic receptor density improves synaptic transmission.
- *Gap junctions:* Gap junctions bridge the pre-and postsynaptic membranes. These gap junctions can transmit impulses at a much faster rate. They are seen in some structures, like the thalamus.
- Synapses provide us with the opportunity to alter the functioning of the nervous system for therapeutic purposes. Examples include:
  - Atropine competitively blocks the muscarinic acetylcholine (ACh) receptors to minimize the parasympathetic side effects of drugs.
  - Donepezil binds to the enzyme cholinesterase. It increases ACh concentrations in the central nervous system synapses and improves the cognition of Alzheimer's Disease patients.
  - Levodopa, unlike dopamine, can cross the BBB and increases dopamine concentrations in the nigrostriatal synapses of patients with Parkinson's Disease to alleviate symptoms.

CHAPTER 1 Cell Biology of the Nervous System

Table 1: Neurotransmitters, their mechanism of action, and their key functions.

Neurotransmitter (NT)	Site of action and physiological effects
Acetylcholine (Ach): Direct via the ACh receptors	Receptors are found in CNS (brain and spinal cord), PNS (glands), ANS, and NMJ. ACh affects many organs. Ach excess can cause Central cholinergic syndrome, e.g., with physostigmine, presents meiosis, diarrhea, diaphoresis, bradycardia, and hypotension. While Anticholinergic syndrome, e.g., with atropine, presents with "hot as a hare, red as a beet, dry as a bone and mad as a hatter"
Norepinephrine (NE): Indirect via the G proteins	CNS (cortex, hypothalamus, brainstem, and spinal cord), PNS (glands), and sympathetic ANS. Affects vigilance, arousal, learning, attention, mood, consciousness, thermoregulation, and pituitary functions. Regulates vascular tone. Stimulant drugs, e.g., cocaine and amphetamines; anti-depressants like SNRIs, inhibit NE uptake
Epinephrine (Epi): indirectly via the G proteins	CNS (thalamus, hypothalamus, mid-brain, and spinal cord); autonomic system to profoundly affect cardiac and respiratory functions. Key role in fight or flight response
Serotonin (Ser): Indirect via the G proteins	CNS (found in the retina, hypothalamus, limbic, cerebellum, and spinal cord), pharmacological modulation of emotion, and effects of psychotropic drugs. Affects bowel mobility, bladder control, and cardiovascular regulation
Dopamine (D): Direct via D1-5 receptors, G-protein coupled	CNS (thalamus and hypothalamus). It plays a critical role in learning, locomotion, controlling pituitary secretions, and modulation effect through reward, emotion, and executive function. Deficiency in the nigrostriatal tract leads to Parkinson's Disease
Glutamate (Glu): Direct via glutamate receptors and indirect via G proteins	Glu receptors include MDA, AMPA, and kainite. It is the key excitatory NT in the retina, cortex, and brainstem. It plays a crucial role in memory and learning. Glu plays a significant role in brain injury and anesthetic neurotoxicity
Gamma amino butyric acid (GABA): Direct and indirect effects	Direct effects via GABA receptors and indirect via the G proteins. GABA-aminergic neurons are located in the cortex, cerebellum, brainstem, and spinal cord. Account for 40% of inhibitory activity in the brain. Role in behavior, cognition, and stress response. Modulate anesthetic drug effects
Glycine: Direct via Glycine receptors	Predominantly found in the retina, spinal cord, and brain stem. It is generally an inhibitory NT. It plays a role in movement, vision, and hearing
Histamine: Direct via H1-4 receptors	Histamine is a NT and a modulator for other NTs. It is widely distributed in the brain and the spinal cord. It affects wakefulness, feeding, and motivation. It plays a significant role in inflammation
Oxytocin: via G proteins	Oxytocin is a NT and a hormone. Receptors in the amygdala, ventromedial nucleus, and hypothalamus. Modulates social behavior, bonding, memory, stress, and anxiety

(NT: neurotransmitter; AMPA: alpha amino propionic acid; ANS: the autonomic nervous system; CNS: the central nervous system; NMDA: N-methyl; D-aspartate; NMJ: neuromuscular junction; PNS: the peripheral nervous system; SNRIs: Serotonin-norepinephrine reuptake inhibitors)

Postsynaptic Response

When the nerve impulse reaches the synapse, it depolarizes the nerve terminal, resulting in an influx of Ca^{++} and the release of neurotransmitters. The density of synaptic vesicles at the terminals and the magnitude of the Ca^{++} influx determines the neurotransmitter release. The magnitude and duration of the postsynaptic response alter the neurocircuitry, both structurally and functionally. The postsynaptic response can lead to *long-acting potentiation or long-acting depression*. When the neurons discharge synchronously (<20 ms), the dendritic connections are reinforced as the density of postsynaptic receptors is increased, and when the discharge is asynchronous (>20 ms), the receptor density is decreased, and dendritic connections are degraded. In this way, the response of neural networks is affected by past conditioning.

The postsynaptic receptors are (1) ionotropic and (2) metabolic.

The *ionotropic* receptors have the following usual characteristics:
- These are membrane-spanning receptors that have five subunits surrounding an ion channel.
- Activation of the receptor opens the ion channel.
- The response is rapid, sub-ms time frame.
- Have a trigger threshold and an "all or none" response pattern.
- Depolarization lasts 1–2 ms.
- *Inotropic receptors can be:*
  - Excitatory (e.g., nicotinic Ach receptors and influx of Na^+ or Ca^{++})
  - Inhibitory (e.g., GABA receptors: GABA receptors are one-third of all postsynaptic receptors in the CNS and inhibited by an influx of Cl^- ions that hyperpolarizes the postsynaptic membrane)

The *metabolic or G-protein-coupled receptors* generally have the following characteristics:
- Slow onset of receptor response.
- They have external ligand-recognizing sites coupled to G proteins linked to inhibitory or activating enzymes.
- A second messenger could be linked to an ion channel downstream.
- Have longer and varied duration of response; depolarization lasts seconds to hours.
- *Metabolic receptors* include dopaminergic, muscarinic, serotoninergic, and glutaminergic receptors.

Key Postsynaptic Receptors in CNS (Table 1)
- *Excitatory glutamate receptors* potentiate neurotransmitter response and play a critical role in synaptic plasticity; N-methyl d-aspartate (NMDA) receptors can alter synaptic functions and lead to long-term potentiation, enabling memory and learning.

Excessive glutamate receptor activation can lead to cell injury in epilepsy, trauma, and ischemic stroke.
- *Inotropic glutamate receptors:*
  - Alpha-amino propionic acid (AMPA) receptors permit Na^+/K^+ and sometimes the Ca^{++} flux. They can cause long-term changes in synaptic functions.

CHAPTER 1 Cell Biology of the Nervous System

- Kainate receptors permit the Na^+/K^+ flux.
- *N-methyl-d-aspartate (NMDA) receptor (NMDAR):* NMDAR is a ligand-activated voltage-controlled receptor that permits a cationic flux. Synaptic NMDAR possibly plays a crucial role in synaptic plasticity, whereas the extrasynaptic receptors play a role in neural injuries. NMDAR modulates the effects of dextromethorphan, phencyclidine, nitrous oxide, and ketamine.
- *Metabotropic receptors:*
  - *GABA and glycine receptors:* These G-protein-coupled receptors affect the milieu of the synaptic neurons, such as intracellular Ca^{++} level, which results in a more prolonged synaptic response. $GABA_A$ and glycine receptor act by modulating the Cl^- flux or by G proteins, whereas $GABA_B$ receptor acts by modulating the K^+ flux. Many anesthetic drugs, including barbiturates, benzodiazepines, and propofol, activate $GABA_A$. Strychnine, a convulsive agent, acts by blocking the glycine receptors in the spinal cord.

TYPES OF NERVE FIBERS

- The axons or nerve fibers **(Table 2)** transmit electrical impulses.
- The myelinated fibers have rapid transmission, as depolarizations that transmit the impulse occur at the nodes of Ranvier.
- Unmyelinated nerve fibers have smaller diameters and slower conduction velocities.
- In general, the diameter and conduction velocity in decreasing order are as follows: *Proprioception:* Aα, Aβ; *mechanoreceptors:* Aβ, Aδ; and *nociceptors and thermoreceptors:* Aδ and C fibers.

Table 2: Classification and characteristics of the nerve fibers.

Fiber type	Sub-type	Num. type	Myelination	Diameter (μm)	Velocity (m/s)	Function	Sensitivity		
							LAA	Hypoxia	Pressure
A	α	Ia	Thick	12–22	70–120	Proprioception and motor	+	++	+++
A	α	Ib	Thick	12–22	70–120	Motor	++	++	+++
A	β	II	Thick	5–12	30–70	Pressure, touch, and vibration	++	++	+++
A	γ	II	Thick	2–8	15–30	Muscle spindles	+++	++	+++
A	δ	III	Thin	1–5	5–30	Sharp pain and temperature	++++	++	+++
B	–	–	Thin	<3	3–15	Preganglionic autonomic	++++	+++	++
C	–	IV	None	0.1–12	0.5–2.3	Dorsal root	++++	+	+
Symp	–	IV	None	0.3–1.3	0.7–2.3	Postganglionic	++++	+	

(LAA: local anesthetic agents)

- The *differential sensitivity of the nerve fibers* to local anesthetic agents, pressure, and hypoxia has clinical implications. For example, local anesthetic agents used for nerve blocks affect autonomic nerves > sensory (sharp pain) > motor. Thus, while testing the onset of the brachial block, the person might move the arm yet not feel the pain. Increasing sensitivity to local anesthetic block is greater for autonomic versus pain versus motor nerve fibers. Consequently, local anesthetics have higher autonomic effects > sensory block > motor block after epidural/spinal anesthesia. Furthermore, lower concentrations of local anesthetic drugs can block pain but spare motor functions.

FURTHER READING

1. Cheon SY et al. Cell Type-Specific Mechanisms in the Pathogenesis of Ischemic Stroke: The Role of Apoptosis Signal-Regulating Kinase 1. Oxid Med Cell Longev. 2018;2018:2596043.
2. Gascoigne DA et al. Early Development of the GABAergic System and the Associated Risks of Neonatal Anesthesia. Int J Mol Sci. 2021;22(23):12951
3. Liu S et al. ketamine inhibits neuronal differentiation by regulating brain-derived neurotrophic factor (BDNF) signaling. Toxicol In Vitro. 2021;72: 105091.
4. Song R et al. Maternal Sevoflurane Exposure Causes Abnormal Development of Fetal Prefrontal Cortex and Induces Cognitive Dysfunction in Offspring. Stem Cells Int. 2017; 2017:6158468.
5. von Bartheld CS. Myths and truths about the cellular composition of the human brain: A review of influential concepts. J Chem Neuroanat. 2018;93:2-15.

Vignette: Brain Size and Function

The human brain weighs about 1,200 g and contains 100 billion neurons and glial cells each. There are about 7000 synapses per neuron, and in all, 1-quadrillion synapses.

While we marvel at the human brain, we overlook the brains of tiny insects. An excellent example of this is the honeybee. Its brain is $1mm^3$ in volume, weighs 1 mg, and has less than a million neurons. Yet, the bees live in large, complex social colonies. They track the time of the day. They travel great distances to find food and then report the route to other bees. They can identify and learn from visual patterns. In the humans, prefrontal cortex is responsible for these functions, while bees have analogous structures called mushroom bodies. The success of the bees shows how tiny insect brains can match the performance of brains that are orders of magnitude larger in size.

Chapter 2

Blood–Brain Barrier

INTRODUCTION

The term blood-brain barrier (BBB) describes the property of the brain to regulate the movement of compounds between the circulating blood and the brain tissue.

The anatomical components of the BBB are endothelial cells (ECs), mural cells, astrocytes, and the basement membrane **(Fig. 1)**. These components constitute a physical barrier to the diffusion of compounds. In addition, a chemical barrier by metabolizing enzymes prevents the entry of specific compounds into the brain tissue.

The permeability of the barrier depends on the following:
- Properties of the compounds (molecular weight, charge, lipid solubility, shape, and size)
- The integrity of barrier components (basement membrane, endothelial and perivascular cells)
- Functional state of transporters, carriers, and metabolizing enzymes..

The barrier is not ubiquitous but relatively deficient in some brain regions. These include nuclei of the third and fourth ventricles, subfornical organs, pineal gland, and area postrema **(Fig. 2)**. The diffusion of molecules across the BBB in these regions is necessary for physiological purposes such as hormonal regulation.

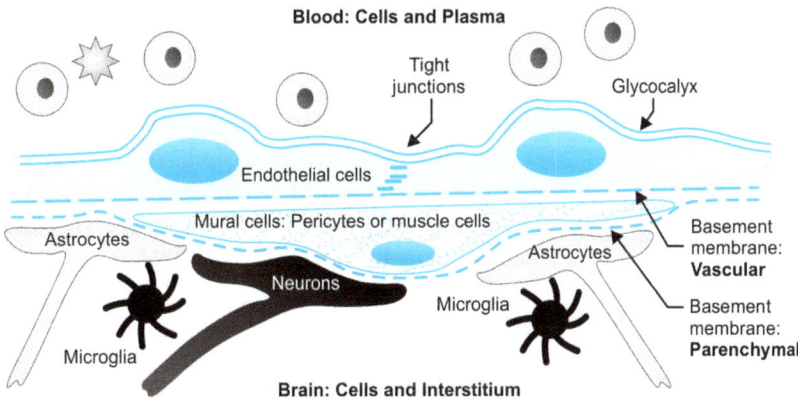

Fig. 1: Components of the blood-brain barrier (blue).

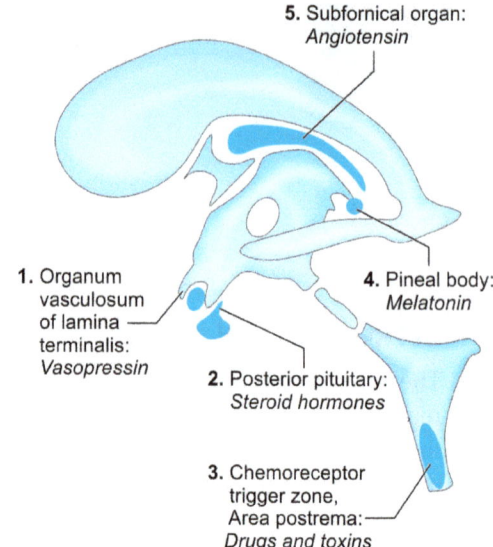

Fig. 2: Regions of the brain where the BBB is deficient.

ENDOTHELIAL CELLS (ECs)

The endothelial cells characteristically are:
- Brain capillary endothelium is about 60% thinner than in other tissues.
- The luminal and abluminal surface membranes are only 1–2 µm apart.
- Usually, single-layered can be multi-layered in larger vessels.
- Form a continuous non-fenestrated network.
- Have low rates of transcytosis.
- Have limited paracellular diffusion due to tight junctions.
- 100-fold greater electrical resistance due to tight junctions.
- Have extensive nutrient-specific transporter systems **(Fig. 3)**.
- Rich in mitochondria, metabolically active.
- Rich in enzymes. Enzymes such as gamma-glutamyl trans-peptidase, aromatic acid decarboxylase, and alkaline phosphatase can metabolize drugs and create an additional "*enzymatic barrier*".
- Luminal surfaces have a low density of leukocyte adhesion molecules.
- In general:
  - Uncharged molecules of about 400 Daltons can cross the BBB.
  - Lipid-soluble compound can bi-directionally cross the BBB.
  - Drugs avidly bound to albumin poorly cross the BBB. However, drugs, such as benzodiazepines, can rapidly dissociate from albumin to cross the barrier.

MURAL CELLS

- Smooth muscle cells and pericytes
- Surround the ECs
- Embedded in the basement membrane

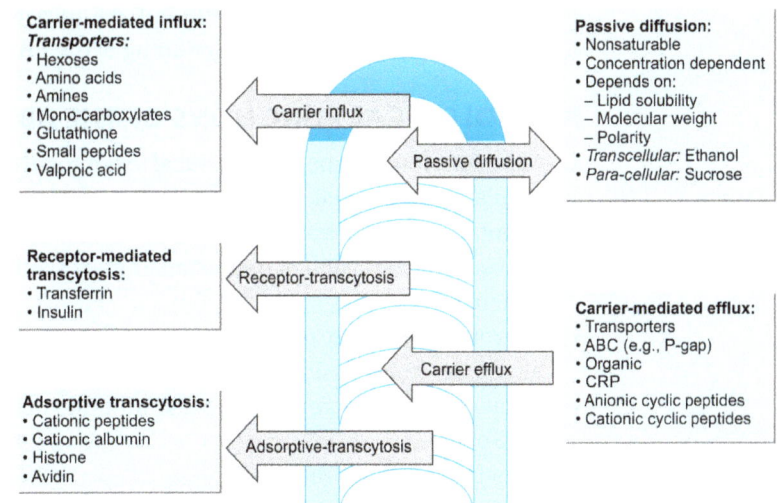

Fig. 3: Transport across the blood-brain barrier.

Pericytes

- They are derived from the neuroectoderm rather than the mesoderm.
- They are identified by staining with platelet-derived growth factor receptor-β and neuron-glial antigen 2.
- In the central nervous system (CNS), the EC: pericyte ratio is 1 to 3:1 compared to 100:1 in other tissues, e.g., muscle.
- They can bridge several endothelial cells.
- They have contractile proteins and can influence the diameter of the capillaries, regulating the blood flow in response to neural activity.
- They play a crucial role in angiogenesis, the deposition of extracellular matrix, and the formation and regulation of the BBB.

BASEMENT MEMBRANE

The basement membrane has two components (Fig. 1):
- The *vascular basement* membrane is secreted by the endothelial cells and the pericytes.
- The *parenchymal basement* membrane is secreted by the astrocytes.
- These two membranes differ in composition.
- Both membranes pose a diffusion barrier.
- Metalloproteases disrupt them.

ASTROCYTES

The astrocytes are glial cells whose end feet completely cover the vascular tube formed by ECs, pericytes, and the basement membrane. The critical functions of the astrocytes include:
- *Regulation of the tissue water content:* They contain specific proteins such as dystroglycan, dystrophin, and aquaporin-4 that regulate the water content of the cells and play a role in developing cerebral edema.

- Regulate the local blood flow through neurovascular coupling.
- Help in the formation and functioning of the BBB.

PHYSIOLOGICAL FUNCTIONS OF THE BBB
- Maintains ionic homeostasis critical to neuronal functioning by actively regulating interstitial Na^+, K^+, Ca^{++}, H^+, and Mg^{++} concentrations.
- Regulates nutrient transport.
- Prevents the diffusion of neurotransmitters synthesized in the nervous system.
- Prevents the influx of potential neurotransmitters like glycine and glutamate from outside the nervous system.
- Limits influx of macromolecules like albumin that can have detrimental CNS effects.
- Protect against neurotoxins.

CONSEQUENCE OF BBB DISRUPTION
- Disruption of ionic homeostasis
- Leakage of albumin into the interstitium
- Increased epileptogenesis
- Increased tissue water content, edema, increased ICP
- Increased non-targeted drug delivery.
- Altered CNS effects of drugs.
- Cellular infiltration
- Hemorrhagic transformation
- Inflammation
- Neuronal death
- Therapeutic BBB disruption has resulted in intractable edema, brain herniation, and death.

PATHOLOGIES WITH LOSS OF BBB FUNCTIONS
- Traumatic brain injury
- Infiltrating/aggressive brain tumors
- *Infections:* Local and systemic
- Ischemic stroke
- Multiple sclerosis
- Alzheimer's disease
- Hypertensive crisis
- Seizures
- Liver failure
- Human Immunodeficiency syndrome
- Severe pain
- Glaucoma
- Lysosomal storage diseases.

IATROGENIC DISRUPTION OF BBB

- Focused ultrasound:
  - It uses transducers configured to target the drug delivery site.
  - Intravenously delivered microbubbles increase the local temperature and enhance BBB disruption.
  - Corrections are made to minimize sound scattering by the skull.
  - Skull implants that minimize beam scattering are currently in development.
- Bradykinin and it's analog (RMP-7) can disrupt the blood tumor barrier via the Bradykinin 2 receptor. Its efficacy is as yet unproven.
- Laser interstitial thermotherapy involves local heating of brain tissue with an implanted optical fiber to disrupt the BBB.
- Non-thermal interstitial electroporation (NTIRE) uses electrical pulses to open the BBB.
- Hyperosmotic BBB disruption:
  - Only clinically used method for brain tumor treatment
  - Requires 90–400 mL of 20–25% mannitol to be injected over 30s.
  - Imposes osmotic stress on the endothelial cells that opens the tight junctions.
  - BBB disruption enhances the delivery of intra-arterial drugs.
  - Increases the cerebral blood flow to enhance the delivery of any circulating drug that is often given intravenously concurrently.
  - The procedure is conducted under general anesthesia.
  - Seizures and cerebral edema can occur after the procedure.
  - Not proven effective in phase III trials.

FURTHER READING

1. Gericke B et al. Similarities and differences in the localization, trafficking, and function of P-glycoprotein in MDR1-EGFP- transduced rat versus human brain capillary endothelial cell lines. Fluids Barriers CNS. 2021;18(1):36.
2. Noe CR et al. Dysfunction of the Blood-Brain Barrier—A Key Step in Neurodegeneration and Dementia. Front Aging Neurosci. 2020;12:185.
3. Pardridge WM. The Isolated Brain Microvessel: A Versatile Experimental Model of the Blood-Brain Barrier. Front Physiol. 2020;11:398.
4. Shin HK et al. Development of blood-brain barrier permeation prediction models for organic and inorganic biocidal active substances. Chemosphere. 2021;277:130330.
5. Watanabe et al. Characterization of a Primate Blood-Brain Barrier Co-Culture Model Prepared from Primary Brain Endothelial Cells, Pericytes, and Astrocytes. Pharmaceutics. 2021;13(9):1484.

Vignette: The Discovery of the Blood-Brain Barrier

Max Lewandowsky first proposed the concept of the blood-brain barrier in 1900. He found that certain compounds did not enter the brain on systemic injections. Paul Ehrlich observed that aniline dyes did not stain the brain or the spine after intravenous injection. Edwin Goldman reported that the neural tissue could be stained when the same dyes were injected into the cerebrospinal fluid. These pioneering experiments demonstrated that a barrier prevented the transfer of compounds from the blood to the brain.

Chapter 3

Applied Anatomy of the Central Nervous System

INTRODUCTION

Most anesthesiologists encounter imaging-verified locations of neurological pathologies by the time they see the patient. It is unlikely that anesthesiologists need to know detailed anatomy. Yet, familiarity with syndromes from pathologies affecting different brain regions could assist them with patient care and to better understand the surgical needs.

The central nervous system (CNS) is divided into three regions: the cortex, deep brain structures, and the spinal cord.

CORTEX

The highly convoluted mammalian cortex is only 2–4 mm thick. It has six layers that receive brain and spinal cord afferent and efferent nerve fibers **(Table 1)**. Injuries to the cortex produce classical symptoms that can help to localize the pathology **(Fig. 1)**. Cortex is divided into four regions frontal, temporal, parietal, and occipital.

Frontal Lobe Syndrome

- The frontal lobe is the largest area of the brain, anterior to the central sulcus.
- Injury can affect motor functions, motivation, planning, social behavior, and language/speech functions. For example:
  - *Premotor cortex* injury produces weakness in the contralateral side.
  - *Broca's and Brodmann's areas* injuries result in non-fluent expressive aphasia.

Table 1: Layers of the cerebral cortex.

Layer	Cell types	Predominant afferent	Predominant efferent
I: Molecular	Dendrites, few neurons	Thalamus (M type), intracortical	Intracortical
II: Ext. Granular	Dense stellate, Small pyramidal	Intracortical, brain stem	Intracortical
III: Ext. Pyramidal	Loose stellate, Medium pyramidal	Intracortical, brain stem	Significant intracortical
IV: Int. Granular	Dense stellate cells only	Thalamus (C type), brain stem	Cortex, thalamus, brain stem
V: Int. Pyramidal	Large. Pyramidal (Betz's cells)	Thalamus, brain stem	Motor, brain stem, spinal cord
VI: Multiform	Mixed pyramidal and other cells	Thalamus, sub-cortex	Thalamus, brain stem, spinal cord

CHAPTER 3 Applied Anatomy of the Central Nervous System

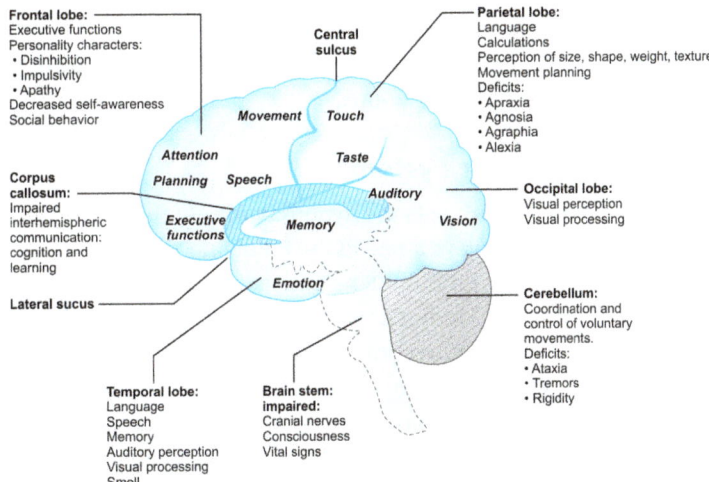

Fig. 1: Functional localization and effects of regional injuries.

Parietal Lobe Syndrome

- *Primary functions are* (1) sensory perception and (2) spatial integration.
- *The left parietal lobe injury results in Gerstmann syndrome:* Writing difficulties (agraphia), computing problems (acalculia), language difficulties (aphasia), and left–right disorientation.
- *The right parietal lobe injury results in* contralateral neglect, impaired drawing abilities, and difficulty constructing objects (constructional apraxia).
- *Bilateral damage—Balint's syndrome:* Ocular apraxia, ocular ataxia, and inability to integrate a visual scene (simultanagnosia).
- *Parietal-temporal lesions:* Memory and personality changes associated with impaired verbal (left) or nonverbal (right) recall.

Temporal Lobe Syndrome

- Its primary functions include comprehending images and sounds, memory and recall, and emotional response.
- *Left-side damage:* Inability to comprehend language or Wernicke (receptive) aphasia.
- *Right-side damage:* Impaired memory for sound/music and inability to sing.

Occipital Lobe Syndromes

- Its primary functions are to process, interpret, integrate, and store visual information.
- Cortical blindness is the inability to see despite normal eyesight.
- *Anton syndrome:* Denial of blindness and visual confabulation with the fabrication of visual information.

DEEP BRAIN STRUCTURES

Deep brain structures include the limbic system, basal ganglia, thalamus, and hypothalamus.

Limbic System

- Connects the hypothalamus to different regions of the cortex
- It plays a role in the following:
  - Emotional response (fear, pleasure, and anger).
  - Memory.
  - Motivational drives (hunger, sex, dominance, and parenting).
- The structures and their functions include:
  - *Hippocampus and parahippocampal gyrus:* Memory
  - *Amygdala:* Fear response/anxiety
  - *Thalamus:* Relays information
  - *Cingulate gyrus:* Emotional response
  - *Septal nuclei:* Pleasure and reward reinforcement
  - *Mammillary bodies:* Memory
  - *Fornix:* Information transfer between mammillary bodies and hippocampus
- Injuries to the limbic system affect memory, emotion, and decision-making.

Basal Ganglia

- It consists of several nuclei, which smoothen movements **(Table 2)**.
- These nuclei include the corpus striatum (the most extensive structure), subthalamic nucleus, and substantia nigra. The corpus striatum is composed of caudate and lenticular nuclei. The lenticular nucleus consists of globus pallidus and putamen.
- Repeated mechanical injuries to the basal ganglia in sports, such as boxing, or exposure to toxins, can result in Parkinson's syndrome.
- Parkinson's syndrome consists of tremors, rigidity, and hypokinesia.

Table 2: Nuclei of the basal ganglia.

Basal ganglia	Significance
Striatum	
Caudate	Primary afferent pathway from the motor cortex to the basal ganglia, relay to substantia nigra
Putamen	
Other nuclei	
Globus pallidus	The primary efferent pathway from basal ganglia via thalamus to cortex and brainstem
Substantia nigra	
Subthalamic nuclei	Inhibitory motor pathway

Hypothalamus
- Hypothalamus is located above the brainstem.
- It exerts control of the autonomic nervous system, modulates the release of pituitary hormones, and synthesizes vasopressin and oxytocin.
- Injuries to the hypothalamus profoundly affect hormonal balance and disturb the milieu interior of the body.

Thalamus
- The afferent fibers to the thalamus are relayed to the cortex.
- All sensory information other than olfaction is relayed to the thalamus.
- Thalamocortical projections permit bidirectional impulse transmission between the cortex and the thalamus.
- The thalamus consists of as many as 50 nuclei.
- Anterior, middle, and posterior cerebral arteries supply the thalamus.
- The perfusion of the thalamus by multiple arteries deep within the brain creates potential watershed zones predisposing to ischemic injuries.
- **Table 3** lists some of the thalamic injuries.

Brainstem
- The brainstem connects the brain to the spinal cord.
- It controls vital functions.
- Injuries to the brainstem are invariably fatal, while one might survive severe cortical injuries.
- The brainstem contains the reticular activating system that affects arousal.

Table 3: Thalamic injuries.

Location	Thalamic nuclei	Key features
Inferolateral injuries (45% of thalamic strokes)	• Ventromedial • Ventrolateral	• Ataxia • Contralateral hemi hypoesthesia, i.e., decreased pain sensitivity • Impaired executive functions
Paramedian Injuries (35% of thalamic strokes)	Dorso-median	• Severe injury results in unconsciousness • Upward gaze paralysis • Apathy, amnesia, motivation
	Intralaminar	• Attention disorders, apathy
Anterior Injuries (15% of thalamic strokes)	Anterior thalamic	• Anterograde amnesia • Episodic and spatial amnesia • Role in Epilepsy, insomnia, prion disease • *Three sub nuclei:* Anteromedial, anterodorsal and anteroventral
	Anteromedial	• Anterograde amnesia with confabulation • Memory impairment in Alzheimer's disease and dementia
Posterior injuries (5% of thalamic strokes)	Pulvinar Nucleus	• 40% of the thalamus with extensive cortical connections • Responsible for visual processing, blindsight • *Injuries cause:* Hemi-spatial neglect, attention deficit, chronic pain, and photophobia

Thalamic pain syndrome: Thalamic injury (stroke, tumor, trauma, or abscess) results in chronic pain, with impaired sensation with dysesthesia (pain with itching, tingling, or burning sensations), or allodynia (pain without an obvious cause), and disturbances of temperature regulation.

To locate the level of brainstem pathology:
- Determine the craniocaudal level by following the cranial nerve rule:
  - Four cranial nerves (CNs) arise in each of the three regions: the midbrain, pons, and medulla oblongata **(Table 4)**.
- Next, determine the location of the injury by assessing the nature of the deficit:
  - *Anterior:* Descending *motor* corticospinal tracts
  - *Lateral:* Pain and *vibration*-transmitting spinothalamic tracts
  - *Posterior:* Touch and *vibration*-conducting posterior spinothalamic tracts.

Cerebellum

- The cerebellum primarily facilitates movement and helps with motor learning. The weight ratio of the cerebrum to the cerebellum in adults is 10:1, while in infants, it is 20:1.
- It has two lateral cerebellar hemispheres and a mid-line vermis.
- These hemispheres have three main parts:
  - Cerebrocerebellums (receive cortical input and initiate movements) have anterior and posterior lobes.
  - Inferiorly is the flocculonodular lobe
  - Mid-line spinocerebellum (gets spinal input and corrects errors in movements)

Cerebellar Injury
- *Tremors:* Contrast from Parkinson's resting tremor that disappears when movement is initiated
- *Ataxia:* Wide-based gait with circumduction of the limb
- *Ataxic dysarthria:* Slurred speech

Table 4: Anatomy of the mid-brain and brainstem.

	Anatomical features	Physiological roles
Mid-brain	Superior colliculi	Visual pathway
	Inferior colliculi	Auditory pathway
	Tegmentum and substantia nigra	Facilitate movements
	CN I–IV	
Pons	Nuclei of CN V–VIII	Sensory to head and face; motor to eyes, face, and mouth; equilibrium and autonomic functions
Medulla oblongata	Respiratory and cardiovascular centers; lower cranial nerve nuclei IX, X, XI, XII; and egress point of upper cranial nerves	Central control of respiratory and cardiovascular responses; roles in swallowing, sneezing, coughing, and vomiting

CHAPTER 3 Applied Anatomy of the Central Nervous System

- *Nystagmus:* Eyes make repetitive, uncontrolled movements
- *Dyssynergia:* Poorly coordinated movements
- *Dysmetria:* Inability to stop at a specified distance.
- *Hypotonia:* Muscle weakness
- *Diadochokinesia* is the inability to execute a rapid alternate movement, such as pronation and supination of the forearm.
- *Classical Romberg's Test is not a test of cerebellar dysfunction:* Romberg's test is tipping over with eyes closed. It can happen with eyes open in patients with cerebellar dysfunction; hence, the test is strictly negative. Romberg's sensory perception test is often confused with cerebellar dysfunction.

FURTHER READING

1. Braunsdorf M et al. Does the temporal cortex make us human? A review of structural and functional diversity of the primate temporal lobe. Neurosci Biobehav Rev. 2021;131:400-10.
2. Kong X et al. Sensory-motor cortices shape functional connectivity dynamics in the human brain. Nat Commun. 2021;12(1):6373.
3. Kullmann S et al. Resting-state functional connectivity of the human hypothalamus. Handb Clin Neurol. 2021;179:113-24.
4. Li K, Fan et al. The human mediodorsal thalamus: Organization, connectivity, and function. Neuroimage. 2022;249:118876.
5. Nano PR et al. Cortical Cartography: Mapping realization using single-cell omics technology. Front Neural Circuits. 2021;15:788560.

Vignette: The Evolution of the Nervous System

The human nervous system is highly complex, and it begs the question: how did such a complex system evolve? Genes for environmentally sensitive ion channels are found in unicellular organisms and some prokaryotes. It is believed that the proto-neurons evolved from cells that had secretory functions. These cells could sense the environment and release chemicals in response. Over time, specialized cells emerged that could coordinate the response throughout the animal. With such cells, it was possible to develop diffuse neural networks. These diffuse networks lacked proper synapses. The networks gave the cnidarians, such as hydra, the ability to catch food and to locomote in response to touch, temperature, and chemical changes. The centralized nervous system first arose in the planarians (flatworms) with a rudimentary bilobed brain-like structure. There were alternate nervous system designs that evolved at the same time. The octopi evolved a radial pattern with a ganglion for each arm and one smaller central ganglion. Though the ganglia function like a brain, they differ from one. The ganglia have a cluster of neurons, but these neurons do not densely communicate with each other. In contrast, the brains have specialized sub-components and a rich network of interneurons connecting them.

In evolutionary timelines, the first brains developed around 521 million years ago; approximately 250 million years ago, the paleomammalian brain developed with the hippocampus, amygdala, and limbic system. The most recent development in the last 200 million years has been the neocortex, corresponding to the pallium in reptiles, fish, and birds. However, of all brain components, it is the neocortex that has dramatically developed in the hominid brain in the last three million years.

Chapter 4

Spinal Cord Anatomy

INTRODUCTION

The spinal cord is the tubular extension of the central nervous system from the medulla oblongata to the conus medullaris. It is encased in the bony vertebral column. From the center outward, it consists of the central canal, gray matter, and white matter. Thus, spinal cord organization is reversed compared to the brain **(Fig. 1)**. Understanding the functional anatomy of the spinal cord is necessary for the anesthetic management of spine surgery cases and in the assessment of neuraxial blocks.

STRUCTURAL ORGANIZATION

- *Size and extent:*
  - The spinal cord is 40–50 cm long and 1–1.5 cm in diameter.
  - It constitutes 2% of the central nervous system (CNS) mass.
  - It extends throughout the length of the spine in embryonic life. However, the vertebral canal growth exceeds the development of the cord; therefore, in adults, the spinal cord ends at L1/2.
- *Segments:*
  - There are 31 spinal segments: *cervical:* 8; *thoracic:* 12; *lumbar:* 5; *sacral:* 5; *coccygeal:* 1.
  - Spinal nerves, except for the C1, exit below the corresponding vertebrae.
  - There are two regions of spinal cord enlargements: (1) Cervical C3-T1 and (2) Lumbar L1-S2.
- *Coverings and support:*
  - It is covered by dura, arachnoid, and pia matter. The cord is tethered to the dura by denticulate ligaments and by the dorsal and ventral roots.

FUNCTIONAL ORGANIZATION

- *Dermatome is an* area of the skin innervated by a single dorsal root.
- *Spinal nerve roots are dorsal* (sensory) and ventral (motor) roots.
- *Gray matter organization:* There are three broad layers **(Fig. 2)**:
  - *Dorsal horn:* Sensory

CHAPTER 4 Spinal Cord Anatomy

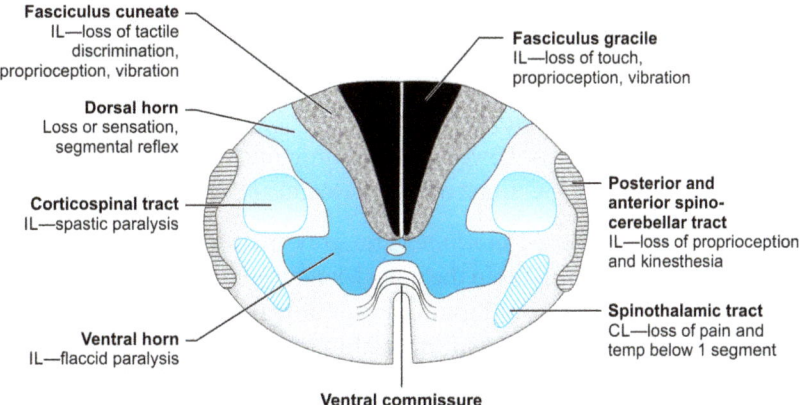

Fig. 1: Spinal tracts and consequences of injuries. (IL: ipsilateral; CL: contralateral; BL: bilateral)

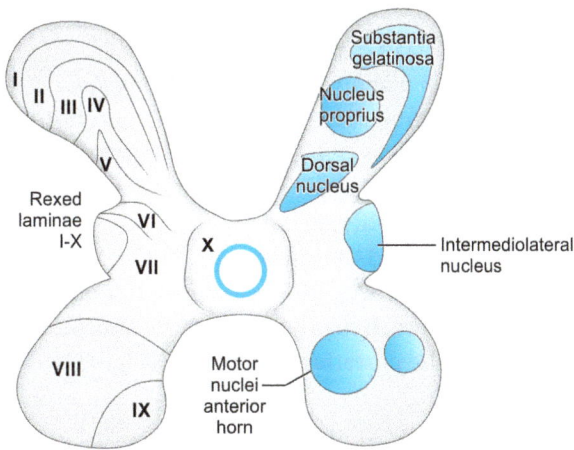

Fig. 2: Organization of the spinal gray matter.

- *Intermediolateral horn:* Visceral
- *Ventral horn:* Motor

Nuclei:
- Dorsal group:
  - *Marginal zone:* Axons to spinothalamic tracts: Pain and temperature
  - *Substantia gelatinosa:* Axons relay to ventral and lateral spinothalamic tracts: Transmit pain, temperature, and light touch impulses.
  - *The nucleus proprius, or* the chief sensory nucleus, contributes to ventral, and lateral spinothalamic tracts: Transmits light touch and pain impulses.
  - *Dorsal nucleus of Clarke (T1-L2):* Located in the lateral funiculus. The afferent dorsal spinocerebellar tracts relay unconscious proprioceptive information from muscle spindles to the cerebellum.

- *Intermediolateral group (C8-L3):*
  - Preganglionic sympathetic fibers relay to the lateral horn to transmit visceral pain.
- *Ventral group:*
  - Lower motor neuron nuclei
  - Innervate the visceral and skeletal muscles.

Rexed laminae: The gray matter of the spinal cord is organized into *laminae* in the dorsal, lateral, and ventral horns. The dorsal horn: Receives sensory input through dorsal nerve roots (laminae I–VI), interoceptive sensations from within the body (I–IV), and proprioceptive sensations (V–VI). The intermediate horn (laminae VII) relays proprioceptive impulses from muscle spindles to the mid-brain and cerebellum. The ventral horn (laminae VIII and IX) relays between motor neurons. Rexed lamina X surrounds the central canal.

SPINAL CORD BLOOD FLOW

Organization of spinal cord blood flow:
- Three spinal arteries, one anterior (ASA) and two posterior spinal arteries (PSA) descend along the length of the spinal cord **(Fig. 3)**.
- The arteries form 6–8 arterial rings, from which branches arise to perfuse the cord radially.
- The ASA perfuses the anterior two-thirds of the gray matter.
- The PSA perfuses the posterior one-third of the gray matter.
- At each segmental level, the radicular arteries augment the anterior and the posterior arterial flow **(Fig. 4)**.

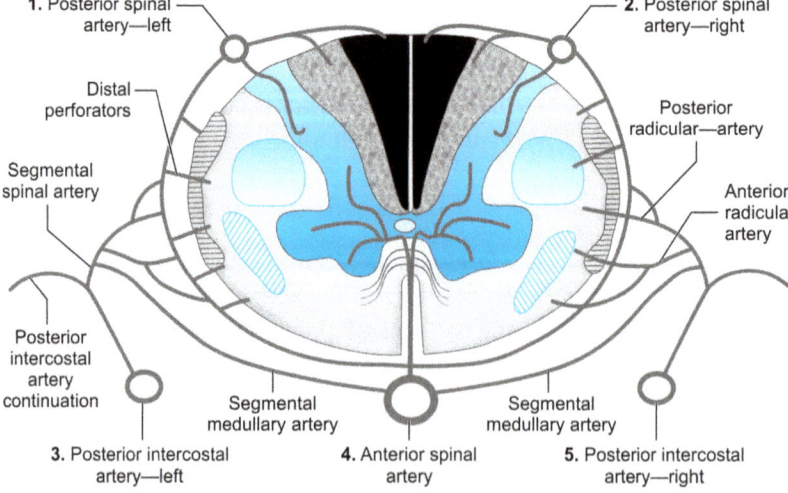

Fig. 3: Segmental spinal cord blood flow with collateral flow from five arteries shown as 1–5.

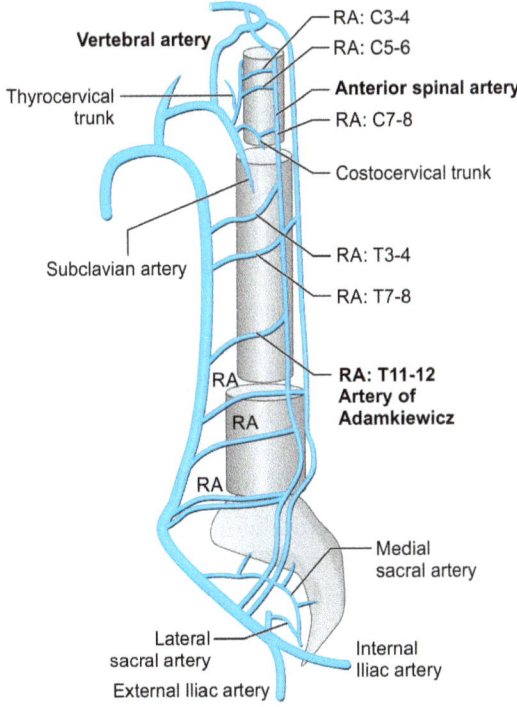

Fig. 4: Arterial supply to the spinal cord. (RA: radicular artery)

Anterior spinal artery:
- It is the dominant artery of the spinal cord.
- It is formed in the cervical region from branches of the vertebral artery that fuse into a single artery at the medulla.
- Descends in the anterior spinal groove, receiving supplementary branches from the segmental arteries.
- At the T10 level, the ASA receives the artery of Adamkiewicz.
- *The artery of Adamkiewicz:*
  - Usually arises from the left posterior intercostal artery at T9 to T 12 levels.
  - In the lower lumbar-sacral region, it is supplemented by several arteries from the pelvis.
  - It is 0.6–1.8 mm in diameter.
  - It provides significant blood supply to the lumbar and sacral cord.
  - Occlusion of the artery results in flaccid paralysis at the level of injury and spastic paralysis below the level; bilateral loss of pain and temperature below the lesion; urinary and fecal incontinence while proprioception, vibration, and touch are spared.
- Occlusion of the ASA can lead to infarction of the spinal cord, and the risk is most significant in the thoracic region.

Posterior spinal arteries:
- They can originate from the vertebral artery, posterior inferior cerebellar, or posterior radicular artery at C-2.
- They descend along the posterior nerve roots.

Pial arterial plexus:
- It arises from the ASAs and the PSAs.
- It encircles the cord. It gives rise to penetrating arteries that supply the outer portions of the spinal cord.

Radicular arteries:
- A pair of radicular arteries at each segmental level, 31 pairs in all.
- They usually do not penetrate the spinal cord.
- They supply blood to the dura, nerve root, and spinal ganglia.

Regulation of Spinal Cord Blood Flow
- Spinal cord blood flow (SCBF) regulation is similar to cerebral blood flow (CBF).
- Of note is the reverse anatomy of the spinal cord compared to the brain, with the white matter outside and the gray matter inside.
- SCBF is higher than CBF.
- The values of SCBF vary between animal species, reflecting arterial supply, venous drainage, and intraspinal pressure differences.
- The spinal cord white matter blood flow is 15–25 mL/100 g/min, and the gray matter blood flow is 100–150 mL/100 g/min.
- SCBF is pressure autoregulated when mean arterial pressure (MAP) ranges between 50 and 135 mm Hg.
- The autonomic nervous system plays a more significant role.
- Like CBF, SCF increases linearly with $PaCO_2$ from 50 to 90 mm Hg.

Preventing Spinal Cord Ischemia
- The gray matter of the spinal cord has a much higher metabolic rate than the white matter, and it is perfused predominantly by the ASA.
- Hypotension, loss of autoregulation, and spinal shock can increase the vulnerability of the spinal cord to ischemic injury.
- Ischemia triggers secondary events such as excitotoxic damage, lipid peroxidation, free radical injury, and inflammation.
- The MAP should be maintained at ≥ 90 mm Hg.
- During aortic clamping, the cerebrospinal fluid (CSF) drain attenuates the rise in intraspinal pressure.
- The benefits of steroid treatment remain unproven and may have adverse effects.
- Hypothermia is beneficial after SCI after cardiac arrest and aortic clamping but is unproven for traumatic cord injuries.

ORGANIZATION OF SENSORY SYSTEM (FIG. 5)

There are two main parts of the sensory system:
1. *Cranial nerves:* Transmit sensation from the head and the face.
2. *Spinal nerves:* Transmit sensation from the rest of the body.

The sensory pathways from the rest of the body also follow two courses:
1. The lateral spinothalamic tracts that cross over to the opposite side at the segmental level.
2. The dorsal column ascends on the same side to cross over at the midbrain level.

Pain and Temperature

The pain and temperature sensations are transmitted via the dorsal root ganglion to the spinal cord via the Aδ and C fibers.
- *Aδ fibers:*
  - The first-order neurons are the Aδ fibers, whose cell bodies are in the dorsal root ganglion. They relay into the spinal cord's posterior

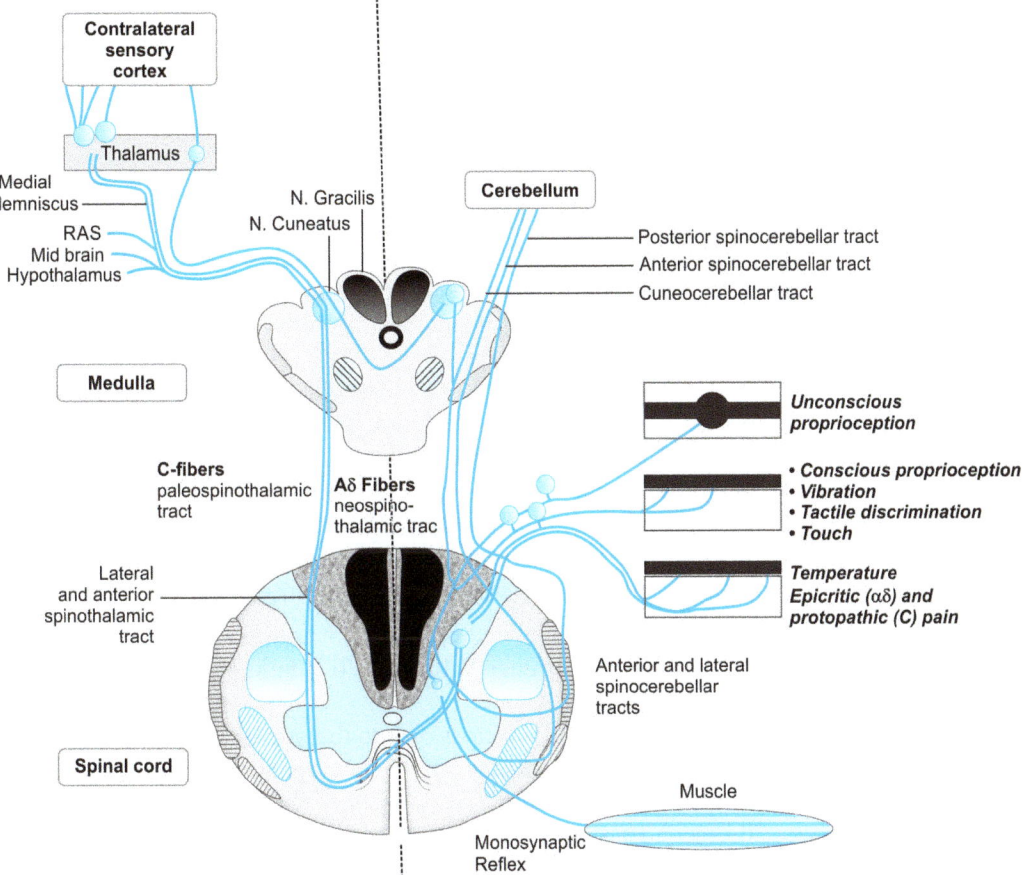

Fig. 5: Organization of sensory pathways.

horn (laminae III and IV). They conduct the sharp/pricking pain sensation, which is well-localized.
- The second-order neurons then cross the mid-line within a segment and relay from the lateral spinothalamic tract to the thalamus. At the pontine level, the tract lies close to the medial lemniscus.
- The third-order neurons then project from the thalamus to the primary and the secondary cortex in areas 3, 1, and 2. A small number of fibers enter the brainstem reticular formation.
- *C fibers:*
  - C fibers are smaller fibers that conduct slow, poorly localized, burning pain.
  - Afferents from the dorsal root ganglia enter the spinal cord. They cross the midline to form the lateral spinothalamic tract. The tract relays to the reticular formation.
  - They project diffusely into the cortex. This pain is poorly localized and has an emotional component.

Touch, Pressure, and Kinesthesia
- The touch sensation can be fine or crude. The fine (epicritic) touch enables subtle discrimination of shapes and textures. The crude (protopathic) touch lacks such qualities.

Epicritic Touch
Mechanoreceptors (proprioceptive and vibratory) located throughout the body constantly report position- and movement-related information to the brain. The proprioceptive end organs are located in the joints and muscle spindles. Most of this information remains in the subconscious realm with minimal awareness.
- The primary fibers from mechanoreceptors ascend in the posterior column and at the mid-brain relay into the nucleus gracilis and cuneatus.
- The second-order neurons, the internal arcuate fibers, then ascend in the medial lemniscus to the thalamus.
- The third-order neurons then project into the sensory cortex.
- Collateral fibers project into the reticular formation and the cerebellum and are responsible for subconscious kinesthesia.

Subconscious proprioception: Proprioceptive information enters the dorsal horn and synapse in laminae V, VI, and VII (Clarke's column). They then ascend by two routes:
1. The second-order fibers cross over to the opposite side and ascend in the *anterior spinocerebellar tract* to the upper pons. They report to the contralateral cerebellum.
2. The second-order medial fibers ascend on the same side to the pons as the *posterior spinocerebellar tract* and project into the ipsilateral cerebellum.

Protopathic Touch

- The primary fibers for protopathic touch relay to the dorsal root ganglia and enter the spinal cord. They cross over to the opposite side within one or two levels. In the spinal cord, they synapse in laminae VI–VIII.
- The second-order neurons then ascend to the thalamus.
- The third-order neurons then project into the sensory cortex.
- Collateral fibers project into the reticular formation, but their significance is relatively unknown.

MANIFESTATIONS OF INJURIES TO THE SENSORY PATHWAYS

- *Peripheral nerve injury (e.g., trauma):*
  - Flaccid paralysis
  - Loss of sensation
  - Loss of muscle tone
  - Loss of reflexes
  - Muscular atrophy
- *Posterior nerve root injury (e.g., disc herniation):*
  - Paresthesia
  - Paroxysmal pain
  - Decreased sensation.
  - Loss of reflexes
  - High stepping gait
  - *Positive Romberg's sign:* Loss of balance with eyes closed due to impaired proprioception.
- *Posterior and lateral funiculus injury (e.g., subacute combined degeneration of the cord).*
  - Loss of proprioception
  - Loss of vibratory sense
  - Muscle weakness
  - Spasticity
  - Hyperactive tendon reflexes
  - Positive Romberg test
  - Positive Babinski test is the dorsiflexion of the great toe with fanning of small ones on stimulation of the lateral aspect of the sole.
- *Gray commissure injury:* Gray matter around the central canal of the spinal cord, lamina X (e.g., syringomyelia)
  - Bilateral loss of pain and temperature at the level of injury
  - No loss of sensations below (sensory disassociation).

SENSORY CORTEX

Primary Sensory Cortex

- It is located in the postcentral gyrus and corresponds to Brodmann areas 3, 1, and 2.
- The area corresponds to a region of dense thalamocortical projections.
- The thalamic neurons project into the IV layer of the cortical cells.
- The cells from this layer project into other cortical layers.
- The projection is vertically stratified into layers of slowly and rapidly adapting neurons.
- The primary sensory cortex is the area of projection of tactile sensation from the contralateral side of the body of the cortex.
- Specifically, the 3B area in the caudal part of the sensory cortex is considered to be critical. It receives most of the thalamic projections, is exceedingly sensitive to somatosensory inputs, and on stimulation, generates sensory effects.
- The area of representation of the sensations is proportional to the density of cutaneous touch receptors. Thus, the face and hand occupy large regions of the homunculus **(Fig. 6)**.
- Injuries to the primary sensory cortex impair the projection of texture, shapes, and size perception by touch.

Secondary Sensory Cortex

- It is located in the parietal cortex and the lateral sulcus.
- It corresponds to Brodmann areas 40 and 43.
- It assists in remembering different tactile shapes and textures.

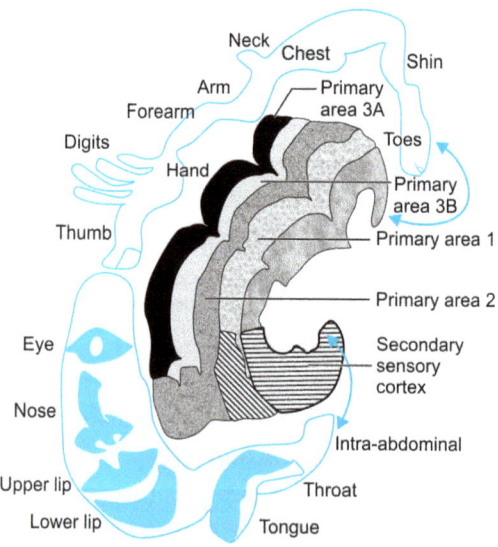

Fig. 6: Sensory cortex with cortical tactile projection in blue.

Common Cortical Sensory Disorders
- *Agraphesthesia* is the difficulty recognizing words written on the skin or the palm.
- *Hemihypesthesia:* Unilateral impairment of tactile sensation
- *Astereognosis:* Inability to recognize the shape of an object with eyes closed.

ORGANIZATION OF THE MOTOR SYSTEM
Motor Cortex
- *Primary motor cortex:*
  - It initiates movements in coordination with other supplementary motor areas.
  - Spontaneous motor tasks are complex. They require synthesizing information from many regions of the brain through many hierarchical feedback loops. For example, lifting a feather or a kettlebell from the exact location requires planning and activation of very different control of the muscles. Furthermore, performing the same task with eyes closed would require very different strategies and muscle control.
  - The primary motor cortex is located in the precentral gyrus, the M1 region.
  - On the motor homunculus, area representation depends on the degree and sophistication of motor control needed for a given body part. Consequently, the areas of the brain controlling the hand and the face dominate the homunculus.
  - These neurons give rise to the corticospinal tracts—the main pathway for controlling voluntary movements **(Fig. 7)**.
- *Premotor complex:*
  - It lies anterior to the primary motor cortex.
  - Functions:
    - Planning of complex movements
    - Sensory guidance of movement
    - It controls movements of the trunk and proximal muscles.
    - It contains fibers to the primary motor cortex and brainstem.
- *Supplementary motor complex:*
  - It is anterior to the primary motor cortex and medial to the premotor cortex.
  - Planning of complex movements
  - Coordinating with bilateral movements
  - It contains fibers to the primary motor cortex and brainstem.
- *Parietal association cortex:*
  - It is located posterior to the sensory cortex.
  - It helps to plan visually guided movements.

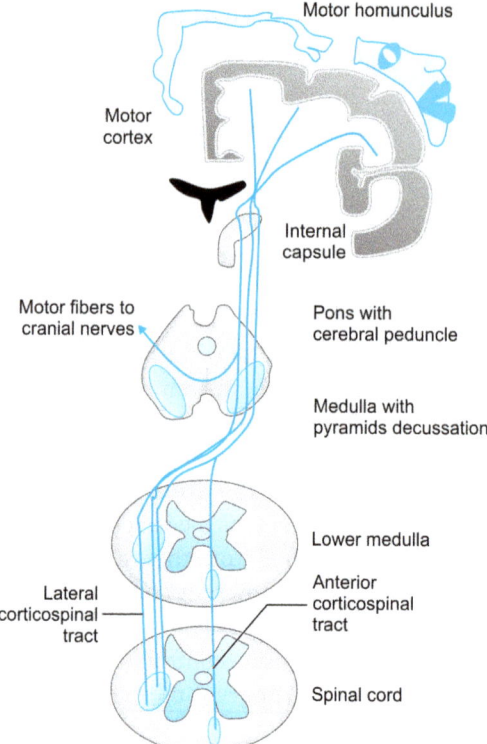

Fig. 7: Organization of motor tracts.

Subcortical Structures

- *Basal ganglia:*
  - Gray matter bodies that lie deep in the cerebral hemispheres
  - Functions:
    - Subconscious control of movement
    - Do not initiate movement.
    - Smoothen-out movement.
    - Affect the movement of the trunk and proximal muscles.
- *Thalamus:*
  - Thalamus lies between the cortex and other structures related to movements that, include the basal ganglia and the cerebellum.
  - Functions:
    - It interacts with these structures to help execute complex movements.
    - It also helps in learning complex motor tasks.

Cerebellum: The principal role of the cerebellum is to smoothen motor movements, e.g., to coordinate with the muscles, increase spatial precision, and control the duration of motor activity.

CHAPTER 4 Spinal Cord Anatomy

Cerebellar damage affects:
- Fine movements
- Balance
- Posture
- Motor learning

Descending Pathways

- *Corticospinal tracts:* Three corticospinal tracts arise from the primary motor cortex but cross over at different levels and are responsible for the conscious control of the innervated muscles.
  - *Corticobulbar tract:* Cross over at the brainstem; terminate on the motor nuclei of the lower cranial nerves at the level of the brainstem
  - *Lateral corticospinal tract:* Cross over at the pyramids of the medulla oblongata; terminate in the lower motor neuron in the anterior spinal horn.
  - *Anterior corticospinal tract:* Cross over at the pyramids of the spinal segment; terminate in the lower motor neuron in the anterior spinal horn.
- *Medial pathway:*
  - *Vestibulospinal tracts* arise from the vestibular nuclei and terminate at the lower motor neurons of the anterior horn. These fibers do not cross. Their role is in the regulation of balance and muscle tone.
  - *Tectospinal tract:* They arise from the tectum (superior and inferior colliculi) to the lower motor neuron in the contralateral anterior spinal horn of cervical segments. They cross over at the brainstem. They control the positioning of the eye, head, neck, and arm in response to visual and auditory stimuli.
  - *Reticulospinal tract:* They arise from the brainstem reticular formation to the spinal lower motor neurons of the same side. They do not cross over. They regulate reflex activity.
- *Lateral pathway:*
  - *Rubrospinal tract:* They arise from the red nuclei in the brainstem to the spinal lower motor neurons of the opposite side. They cross over at the brain stem. They regulate upper limb muscle tone and movement.

Motor Pathway Injuries

- *Anterior horn injury (e.g., poliomyelitis) leads to:*
  - Flaccid paralysis
  - Loss of muscle tone
  - Loss of reflexes
  - Muscular atrophy

Table 1: Upper versus lower motor neuron lesions.

Paralysis type	Upper motor neuron	Lower motor neuron
Weakness	*Arm:* Extensor > flexors *Legs:* Flexors > extensors	In a specific nerve root distribution
Wasting	Minimal	Significant, focal
Reflexes	++++	Impaired
Clonus	++++	Absent
Spasticity	++++	Flaccid
Fasciculation	None	+++
Babinski's sign	+	N/A
Hoffman's sign	+ but not specific	N/A
Pronator drift	+	N/A

- Anterior horn and lateral corticospinal tract injuries (e.g., amyotrophic lateral sclerosis) lead to:
  - Muscle weakness
  - Fasciculation
  - Spastic paralysis
  - Muscular atrophy

Upper versus Lower Motor Neuron Lesion

Upper versus lower motor neuron lesions are compared in **Table 1**.
- *Babinski's sign* indicates fanning out of the toes when the sole is stimulated. It usually disappears by two years of age, as with other reflexes such as grasping, sucking, and rooting.
- *Hoffman's sign:* It indicates flexion of the thumb and the fingers with the flicking of the distal phalanx of the middle finger.
- *Pronator drift:* With an upper motor neuron lesion, the extended arms show progressive pronation when the eyes are closed.

AMERICAN SPINAL INJURY SCORING (ASIA)

- *Complete spinal cord injury:* Bilateral loss of motor/sensation functions below injury
- *Incomplete spinal cord injury:* Preserves some functions below the injury.
- American spinal injury score:
  - *Grade A:* No function
  - *Grade B:* Sensory but no motor function
  - *Grade C:* Sensory with motor strength grade 3 or less
  - *Grade D:* Sensory with motor strength greater than grade 3
  - *Grade E:* No deficits

CHAPTER 4 Spinal Cord Anatomy

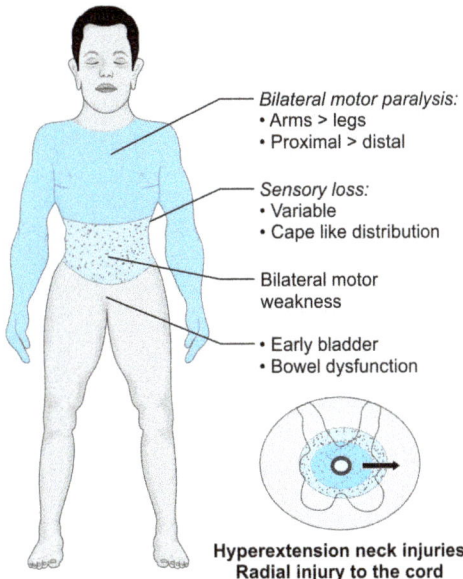

Fig. 8: Central cord syndrome.

SPINAL CORD SYNDROMES

Syndromes listed in order of their clinical frequency are:
- *Central cord syndrome* **(Fig. 8)**
  - Most common spinal cord injury (SCI), accounting for 45% of all classified injuries
  - Usually, in the elderly >50 years, often with degenerative spine disease
  - Typically, due to hyper-extension of the cervical spine
  - Results in:
    - Weakness of the arms more than the legs
    - Partial sensory loss below the level of injury
    - Cape-like sensory loss:
      - Affecting the arms and trunk
      - Pain and temperature sensations lost.
      - Light touch and proprioception are preserved.
    - Urinary retention and incontinence
    - Recovery possible
- *Cauda equina syndrome* **(Fig. 9)**
  - About 25% of the classified SCI
  - Besides trauma, it can be due to tumors, hematoma, and infection (abscesses)
  - Injury to the nerves emerging from conus medullaris.
  - Lumbar symptoms earlier than sacral symptoms

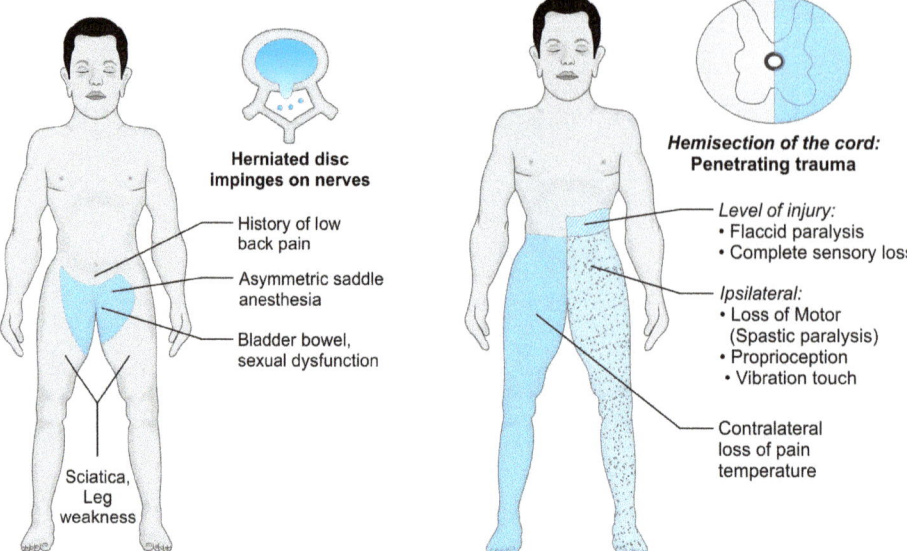

Fig. 9: Cauda-equina syndrome. **Fig. 10:** Brown–Séquard syndrome.

- Results in:
  - Back pain is less than with conus medullaris syndrome.
  - Gradual and unilateral radiculopathy
  - Saddle anesthesia is asymmetric.
  - Incontinence of the bowel is late.
  - Urinary retention is late.
  - Sexual dysfunction less frequent than conus medullaris
- *Brown–Séquard syndrome (20%)* **(Fig. 10)**
  - Hemi-section of the spinal cord
    - Typically, it is caused by penetrating trauma, stabbing, or gunshot injury. Other causes include tumors, ischemia, infection, inflammation, and bends.
  - *Results in:*
    - *At the level of injury:*
      - Flaccid paralysis
      - Loss of sensation
    - *On the side of injury below:*
      - Spastic paralysis
      - Hyperreflexia
    - Impaired sensations
    - Proprioception
    - Vibration
    - Fine touch

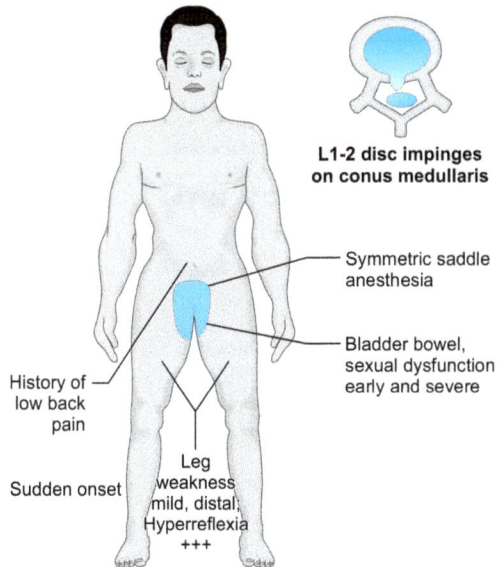

Fig. 11: Conus medullaris syndrome.

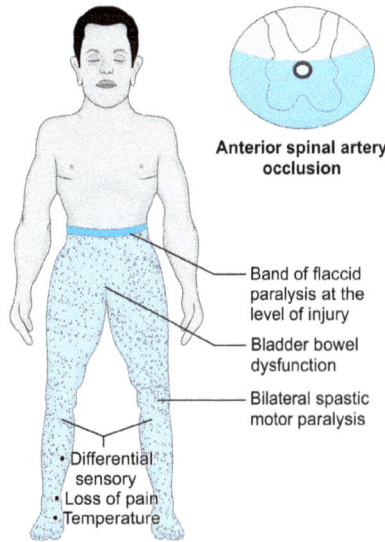

Fig. 12: Anterior spinal syndrome.

- *On the opposite side*:
  - Usually, one to two levels below as the fiber cross-over requires one to two segments.
  - Loss of pain and temperature
- Conus medullaris syndrome **(Fig. 11)**
  - It accounts for about 10% of the classified SCI.
  - Usually due to compression of the conus because of T12-L2 injury
  - Clinical features as with cauda equina syndrome but with sacral dominance
  - *Results in:*
    - Back pain is frequent.
    - Symmetric saddle anesthesia
    - Bowel incontinence occurs early.
    - Urinary retention occurs early.
    - Sexual dysfunction is frequently seen.
    - Pain radiating down the legs, ankle jerk is lost
- Anterior spinal injury syndrome **(Fig. 12)**
  - Seen in 5% of spinal cord injuries.
  - The most common partial injury.
  - After high-velocity impact with flexion and rotation of the spine.
  - Usually, due to ischemic injury to the anterior cord
  - *Results in:*
    - Complete motor paralysis below the lesion
    - Loss of pain and temperature below the lesion

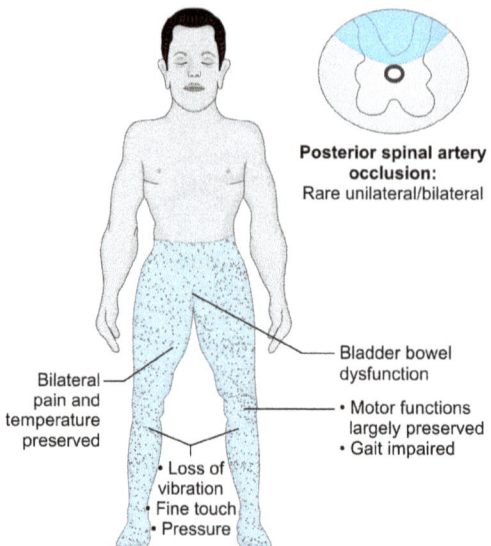

Fig. 13: Posterior spinal syndrome.

- Dorsal column sensation (vibration and proprioception) intact
- Bowel incontinence and urinary retention
- Hypotension due to autonomic dysfunction
- *Posterior spinal injury syndrome* **(Fig. 13)**
    - Rare type of SCI—<1%
    - Due to hyperextension spine injury, tumors, vitamin B_{12} deficiency, and infections (syphilis)
    - *Results in:*
        - Ipsilateral/bilateral loss of:
            - Proprioception
            - Vibration
            - Fine touch
            - Pressure
            - Motor power preserved.
        - Impaired reflexes and extreme paralysis

FURTHER READING

1. Ahuja CS et al. Spinal cord injury-What are the Controversies? J Orthop Trauma. 2017;31(Suppl 4):S7-13.
2. Cadotte DW et al. What has been learned from magnetic resonance imaging examination of the injured human spinal cord: A Canadian perspective. J Neurotrauma, 2018;35(16):1942-57.
3. Parthiban J et al. Outcomes of spinal cord injury: WFNS spine committee recommendations. Neurospine, 2020;17(4):809-19.

4. Powers JM, et al. Ten key insights into the use of spinal cord fMRI. Brain Sci. 2018;8(9):173.
5. Wei ZX et al. Spinal cord magnetic resonance imaging: methods and applications. Sheng Li Xue Bao, 2021;73(3):369-88.

Vignette: Santiago Ramon Y Cajal: The Man Who Mapped the Neurons

Santiago Ramon Y Cajal was a pioneering neuroscientist whose brain and spinal cord illustrations have been used for nearly a century. Cajal applied the Golgi method to stain dendrites and axons with potassium dichromate and silver nitrate. The method permitted imaging of frail structures beyond conventional microscopy. The technique revealed the complex and highly organized dendritic networks within and between various brain structures that were also very aesthetic. Cajal's biography is exceptional in many ways. It includes the 1906 Nobel Prize for medicine and imprisonment at a very young age. At the age of 11 years, he was arrested after he blew up his neighbor's farm gate with a homemade cannon. He was declared to be a poor student at school. Allegedly lacking in discipline, he started as an apprentice to a cobbler. He was introduced to anatomy while digging bodies with his father, who was an anatomy instructor. Cajal was, however, a precocious talent who excelled in athletics, arts, and the sciences. He died in 1934 at the age of 82 years.

Chapter 5

Visual Pathway

INTRODUCTION

The visual pathway represents structures extending from the cornea to the cortex that convert light energy into electrical signals that the brain can interpret.

FUNCTIONS OF THE VISUAL SYSTEM

- *Image-forming functions:*
  - Create an image of the environment by perceiving light, recognizing shape and color, and perceiving depth and distances.
  - Perception of motion
  - To guide movement.
- *Nonimage-forming functions:* Include pupillary light reflex and circadian rhythm.

ORGANIZATION OF THE VISUAL SYSTEM

Cornea

Avascular structure accounts for 80% of the focusing power of the eye.

Pupil

- The Iris controls the pupillary diameter, which is 3–7 mm in size, depending on the light intensity. The pupillary area can vary by as much as five-fold.
- *Stiles–Crawford effect:* Central stimulation results in a brighter image than with marginal stimulation of the retina.
- With low light, when the pupillary diameter increases, vision is maintained even when illumination is decreased by ten-fold.

Lens

The lens provides 20% of the focusing power but adjusts dynamically. Ciliary muscles control the lens curvature. *Accommodation* is the power to focus on objects at different distances. Myopia is impaired distant vision. *Presbyopia* is impaired near vision.

   Myopia or near-sightedness, is impaired distant vision. *Presbyopia* is age-related inability to focus images on the retina due to changes in refractiveness of the lens increased lens rigidity or poor ciliary muscle control of lens curvature. It is an aging related problem. *Hypermetropia* or hyperopia is far-sightedness due to the image forming behind the retina. Unlike presbyopia is not age related and can be due to development defects, trauma, or malignancy. Hypermetropia presents with blurry vision, photophobia, intorsion of the eyes, fatigue, watery eyes, and headaches.

Retina

- It is the photosensitive layer of the eye.
- The receptors are oriented toward the pigment layer.
- The 6–7 million cones for color vision are densely located in the rod-free fovea centralis. The three types of cones have peak light absorption wavelengths at 420–440, 530–550, and 560–580 nm, respectively. They have higher spatial resolution and are responsible for visual acuity. Cones function across a narrow band of light intensity whereas the rods perform across a much wider band of intensity.
- The 120 million rods for dim light vision are distributed widely.
- The pigment layer absorbs light, prevents backscattering, and provides nutrition to the retinal receptors.
- Retinal signals are passed through four transparent layers of cells: (1) amacrine, (2) bipolar, (3) horizontal, and (4) ganglion. The ganglion cells relay through the blind spot that is devoid of receptors.

Neural Circuits

- Image processing takes place in the retina, where the ganglion cells process the signal generated from the retina, and the information is passed to the optic nerve **(Fig. 1)**.
- The optic nerve fibers from the temporal and medial sides separate at the chiasma and cross over to the opposite side of the lateral geniculate body.
- The lateral geniculate receives 90% of the optic tract fibers, while the superior colliculus, pretectum, and hypothalamus receive 10%.
- The superior colliculus receives information about eye movements. The pretectum controls the pupillary responses. The visual input to the hypothalamus plays a role in the perception of circadian rhythms.
- However, visual information is controlled by the lateral geniculate body, which also receives descending signals from the visual cortex, thalamus, and brainstem.
- The lateral geniculate is organized in six layers, with alternate bands receiving information from the ipsilateral and contralateral eyes.
- From there, the information is transmitted to the striate cortex. The striate cortex interacts with the temporal and parietal lobes to generate meaningful information.
- **Table 1** lists the abnormalities in the visual fields due to injuries along the visual pathway.

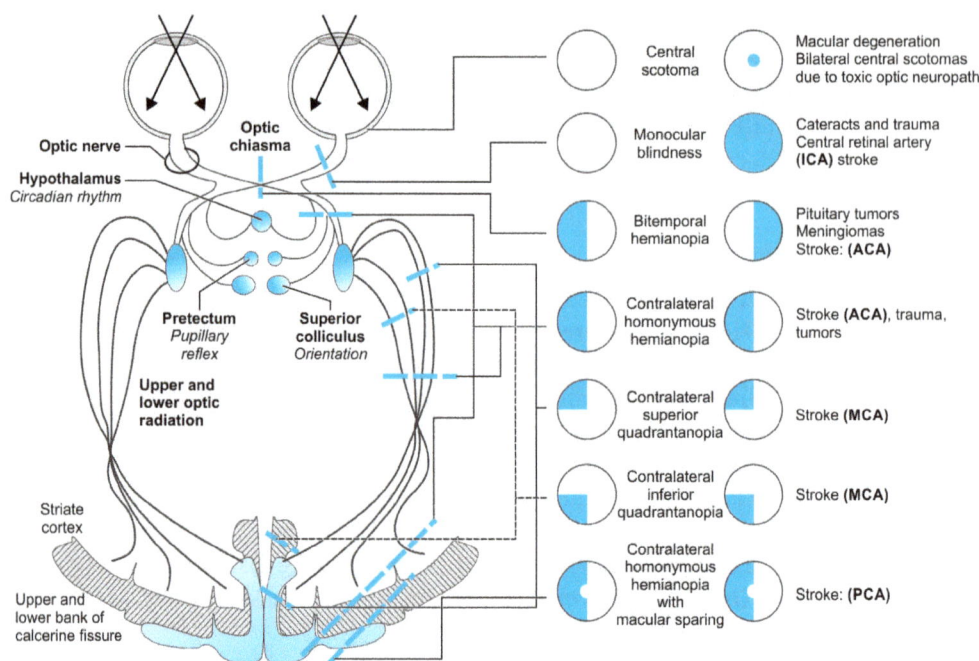

Fig. 1: Optical pathway, visual field defects, and vascular territories. (ICA: internal carotid artery; ACA: anterior cerebral artery; MCA: middle cerebral artery; PCA: posterior cerebral artery).

Table 1: Injuries to visual pathway.		
Component and function	**Visual field anomaly**	**Etiology**
Retina: Rods (scotopic vision) function in relative darkness, while cones function in light for color vision (photopic vision)	Central scotoma	Retinal degenerative diseases, detachment, and ischemic retinopathy
Optic nerve: Links retina to the cortex, pupillary, and accommodative reflex	Mono-ocular blindness, impaired pupillary, and accommodative reflexes	Optic neuritis or atrophy, ischemia or emboli of retinal artery, and papilledema
Optic chiasma: Crossover of nasal and temporal fibers	Mid-line crossing fibers interruption: Bitemporal heteronymous hemianopsia	Pituitary adenoma, craniopharyngioma, internal carotid artery aneurysm, and meningiomas
Optic tracts: Project into the lateral geniculate, superior colliculi, and the suprachiasmatic nuclei	Contralateral homonymous hemianopsia	Middle cerebral artery stroke
The lateral geniculate nucleus transmits via optic radiations to the cortex	Contralateral homonymous hemianopsia	Middle cerebral artery stroke
Optic radiations: Lateral bundle or Meyer's track and medial bundle	Lateral bundle: Contralateral upper homonymous quadrantanopia; medial bundle: contralateral lower homonymous quadrantanopia; both: contralateral homonymous hemianopsia	Middle cerebral artery stroke, upper deficit temporal stroke, and lower deficit parietal stroke
Visual cortex	Contralateral homonymous hemianopsia with macular sparing	Posterior cerebral artery stroke

CHAPTER 5 Visual Pathway

FURTHER READING

1. Bridge H et al. Structural and functional brain reorganization due to blindness: the special case of bilateral congenital anophthalmia. Neurosci Biobehav Rev. 2019;107:765-74.
2. Najarpour Foroushani A, et al. Cortical visual prostheses: from microstimulation to functional percept. J Neural Eng. 2018;15(2):021005.
3. Pitcher D, et al. Evidence for a third visual pathway specialized for social perception. Trends Cogn Sci. 2021;25(2):100-10.
4. Sellal F. Anatomical and neurophysiological basis of face recognition. Rev Neurol (Paris). 2021.
5. Sims JR et al. Role of structural, metabolic, and functional MRI in monitoring visual system impairment and recovery. J Magn Reson Imaging. 2021;54(6): 1706-29.

Vignette: The Roach Leads the Pack

Light perception threshold: Human beings: 1 lux, cats: 0.125 lux, tarsier: 0.001 lux, dung beetle: 0.001–0.0001 lux, the social sweet bee: 0.00063 lux, carpenter bee: 0.000063 lux, but the most sensitive light perception is by the cockroach whose receptors can respond to a few as -1photon/10 s. The extreme sensitivity of the roach's eyes is because they have abundant photoreceptors and temporarily synthesize information from different receptors to recreate the image—similar to time-lapse photography.

Vignette: Use it or Lose it

Cave animals like crustaceans and fish that live in perpetual darkness lose their eyesight. The eyes lose the pigmentation, and the lens fails to form, eventually the eyes atrophy. Downregulation of the PAX 6 gene plays a critical role in ocular regression. Conversely, in fruit flies, the overexpression of PAX 6 can induce the development of additional ectopic eyes. PAX 6, in conjunction with the SOX2 gene, plays a critical role early development of the eyes, particularly the lens. These genes are similar in developing mammalian eyes and ocular degenerative diseases. Creatures with extra eyes are the subject of many mythological tales. Many animals have more eyes than we can see. The insects, for example, have two large compound eyes, but there are three other minor simple eyes.

Chapter 6

Auditory Pathway

INTRODUCTION

The auditory system includes the ear and the auditory pathway.

The ear consists of the external, middle, and internal ear. The external ear consists of the pinna, the external auditory canal, and the eardrum. The middle ear contains three bones, malleus, incus, and stapes.

The inner ear consists of the utricle, saccule, and cochlea. The auditory pathway extends from the cochlea (Organ of Corti) to the cortex. The ear converts mechanical sound signals into electrical impulses. The auditory pathways transmit the impulses to the cortex and decode them as meaningful sounds.

FUNCTIONS OF THE AUDITORY SYSTEM

- *Hearing:* The perception and decoding of sound signals.
- Equilibrium
- Motion perception
- Arousal response.

ORGANIZATION OF THE AUDITORY SYSTEM

- The pinna, or the auricle, is the externally visible part of the ear. It is a helical structure that gathers and redirects sound waves to the external auditory meatus and the ear canal. It amplifies low-frequency conversational sounds by 10–15 folds. It also has an upward directional bias that can help localize the source of sound vibrations. The sound vibrations travel through the canal to the eardrum to vibrate the ossicular chain **(Fig. 1)**.
- The ossicular chain consists of malleus, incus, and stapes. Together, they amplify sound about 20-fold while transmitting it to the inner ear. The chain can also dampen loud sound signals.
- The inner ear consists of the vestibular apparatus and the cochlea. The vestibular apparatus consists of the three semi-circular canals, the utricle, and the saccule, that help with orientation and balance, while the cochlea is the organ of hearing. Common to the vestibular and the auditory systems are the hair cells that can sense the subtle disturbances of the endolymph that bathes them.

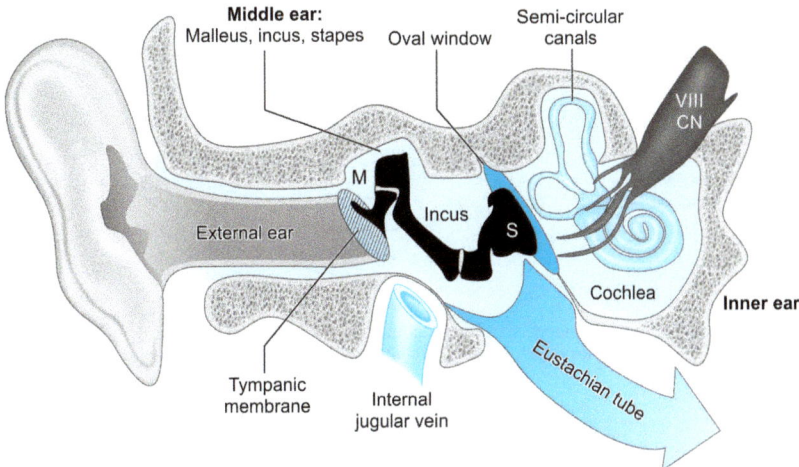

Fig. 1: Anatomy of the ear.

- There are two types of hair cells in the cochlea: (1) inner (3,500) and (2) outer (12,000). The hair in the cells extends 2–5 micrometers in length. The largest hair cells embed in a membranous structure, the tectorial membrane. The hair cells and the tectorial membrane amplify the mechanical signals to depolarize and generate nerve impulses **(Fig. 2)**.
- *Cochlear pathway:* The vibrations in the endolymph are sensed by the hair cells. Tufts of hair cells translate mechanical movements to electric impulses through Ca^{++}-gated voltage channels. The electric pulses are then transmitted via the auditory part of the VIII cranial nerve (VIII CN).
- *Vestibular pathway:* It consists of three perpendicularly oriented (lateral, superior and posterior) semi-circular canals, utricle, and saccule sense balance, movement, and acceleration. Hair cells and otoliths can sense the displacement of the endolymph during movement. These hair cells are located in the ampullae at the base of the semi-circular canal. The otoliths are located in the utricle and the saccules. The impulse generated is transmitted to the vestibular part of VIII CN.

Auditory Pathway

- It consists of two main components: (1) Lemniscal or primary and (2) Non-lemniscal (also known as the non-primary pathway or the reticular sensory pathway), as shown in **Figure 3**.
- *Lemniscal pathway:*
  - *First-order neurons:* In the auditory nerve, pass via the internal auditory meatus to the cochlear nucleus.
  - *Second-order neurons:* These cross the mid-line relay to the superior olivary complex.
  - *Third-order neurons:* Terminate at the inferior colliculus.

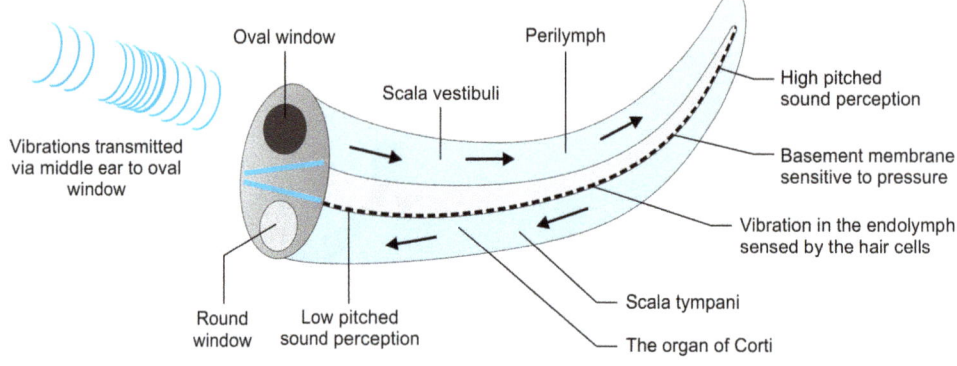
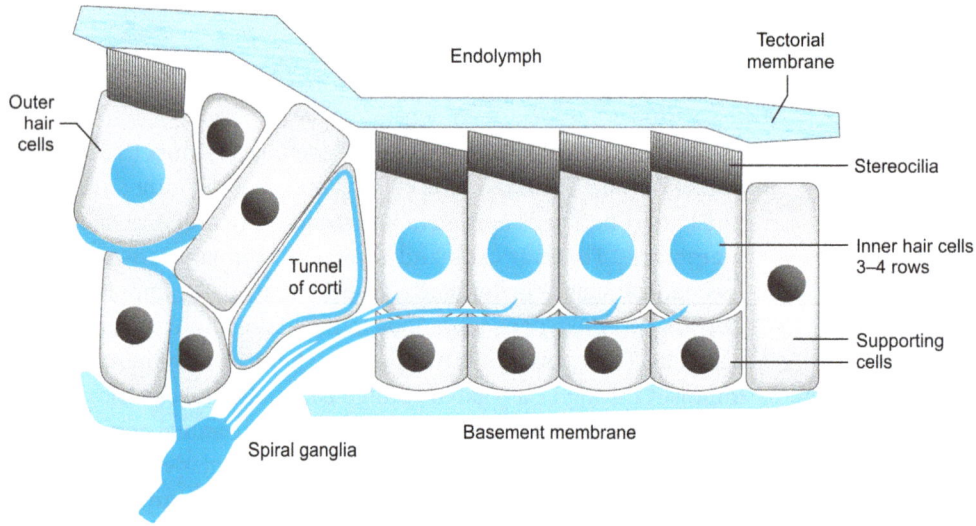

Fig. 2: The mechanism of hearing.

- Fourth-order neurons: These relay to the medial geniculate body from where fibers project into the auditory cortex.
- *Nonlemniscal pathway:*
  - Fibers of this pathway also traverse to the cochlear nucleus. The small fibers from the cochlear nucleus join the reticular formation. The reticular formation extends upward and nonspecifically projects into the thalamus. The thalamic fibers project into the polysensory cortex.

TESTS FOR THE VIII CRANIAL NERVE
- *Audiometry:* Detects the frequency range and severity of hearing loss
- Brain stem auditory evoked response (BAER), **(Fig. 3)**.
- *Video electronystagmography:* Nystagmus during tracking of the moving target

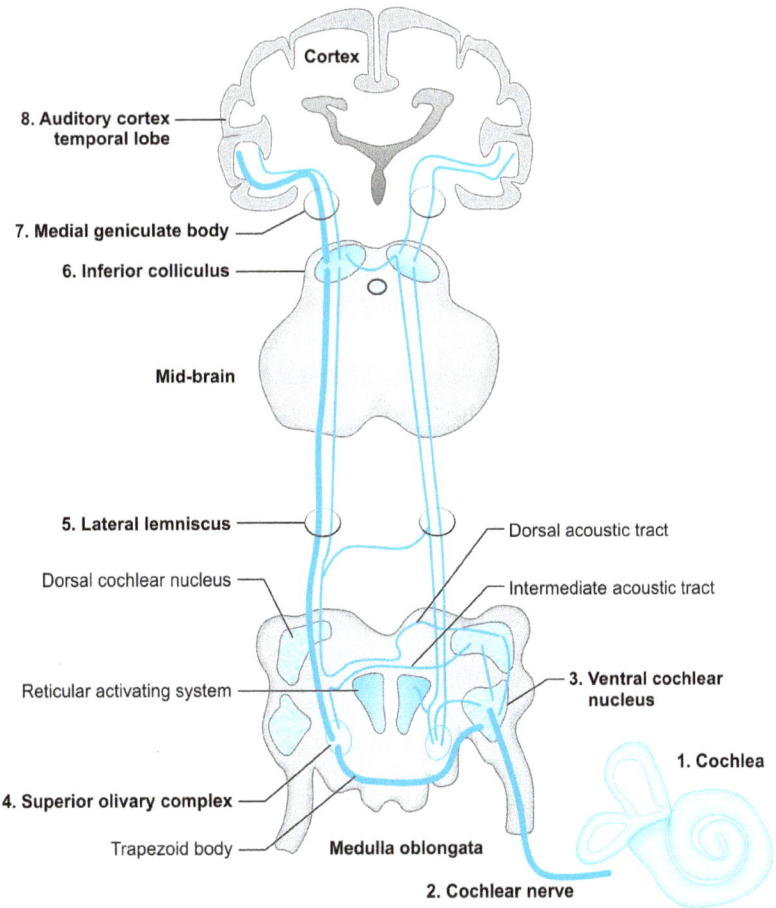

Fig. 3: Auditory Pathway and the origin of waves seen in the brain stem auditory evoked responses (BAER).

- *Rotational chair:* The patient is rotated in a chair, and the eye movements are tracked to test vestibular response.
- *Dynamic visual acuity testing:* Determines the effect of motion on visual acuity.
- *Computerized posturography* for assessment of balance.

DEAFNESS

- *Incidence:* The incidence in the general population is 2% <18 years, 10% are 18–65 years, and 30% are >65 years
- *External ear:* Trauma and wax
- *Middle ear:* Trauma, fluid, otosclerosis, and cholesteatoma
- *Inner ear:* Trauma, infection, and Meniere's disease
- *Meniere's disease:* Recurrent episodes of headache, fullness in the ear, vertigo, tinnitus, and low- to mid-frequency hearing loss; may be associated with autonomic disturbances.

- *Auditory pathway, VIII CN, and beyond:* Viral infections (measles, mumps, herpes, Epstein–Barr, HIV, and West Nile), meningitis, tumors (cerebellopontine angle tumors and acoustic neuroma), and multiple sclerosis.

Cochlear Implants

Implants are used to treat moderate-to-severe sensorineural deafness. They have a soft, flexible electrode implanted within the entire length of the cochlea. The electrode directly stimulates the auditory nerve across a wide range of frequencies. The external device has a microphone and a processing unit that generates electrical impulses. The impulses are transcutaneously transmitted to the cochlear electrode. With congenital deafness, cochlear implant surgery is best performed in early childhood to encourage normal speech development.

FURTHER READING

1. Botto C et al. Progress in gene editing tools and their potential for correcting mutations underlying hearing and vision loss. Front Genome Ed. 2021; 3:737632.
2. Chaudhry D et al. Cochlear implantation outcomes in postsynaptic auditory neuropathies: a systematic review and narrative synthesis. J Int Adv Otol. 2020;16(3):411-31.
3. Plack CJ et al. Pitch coding and pitch processing in the human brain. Hear Res. 2014;307:53-64.
4. Romano DR et al. Deafness-in-a-dish: modeling hereditary deafness with inner ear organoids Hum Genet. 2022; 141(3-4):347-62.
5. van der Jagt MA et al. Visualization of human inner ear anatomy with high-resolution MR imaging at 7 T: initial clinical assessment. Am J Neuroradiol. 2015;36(2):378-83.

Vignette: The Superb Hearing of the Bats!

The ear of bats can process sound with 10× higher frequencies than the human ear. Bats have a very dense concentration of hair cells and can detect frequency changes in the range of 0.001 kHz. However, cave-dwelling bats need superb hearing to echolocate. Echolocation involves generating an outgoing sound and processing the returning signal. To do this, some bats can coordinate their laryngeal muscles with the ossicles in the middle ear. During phonation, the stapedius muscle of the ear contracts shortly before the cricothyroid muscle in the larynx. The contraction dampens the reception of the sound by the ossicles while the sound is being generated. The hearing soon returns after the sound has been emitted. Bats can detect an insect at one meter. Considering that the sound travels in air at 343 m/s, so the bats get an exceedingly short time to catch their meal!

Chapter 7

Cerebral Circulation: Anatomy

INTRODUCTION

The brain lacks the capacity for anaerobic metabolism, requiring constant blood flow. It accounts for 2% of body weight, 20% of cardiac output, and 20% of body glucose metabolism in adults.

The brain/body weight ratio is much greater during early childhood than in adults. Brain glucose metabolism increases from birth to as much as 66% of the body's metabolism by year 5. High brain metabolism increases the risk of ischemic injury in children. Thus, the need to ensure adequate cerebral perfusion is even greater in children than in adults.

MECHANISMS TO ENSURE CONSTANT BLOOD FLOW TO THE BRAIN

- The brain is perfused by multiple arteries (35% each internal carotid artery and 15% each vertebral artery). These arteries form the Circle of Willis that ensures distal perfusion should one of the arteries be occluded.
- The brain is suspended in cerebrospinal fluid. The buoyancy of the brain in CSF minimizes the effect of posture on blood flow.
- Multiple regulatory mechanisms exist for tonic and dynamic control of blood flow.
- Robust autoregulatory control of flow across a range of perfusion pressures.
- Robust metabolic control via flow-metabolism coupling
- The brain receives surplus flow:
  - The baseline blood flow is 3–4× of the ischemic injury threshold.
  - The 2% body weight of the brain gets 20% of the cardiac output.
  - Metabolically active gray matter is 4× better perfused and has 3× capillary density compared to white matter.
- The brain is preferentially perfused during shock.
- Adaptive neovascularization during cerebral ischemia is possible but can lead to hemorrhages (e.g., Moyamoya disease).
- In some animals, such as pigs, there are communications between the external and internal carotid arteries *(rete mirabile)*. In other animals (such as rabbits), the distal pial precapillary arteries communicate with each other *(the Circle of Duret)*.

CEREBRAL BLOOD FLOW THRESHOLDS

- *Normal: 50 mL/100 g/min*
- *Impaired EEG/cortical failure: 25 mL/100 g/min*
- *Progressive EEG slowing with decreasing blood flow:*
  - Normal: 35 mL/100 g/min
  - Loss of beta (13–20 Hz): 25 mL/100 g/min
  - Loss of alpha (8–13 Hz): 20 mL/100 g/min
  - Loss of theta (4–7 Hz): 15 mL/100 g/min
  - Loss of delta (1–4 Hz): 10 mL/100 g/min
  - EEG Silence/injury: 5 mL/100 g/min
- *Loss of evoked responses:* 20 mL/100 g/min
- *The injury threshold:* 5–10 mL/100 g/min
- Sudden complete cessation of the blood flow leads to loss of consciousness in 20 seconds.

VARIATIONS IN THE ORIGINS OF THE CAROTID ARTERIES

Two-thirds of the cerebral blood flow is through internal carotid arteries, and one-third is through vertebral arteries. There are several variations in the origin of the arteries from the aortic arch. Some of these variations can increase the difficulty of performing angiographic procedures. Also, the anatomy of the cerebral arteries could affect the consequences of arterial occlusion. In 7-27% of the patients, both common carotids could arise from a common brachiocephalic trunk **(Figs. 1A to D)**.

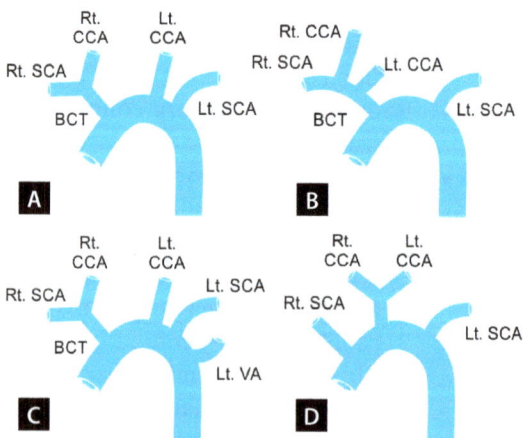

Figs. 1A to D: Variations in the origin of intracranial arteries. (A) Typical origin of arteries and (B to D) three common variations. (BCT: brachiocephalic trunk; Rt. SCA: right subclavian artery; Rt. CCA: right common carotid artery; Lt. CCA: left common carotid artery; Lt. SCA: left subclavian artery; Lt. VA: left vertebral artery)

VARIATIONS IN THE ARTERIES FORMING THE CIRCLE OF WILLIS

An evenly balanced Circle of Willis is seen in 20% of individuals (**Figs. 2A and B**). In most people, the circle has one or more hypoplastic segments. At the normal cerebral perfusion pressure, despite the COW, there is little blood mixing within the major arterial distributions and much less with the contralateral side.

The clinical consequences of the anatomical variations of the COW are as follows:
- Different effects of the occlusion of the same artery by a clot or during surgery
- Difficulty in sonicating arteries during Transcranial Doppler ultrasound
- Predisposition to aneurysm formation
- Predisposition to thrombosis
- Malformation might show a familial cluster.
- *Balloon test occlusion:* When the internal carotid artery has to be sacrificed during planned surgery, a balloon test occlusion is undertaken with or without concurrent hypotension to test for the collateral blood flow and vascular reserve.

CEREBRAL VENOUS DRAINAGE

- The cerebral venous system has veins and sinuses (**Figs. 3 and 4**).
- The sinuses lie between the periosteum and the dura matter.
- They are lined by endothelial cells.
- The sinuses, unlike the veins, lack a muscular layer.

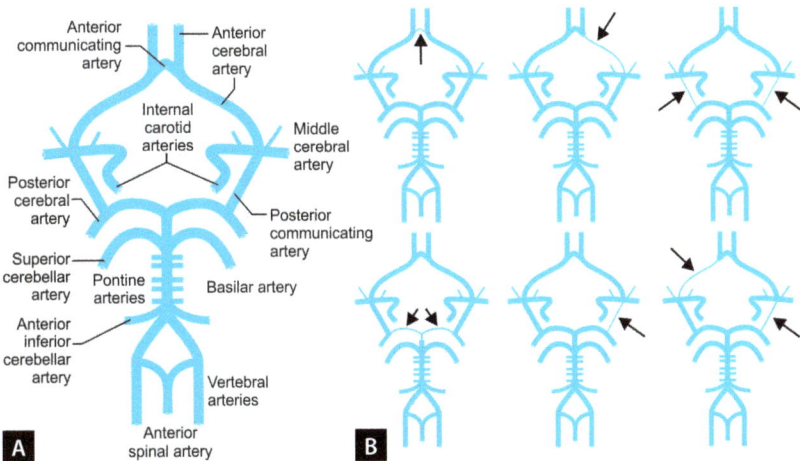

Figs. 2A and B: (A) Normal balanced Circle of Willis is seen in 20% of the population; (B) In most other cases, the black arrows indicate that one or more component vessels may be hypoplastic.

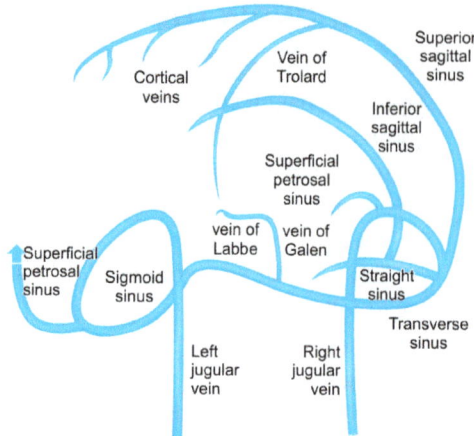

Fig. 3: Superficial venous drainage of the brain.

- The walls contain arachnoid granulations.
- The blood flow in the cerebral venous system can be bidirectional.
- Cerebral veins and sinuses have no valves.
- They do not follow the arterial blood flow pattern. Hence, clinical presentations of arterial and venous ischemic strokes are different.

ARRANGEMENT OF THE VENOUS SYSTEM

Intracranial veins and sinuses are shown in **Figures 3 and 4**:
- Dural venous sinuses.
  - Anteroinferior group
    - Cavernous sinus
    - Superior and inferior petrosal sinuses
    - Basal venous plexus
    - Spheno-parietal sinus
  - Posterosuperior group
    - Superior and inferior sagittal sinuses
    - Straight sinus
    - Transverse sinus
    - Sigmoid sinus
    - Jugular bulb
- Cerebral veins
  - Superficial cortical veins
    - Superior, middle, and inferior cortical veins
  - Deep cerebral veins
    - Medullary veins
    - Subependymal veins

- Deep paramedian veins
- Brainstem and posterior fossa venous system
  - Galenic group
  - Petrosal group
  - Posterior fossa group.

APPLIED ANATOMY

- There is a mixing of the venous blood draining the left and right sides; superficial and deep structures; and extracranial and intracranial venous blood, such as through the emissary veins.
- The increased risks of venous air embolism during craniotomy can be due to the lack of valves in the cerebral veins, the inability of venous sinuses and emissary veins to retract, and the need to elevate the head above the level of the heart during surgery to obtain a clear field.
- Superficial venous sinus injury is a significant risk during mid-line, and occipital craniotomies can lead to massive bleeding and air embolism. Deep venous sinus, such as the cavernous sinus, can be perforated during transsphenoidal surgery as the pituitary gland lies between the two cavernous sinuses **(Fig. 4)**.
- The cavernous sinus also receives the venous return from the pituitary, which can be sampled by blood drawn from the petrosal sinus.
- Blood flow through cerebral sinuses can be significantly increased by arteriovenous fistulae leading to an intracranial bleed, raised intracranial pressure, and congestive heart failure.

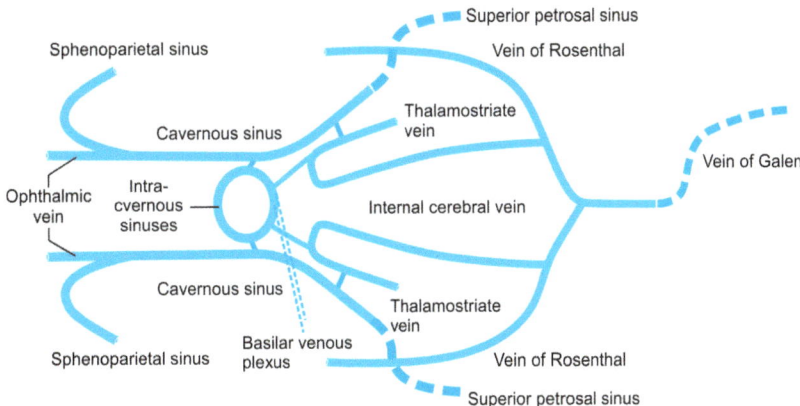

Fig. 4: Deep venous drainage of the brain.

- Generally, the internal jugular vein drains about two-thirds of blood from the ipsilateral hemisphere. The remaining venous return is from the contralateral side.

FURTHER READING

1. Bernier M et al. The morphology of the human cerebrovascular system. Hum Brain Mapp. 2018;39(12):4962-75.
2. Keelan J et al. Development of a globally optimized model of the cerebral arteries. Phys Med Biol. 2019;64(12):25021.
3. Klimont M et al. Deep learning for cerebral angiography segmentation from non-contrast computed tomography. PLoS One. 2020;15(7):e0237092.
4. Liu J et al. A comparative analysis framework of 3T and 7T TOF-MRA based on automated cerebrovascular segmentation. Comput Med Imaging Graph. 2021;89:101830.
5. Yao JF et al. Cerebral circulation time derived from fMRI signals in large blood vessels. J Magn Reson Imaging. 2019;50(5):1504-13.

Vignette: Does a Siphon Augment Cerebral Blood Flow?

Siphons provide a mechanism to overcome height while delivering fluids from a higher to a lower level. So, imagine if a column of blood extended from the thoracic aorta to the right heart that perfuses the brain at a significantly greater height. Could the siphon mechanism augment cerebral blood flow? The siphon effect has been an area of controversy. Experiments show that the siphon mechanism does not affect cerebral circulation. The problem is that the veins in the neck collapse easily, and when they close down, the column of blood is interrupted, and the siphoning effect, if any, fails. It is unlikely that the siphon mechanism works in clinical situations, such as in a sitting position.

Chapter 8

Cerebral Blood Flow Regulation

INTRODUCTION

The human brain receives 20% of the cardiac output, although it amounts to 2% of body weight. The average blood flow to the brain is about 50 mL/100g/min. However, the brain is exceedingly well perfused; due to its high metabolic needs and the lack of anaerobic reserves, it remains venerable to ischemic injury. Understanding and manipulating cerebral blood flow during surgery is vital to neuroanesthesia practice.

HAGEN–POISEUILLE FORMULA

Hagen–Poiseuille formula (HPF) describes flow (ΔQ) in a blood vessel. Where P is the perfusion pressure, R is the radius, L is the length, and η is the coefficient of viscosity:

$$\Delta Q = \pi P R^4 / 8\, \eta L$$

There are several erroneous assumptions in this formula:
- Arteries are assumed to be uniform rigid tubes rather than dynamically reacting branching biological entities.
- Blood is a Newtonian fluid. As a Newtonian Fluid, blood viscosity should not change with shear rates. However, blood is a non-Newtonian fluid. Blood cells clump at low shear rates; hence the viscosity is not linearly related to the shear rate.
- The properties of blood are homogeneous throughout the tube.
- The pressure gradient is constant. However, the perfusion pressure is usually pulsatile.
- There are no pathological changes in the vessel diameter.
- Flow in the blood vessels is laminar throughout, but the flow in the arteries can be turbulent manifesting as bruit on clinical exam.

Thus, the underlying assumptions of the HPF are not always valid. A more accurate approximation of the HPF is to describe flow as a function of $R^{2.4}$ instead of R^4. However, the formula provides a valuable conceptual framework for understanding critical issues related to blood flow. Clinically relevant implications of HPF include:
- Vascular resistance is mainly due to distal arteries and arterioles and not due to large vessels.

- Reduction of viscosity by hemodilution decreases resistance and improves blood flow during cerebral vasospasm.
- Reduction of viscosity decreases endothelial stress, resulting in vasoconstriction and a decrease in ICP with mannitol treatment.

COMPLEX BIOMECHANICS OF ARTERIAL BLOOD FLOW

- The HPF provides a simple construct for describing the blood flow that completely ignores the properties of the arterial wall. A better understanding of arterial flow, including biomechanics of vessel walls, is needed in clinical situations. The arterial blood pressure tracing, for example, is a result of the interaction of two waves:
- *Percussion wave:*
    - Isometric contraction of the heart generates a percussion wave.
    - The percussion wave is a seismic wave transmitted along the arterial wall at a rate determined by sympathetic tone and the rate of rise of pressure in the heart.
    - This percussion wave determines the upstroke angle of the pressure pulse.
    - It determines the slope and height of the arterial pressure tracing, affecting the systolic blood pressure value.
- *Tidal wave:*
    - The percussion wave is followed by the tidal wave generated by the opening of the aortic valve and the ejection of blood.
    - The tidal wave is a function of the stroke volume, the elasticity of the aorta, and the systemic vascular resistance.

The percussion and the tidal waves are shown in **Figure 1**. The example illustrates changes in hypovolemic shock where there is intense sympathetic activity. During shock, myocardial contraction is forceful, and there is systemic vasoconstriction. Both lead to a strong percussion

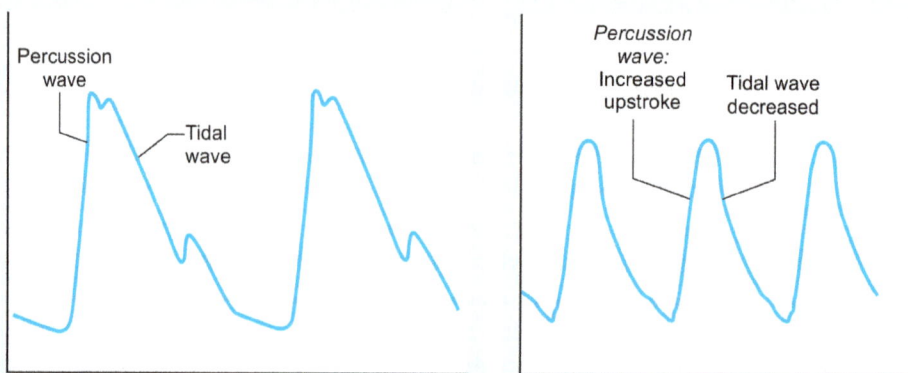

Fig. 1: The biomechanics of the arterial wall affects the arterial blood pressure recording. Compared to the normal arterial pressure recording (left), the slope of the arterial pressure upstroke (percussion wave) is increased in hemorrhagic shock, and the amplitude of the tidal wave is decreased (right).

CHAPTER 8 Cerebral Blood Flow Regulation

wave. However, the decreased blood volume leads to a small tidal wave. The arterial pressure has a rapid upstroke and a rapid collapse leading to an overestimation of systolic and possibly an underestimation of diastolic blood pressure.

CEREBRAL PERFUSION PRESSURE

It has several definitions:
- CPP = MAP – mean ICP.
- CPP = MAP – (mean ICP or mean JVP, whichever is greater).
- CPP = (MAP – pressure zero flow) – (mean ICP or mean JVP, whichever is greater).
- *Pressure zero flow:* Pressure is required to open the vessel lumen before blood flow can be established. Modeling data suggest that in the cerebral circulation, it is about 17 mm Hg *(see* **Fig. 2**).
- *No reflow phenomenon:* It is a similar but different concept. Following circulatory arrest lasting 5 minutes or more, not all capillary perfusion is restored, irrespective of the increase in pressure.

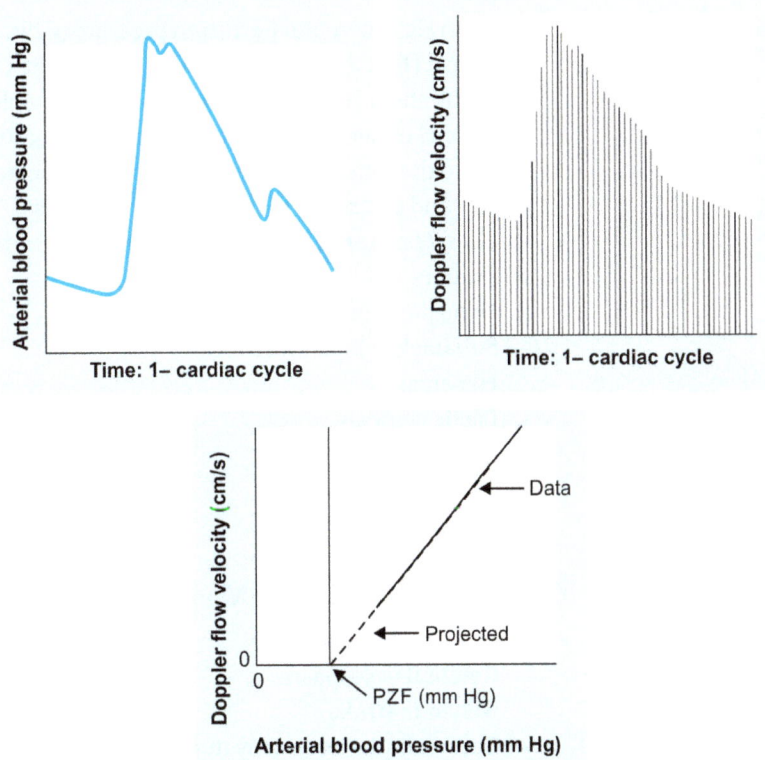

Fig. 2: Pressure zero flow (PZF) can be determined by plotting instantaneous blood flow velocity as determined by transcranial Doppler against arterial pressure value for a given cardiac cycle. PZF is the minimum pressure needed to start the flow in a vessel.

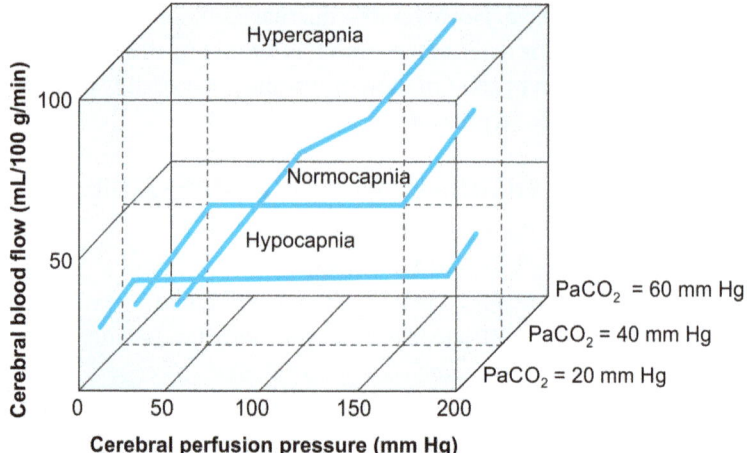

Fig. 3: Cerebral autoregulation during normo-, hypo-, and hypercapnia.

Pressure Autoregulation

- Cerebral blood flow (CBF) is maintained constantly between 50 and 150 mm Hg of cerebral perfusion pressure (CPP) by a dynamic vascular response **(Fig. 3)**. The endothelial cells of the cerebral arteries transduce the shear stress as a servo control of vascular tone.
- In chronic hypertension, adaptive remodeling shifts the autoregulatory curve to the right such that the lower limit of cerebral autoregulation is higher and can result in ischemia even with a CPP of 50 mm Hg.
- *Impaired pressure autoregulation can be seen with the following:*
  - Trauma
  - Hypoxia, ischemia, stroke
  - Subarachnoid hemorrhage
  - Hypercarbia
  - Lactic acidosis
  - Infections
  - Tumors
  - Pain.

Clinical Blood Pressure Manipulation

- *Induced hypertension:*
  - Cerebral vasospasm
  - Ischemic stroke
  - Carotid endarterectomy during internal carotid artery occlusion
  - Test the integrity of the vascular bed after arteriovenous malformation (AVM) resection.
  - During temporary arterial occlusion with aneurysm clipping.

CHAPTER 8 Cerebral Blood Flow Regulation

- *Induced hypotension:*
  - Decreases blood loss during tumor and spine surgery.
  - Facilitates aneurysm dissection during surgery.
  - Decreases blood flow during embolization of high-flow AVMs.
  - Prevents hyperperfusion syndrome after clamp release during carotid endarterectomy.
  - As a temporary measure during intraoperative aneurysm rupture while securing the aneurysm.

Carbon-dioxide

- CO_2 is the most potent vasodilator. Between 20- and 80-mm Hg, CBF increases by about 2% for every mm Hg increase in $PaCO_2$.
- *Interaction between pressure autoregulation and CO_2 autoregulation:* Hypertension accentuates CO_2 response while hypotension attenuates it. Conversely, hypercapnia attenuates pressure autoregulation, and hypocapnia accentuates pressure autoregulation response. Hyperventilation can also attenuate cerebral vasodilation by volatile anesthetic agents.

Pros and Cons of Hyperventilation in Neuroanesthesia

Pros

- Rapid reduction of CO_2 is possible and can decrease ICP quickly.
- A decrease in ICP improves CPP.
- Offsets the vasodilator effects of volatile anesthetic agents.
- Enhances autoregulatory pressure response.
- Improves systemic oxygenation, decreasing chances of hypoxic brain injury.
- Increases blood flow to regions of impaired autoregulation (tumors/trauma) due to cerebral steal phenomenon.
- Steal can preferentially deliver drugs to brain tumors while decreasing delivery to healthy tissues.

Cons

- The effect of hyperventilation is temporary.
- It decreases blood flow to healthy regions of the brain and can lead to ischemia.
- Alkalosis shifts the oxygen-hemoglobin dissociation curve to the left and decreases tissue oxygen extraction.
- Luxury perfusion of tumors may increase blood flow and tumor volume.
- It increases positive pressure ventilation, intra-thoracic pressure, and ICP while decreasing venous return, cardiac output, and blood pressure.
- A decrease in ICP increases transmural pressure and can increase the chances of aneurysmal bleeding.
- Worsens ischemia due to cerebral vasospasm.

Oxygen

Hypoxia with PaO_2 <40 mm exponentially increases CBF, but it decreases the flow when PaO_2 is >250 mm Hg.

METABOLIC REGULATION

Metabolic regulation is mediated by metabolites such as adenosine, hydrogen ions, and local neurogenic mechanisms:
- Flow metabolism coupling matches blood flow to the metabolic needs of the tissue.
- *Increased metabolic activity:* Cortical activation, analeptic drugs, and seizures.
- *Decreased metabolic activity:* Hypothermia (decreases by 6% per °C) and anesthetic drugs.

Autonomic regulation through cervical sympathetic and parasympathetic.

Pharmacological modulation is formed through the:
- Anesthetic drugs **(Table 1)**
- Cerebral vasodilators and constrictors

Cellular Mechanisms of Cerebral Blood Flow Regulation

- *K^+ channels* mediate the effects of PGI2, cGRP, VIP, β agonists, and endothelin- derived hyperpolarizing factor.
- *cAMP:* It mediates vasodilation by adenosine, methyl-xanthine, PGI2, PFE2, β agonists, adrenomedullin, and pituitary adenylate cyclase.
- *C-GMP:* It mediates nitric oxide, BNP, carbon monoxide, AMP, and c-natriuretic peptide.

Methods to Assess Cerebral Blood Flow

Table 2 lists various methods to measure blood flow. However, a safe method that can permit real-time, safe, convenient measurements of absolute blood flow still eludes us.

Table 1: Anesthetic drugs and CBF.

Parameter	Increased	Decreased	Preserved
Cerebral blood flow	Volatile agents and ketamine	All intravenous agents (except ketamine) and Xe	Narcotics/ benzodiazepines
Cerebral metabolism	Ketamine	All volatile and IV anesthetics	
Cerebral autoregulation	Hyperventilation/ hypocapnia	Impaired at >1 MAC Desflurane and isoflurane worse than sevoflurane; hypercapnia	IV anesthetics
Flow metabolism coupling			Propofol, Pentobarbiturate

Table 2: Methods to assess cerebral blood flow.

Method	Parameters assessed, the underlying concept	Advantages	Disadvantages
Require jugular bulb cannulation			
Kety–Schmidt method	A-V difference during 15% nitrous oxide inhalation	Bedside possible	Assumes steady-state blood flow and N_2O extraction, requires time
Jugular venous oximetry	The difference in arterial and jugular venous blood oxygen content	Bedside, real-time monitoring is possible with oximetric catheters in the jugular venous bulb	Invasive, facial vein contamination, cerebral oxygen consumption assumed constant
Require intracranial (surface/brain parenchymal) probes			
Thermal diffusion	Local CBF by heat diffusion	Real time	Invasive placement of an intra-cranial probe
Laser Doppler	Local CBF, by optically determined blood cell velocity	Real time	Invasive placement of an intra-cranial probe
Hydrogen clearance	Local CBF	Real time	Invasive placement of an intracranial probe
Noninvasive			
Transcranial Doppler	Blood flow velocity	Bedside, ease of use, real-time monitor, can detect emboli	Measure flow velocity, not net flow; difficult to interpret if vessel diameter changes, e.g., vasospasm
Perfusion CT	Measure regional and global CBF, CBV, and MTT	Ease of use	Snapshot data, transport to the scanner, allergic reaction to iodinated contrast
Xe CT	Measure regional and global CBF	Possible during CT scan by inhaling 30% Xe	Snapshot data, transport to the scanner, Xe is a viscous gas, ventilation may be difficult; Xe can affect CBF $CMRO_2$
133Xe washout	Measure regional and global CBF	It can be done by inhalation, IV, or arterial 133Xe delivery gives gray and white matter blood flows	Radioisotope uses limited applications, snapshot data, 2D data, possible cross talk from the other hemisphere
Perfusion weighted MRI	Assess regional and global CBF, CBV, and MTT	No radiation risk, several methods such as, spin labeling, time of flight	Snapshot data, transport to the scanner, requires normalization of data
Positron emission tomography (PET)	• Measures CBF and CBV; $CMRO_2$ • CMRglu, and oxygen extraction fraction	3D perfusion mapping but with poor anatomical resolution	Radiation hazard, isotope preparation facility needed, snapshot data, transport to scanner
Single-photon emission tomography (SPECT)	CBF	^{99m}Tc HMPAO and ^{99m}Tc ECD used for 3D perfusion mapping	Radiation hazard, snapshot data, transport to the scanner, poor spatial resolution

(CBF: cerebral blood flow; CBV: cerebral blood volume; ECD: ethylcysteinate dimer; HMPAO: hexamethylpropyleneamine oxime; MTT: mean transit time)

Pathological Vasoconstriction

The pathology of cerebral vasospasm is complex. The mechanisms invoked include potent vasoconstrictors such as endothelin or a lack of vasodilators such as nitric oxide.

- Typically, it occurs 1–2 weeks after subarachnoid hemorrhage. The cerebral arteries narrow to reduce blood flow, resulting in new neurological deficits.
- Cerebral vasospasm is directly related to the amount of blood in the subarachnoid space.
- Cerebral vasospasm is associated with a narrowing of the large arteries on angiography and a corresponding increase in the blood flow velocity when assessed by doppler ultrasound.
- The vasospasm can also affect the distal cerebral arterioles resulting in a delay in clearing the contrast agents during angiography.
- The treatment requires increasing cerebral perfusion pressure by increasing the systolic arterial pressure to 180–200 mm Hg. Such hypertensive treatment requires the early clipping of ruptured aneurysms. However, intra-arterial vasodilators and stenting may be needed when medical treatment fails to reverse the arterial narrowing.

CEREBRAL HYPERPERFUSION SYNDROME

- Sometimes seen after carotid surgery due to a substantial increase in CBF, even at normal blood pressure. It manifests with headaches, hypertension, neurological symptoms, and sometimes seizures.
- With carotid stenosis, the distal cerebral circulation adapts to a lower regional perfusion pressure. Once the lumen is restored, it cannot adapt to the increased perfusion pressure. Prevention of hyperperfusion syndrome requires meticulous blood pressure control after endarterectomy at 10–20% below baseline pressures.

FURTHER READING

1. Caldwell HG et al. Acid-base balance and cerebrovascular regulation. J Physiol. 2021;599(24):5337-59.
2. Hamner JW et al. Revisiting human cerebral blood flow responses to augmented blood pressure oscillations. J Physiol. 2019; 597(6):1553-64.
3. Herthum H et al. Real-Time Multifrequency MR Elastography of the Human Brain Reveals Rapid Changes in Viscoelasticity in Response to the Valsalva Maneuver. Front Bioeng Biotechnol. 2021;9:666456.
4. Tamayo A et al. Regulation of blood flow in the cerebral posterior circulation by parasympathetic nerve fibers: physiological background and possible

clinical implications in patients with vertebrobasilar stroke. Front Neurol. 2021;12:660373.
5. Wieronska JM et al. Nitric oxide-dependent pathways as critical factors in the consequences and recovery after brain ischemic hypoxia. Biomolecules, 2021;11(8):1097.

Vignette: Regulating the Cerebral Blood Flow of a Giraffe

Perhaps the animal that poses the most significant challenge to its cerebral circulation is the giraffe. It seems that the cerebral hemodynamics of the animal would change dramatically when it raises or lowers its head, often in a matter of seconds. The net change in height can be 2–3 meters. When the animal is erect, the mean arterial pressure of the animal is about 200 mm Hg, the carotid artery pressure is about 130 mm Hg, the jugular veins are in a collapsed state, and there is hardly any venous volume. However, when the head is lowered, the jugular vein dilates. As the head is lowered, almost a liter of blood pools in the vein. The cardiac output drops by 30%, and the mean arterial pressure decreases significantly by 70 mm Hg. The brain autoregulates to maintain cerebral blood flow. Thus, cerebral hemodynamics is relatively immune to the position of the animal's head.

Chapter 9

Brain Metabolism and Flow Metabolism Coupling

INTRODUCTION

Understanding brain metabolism and its modulation by anesthetic drugs is a foundation of neuroanesthesia practice. It was generally believed that the brain tissue was incapable of anaerobic glucose metabolism. In the late 1900s, blood oxygen level-dependent (BOLD)-functional magnetic resonance imaging (fMRI) revealed that brain stimulation results in a more significant increase in glucose utilization and blood flow than oxygen consumption. Animal studies have shown that brain stimulation increases glucose consumption with substantial increases in tissue lactate concentrations. The lag in oxygen consumption during neuronal activation is due to the ability of the astrocytes to rapidly metabolize glucose to lactate and transfer it to the neurons. The neurons can further metabolize lactate to generate energy. Thus, neurons benefit from some degree of anaerobic metabolism via astrocytes. Monitoring and modulating brain metabolism by drugs and hypothermia are critical to improving the outcome of neurosurgical interventions.

BRAIN METABOLISM OVERVIEW

- The brain accounts for 2% of body weight and 20% of total body oxygen consumption. About 80% of the brain's total energy consumption is by the neurons. Most of that energy is used for repolarization of the cell membranes, synaptic transmission in synthesizing and recycling neurotransmitters, and for axonal transport.
- Brain metabolism is tightly coupled to neuronal activation. Regional blood flow is spatially and temporarily linked to neuronal activation. Regions of the cortex are usually quiescent unless activated when they show a dramatic increase in metabolism and blood flow. Although some regions of the brain, such as the hippocampus, are constantly active.
- About 50% of total brain metabolism is due to synaptic activity secondary to neuronal activation, while 50% is for maintaining cell processes needed to ensure viability. The former is depressed with anesthetic drugs, but the latter is not. In contrast, hypothermia depresses both.

CHAPTER 9 Brain Metabolism and Flow Metabolism Coupling

- The bulk of synaptic metabolism is glutaminergic pathways (80%). A small portion reflects GABA-aminergic pathways (10%).
- Although glucose is the primary nutrient substrate for the brain, during neuronal activation, lactate is transferred to the neurons from the astrocytes (astrocyte-neuron transport shuttle).
- Cerebral metabolism is often assessed by quantifying the utilization of substrates. The typical values are:
  - *CMRglu (cerebral metabolic rate for glucose):* 5 mg/100 g/min
  - *$CMRO_2$ (cerebral metabolic rate for oxygen):* 3.5 mL/100 g/min
  - *CMR lactate (cerebral metabolic rate for lactate):* 0.5 mg/100 g/min

METHODS TO ASSESS BRAIN METABOLISM

Methods to assess cerebral metabolism can broadly be divided into two broad groups: Those that can be used on the bedside and those that use magnetic or isotopic imaging in a dedicated facility.

- *Bedside method to assess cerebral metabolism* **(Table 1)**:
  - *Electroencephalography (EEG):* Provides indirect assessment of cerebral metabolism as it assumes a linkage between the neuronal activity being monitored and the underlying metabolism. EEG silence provides a target for the dosing of anesthetic drugs for neuroprotection. It is useful mainly because of its ease of use and wide availability.

Table 1: Bedside methods to assess cerebral metabolism.

Method	Parameters assessed, the underlying concept	Advantages	Disadvantages
Jugular venous oximetry	Difference between the arterial and jugular venous blood oxygen content	Bedside, real-time monitoring is possible with oximetric catheters in the jugular venous bulb	Invasive, facial vein contamination; CBF has to be assumed constant
Near-infrared spectroscopy	Oxygen saturation of brain tissue, usually in the frontal lobes	Noninvasive, real-time; new devices with time-of-flight measurements are expensive but have a high spatial resolution	The two-channel clinical device offers only crude reflection on cerebral metabolism; deep cortex and white matter remain inaccessible
Tissue oximetry	The local partial pressure of oxygen in tissue	Real-time data	Invasive technique, site-specific changes
Microdialysis	Local metabolites (glucose/lactate/pyruvate/glycerol/and glutamate)	Early detection of injury	Invasive samples have to be processed, and labor and time intensive

- Arterial to "cerebral" venous blood gradients for metabolites such as lactate. Sustained elevation of lactate may be seen with transient cerebral ischemia. The accuracy of the method improves by sampling veins draining the ischemic region.
- Jugular venous oximetry can measure oxygen extraction by brain tissue and has been clinically used to optimize blood pressure and ventilation in critical care settings.
- *Near-infrared spectroscopy:* The ability of near-infrared light to penetrate the skull and the brain tissue, allowing it to assess tissue hemoglobin saturation. NIRS can be used for comparing change on either side by paired frontal optodes when a unilateral ischemic injury is suspected/likely. The whole brain of a neonate can be mapped with an array of optodes. Optode arrays are used for research purposes in adults with better spatial resolution.
- *Tissue oximetry:* Using implantable sensors, tissue oxygen tension can be measured in real-time.
- *Micro-dialysis:* Lactate, pyruvate, glutamate, and glucose can all be monitored using micro-dialysis to assess tissue metabolic state.
- *Brain metabolism imaging:*
  - *Magnetic resonance imaging (MRI) and spectroscopy (MRS):*
    - MRI/S methods are relatively safe and tissue noninvasive. They can also provide detailed anatomical definitions.
    - *fMRI:* Fully oxygenated hemoglobin molecule is inert in the magnetic field. However, deoxyhemoglobin generated by increased metabolism due to oxygen extraction after neuronal activation is paramagnetic and disrupts the magnetic field. The paramagnetic signal generated by deoxyhemoglobin is the basis of the blood oxygen level-dependent (BOLD) signal used in fMRI to map neuronal activity. It provides a useful method to assess changes in tissue metabolism.
    - Common elements with an odd number of neutrons and protons that are either endogenous or can be introduced for imaging purposes and can be used for MRS and NMR applications to track brain metabolism. These include:
      - ^{17}O for tracking oxygen utilization
      - ^{31}P for ATP synthesis
      - ^{13}C for tracking glutaminergic neurotransmission
      - ^{19}F-for tracking cytosolic glucose metabolism
  - *Positron imaging technology (PET):*
    - PET uses radioisotopes that spontaneously decay to release a positron. The radioisotopes such as $^{15}O_2$ are used either alone or as radioligands, such as., ^{18}F-fluoro-deoxy-glucose, ^{18}F-FDG. The positron travels a distance of about 1-3 mm before interacting

CHAPTER 9 Brain Metabolism and Flow Metabolism Coupling

with an electron. The encounter annihilates both particles and releases two photons in the gamma range in the opposite direction. Two opposite scintillation detectors in the surrounding circular array, sense the gamma emissions, and localize the point of positron annihilation in the 3D space. The emission point is then co-registered in a corresponding anatomical image, either an X-ray, computed tomography, or MRI scan.

- The limitation of PET techniques is the logistics of isotope production because the half-life of these isotopes can be exceedingly short, and on-site production might be necessary.
- Furthermore, PET imaging lacks spatial resolution. PET data has to be co-registered with another imaging modality.
- PET is a highly versatile technology due to the wide range of radioligands available. Two specific PET applications for brain metabolism imaging are:
  - ^{18}F-FDG is the most widely used PET ligand. It has a half-life of 110 min. It is used for assessing glucose metabolism in the brain and for malignant and metastatic tumor localization.
  - $^{15}O_2$: The isotope's half-life is exceedingly short, about 2 min. It is used to determine $CMRO_2$ and oxygen extraction fraction to assess brain metabolism. It has been injected directly into arteries and combined with targeting molecules that are used as radioligands.

ANESTHETIC PHARMACOLOGY

Effects of Narcotics

Narcotics have direct and indirect effects on cerebral blood flow (CBF). Some of these effects are doses and species related.

- High-dose narcotics decrease CBF more than they reduce the $CMRO_2$.
- They increase intracranial pressure (ICP) independent of the indirect effect through hypercapnia. Since narcotics decrease the mean arterial blood pressure, their net effect is a decrease in cerebral perfusion pressure (CPP).
- While small doses of narcotics are safely tolerated in healthy patients, high doses should be used with caution in patients with a suspected increase in ICP.

Effects of Lidocaine

- Lidocaine decreases CBF and $CMRO_2$ with a net improvement in tissue oxygenation. It prevents the rise in ICP associated with intubation.
- Unlike most sedative-hypnotics, lidocaine decreases the cell's "metabolic" needs.

- Lidocaine is metabolized into active metabolites monoethylglycinexylidide and glycinexylide, which are pro-convulsive compounds that accumulate in renal failure.

Effects of Intravenous Anesthetics (Table 2)

- Most intravenous anesthetics decrease CBF, decrease $CMRO_2$, and decrease ICP, except ketamine.
- *$CMRO_2$:* Intravenous anesthetics decrease $CMRO_2$; however, the decrease is only related to the suppression of synaptic activity. If the background electroencephalogram (EEG) is already depressed due to loss of excitability, such as hypothermia or injury, the decrease in $CMRO_2$ is attenuated. Anesthetics do not decrease the in-house cerebral metabolic requirement of the neurons in contrast to hypothermia.
- *Cerebral blood flow:* Intravenous anesthetics decrease CBF and increase cerebrovascular resistance. They can redistribute regional blood flow to ischemic regions.
- *Volatile versus IV anesthetics:* 1.5–2 MAC causes EEG silence and the maximum reduction of $CMRO_2$. Doses >1 MAC of volatile anesthetic affect the CO_2 response. Between 0.5 and 2 MAC anesthetic concentrations, there is a linear increase in CBF and ICP. Therefore, limiting

Table 2: Effects of anesthetics on the cerebral blood flow and related parameters.

	CBF	$CMRO_2$	Autoregulation	CO_2 response	ICP
Volatile agents					
Sevoflurane	++	–	–	0	+
Desflurane	+++	–	–	0	++
Isoflurane	+	– –	–	0	+
Nitrous oxide	+++	++	–	0	++
Intravenous agents					
Opioids	–	+	0	0	0
Benzodiazepines	– –	–	0	0	–
Propofol	– – –	– – –	0	0	– –
Etomidate	– – –	– –	0	0	– –
Ketamine	+++	++	0	0	++
Barbiturates	– – –	– – – –	0	0	– –
Miscellaneous agents					
Xe (30%)	–	– –	0	0	–
CO_2 (5%)	+++++	–	–	N/A	+++

(CBF: cerebral blood flow; $CMRO_2$: cerebral metabolic rate for oxygen; ICP: increased intracranial pressure)

CHAPTER 9 Brain Metabolism and Flow Metabolism Coupling

volatile anesthetics to 1 MAC is helpful to avoid an increase in CBF and ICP. With intact autoregulation, hyperventilation can attenuate the vasodilator effects of volatile anesthetics. High doses of volatile agents (2–3 MAC, isoflurane) have been used to suppress refractory seizure activity but result in hypotension and cardiac arrhythmias.
- Most intravenous agents, except ketamine, have opposite effects of decreasing blood flow and ICP and sparing autoregulation. As a general rule, when in doubt, go for total intravenous anesthesia (TIVA) while optimizing the CPP.

Pros and Cons of Nitrous Oxide Use

Pros
- Rapid onset and offset of effect
- Potent analgesic
- Extensive history of clinical use.

Cons
- Increases CBF, ICP, and $CMRO_2$
- Increases the risk of vascular air embolism (VAE)
- Expands volumes of trapped air in head trauma—pneumocephalus
- Interferes with electrophysiological monitoring.
- May contribute to postoperative nausea and vomiting.

Pros and Cons of Using Volatile Agents

Pros
- Excellent controlled hypnosis
- Easily monitored by expired gas analysis
- Do not require intravenous access.
- They can be used for rapid single-breath induction.
- Hyperventilation can offset some vasodilator effects.
- At <1 MAC, cerebrovascular effects are usually acceptable.

Cons
- Modern volatile agents lack sufficient analgesic properties.
- Increase CBF, CBV, and ICP
- Impair cerebral blood flow autoregulation.
- Impair flow metabolism coupling.
- Impairs evoked responses.
- It can alter regional blood flow to cause cerebral steal.
- Cause hypotension, increase ICP to decrease CPP.

- Toxic to personnel requires scavenging of waste gases.
- Harmful to the environment, halogenated compound damage the ozone layer.

Pros and Cons of Propofol—Total Intravenous Anesthesia

Pros

- Extensive track record of safety
- Decreases $CMRO_2$, CBF, ICP
- Preserves autoregulation.
- Preserves flow metabolism coupling.
- Smooth induction, easy maintenance, and prompt emergence
- Processed EEG can enable depth of anesthesia monitoring
- Does not impair evoked response monitoring
- Hypotension manageable
- Anticonvulsant
- Anti-emetic properties

Cons

- Require set-up time and equipment
- Requires additional EEG/processed EEG monitoring for precise control
- Pain during infusion
- Can cause hypotension
- High doses can cause propofol infusion syndrome
- Rarely causes diabetes insipidus.

Alternatives to Propofol

- *Dexmedetomidine* is better for maintaining the airway and provides analgesia. The hypotension is easily titratable. It can be used independently or supplement propofol TIVA.
- *Etomidate:* Limitations: infusion suppresses adrenals, pain on injection, excitatory movements.
- *Ketamine:* Limitations: Increases ICP, $CMRO_2$ and has potential psychogenic side-effects.

FURTHER READING

1. Claassen JAHR et al. Regulation of cerebral blood flow in humans: physiology and clinical implications of autoregulation. Physiol Rev. 2021;101(4):1487-1559.
2. Kakimoto A et al. Age-Related Sex-Specific Changes in Brain Metabolism and Morphology. J Nucl Med. 2016;57(2):221-5.
3. Mattos JD et al. Human brain blood flow and metabolism during isocapnic hyperoxia: the role of reactive oxygen species. J Physiol. 2019;597(3):741-55.

4. Pilli VK et al. Objective PET study of glucose metabolism asymmetries in children with epilepsy: Implications for normal brain development. Hum Brain Mapp. 2019;40(1):53-64.
5. Sertbas M et al. Unlocking Human Brain Metabolism by Genome-Scale and Multiomics Metabolic Models: Relevance for Neurology Research, Health, and Disease. OMICS. 2018;22(7):455-67.

Vignette: Flow Metabolism Coupling in the Brain—the Very First Studies

In 1879, an Italian physiologist, Angelo Masso, investigated the brain pulsations of three patients (Benito, Thorn, and Catherina) with skull defects. Through the defects, Angelo was able to feel and monitor these pulsations. He could record the brain pulsations by attaching a lever to the skin, sometimes for hours. He observed that the amplitude of brain pulsation was affected by breathing, waking up from sleep, calling the subject's name, ringing the church bells, and even convulsions. Masso observed that administering chloral hydrate, which induced deep sleep, decreased the pulsations. Masso therefore was the first researcher to investigate the effects of anesthetic drugs on cerebral blood flow.

Chapter 10: Cerebrospinal Fluid Formation and Circulation

INTRODUCTION

Cerebrospinal fluid (CSF) is the clear, colorless fluid surrounding the brain and the spinal cord. CSF is contained in the subarachnoid space. Three layers of meninges encase the brain. The outermost meningeal layer is the dura mater (mater: Latin māter, mother) which provides a tough yet flexible tissue that mechanically holds the CSF and protects the brain. Beneath it is the arachnoid layer that lines the dura mater. While the pia mater tightly invests the brain. CSF is contained in the space between the arachnoid and pia mater.

CEREBROSPINAL FLUID

- CSF is an ultrafiltrate of plasma with some secreted molecules.
- It is usually devoid of cells.
- The buoyancy of the brain in CSF decreases its weight from 1,500 to 50 g.
- CSF accounts for 5% of the intracranial volume.
- The total volume of CSF is about 135 mL (75 mL in the spinal cord, 35 mL in the ventricles, and 25 mL in the subarachnoid space).
- The CSF volume is replaced four to five times each day.

Functions

- CSF plays a crucial role in the embryologic development of the brain.
- The essential function of the CSF is to provide buoyancy to the brain tissue. Buoyancy decreases pressure on neural and vascular structures, enabling them to function effectively.
- This hydraulic support dissipates any pressure due to postural changes.
- CSF is the shock absorber that protects against mechanical injuries.
- CSF provides a pathway for waste disposal.
- It provides a pathway for nutrients through the choroid plexus.
- The blood-CSF barrier provides chemical protection.

Formation

- The choroid plexus and ependymal lining of the ventricle secrete the CSF.
- Choroid plexus cells are modified ependymal cells with dense and elongated villi and tight junctions between the cells.

CHAPTER 10 Cerebrospinal Fluid Formation and Circulation

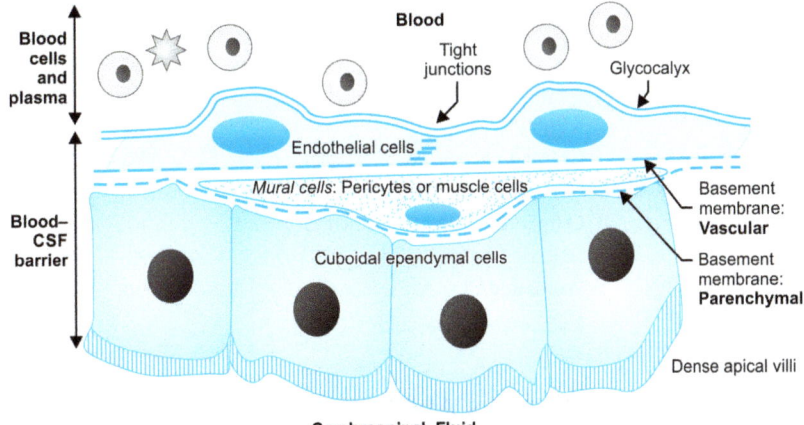

Fig. 1: Choroid plexus cells and the blood–CSF barrier.

- The tight junctions prevent the transfer of macromolecules and cells.
- Analogous to the blood-brain barrier is the blood-CSF barrier **(Fig. 1)**.
- A 5-mV potential across the ependymal cells facilitates the Na^+ transport.
- Water is freely diffusible into the CSF via the aquaporin-1 channels.
- *Mechanism:* Primarily by the secretion of Na^+, Cl^-, and HCO_3^- and plasma ultrafiltration.
- *Rate of CSF formation:* Approximately 0.35 mL/min.

Characteristics

- pH 7.4
- *Proteins:* 0.015–0.05 mg/dL
- *Pressure:* 5–15 mm Hg in the lateral position and 30–50 mm Hg in the sitting position.
- *The density of CSF:*
    - CSF density is 1.003–1.0007 g/mL in adults
    - CSF density decreases in pregnant patients
    - Adding dextrose can alter the density of local anesthetic drugs.
    - The density of isobaric bupivacaine is 0.999 compared to CSF 1.003 g/mL
    - The density of hyperbaric bupivacaine is 1.022 compared to CSF 1.003 g/mL
- *The viscosity of CSF:*
    - CSF, unlike blood, is a Newtonian fluid.
    - At 37°C, CSF viscosity is 0.7 to 1 centipoise.
    - Clinically, cells and proteins do not affect CSF viscosity.
    - Changes in CSF viscosity could affect shunt performance.
- The composition of CSF, lymph and serum is listed in **Table 1**.

Table 1: Composition of CSF, lymph, and serum.

	CSF	Lymph	Serum
Na (mEq/L)	138	136	140
K (mEq/L)	3.0	3.5	4.0
Ca (mEq/L)	2.5	4.0	4.6
Mg (mEq/L)	2.7	1.7	1.8
Cl (mEq/L)	125	100	100
Glucose (mg/dL)	60	95	90
Proteins (g/dL)	<0.05	5.0	7.0

(CSF: cerebrospinal fluid)

FACTORS AFFECTING CSF FORMATION

- A significant reduction of the choroidal perfusion pressure or increased intraventricular pressure can decrease CSF formation.
- *The core temperature has a significant effect:*
  - 11% decrease in CSF formation for each °C decrease in temperature
  - CSF formation ceases at 15°C
  - A 5-8°C decrease in temperature decreases CSF formation by 50%.
- Carbonic anhydrase inhibitors decrease CSF production by as much as 40%.
- Steroids decrease CSF formation by 50%.

CSF CIRCULATION

- Due to the relatively slow movement of fluid, CSF circulation is more akin to the recycling of the fluid, unlike the volume flow changes seen with blood circulation **(Figs. 2 and 3)**.
- The bulk flow of CSF is probably due to cardiac pulsation and respiratory pressure changes.
- *CSF is contained in the following:*
  - *Subarachnoid space around the brain and the spine:* About 100 mL
  - *Ventricles:* About 35 mL
  - *Cisterns* are dilated subarachnoid spaces containing CSF.
    - These include:
      - *Cisterna magna,* which is the largest cistern. Communicates with the fourth ventricle via the foramen of Magendie. It contains:
        - About 5–10 mL of CSF
        - Lower four cranial nerves: IX, X, XI, and XII
        - Vertebral and the posterior inferior cerebellar artery
      - *Other cranial cisterns, which are in a craniocaudal sequence:*
        - Pericallosal cistern
        - Quadrigeminal cistern
        - Cisterna chiasmaticus

CHAPTER 10 Cerebrospinal Fluid Formation and Circulation

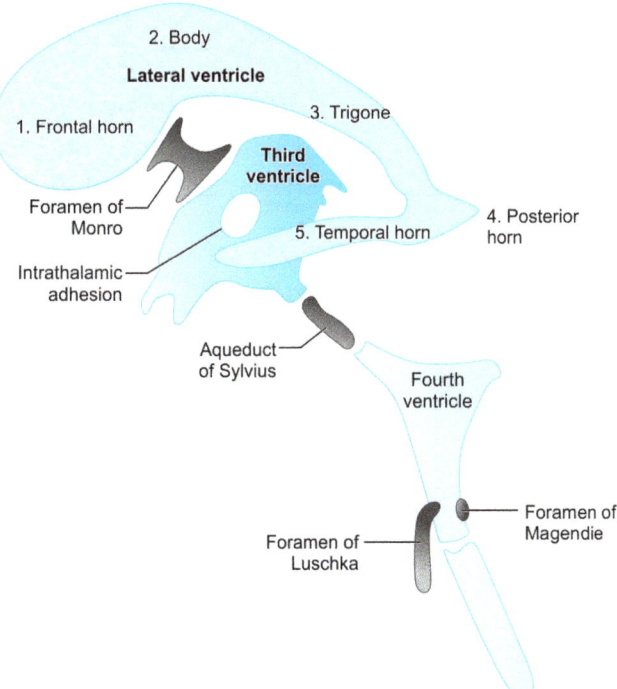

Fig. 2: The ventricular system: exploded diagram.

- ◆ Cisterna ambiens
- ◆ Cisterna interpeduncular
- ◆ Cisterna pontis
- *Lumbar cistern:*
  - ◆ Extends from conus medullaris to the sacrum.
  - ◆ Contains cauda equina nerve roots and filum terminalis.
  - ◆ It is the site of CSF withdrawal and lumbar spinal drug delivery.

Lateral Ventricles

- The lateral ventricles are paired structures.
- Each ventricle is divided into five regions:
  - Frontal horn
  - Body
  - Trigone
  - Temporal horn
  - Posterior horn.
- 80% CSF is formed by the choroid plexus of the lateral ventricles.
- The size of the lateral ventricles increases with the following:
  - Age

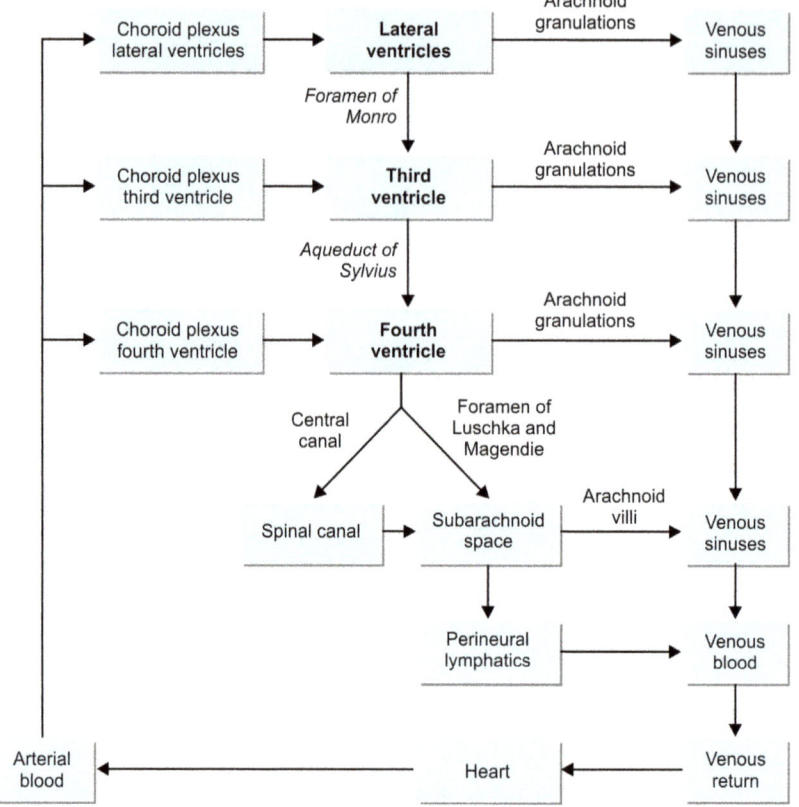

Fig. 3: The formation and circulation of cerebrospinal fluid.

- Contra-lateral to the dominant hemispheric
- Hydrocephalus.

Foramen of Monro

These are:
- Paired structures drain the lateral ventricles into the third ventricle.
- Crescent-shaped openings.
- Located behind the thalamus.
- Lined with choroid plexus.
- Tumors, trauma, and infections can obstruct the foramen.

Third Ventricle

- The choroid plexus lines the roof of the third ventricle.
- The ventricle floor is shaped as a funnel that forms the infundibulum, investing in the hypothalamus.
- During the third ventriculostomy, the third ventricle floor, near the mamillary bodies, is incised. The opening is dilated to drain CSF into the basal cistern.

Aqueduct of Sylvius
- It permits the flow of CSF between the third and the fourth ventricles.
- It is located between the pons and the cerebellum.
- It is surrounded by periaqueductal gray matter.
- It is the most common site of obstruction in congenital hydrocephalus.
- Obstruction leads to non-communicating hydrocephalus.

Fourth Ventricle
- It is a tent-shaped structure.
- The apex of the tent is in the cerebellum.
- The base is the pons and medulla.
- CSF drains into the ventricle via the aqueduct of Sylvius.
- The CSF outflow from the ventricle happens by four possible routes:
  - Via the obex into the central canal of the spinal cord
  - Via the midline foramen of Magendie into the cisterna magna
  - Via the two lateral foramen of Luschka into the cerebellopontine cistern.
- Tumors in the IV ventricle can obstruct CSF flow.

Routes of Cerebrospinal Fluid Reabsorption
- Via cranial and spinal arachnoid villi
- Via extracranial lymphatics along spinal nerve roots
- Via lymphatics that drain the Virchow–Robin space
- Direct absorption through intracranial veins
- Via lymphatics along the ophthalmic nerve through the cribriform plate.

Intracranial and spinal subarachnoid granulations and villi:
- Arachnoid granulations and villi function as non-return valves that drain CSF into the venous sinuses.
- The pia mater of the brain protrudes into the venous sinuses.
- Though arachnoid granulations are sufficiently large to be seen by the naked eye, the villi, on the other hand, are microscopic structures.
- The mechanism which prevents the non-return of CSF is probably due to vacuoles and unidirectional delivery of CSF.

ABNORMALITIES OF CSF CIRCULATION

Hydrocephalus
Hydrocephalus can be due to excessive formation, obstruction of circulation, or inadequate drainage of CSF.

Presents with:
- In adults:
  - Headaches
  - Nausea and vomiting

- Cognitive impairment
- Bladder and bowel dysfunction
- In infants:
  - A high-pitched cry
  - Increased head circumference in infants and children.
  - Failure to thrive and delayed milestones in infants
- With Features of raised intracranial pressure (ICP):
  - Headache
  - Bradycardia
  - Hypertension, increase pulse pressure
  - Irregular respiration
  - Convulsions

Hydrocephalus can be communicating or non-communicating:
- *Communicating hydrocephalus:*
  - CSF flow between the ventricles is not obstructed.
  - All ventricles are dilated, and the dilation is symmetrical
  - The obstruction at the skull's base prevents CSF drainage into the subarachnoid space.
  - Etiology:
    - Subarachnoid hemorrhage (SAH)
    - Meningitis.
- *Non-communicating hydrocephalus:*
  - CSF flow obstructed at the foramen of Monro or aqueduct of Sylvius.
  - The lateral and third ventricles are dilated.
  - Compressed or normal fourth ventricle
  - Ventricles may be asymmetric on imaging.
  - Etiology:
    - *Mass lesions:* Tumor, hemorrhage, and cysts
    - Stenosis of the CSF drainage pathways
    - IVH.
- *Lumbar puncture (LP):*
  - To be done with care when raised ICP is suspected.
  - The sudden release of pressure can lead to brain herniation.
  - Avoid LP in patients with non-communicating hydrocephalus.
- *Treatment strategies:*
  - Treatment of underlying causes, such as tumor
  - Ventriculoperitoneal or ventriculo-atrial shunt
  - Intracranial drainage, e.g., third ventriculostomy
  - Ablation of choroid plexus.

Cerebral Hypotension
- A leak of CSF can lead to cerebral hypotension.
- Inadequate CSF leads to the loss of buoyancy of the brain tissue.
- It results in traction on the meninges and the cranial nerves.

- *Presents as:*
  - Postural headache
  - Neck stiffness
  - Nausea and vomiting.
- *MRI imaging reveals:*
  - Increased intracranial venous volume.
  - Pituitary hyperemia
  - Prominent pachymeninges
  - Sagging of brain structures.
- *Treatment strategies:*
  - Medical management with:
    - Bed rest
    - Fluids
    - Analgesics
    - Caffeine
  - Blood patch
  - Surgical correction.

Pseudotumor Cerebri or "False Brain Tumor"

- A rare condition with symptoms of raised ICP without any apparent cause and with normal ventricular size.
- *Etiology unknown:* Probably due to failure of CSF reabsorption.
- *Associated risk factors:*
  - In adults, 10× more in females
  - Child-bearing age, 20–44 years
  - Obesity
  - Anemia
  - Polycystic ovary syndrome
  - Renal failure
  - Growth hormone treatment
  - *Drugs:* Minocycline and other tetracyclines, Vitamin A overdose, and steroid withdrawal.
- *Presents with:*
  - Headaches
  - Nausea
  - Tinnitus
  - Diplopia, visual field cuts, and visual loss.
- *On examination:*
  - *Fundoscopy:* Papilledema
  - *CSF pressure:* >20 mm Hg water.
- *Treatment strategy:*
  - Loss of vision is a significant concern.
  - Medical management with acetazolamide

- A shunt might be indicated.
- Decompression of optic nerve.

Meningitis

- *Meningitis:* Inflammation of the meninges. It can be bacterial or aseptic.
- *Bacterial meningitis:*
  - More dangerous
  - *Common bacterial pathogens: Streptococcus pneumonia, Neisseria meningitides, Haemophilus influenzae, Listeria monocytogenes, Group B streptococci,* and *Escherichia coli.*
- *Aseptic meningitis:*
  - Common pathogens:
    - *Fungi:* Cryptococci, histoplasma, blastomyces, and coccidiosis
    - *Viral:* Enterovirus, coxsackie, echovirus, herpes, mumps, and HIV
    - *Bacterial:* Mycoplasma, brucella, and treponema
    - *Parasites:* Toxoplasma and cysticercosis
  - *Malignancy:* Lymphoma and carcinomatosis
  - *Autoimmune diseases:* Sarcoid and vasculitis
  - *Drugs:* Nonsteroidal anti-inflammatory drugs (NSAIDs), anti-microbial, and intrathecal chemotherapy.
- *Presentation:*
  - Fever
  - Neck rigidity
  - Photophobia
  - Altered mental status
  - Seizures
  - Focal signs.
- *Diagnosis:*
  - *CSF:* The presence of infection is usually indicated by leukocytes. Normal CSF has ≤5/mm^3; 5–10 WBCs/mm^3 is suspicious, while ≥10 WBCs/mm^3 is abnormal in the absence of red blood cells (RBCs)
  - *Bacterial meningitis:* Turbid CSF with low CSF glucose
  - *Viral meningitis:* Polymerase chain reaction (PCR) diagnostic.
- *Treatment strategy:*
  - *Bacterial meningitis:* Initially broad spectrum but later based on culture sensitivity.
  - *Aseptic meningitis:* Usually symptomatic treatment.

Subarachnoid Hemorrhage

- Hemorrhage into the subarachnoid space results in severe neurological complications with a grave prognosis.

- SAH is usually due to the rupture of a cerebral aneurysm. Other causes include traumatic brain injury, rupture of an arteriovenous malformation, or impaired blood coagulation.
- *Presents with:*
  - Sudden severe headache
  - Neck rigidity
  - Photophobia
  - Nausea
  - Vomiting
  - Double or decreased vision
  - Confusion or irritability
  - Seizure
  - Unconsciousness.
- *Diagnosis:*
  - *CSF:* With traumatic SAH, the CSF samples the blood clears over time. In contrast, in the case of nontraumatic hemorrhage, the CSF does not clear, and samples remain blood-tinged. With aneurysmal SAH, the CSF does not clot. It has abundant RBCs and white blood cells (WBCs). It is usually xanthochromic after 6–12 hours following the bleed.
  - *MR imaging and angiography* show vascular abnormality. It can detect and quantify the volume of blood to assess the outcome.
  - *CT scan and CT angiography:* Similar to MRI, it helps diagnose and quantify the lesion.
  - *Cerebral angiography* is the gold standard. It helps identify and guide treatment.
- *Treatment strategy:*
  - SAH is a medical emergency.
  - Treatment depends on the etiology and severity of the bleed:
    - Due to the likelihood of rebleeding from an aneurysm, early surgical clipping or coiling is needed.
    - Arteriovenous malformation hemorrhages are rarely subarachnoid and are less likely to rebleed. They can be treated by excision or embolization.
  - Ventricular drain to diagnose and treat increased ICP.
  - Traumatic SAH
  - Coagulation defects have to be corrected.

FURTHER READING

1. Korzh V. Development of brain ventricular system. Cell Mol Life Sci. 2018; 75(3):375-83.
2. Lokossou A et al. ICP monitoring and phase-contrast MRI to investigate intracranial compliance. Acta Neurochir Suppl. 2018;126:247-53.

3. Unnerback M et al. Validation of a mathematical model for understanding intracranial pressure curve morphology. J Clin Monit Comput. 2020;34(3):469-81.
4. Yamada S. Cerebrospinal fluid dynamics. Croat Med J. 2021;62(4):399-10.
5. Yan J et al. Cerebrospinal fluid metabolomics: detection of neuroinflammation in human central nervous system disease. Clin Transl Immunology. 2021;10(8):e1318

Vignette: Cerebrospinal Fluid History

Fluid leaking from the brain after skull fracture was described in the Edwin Smith papyrus dated 1550 BCE. Edwin Smith's papyrus was believed to be a copy of an older manuscript. The manuscript has recently been sourced to Imhotep, who lived around 2700 BCE and was a renowned scholar, architect, and healer. The classical Greeks knew about the fluid in the brain. Hippocrates thought that the animal spirit lived in the ventricles. Galen believed that CSF was a vaporous fluid that provided energy to the whole body. An Italian anatomist, Nicolo Massa, provided the modern description of CSF in 1536.

Chapter 11: Hypothalamus—Pituitary Axis

INTRODUCTION

The hypothalamus and pituitary act in concert to maintain homeostasis, control bodily functions, and enable the body to cope with stress. These glands interact with other organs, such as the adrenals, thyroid, and gonads, to form hypothalamic-pituitary-adrenal, hypothalamic-pituitary-thyroid, and hypothalamic-pituitary-gonadotropic axes, respectively. The hypothalamus and pituitary glands represent the most important endocrine organs, which are critical to the survival of an individual.

HYPOTHALAMUS

Anatomy

- The hypothalamus weighs about 2.5 g.
- Hypothalamic boundaries (**Figs. 1 and 2**):
  - *Superiorly:* Hypothalamic sulcus separates it from the thalamus
  - *Inferiorly:* Tuber cinereum and the infundibulum that extends into the pituitary
  - *Anteriorly:* Optic chiasma and the lamina terminalis
  - *Posteriorly:* Mammillary bodies
  - *Laterally:* Optic tract and internal capsule
  - *Medially:* Third ventricle.

Functions

- The hypothalamus plays a critical role in maintaining homeostasis and ensuring survival. Its functions include:
  - *Endocrine functions:*
    - Supraoptic and paraventricular nuclei secrete hormones vasopressin (antidiuretic hormone, ADH) and oxytocin.
    - Preoptic, ventromedial, and arcuate nuclei secrete pituitary hormones releasing peptides.
  - Temperature control
  - Diet control
  - *Behavior:* Defensive behavior.

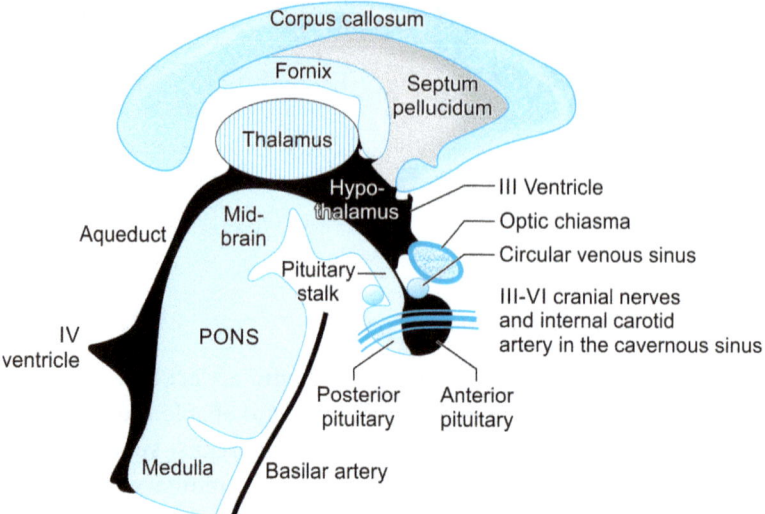

Fig. 1: Pituitary anatomy: Key structures—sagittal plane.

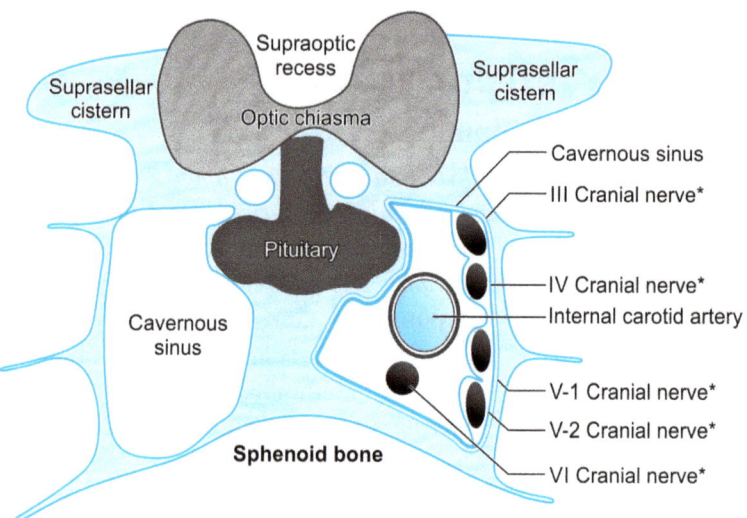

Fig. 2: Pituitary anatomy: Key structures—coronal plane. Cranial nerves III, IV, V-1, and V-2 [*] are located in the sinus wall.

Hypothalamic Hormones

- *Via the neural hypothalamic–hypophyseal tract to the posterior pituitary:*
  - Oxytocin
  - Vasopressin (ADH)
- *Via the hypothalamic–hypophyseal portal system to the anterior pituitary:*
  - Corticotropin-releasing hormone (CRH)
  - Thyrotropin-releasing hormone (TRH)
  - Growth-hormone-releasing hormone (GHRH)

- GHRH and inhibiting hormone (somatostatin)
- Prolactin-releasing hormone (postulated)
- Dopamine–Prolactin release inhibiting hormone.
- Gonadotropic-releasing hormone

The pituitary gland, also known as hypophysis:
- It weighs 0.5 g, is a pea-sized structure
- It is a midline structure located on the sphenoid apex.
- It lies in the hypophyseal fossa.
- It lies in a depression in the skull base called sella turcica (Turkish saddle).
- The sella turcica is surrounded by several identifiable structures **(Fig. 2)**:
    - *Superiorly:* Diaphragma sellae separate it from the hypothalamus
    - *Inferiorly:* Sphenoid bone and sphenoid air sinuses.
    - *Laterally:* The cavernous sinus which contains:
        - The cavernous portion of the internal carotid artery
        - The III-VI cranial nerves.
- The pituitary is divided into two main lobes with an intermediate lobe:
    - *The intermediate lobe* of the pituitary secretes the melanocyte-stimulating hormone (MSH). The pale color, a symptom of Addison's Disease, is due to a lack of MSH.
    - Anterior pituitary, pars-distalis, or adenohypophysis:
        - *Ectodermal:* Develops from the primitive pharynx called Rathke's pouch
        - *Main hormones:* Follicle-stimulating hormone (FSH), adrenocorticotropin hormone (ACTH), thyroid-stimulating hormone, and luteinizing hormone (LH)
        - On histological staining, five types of cells are identified in the anterior pituitary **(Table 1)**.
        - The key to the functioning of the anterior hypothalamus is the *hypothalamic–hypophyseal portal system* **(Fig. 3)**. A hypophyseal artery branch forms capillaries in the lower hypothalamus. Tropic factors can diffuse through the capillaries into the portal

Table 1: Cells of the adenohypophysis.

Cell type	Hormone secreted	% Total cells
Somatotropes	Human growth hormone	50%
Corticotropes	Adrenocorticotropin hormone	20%
Thyrotropes	Thyroid-stimulating hormone	5%
Gonadotropins	Luteinizing hormone and follicle-stimulating hormone	5%
Lactotropes	Prolactin	5%

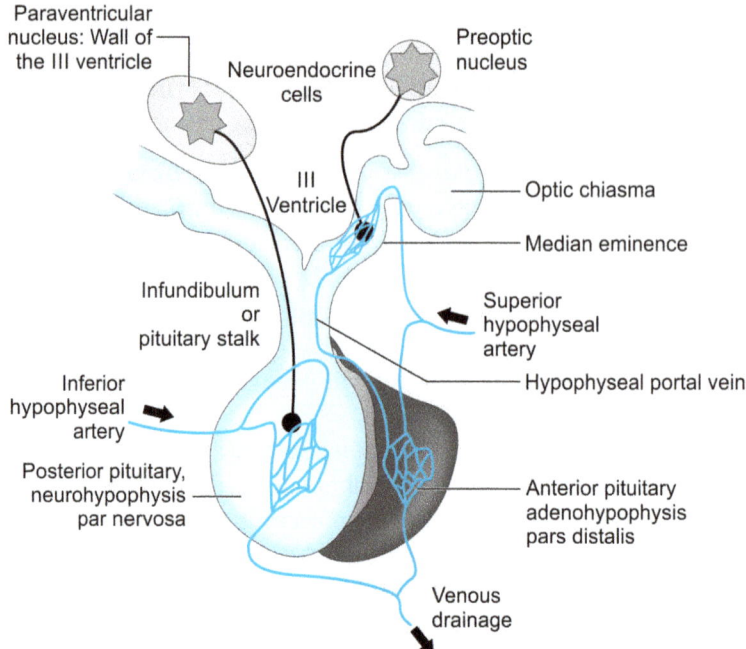

Fig. 3: Pituitary anatomy and the hypophyseal portal system.

system to reach the adenohypophysis. In adenohypophysis, they form another capillary from which these controlling hormones can diffuse out. Hypothalamic tropic factors reach the anterior hypophysis rapidly in high concentrations through the portal system. The system avoids exposure to the systemic circulation that would dilute the factors and delay the response.

- *Posterior pituitary or neurohypophysis* **(Table 2):**
  - It is an extension of the hypothalamus
  - Neural down growth consists of the pituitary stalk and infundibular process (the posterior lobe)
  - The axons of the hypothalamus descend in the pituitary stalk into the posterior portion of the gland
  - *Main hormones:* Oxytocin and vasopressin.

Blood Supply

- *Arterial:* Superior and inferior hypophyseal arteries.
- *Venous drainage:* The hypophyseal veins drain into the cavernous sinus.

PITUITARY SYNDROMES

- *Multiple endocrine neoplasia type 1 (MEN1) syndrome:*
  - Also known as Werner syndrome, autosomal dominant disease

Table 2: Hypothalamic–pituitary hormones.

Hypothalamic-releasing hormone	Pituitary hormone	Target organ	Effect
Posterior pituitary hormones			
Antidiuretic hormone (ADH)	ADH stores	Renal, sweat, and vascular bed	Water balance and vascular resistance
–	Oxytocin	Uterus	Uterine contractions
Anterior pituitary hormones			
Gonadotropin-releasing hormone (GnRH)	Luteinizing hormone (LH)	Gonads	Sex hormone production
Gonadotropin-releasing hormone (GnRH)	FSH	Gonads	Egg or sperm production
Thyrotropin-releasing hormone (TRH)	Thyroid-stimulating hormone	Thyroid gland	Releases thyroid hormones
Dopamine (prolactin-inhibiting hormone, PIH)	Prolactin-releasing hormone	Mammary gland	Milk secretion
Growth-hormone-releasing hormone (GHRH)	Growth hormone	Bone, muscles, and organs	Stimulates growth release of insulin-like growth factor
Corticotropin-releasing hormone (CRH)	ACTH	Adrenal glands	Corticosteroid release

- *Incidence:* 1:30,000
- Common tumors of the parathyroid, islet cells of the pancreas, and pituitary
- *Less frequent tumors:* Adrenal cortical tumors, neuroendocrine (carcinoid) tumors, and pheochromocytomas
  - *Nonendocrine tumors:* Facial angiofibromas, collagenoma of the skin, lipomas, leiomyomas, and meningiomas
- *Familial isolated pituitary adenoma:*
  - 2% of pituitary adenomas have a familial disease
  - It affects some 200 families.
  - It affects the aryl-hydrocarbon interacting (AIP) gene on the long arm of chromosome 11.
  - Associated with nonmalignant tumors of the brain.
  - *The adenomas can be:*
    - Prolactinomas
    - Somatotropinomas
    - Somatolactotropinomas
    - Adrenocorticotropic-hormone-secreting tumors
    - Nonfunctioning adenomas.

- *Acromegaly and Gigantism: Excess of growth hormone*
  - Incidence 1:10,000 population.
  - *Children:* Excessive growth with increased height, gigantism.
  - *Adults:* When epiphyses have sealed: Acromegaly
  - Enlargement of hands and feet (acral parts)
  - Prognathism
  - Visual field cuts, classically bitemporal hemianopia.
  - Weight gain
  - Increased bone weight
  - Hypertension and cardiomegaly
  - Diabetes.
- *Cushing's disease: Excess of adrenocorticotropin hormone*
  - *Incidence:*
    - 10 per million population
    - Greater in females.
- *Clinical features:*
  - *General:*
    - Weight gain with truncal obesity, moon face, and buffalo hump
    - *Skin changes:*
      - Thin, fragile, easy bruising.
      - Acne
      - Striae or pigmented stretch marks on the trunk, arms, thighs, and breast
    - Fatigue and muscle weakness
    - Hypertension
    - Headache, emotional changes, and cognitive difficulties
    - Increased skin pigmentation
    - Bone loss
    - *Gender-specific:*
      - *Females:*
        - Irregular and absent menstrual periods.
        - Hirsutism.
      - *Males:*
        - Decreased libido.
        - Erectile dysfunction.
- *Prolactinomas: Excess of prolactin*
  - *Incidence:*
    - *Incidence:* 5/100,000/year; prevalence: 50/100,000
    - Tumors are larger and more aggressive in males.
  - *Clinical features:*
    - *Children:* Delayed growth, delayed puberty, headaches, visual changes, and amenorrhea in girls

CHAPTER 11 Hypothalamus—Pituitary Axis

- Adults:
  - *Female:* Amenorrhea, galactorrhea, infertility, acne, decreased bone mass, and neurological effects
  - *Males:* Decreased libido, erectile dysfunction, oligo- or azoospermia, decreased bone mass, and neurological effects.
- *Secondary adrenal insufficiency: lack of adrenocorticotropin hormone*
  - *Incidence:*
    - *Prevalence:* 300/million population
    - Typically, seen in the sixth decade.
    - Iatrogenic, due to steroid treatment or withdrawal
    - Panhypopituitarism
    - ACTH deficiency.
  - *Clinical features:*
    - The main difference from primary adrenal insufficiency is the absence of skin pigmentation.
    - Fatigue
    - Weakness
    - Weight loss
    - Nausea
    - Vomiting
    - Diarrhea
- *Pituitary apoplexy*
  - *Incidence:*
    - Over incidence in the general population: 5/100,000
    - People with pituitary tumors have a 1–10% chance of apoplexy.
    - Without pituitary tumors, apoplexy is exceedingly rare.
  - *Etiology:*
    - Tumor infarction
    - Tumor hemorrhage
    - *Can be associated with:*
      - Hypertension
      - Stress
      - Infection
      - Pregnancy
  - *Clinical presentation:*
    - Acute-onset headache
    - Vomiting
    - Visual defects
    - Sensory changes
    - Endocrinopathy
    - Presenting feature of an underlying adenoma
- *Craniopharyngiomas arise from the remnants of Rathke's pouch.* It is an invagination of the primitive stomodeum toward the neuroectoderm.

The pouch is the progenitor of the adenohypophysis. In some instances, there is development arrest, and cells from the primitive stomodeum are trapped along the migratory path, resulting in the formation of tumors or craniopharyngioma. Thus, in location, craniopharyngiomas can be infrasellar, sellar, infundibular, or suprasellar.
- *Incidence:*
  - *Overall incidence:* 2/million population/year
  - 1% of all brain tumors and 13% of all suprasellar tumors
  - The bimodal age distribution curve peaks at 5–14 years and after 65 years
  - In children, they represent 60% of all suprasellar tumors and carry a better prognosis.
- *Clinical features:*
  - Headaches and vomiting
  - *Visual disturbances:*
    - Visual field cuts
    - Decreased visual acuity.
  - *Endocrinopathies:*
    - Growth retardation
    - Delayed puberty
    - Diabetes insipidus and excessive thirst
    - *Sexual dysfunction:* Hypogonadism.
  - *Hyperprolactinemia:*
    - *Females:* Amenorrhea syndrome and infertility.
    - *Males:* Impotence, decreased libido, and erectile dysfunction
- Cognitive impairment, emotional changes, and disturbances of circadian rhythm
- Hydrocephalus.

FURTHER READING

1. Deopujari CE et al. Evolution of Pituitary Surgery. Neurol India. 2020; 68(Supplement): S33-8.
2. Herman JP The neuroendocrinology of stress: Glucocorticoid signaling mechanisms. Psychoneuroendocrinology. 2021;137:105641.
3. Serioli S et al. Pituitary Adenomas and Invasiveness from Anatomo-Surgical, Radiological, and Histological Perspectives: A Systematic Literature Review. Cancers (Basel). 2019;11(12):1936.
4. Solari D et al. Pituitary Adenomas: What Are the Key Features? What Are the Current Treatments? Where Is the Future Taking Us? World Neurosurg. 2019;127:695-709.
5. Wu X et al. Pituitary adenoma with posterior area invasion of cavernous sinus: surgical anatomy, approach, and outcomes. Neurosurg Rev. 2021; 44(4):2229-37.

CHAPTER 11 Hypothalamus—Pituitary Axis

Vignette: The Tallest Human Being

In 1940, Robert Wadlow measured 242 cm or 8 feet and 11.1 inches. He is reported to be the tallest human being ever. He was diagnosed with pituitary hyperplasia. Wadlow weighed 500 lbs at his peak. At birth, he was a normal infant who weighed 8.7 lbs. At the age of 5 years, Wadlow was 163 cm tall and weighed 108 lbs. He continued to grow throughout his life. His daily diet averaged 8,000 calories. His shoe size was 47 cm, but he did not have to buy those shoes under an advertising contract with a shoe company. He died from sepsis following a minor foot injury while testing a new brace at the age of 22 years.

Chapter 12

Electrophysiological Monitoring

INTRODUCTION

Electrophysiological (EP) monitoring is the standard of care for specific neurosurgical interventions such as corrective spine surgery. However, the role of EP monitoring in guiding other surgeries, such as brain and spine tumor resection, is less established.

A range of EP monitoring devices are a part of modern neuroanesthetic practice, and their role is likely to expand as minimally invasive procedures advance.

OBJECTIVES OF EP MONITORING

The objectives of electrophysiological monitoring are:
- To prevent injury during surgery.
  - Direct injury to the spine or a peripheral nerve.
  - Guide tumor resection in eloquent areas of the brain.
  - Assess the safety of vascular occlusion, e.g., carotid surgery and aortic clamping.
- Monitor and prevent ongoing neurological injury, e.g., during cerebrovascular surgery or aortic surgery.
- To assess and monitor the depth of anesthesia to control anesthetic drug dosing.
  - Avoid intraoperative awareness.
  - Ensure rapid emergence for anesthesia.
  - Provide a target for pharmacological neuroprotection.
- To guide surgery such as facial nerve monitoring in head and neck surgeries or evoked potential monitoring during minimally invasive spine surgeries **(Table 1)**.

ELECTROENCEPHALOGRAPHY

Electroencephalography (EEG) is the sum of the electrical activity of the neurons recorded by surface electrodes. Most of the signals arise from the pyramidal cells in the 3rd to 6th layers of the cortex. Individual neurons have a membrane potential of −60 mV. Neuronal activation can affect the surface charge by hyperpolarizing or depolarizing the cell membranes.

CHAPTER 12 Electrophysiological Monitoring

Table 1: Electrophysiological monitoring during neurosurgery.

Surgery	Monitoring methods	Others
Spine		
Scoliosis	SSEP, MEP, and wake-up test	Processed EEG (BIS)
Spine tumor	SSEP and MEP	Processed EEG (BIS)
Spine trauma	SSEP and MEP	Processed EEG (BIS)
Vascular		
Carotid surgery	EEG, SSEP, awake surgery under regional	TCD, NIRS, processed EEG (BIS)
Aneurysm clipping	EEG and processed EEG (BIS)	SSEP and MEP
Decompression		
Trigeminal	BAER, Facial nerve	Processed EEG (BIS)
Facial	BAER and facial nerve	Processed EEG (BIS)
Spinal stenosis	SSEP and MEP	Processed EEG (BIS)
Tumors		
Supra-tentorial	Cortical EEG, SSEP, and MEP	Awake craniotomy
Infra-tentorial	BAER, SSEP, MEP, and facial nerve and X CN (vocal cords)	Processed EEG (BIS)
Spine	SSEP and MEP	Processed EEG (BIS)

(BAER: brainstem auditory evoked responses; NIRS: Near Infrared Spectroscopy; BIS: bi-spectral index; EEG: electroencephalography; EMG: electromyography; SSEP: somatosensory evoked potential; TCD: transcranial Doppler)

- *Indications:*
  - Monitoring the depth of anesthesia
  - Monitoring of brain injury during surgery, e.g., carotid endarterectomy
  - Assisting the resection of epileptic foci
  - As a part of somatosensory evoked potential (SSEP) monitoring during:
    - Spine surgery
    - Nerve decompression
- *Techniques:*
  - *EEG montages:*
    - *Two-channel bilateral frontal EEG* is used to grossly monitor the brain's electrical activity as part of processed EEG monitoring or during electroconvulsive therapy. Such measurements help monitor the depth of anesthesia, convulsions, global reduction in cerebral blood flow, or drug-induced EEG silence but cannot reliably detect focal injury.
    - *Simplified eight-lead EEG* is clinically used to monitor the electrical activities in the major cerebral arterial distributions. It crudely monitors the regional cortical function.

- EEG leads using 10-20 leads monitor the brain regions 2-3 cm wide. This lead system is sufficient to monitor abnormal excitatory (epilepsy) or inhibitory (stroke/ischemia) focal activity with a clinically accepted spatial resolution. This montage is most widely used in clinical neurology.
- Dense EEG recordings with 64 or 128 electrodes are done for research purposes and in thought-controlled devices.
- Direct cortical recording with surface leads is done during epilepsy focus localization.
- Dense needle recording of EEG activity with cell cluster level resolution in specific regions is done for brain-computer interfaces.
- *EEG spectrum:* Frequency bands arise from rhythmic activity in the thalamus.
    - *Delta:* 0–4 Hz seen in deep anesthesia, brain injury
    - *Theta:* 4–8 Hz
    - *Alpha:* 8–12 Hz
    - *Beta:* 12–24 Hz
    - *Gamma:* >24 Hz
- *Processed EEG:*
    - *Time domain:* It displays voltage changes over time.
        - Average power is the square of voltage amplitude.
        - Burst suppression ratio: % time in EEG silence.
    - *Frequency domain:* Using the Fourier analysis, the EEG spectrum is fractionated into component waves and presented as a frequency distribution graph.
        - *Compressed spectral array:* It gives the frequency distribution over time.
        - *Density spectral array:* It shows amplitude over time.
        - *Spectral edge frequency* shows the threshold frequency beyond which little power is evident.
        - *The bi-spectral analysis* looks at the phase difference with a frequency band.
- **Effect of anesthetic on EEG:**
    - *Typical EEG shifts under anesthesia:*
        - Alpha and beta activity is evident in the frontal cortex.
        - The alpha activity occurs in the posterior cortex.
        - The posterior activity pattern shifts forward while frontal activity goes back.
        - Homogenization of EEG activity: Cortical synchrony
        - Increase in slow theta delta activity.
        - Decrease in amplitude.
        - Burst suppression pattern.
        - Silence.

- *Notable patterns:*
  - Volatile anesthetics produce burst suppression at 1.5 MAC concentrations.
  - Nitrous oxide is an exception, as it increases EEG activity.
  - IV anesthetic agents decrease EEG amplitude and produce burst suppression; the pattern shifts occur characteristically in different brain regions.
    - *Barbiturates:* Produce classic burst suppression pattern. Typically, a 10:1 silence-to-burst suppression ratio is desired for neuroprotection. However, pharmacological burst suppression has not been proven neuroprotective in clinical trials.
    - *Propofol* produces maximum power and coherence at 11 Hz. Frontal leads show high amplitude spindles with slow oscillations.
    - *Dexmedetomidine* produces maximum power and coherence at 13 Hz. Poorly suppresses EEG activity in posterior leads.
    - *Ketamine* increases theta activity in the frontal and posterior lobes, while alpha remains localized in the posterior regions. Ketamine can cause seizure-like activity.
    - *Opioids* can increase EEG activity.
- To increase seizure activity during electrocorticography, consider the following:
  - Hyperventilation
  - Ketamine, etomidate, and methohexital infusions.
  - Enflurane and sevoflurane.

ELECTROMYOGRAPHY

- *Indications:*
  - Assessment of neuromuscular block
  - Motor nerve monitoring during lower cranial nerve surgery
  - Guiding minimally invasive spine surgery
  - Nerve decompression and repair
  - Non-neurosurgical operations:
    - Thyroid, parathyroid, facial, mandibular, and high cervical surgeries
    - Management of cases with myopathies, polymyositis, and myotonic dystrophies.
- *Technique:*
  - Electromyography (EMG) recording for a given muscle is best done by placing three leads: (1) at the motor point, (2) at the most distal region of the muscle, and (3) at a remote ground. The response is recorded as a voltage or in the operating room, converted to recognizable sound.

- Besides monitoring the muscle, it also monitors the motor nerve and the neuromuscular junction.
- *There are three patterns of nerve injury seen with motor nerve monitoring, such as the facial nerve:*
  - Background continuous low-amplitude activity with spikes
  - Neurotonic burst due to mild irritation, traction, remote electrical stimulation, or nerve contact. It is reversible if the cause is promptly relieved.
  - A sustained neurotonic burst or a repetitive pattern suggests greater chances of injury.
- *Compound muscle action potential (CMAP):*
  - The compound motor action potential represents the net response of the motor endplate to nerve stimulation.
  - The net muscle contraction is a composite of three components: (1) Motor plate potential, (2) muscle depolarization, and (3) the H reflex, which is the segmental response to stimulation.
  - CMAPs are increased with muscle exercise.
  - CMAPs are prolonged with recumbency and myopathy.
  - Anesthetics decrease CMAPs and attenuate the EMG response.
- *Commonly monitored cranial motor nerves:* Facial, vagus (recurrent larynges nerve), spinal accessory, and hypoglossal nerves.

- *EMG for monitoring paralysis:*
  - Neuromuscular monitoring for muscle paralysis is routinely used by anesthesiologists using tactile or visual inspection. However, such monitoring can be challenging in spine cases due to limited access. EMG could be used as an alternative means of monitoring paralysis. However, EMG based neuromuscular monitoring devices are not widely available. Electrophysiologists routinely use the EMG for monitoring paralysis during surgery and, when needed, could assist with anesthetic management.
  - Indications for monitoring neuromuscular functions during anesthesia:
    - Determine optimum intubating conditions.
    - Ensure immobility during surgery.
    - Permit mechanical ventilation.
    - Enable safe monitoring with sub-paralytic doses of muscle relaxants:
      - Improve SSEP monitoring by decreasing muscle artifacts.
      - Prevent gross motor response during MEP monitoring.
    - Determine safe conditions for the reversal of muscle paralysis.
    - Assess postoperative muscle weakness.
    - Management of paralytic drug dosing in disease conditions:
      - Neuromuscular diseases
      - Resistance to muscle relaxants due to anticonvulsant drugs

- *Advantages of EMG versus mechanical response assessment:*
  - Independent of factors that affect the motor response, such as:
    - Preload
    - Certain myopathic conditions
  - It does not require visual inspection for:
    - Motor response
    - Accelerometer displacement.
- *Disadvantages:*
  - Unfamiliarity and limited availability
  - Electrical interference.

SOMATOSENSORY EVOKED RESPONSES

- *Indications:*
  - Spine surgery
  - Posterior fossa surgery
  - *Detect intraoperative complications:* Loss of signals due to positioning, hypoxia, hypotension, and hypothermia.
  - *Determining the adequacy of perfusion:* Carotid endarterectomy, aortic surgery, and spines surgery.
- *Technique:*
  - SSEP helps monitor the spinal pathways from arms and legs, which are sufficiently long and superficial to stimulate with subcutaneous electrodes (**Fig. 1**). The resulting EEG signals with SSEP signals are in the 10-µV range, while background EEG signals are in the 10–100-µV range. The SSEP response is extracted from the background EEG activity by stimulating the nerve 100–250 times at 2–5 Hz. The cortical response is aggregated such that background EEG noise is eliminated. The SSEP signal is assessed for amplitude and latency. A significant change is a 50% decrease in amplitude and a 10% increase in latency (**Fig. 2**).
  - *SSEP tracings:* SSEP data appears as a series of positive (P) and negative (N) waves at specific time points (designated by the number of milliseconds elapsed after stimulation). For example, P20 is a positive wave 20 milliseconds after stimulation.
  - The most common sites of stimulation for SSEP are C5-6 (median nerve), C8-T1 (ulnar nerve), L4-S3 (tibial nerve), and L4 S2 (common peroneal nerve).
  - *Pathway:* Fibers ascend in the posterior column (proprioception and vibration sensations). First synapse at the cervical level: For the upper extremity, it is the nucleus cuneatus, while for the lower extremity, it is the nucleus gracilis. Crossover to the contralateral side: The second synapse is at the ventroposterolateral nucleus of the thalamus. The third-order neurons then project into the cortex,

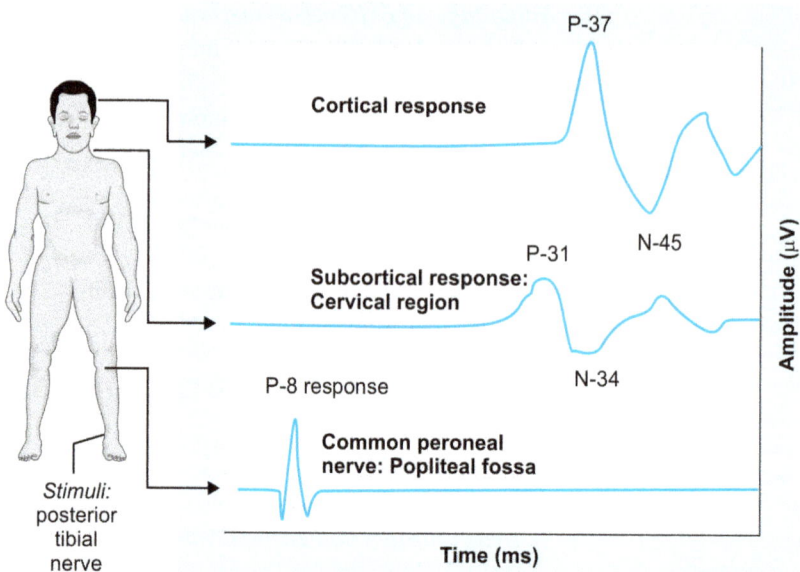

Fig. 1: Example of somatosensory response recorded after stimulating the posterior tibial nerve. The response shown here is designated as P-8, P-31, or P-37 for the positive waves. N-34 and N-35 negative waves follow the latter two. The numbers designate the time lapse in ms after the stimuli.

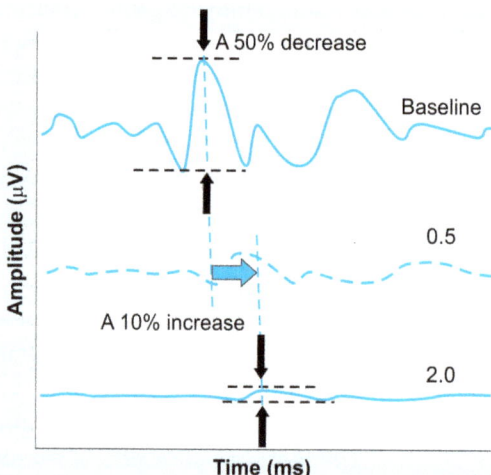

Fig. 2: : The effect of increasing end-tidal anesthetic concentrations on somatosensory evoked potentials on the response's amplitude and latency. During monitoring, a 50% decrease in amplitudes or a 10% increase in latency is considered significant

and the lower limb is projected into the interhemispheric sulcus (anterior cerebral artery irrigation). In contrast, the upper limb is projected into the parietal cortex and is easier to monitor (middle cerebral artery irrigation).

- *Effects of anesthetic drugs:*
  - *Intravenous drugs:*
    - Propofol/opioid intravenous anesthesia is usually combined during electrophysiological monitoring. However, propofol decreases amplitude and increases the latency of SSEPs.
    - *Dexmedetomidine:* It offers the benefits of sedation, anxiolysis, analgesia, and less respiratory depressant effects. Dexmedetomidine is a safe supplement to propofol/opioid or volatile agent/opioid anesthesia because it minimally interferes with SSEP monitoring. It has been combined with ketamine to provide an alternative to propofol/narcotic-based TIVA.
    - *Etomidate:* Etomidate can increase cortical amplitudes; however, prolonged etomidate infusion can lead to adrenal suppression due to the suppression of 11-beta-hydroxylase, a key enzyme in steroid synthesis.
- Volatile agents suppress evoked responses in a dose-dependent manner. However, 0.5 MAC can be tolerated. Low (0.25 MAC) MAC anesthesia can prevent recall or decrease excessive propofol requirements. Any use of volatile agents has to be in consultation with the electrophysiologists, who should be notified regarding any change in inhaled concentrations during use.
  - Muscle relaxants in sub-paralytic doses can improve SSEP recordings by decreasing movement artifacts.

BRAINSTEM AUDITORY EVOKED RESPONSES

- *Indication:*
  - VIII cranial nerve monitoring for posterior fossa tumor surgery
  - Monitoring brainstem functions, e.g., V and IX CN microvascular decompression.
- *BAER Technique:*
  - One to two thousand auditory clicks are delivered at 1–4 kHz by earphones to elicit the BAER response.
  - Hearing from both ears is integrated in the pons; therefore, BAER might be helpful even with unilateral disease.
  - Brainstem auditory evoked responses (BAER) typically have eight peaks: Of these peaks, I–V are resistant to anesthetic effects and are most consistently monitored **(Table 2)**.
- *Effect of anesthetic drugs:*
  - BAER is relatively resistant to anesthetic drugs.
  - Peaks I–V are immune to the effects of anesthetic drugs **(Fig. 3)**
  - Nitrous oxide can increase the middle air pressure, decrease hearing, and impede BAER monitoring.

Table 2: Peaks observed during brainstem auditory evoked responses.

Peak	Anatomical location	Clinical significance
I	Cochlear nerve	Ipsilateral component/resistant to anesthetics
II	Cochlear nucleus	
III	Superior olivary complex	Bilateral component/resistant to anesthetics
IV	Lateral lemniscus	
V	Inferior colliculus	
VI	Medial geniculate nucleus	Low-amplitude waves/affected by anesthetics
VII	Thalamocortical projections	
VIII	Cortex	

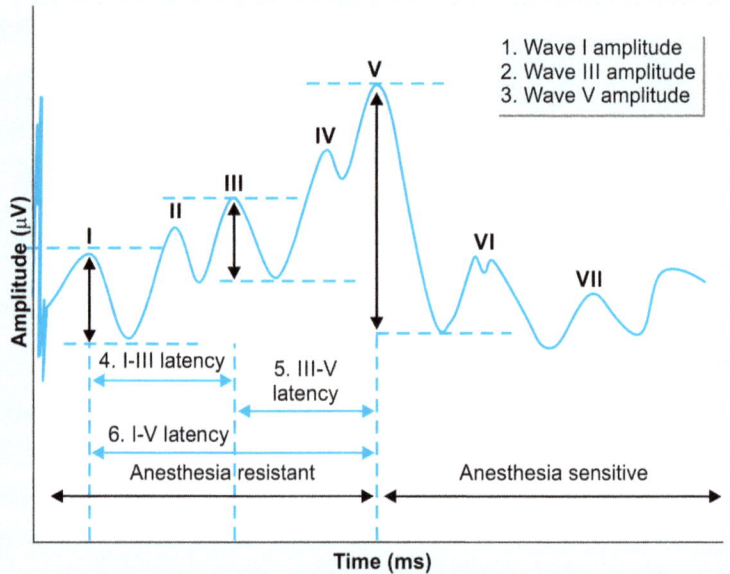

Fig. 3: Six parameters (1-6) monitored during brainstem auditory evoked responses.

VISUAL EVOKED RESPONSES

- *Indications:*
  - Extrasellar pituitary surgery
  - Injury to chiasma
- *Technique:*
  - The altering checkerboard elicits the best response.
  - Flashing LED lights can be used during surgery.
  - With increasing cycle frequencies, the waves become attenuated, and the response becomes sinusoidal with limited clinical application **(Fig. 4)** lower trace.

CHAPTER 12 Electrophysiological Monitoring

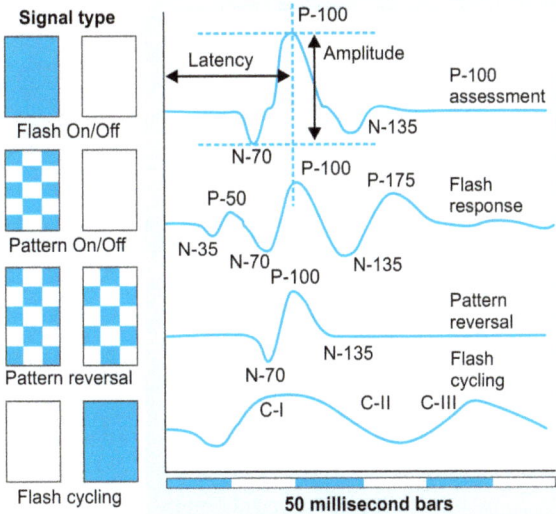

Fig. 4: Visual evoked responses depend on the type of signal and cycling frequency. Primary assessment is by the amplitude and latency of the N 100 or C2 wave.

- The primary signal monitored with flashing lights is N70 (negative signal at 70 milliseconds) and P100 (positive wave at 100 milliseconds).
- The latency and amplitude of these signals **(Fig. 4)** are tracked and compared to the other side
    - *Factors affecting amplitude:*
        - Nerve compression (pituitary tumors/surgery)
        - Optic atrophy
        - Toxic nerve injury
        - Amblyopia
    - *Factors affecting latency:*
        - Aging
        - Glaucoma
        - Demyelinating diseases
    - *Both:*
        - Refractive errors
- *Limitations:*
    - Technical execution becomes difficult during surgery.
    - Highly susceptible to anesthetic drugs.

MOTOR EVOKED RESPONSES

- *Indications:*
    - Spinal instrumentation
    - Intramedullary spine surgery
    - Tumors on the motor cortex

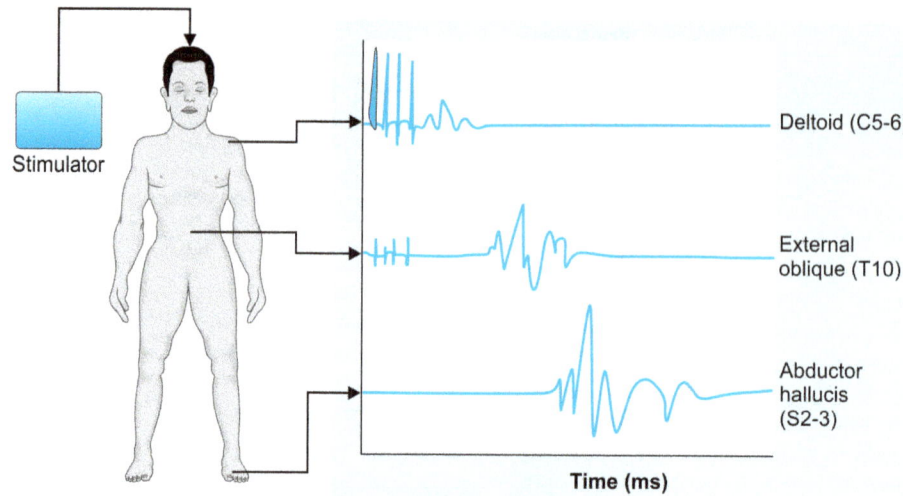

Fig. 5: Transcranial motor evoked responses.

- Carotid surgery
- Possibility of direct or indirect (vascular) brainstem injury
- Aortic surgery.
- *Technique:*
  - *Anatomy:* From the motor cortex, the motor pathways descend through the internal capsule to cross over at the pyramid to the lateral corticospinal tracts. The uncrossed fibers descend in the anterior spinothalamic tracts to cross over at the segmental level. The fibers converging on the anterior horn cell supply the motor nerve **(Fig. 5)**.
  - *Stimulation method:* Transcranial motor cortex stimulation can be done electrically or by magnetic stimulation. Magnetic stimulation is not practical in the operating room.
  - *Cortical stimulating electrode:* Skin-penetrating corkscrew or surface electrodes are placed across the mid-line over the motor cortex. Since the lower limb regions are close to the mid-line chest, arm in the middle, and face and tongue laterally, it is easy to stimulate the lower limb. The stimulating electrodes must be placed more laterally to stimulate the upper limb. Lateral stimulation can lead to masseter contractions and greater chances of tongue bite and jaw pain.
  - *Electrical stimulation parameters:* Stimulation consists of 5–10 impulses of 100–400 V with a maximum of 1,000 V. The stimulation involves a group of pulses, typically with three stimuli per train and 3–4 trains per stimulatory sequence. The stimulus pattern is typical of assessing distal MEPs, but if the D waves are monitored, then single stimuli may suffice.

CHAPTER 12 Electrophysiological Monitoring

Table 3: Commonly monitored muscles and their roots.

Muscles monitored	Nerve root
Trapezoid and sternocleidomastoid	C2–4
Biceps and deltoid	C5–6
Flexor carpi radialis	C6–7
Adductor pollicis brevis and abductor digiti minimi	C8–T1
Rectus abdominis:	
– Subcostal	T5–6
– Upper	T7–8
– Middle	T9–10
– Lower segments	T11–12
Adductor longus	L2
Vastus medialis	L2–4
Tibialis anterior	L4–S1
Peroneus longus	L5–S1
Gastrocnemius	S1–S2
Abductor hallucis	S1–3
Anal sphincter	S2–S4

- *Response patterns:*
    - The muscles commonly monitored during motor-evoked response testing are listed in **Table 3**.
    - *Stimulation artifacts:* Stimulation can result in electrical and motor artifacts that limit observation.
    - *D waves:* D waves are due to the direct activation of the pyramidal cells of the corticospinal tracts. They require the placement of subdural or epidural electrodes. They have consistent discrete peaks that are easy to interpret. They are resistant to anesthetic drugs. Multiple stimuli are not required for monitoring D waves.
    - *I wave:* I waves are due to indirect activation of the interneurons and have multiple equally spaced peaks. Anesthetic drugs abolish them.
    - *M waves:* M waves are due to compound muscle action potentials. These are complex waves, and a burst of stimuli is needed to assess the response.
- *Assessing MEPs:* The amplitude of MEP response is usually evaluated, and a 50% reduction is considered significant enough to alert the surgeons. If the motor response decreases, the surgeons can be alerted with incremental changes such as at 60, 70, 80, and 90% decrease until there is no response.
    - *Actionable threshold changes during MEP testing:*
        - Decrease in amplitude by 50%
        - Motor response lost.
        - A unilateral decrease
        - Increase voltage requirement for stimulation if greater than 100 V.

Complementary nature of MEPs and SSEPs:
- MEPs are more sensitive to the effects of anesthetic drugs compared to SSEPs. If a change is noticed during surgery, their combined use could help assess the role of anesthetic agents.
- MEPs depend on anterior spinal horn cells. The anterior spinal artery perfuses this region of the cord. Segmental branches supplement the anterior spinal artery at different levels. These vary in size; therefore, MEPs are vulnerable to ischemia. While the SSEPs monitor the posterior portions of the cord, thereby complementing the MEPs.
- MEPs are more useful in monitoring extramedullary tumors, while SSEPs are more useful for intramedullary tumors.

Complications of motor-evoked response monitoring:
- Avoiding muscle relaxants requires a deeper level of anesthesia.
- Due to lack of paralysis, the patient can cough or buck during positioning.
- Gross movement can interfere with surgery that may require some degree of muscle paralysis.
- Temporalis muscle contractions:
  - Tongue injury:
    - Jaw fracture
    - Endotracheal tube puncture
- Seizures have been reported in the past, but a history of seizures is not a contraindication for MEP monitoring.
- *Effect of anesthesia on MEPs:*
  - Similar but more sensitive than SSEPs,
  - Avoid volatile agents.
  - Intravenous agents are safe, but high doses can inhibit the motor response.
  - TIVA with propofol/dexmedetomidine and narcotics optimum
  - Ketamine can enhance MEPs.

CONSIDERATIONS IN PEDIATRICS EVOKED POTENTIAL MONITORING

- Brain development is ongoing at birth; myelination is not complete until three years.
- *EEG:* Pediatric EEG shows age-related changes in dominant waves:
  - *<3 months:* 3-4 Hz
  - *6 months:* 5 Hz
  - *24 months:* 8 Hz
  - *9 years:* 9 Hz
  - *12 years:* 10 Hz
  - *11-15 years:* Adult EEG

CHAPTER 12 Electrophysiological Monitoring

- EMG is difficult due to subcutaneous fat and immature NM junction.
- *SSEP:* Due to ongoing myelination SSEPs, amplitudes increase, and latency decreases <4 years. Cortical signals are weak, and ketamine could help augment SSEPs.
- *MEPs:* They are difficult as cortical tracts are immature, nerve myelination is incomplete, neuromuscular junctions are immature, and muscle mass is relatively small. Landmarks are also smaller to target. Ketamine could help improve signal quality.

FURTHER READING

1. Charalampidis A et al. The Use of Intraoperative Neurophysiological Monitoring in Spine Surgery. Global Spine J. 2020;10(1 Suppl):104S-114S.
2. Halsey MF et al. Neurophysiological monitoring of spinal cord function during spinal deformity surgery: 2020 SRS neuromonitoring information statement. Spine Deform. 2020;8(4):591-96.
3. Kondo T et al. Intraoperative responses of motor evoked potentials to the novel intravenous anesthetic remimazolam during spine surgery: a report of two cases. JA Clin Rep. 2020;6(1):97.
4. Perera et al. A pilot study to determine whether visually evoked hemodynamic responses are preserved in children during inhalational anesthesia. Paediatr Anaesth. 2015;25(3):317-26.
5. Shields CB et al. BAER suppression during posterior fossa dural opening. Surg Neurol Int. 2015;6:57.

Vignette: The Gruesome Roots of Electrophysiology during the French Revolution

The use of the guillotine for capital punishment was made famous during the Reign of Terror that followed the French Revolution. Guillotine-like devices were used in Europe. At that time, the heads were placed on pikes in public places. It was a method for the royals to show their power over the subjects. The guillotine was invented by a French freemason and physician named Joseph-Ignace Guillotin. It was designed for swift, humane capital punishment. What is startling is that after beheadings, the heads would be collected. Close to the guillotine were physicians, and certainly quacks, who experimented with the severed heads. It was observed that the decapitated heads could respond to verbal commands for a few minutes after being severed. A laboratory was close to the execution site for experiments on fresh corpses using electricity generated by a large phosphorus wheel. Fresh corpses were transported to the lab, and motor responses were elicited by applying current. These macabre experiments with "galvanism" partly inspired Mary Shelley's novel, "Frankenstein," first published anonymously in 1818.

Chapter 13: Neurological Monitoring and Imaging

INTRODUCTION

This chapter describes monitoring devices and imaging techniques used during neurosurgery and critical care. These techniques help improve patient care by localizing and characterizing the pathology and assessing its functional impact. Electrophysiological monitoring is not included in this chapter.

BRAIN TISSUE OXYGEN TENSION MONITORING

- Implantable oxygen electrodes can continuously monitor the partial pressure of oxygen in the brain tissue.
- *The oxygen cascade:* The partial pressure of oxygen gradually decreases from the atmosphere to the mitochondria, as shown in **Figure 1**. Mitochondria require 2 mm Hg corresponding to the brain tissue partial pressure of oxygen of 15–20 mm Hg.
- *Brain tissue oxygen monitoring:*
  - The technique involves the placement of either a fiberoptic O_2 sensor or a small Clark electrode.

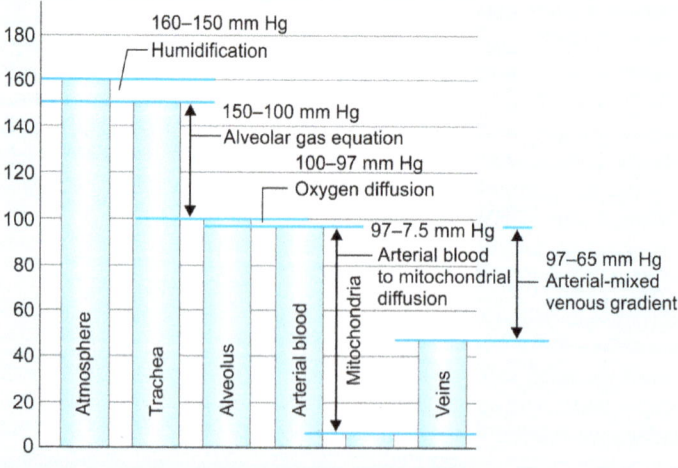

Fig. 1: The oxygen cascade showing gradient in the partial pressure of oxygen (mm Hg) from the atmosphere to the mitochondria.

CHAPTER 13 Neurological Monitoring and Imaging

- The technique can detect changes in tissue oxygenation, but it is tissue invasive
- Therefore, it carries risks of bleeding and infection
- The hypoxic threshold is 20 mm Hg.
- Low tissue PtO_2 can be due to the following:
  - *Decreased O_2 availability:* Systemic hypoxia, hypotension, or raised intracranial pressure (ICP)
  - *Increased O_2 demand:* Hyperthermia and seizures.
- The partial pressure of oxygen values in the brain tissue are:
  - *Normal:* 25–35 mm Hg
  - *Hypoxia:* 20 mm Hg and treatment threshold
  - *Moderate hypoxia:* 15 mm Hg
  - *Severe hypoxia:* 10 mm Hg
  - *Injury:* 5 mm Hg.

TRANSCRANIAL DOPPLER ULTRASOUND

Transcranial Doppler (TCD): The Doppler technique relies on the frequency change in the reflected ultrasonic sound wave after contact with moving particles (such as the red blood cells) that can be used to determine the blood flow velocity.

- *Indications:*
  - Assessment of cerebral blood flow (CBF)
  - Assessment of autoregulation
  - Detection of cerebral vasospasm
  - Detection of emboli
  - Stenosis
  - Detection of brain death.
- *Technique:*
  - Piezoelectric crystals are used to generate and sense ultrasonic waves
  - 2–18 MHz ultrasound waves are generally used for medical applications. Typically, 2 MHz is used for TCD purposes.
  - Higher frequencies improve resolution but limit penetration
  - *Types:*
    - Velocity measurements based on phase shift (**Fig. 2**)

$$V = \frac{C \times F_{(d)}}{2 \times F_{(t)} \cos\theta}$$

  - Here, V is the flow velocity, C is the velocity of the ultrasonic wave in the tissue, $F_{(d)}$ is the shift in the Doppler frequency, and $F_{(t)}$ is the transducer frequency. $\emptyset$ is the angle of insonation to the direction of blood flow:
    - *B mode* for cross-sectional scans. Duplex scans are cross-sectional scans with velocity measurements
    - *M (Motion) mode* multiple velocities from a range of depths.

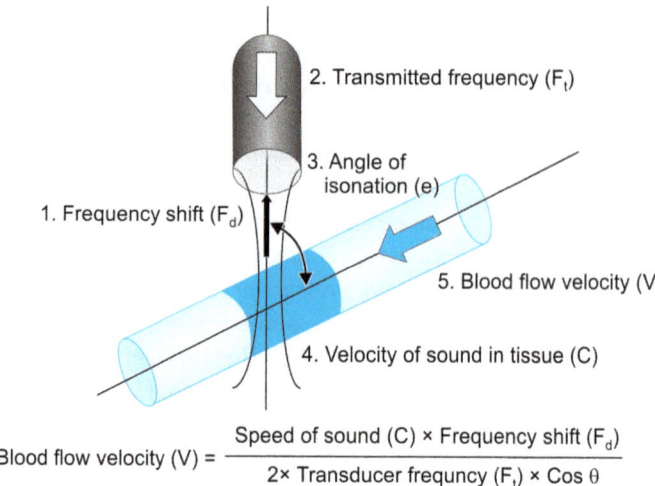

$$\text{Blood flow velocity (V)} = \frac{\text{Speed of sound (C)} \times \text{Frequency shift (F}_d)}{2\times \text{Transducer frequncy (F}_t) \times \cos \theta}$$

Fig. 2: Measurement of blood flow velocity with Doppler ultrasound.

- *Pros and cons of TCD:*
  - *Pros:*
    - Noninvasive
    - Safe
    - Relatively simple
    - Real-time measurement of flow velocity.
  - *Cons:*
    - Measures flow velocity, not absolute flow
    - If used for CBF assessment, the diameter of the vessel is assumed to be constant.
    - Insonation of intracranial arteries is not always possible due to the lack of sonication windows.

JUGULAR VENOUS (JV) OXIMETRY

- *Indications:*
  - *Traumatic Brain Injury:* Detection of ischemia and optimization of ventilation and resuscitation.
  - Cerebral vasospasm after subarachnoid hemorrhage
  - Intraoperative monitoring of cerebral perfusion during cardiac and neurosurgery, e.g., to determine the need for hyperventilation
- *Technique:*
  - *Anatomy:*
    - The jugular bulb is the dilation of the vein as it emerges from the skull.
    - Two-thirds of the blood is from the ipsilateral, and one-third is from the contralateral hemisphere
    - Furthermore, subcortical areas drain on the left and the cortical regions on the right.

- *Physiology:* CMRO$_2$ = CBF × (CaO$_2$ − CjvO$_2$)
  Where CMRO$_2$ is the cerebral metabolic rate for oxygen; CaO$_2$ is the oxygen content of the arterial blood; and CjvO$_2$ is the oxygen content of the jugular venous blood.
  - Normal JV blood oxygen saturation = 55–75%
  - Corresponds to arterial-to-JV blood oxygen content difference of 4–8 ml/dL.
  - *Technique:* Requires retrograde placement of oximetric catheter under fluoroscopic control **(Fig. 3)**.
- *Normal values:*
  - *Hb saturation values for JV blood:*
    - Ischemia: <40%
    - Hypoperfusion <50%
    - Normal range: 55–75%
    - Hyperemia: >75%
  - Difference between the oxygen content of arterial and JV blood—(A-JV) DO$_2$ thresholds:
    - Low flow >7.5%
    - Normal range: 5–7.5%
    - Hyperemia <5%.
- *Interpretation:* The facial vein drains into the JV, and facial blood can contaminate the jugular venous return. Before the interpretation of the data, the position of the catheter needs to be verified:
  - *Increased CJVO$_2$:*
    - *Increased blood flow:* Hyperemia with IA vasodilators, excessive CO$_2$, and AV shunts

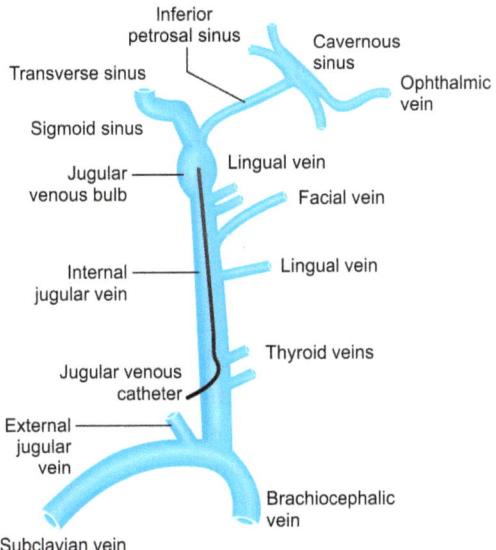

Fig. 3: Placement of oximetry catheter in the jugular bulb.

- *Decreased brain metabolism:* Excessive sedation, hypothermia, and brain death.
- *Decreased CJVO$_2$:*
  - *Decreased CaO$_2$:* Inadequate ventilation, decreased cardiac output.
  - *Decreased cerebral blood flow:* Hyperventilation, inadequate resuscitation, and vasospasm
  - Increased ICP
  - *Increased metabolic demand:* Hyperthermia, seizures, shivering, pain, and anxiety.
- *Contraindication:*
  - Local surgery or trauma
  - Pre-existing ante-grade catheter
  - Thrombosis
  - Coagulopathy
- *Complications:*
  - Placement injuries
  - Jugular venous thrombosis
  - Hematoma
  - Carotid injury
  - Infection

INTRACRANIAL PRESSURE MONITORING

- *Indication for ICP monitoring:*
  - Severe head injury with GCS of ≤8 with an abnormal CT scan
  - Severe head injury but with normal CT scan and a combination of two of the following three:
    - Age >40 years
    - Hypotension (SBP <90 mm Hg)
    - Decerebrate/decorticate positioning
  - Impaired consciousness with comorbidities such as:
    - Stroke
    - Vasospasm
    - Metabolic disorders like:
      - Diabetic ketoacidosis
      - Fulminant liver failure.
  - Postoperative management of patients after removal of a sizeable intracranial mass.
- *Contraindications to ICP monitoring:* Coagulopathy.
- *Technique:* The most accurate, commonly used, and cost-effective method of monitoring the ICP is through a ventricular drain.

CHAPTER 13 Neurological Monitoring and Imaging

Table 1: Intracranial pressure (ICP) monitoring methods.

Technique	Advantages	Disadvantages
Intraventricular catheter	• Gold standard • Most commonly used • Permits draining of CSF • It can be easily be calibrated	• Tissue invasive • Risk of bleeding and infection • Insertion is difficult when ventricles are collapsed • Overdrainage and blockage are possible
Intraparenchymal probe	Simpler placement	• Measures tissue pressure • Drifts overtime
Subdural bolt	• Easy placement • Brain tissue noninvasive • Low complication rate	• Blockage frequent • High failure rate • Limited accuracy
Subdural catheter	Brain tissue noninvasive	• Blockage frequent • High failure rate • Limited accuracy and overestimates
Epidural bolt	• Easy insertion • Low complication rate	Limited accuracy
Lumbar puncture	• Technically easy • Extracranial location	• Postural dependency makes it unsuitable for monitoring • It can lead to brain herniation • Infection and over-drainage are possible
Tympanic membrane displacement	Noninvasive	Approximation of ICP
TCD PI index	Noninvasive assessment of blood flow	Indirect inferential assessment

(TCD PI: transcranial Doppler pulsatility index)

Alternately, subdural catheters, epidural and subarachnoid bolts, and intraparenchymal pressure sensors can measure ICP **(Table 1)**. In infants, where the fontanelles are open, fontanometry is possible.

- *Direct methods:*
  - *The intraventricular catheter* is the gold standard for ICP monitoring:
    - Ventricular drain permits the cerebral spinal fluid (CSF) to drain when needed. For transducing purposes, the drain has to be zeroed at the external auditory meatus or the base of the skull
    - *The problems with the drain include:* Difficulty in placement if the ventricles are compressed, displacement of the drain requiring surgical repositioning, and infection.
    - *Intraparenchymal:* Using a pressure sensor on a wire tip or a fiber-optic cable
    - *Subarachnoid:* Bolt tip placed 1 mm below the dura from where the pressure is directly transduced.
    - *Subdural catheter* unreliable overestimates.
- *Indirect methods:*
  - Transcranial Doppler pulsatility index

- Optic nerve sheath diameter by ultrasound
- Tympanic membrane displacement.

Intracranial Pressure Values

- *Infants:* 3-7 mm Hg
- *In children and adults:* >10 and <15 mm Hg.
- *An increase in children and adults is a value* >20-25 mm Hg.
- *Risk of injury, an ICP* >40 mm Hg.

Clinical Signs of Raised Intracranial Pressure (Table 2)

- Headache, vertigo, restlessness, perceived roaring, excitement, delirium, or unnatural sleep.
- *Stage 1:* ↑BP, ↓HR, respiratory irregularity (Cushing's triad), and rhythmic pupillary dilation.
- *Stage 2:* ↓BP, ↓, or an irregular HR, coma, pupillary dilation, and loss of muscle tone.
- *Stage 3:* Cardiorespiratory arrest.

Dynamic Assessment of Intracranial Pressure

- *Volume-pressure response:* Increase in ICP with 1 mL increase in volume (**Fig. 4**).
- *Pressure-volume index* is calculated from the formula.

$$PVI = \frac{\delta V}{\text{Log} \frac{P_o + \delta P}{P_o}}$$

PVI: Pressure volume index
δV: Added IC volume
δP: Increase in ICP
P_o: Baseline ICP

- On the bedside, jugular vein compression can demonstrate an increase in ICP (**Fig. 5**).

Table 2: Clinical features of increased ICP.

Range	Normal ICP	Mild increase in ICP	Moderate increase	Severe increase
ICP	<20 mm Hg	20–30 mm Hg	30–40 mm Hg	>40 mm Hg
Symptoms	Postural headache, and nausea	Persistent headache, projectile vomiting, and blurred vision	Agitation, confusion, coma, lethargy, seizures, and focal weakness	Unconsciousness, decerebrate posturing, seizures
Vital signs	Hypertension, tachycardia	Hypertension tachycardia	Hypertension tachycardia and spontaneous hyperventilation	Hypertension-bradycardia/hypotension; abnormal respirations
Ocular signs	Fundus: Normal	Fundus: Venous congestion and papilledema	Impaired pupillary response	Asymmetric pupils; tonic eye response (sunset sign)

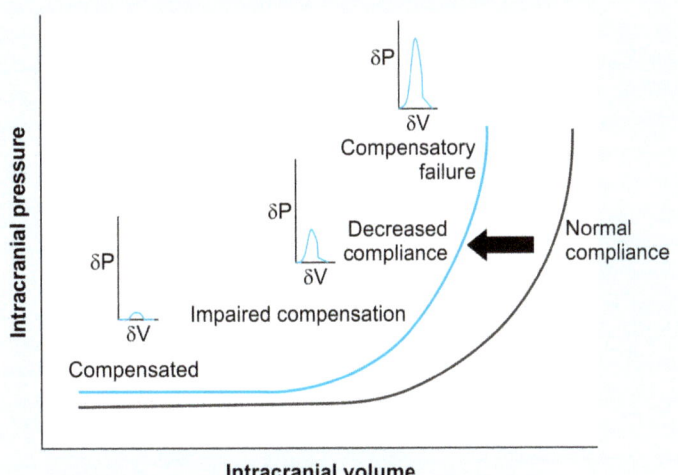

Fig. 4: Intracranial pressure-volume relationship.

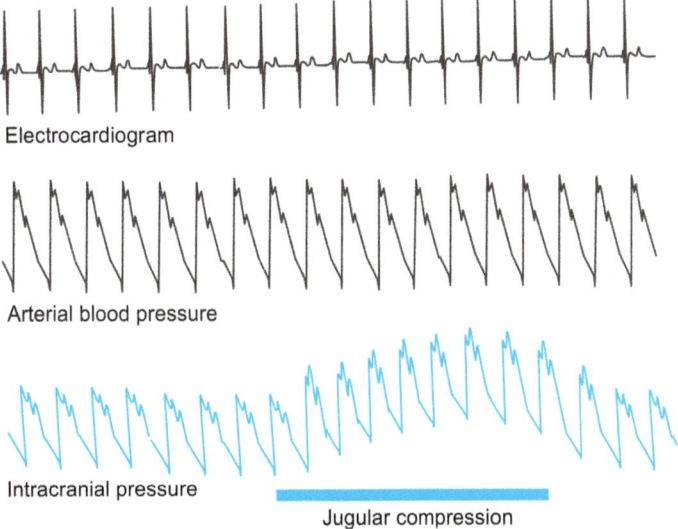

Fig. 5: Effect of jugular compression on the ICP waveform.

Intracranial compliance curve: Intracranial pressure-volume relationship is a mono-exponential curve demonstrating somewhat greater compliance when measurements are made in the lumbar region than direct intracranial measurements. Being a mono-exponential curve, the ICP rise typically occurs around 20 mm Hg.

Intracranial pressure waves generally have three components: P1 is the percussion wave, representing the initial systolic component of the arterial pulse. P2 is the tidal wave, which reflects intracranial compliance. P3 is the

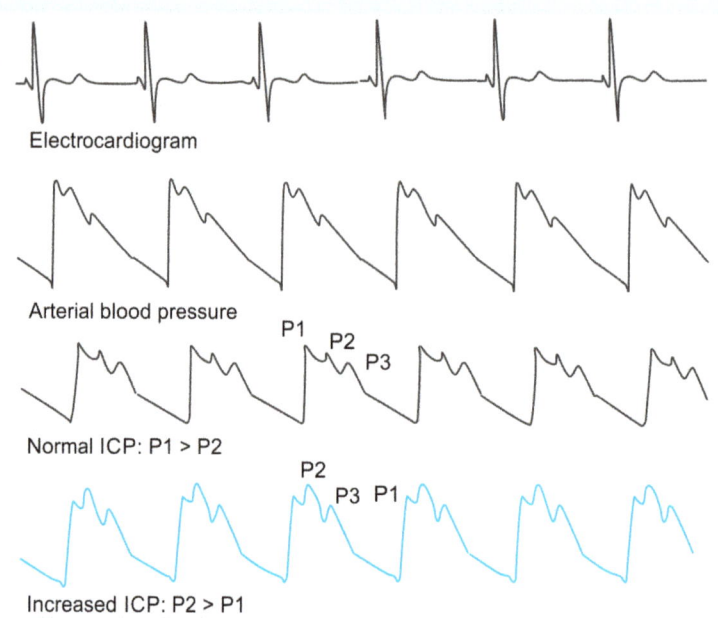

Fig. 6: Normal and increased ICP waveforms.

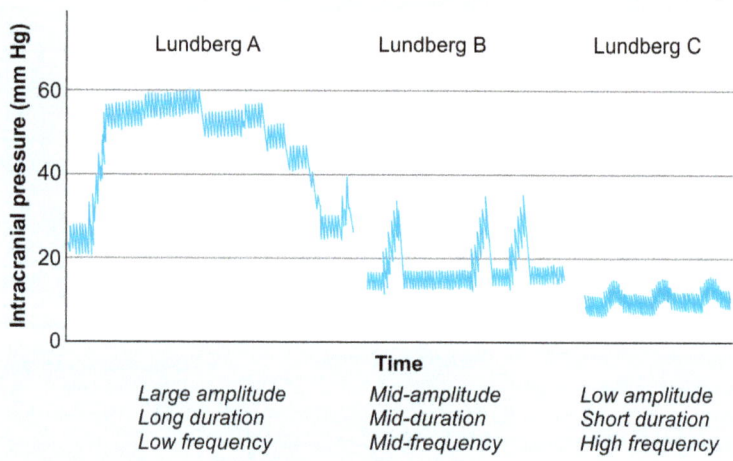

Fig. 7: Pathological ICP waves.

dicrotic wave, which flows after the aortic valve closure. Normally P1 > P2 > P3. If P2 > P1, it suggests intracranial hypertension **(Fig. 6)**.

Pathological waves (Fig. 7):
- A-waves or plateau waves are irregularly occurring, large amplitude (50–100 mm Hg) waves that last for 5–10 minutes and have a low frequency (every 5–20 minutes). They are unrelated to any hemodynamic trigger.

Clinical symptoms include headache, restlessness, incontinence, a marked decrease in consciousness, decerebration, apnea, or respiratory arrest. A-waves are suggestive of impending herniation.
- *B-waves:* Frequent waves (0.5–2 per minute) associated with a decrease in consciousness. Probably, they represent cerebral vasospasm as they are associated with increased blood flow velocity on TCD.
- *C-wave:* Traube–Herring Mayer's waves have a frequency of 4–8 per minute. These are seen in healthy individuals due to a compound effect of cardiovascular and respiratory cycles. C waves may also be imposed over the A waves in a patient with impending herniation.

COMPLICATIONS OF ICP MONITORING

- *Obstruction:* Drain blockage or kinked tubes.
- *A damped ICP wave* may require careful flushing but with herniation risk.
- *Infection is more likely with:*
  - Systemic infection
  - CSF leak at the site
  - Repeat sampling
  - Depressed fracture
  - Prolonged placement.
- Colonization is more frequent than infection, but prophylactic antibiotics and periodic exchange are not recommended.
- Hemorrhage
- Over-drainage
- Malfunction
- Displacement of catheter or sensor
- ICP monitoring may be needed for days until there is a response to treatment.

Concerns with CSF drains
- *At placement:*
  - Difficulty in localizing the ventricle due to compression/displacement.
  - Brain tissue invasive
  - Hemorrhage.
- *During use:*
  - Rapid decrease in ICP
  - Hemorrhage from an aneurysm
  - Upward herniation.
- Need to calibrate "zero" pressure with postural changes.
- Establishing the ICP waveform can take time up to 30 seconds.
- *Sampling errors:*
  - CSF samples for counts and cultures are obtained directly from the catheter and not the bag to avoid contamination.
  - Cloudy CSF indicates potential infection.

BRAIN IMAGING

Ultrasound Imaging

Due to the scattering of ultrasound waves by the skull, the applications of imaging the brain with ultrasonic devices are limited. However, ultrasonic probes can image brain tissue once the skull is removed, such as during surgery. Brain tumors are acoustically denser, while cystic lesions are lighter than brain tissue. Ultrasound imaging helps identify tumor remnants during surgery. The classical B mode ultrasonic imaging has been replaced by 3D imaging. The 3D images can also assess blood flow. They are seamlessly co-registered with preoperative MRI images. These advances expand the application of ultrasound imaging during surgery.

X-Ray Imaging

In general, soft tissue imaging is not possible by X-rays. However, the tissue distortion may be evident in contrast studies such as myelograms. Calcified lesions can also be seen on plain X-rays of the skull. However, newer approaches, such as phase contrast X-rays, are being developed for tissue imaging by X-rays.

Diffuse Optical Spectroscopy

The ability of near-infrared (NIR) light to penetrate the skull and the superficial layers of the cortex is used for cerebral oximetry. An optodes array monitors backscattered infrared light to map oxygen saturation changes in the cortex's superficial regions. However, this method cannot assess the deeper regions of the brain and its undersurface. Using time-of-flight measurements, one can undertake the mapping of cortical functions. Diffuse NIR spectroscopy can be used to detect subdural hematomas.

CT Scan

Computed tomography scans integrate data from several two-dimensional images acquired around a central axis of rotation into a combined 3D data set that can produce cross-sectional images. The anatomical resolution of the images can be further enhanced by contrast injection.

Non-contrast CT: In this method, no preparation is necessary. It can diagnose gross bony and soft tissue abnormalities, edema, and hemorrhages as they have different relative CT intensities.

Relative CT intensities: Air (–1000 HU), fat (–40 HU), water (0 HU), CSF (5 HU), edema (10 HU), thecal sac (20 HU), white matter (30 HU), gray matter (40 HU), disk (60 HU), a blood clot (80 HU), calcified vessels (100 HU), bone (500 HU), and dense bone (1000 HU). Calcium >>> water > fat.

Contrast-enhanced CT: Contrast can be given orally or by IV as needed for imaging. Contrast-enhanced CT is not accurate near clots, or imaging ends on vessels.

CHAPTER 13 Neurological Monitoring and Imaging

CT perfusion scan: Regions of interest (ROIs) identified, 5 mL/s contrast IV for 8s, images q 2s for 1 minute. Parameters calculated: Time to peak, cerebral blood volume, mean transit time, and cerebral blood flow (CBV/MTT). Perfusion CT scans are better than perfusion-weighted MRIs as they scan the whole brain and have fewer artifacts.

Acetazolamide perfusion scan: Baseline scan with IV contrast (5 mL/s, for 8 seconds) with ACZ 1000 mg IV and contrast scans q 15 minutes. Additional to the CT perfusion scan: Cerebral vascular reserve (ability to increase blood flow) and redistribution of regional blood flow due to cerebral steal.

MRI Scans

Atomic nuclei, mostly protons in water and fat molecules, orient themselves along the field of the powerful MRI magnet, but their magnetic signals cannot be detected. However, when a radiofrequency pulse is applied, the protons realign themselves away from the magnet's field. When the radiofrequency pulse is turned off, the protons realign with the magnet's field at varying rates. The process of proton realignment generates detectable magnetic signals that are used to create MR images.

Types of MRI Scans

MRI imaging protocols have been optimized for specific applications:
- *T1-weighted scan:* CSF = dark; fat = white; bone= dark.
- *T2-weighted scan:* Edema = white; fat = dark; bone = dark (To remember: H_2O on T2 is bright two)
- Spin echo MRI for demyelinating diseases
- Fluid-attenuated inversion recovery (FLAIR: *SAH and infracted brain imaging*).
- Echo train (Reduced scan time)
- Gradient echo (Imaging blood)
- Short Tau Inversion Recovery (STIR, spine imaging).
- Magnetic resonance angiography (MRA) with gadolinium contrast for aneurysm screening.
- *Diffusion-weighted imaging:* Detects ischemia and abscesses.
- *Perfusion-weighted scans:* Detects ischemia, technically challenging.

Magnetic resonance spectroscopy (MRS): MRS permits the determination of the concentration of certain chemicals in ppm. The technique helps diagnose tumors by differentiating them from infection, infarction, and pseudoprogression. In contrast to the normal brain:
- *Brain tumors* have increased lactate, lipid, and choline. Choline concentrations decrease with an infarction. Tumors also have decreased N- acetyl aspartate (NAA).

- *Infarction:* Low choline; however, lactate is increased for several months after stroke.
- *Abscess:* Decreased NAA and choline; increased succinate and acetate (atypical).
- *Multiple sclerosis:* Attenuated concentrations of most chemicals but with increased lactate and lipids.

MRI Contrast: Gadolinium-based. Problems with MRI contrast:
- Allergic reactions 1:200
  - Preventive steroid regime similar to iodinated contrast agents
- Nephrotoxicity
- Contraindicated in pregnancy.

Contraindication to MRI:
- Ferromagnetic implants can move and/or heat up: The manufacturer can verify the compatibility of a metallic object with MRI.
  - Certain but not all aneurysm clips
  - Pacemakers, stimulators, infusion pumps, and cochlear implants
  - Metal fragments
  - Stents, coils, and filters
  - Swan–Ganz catheters
  - Shunts with programmable valves.
- Very sick patients
- Morbidly obese patients
- Claustrophobic patients
- Pregnant patients:
  - MRI best avoided throughout—Fetal effects unknown
  - Contrast contraindicated in the first trimester.

Positron Emission Tomography

Positron emission tomography (PET) imaging uses positron-emitting radiotracers such as Fluorine-18 with a very short half-life; in the case of F-18, it is about 110 minutes. The radio-tracers are incorporated into molecules (radio ligands) to locate specific molecules or track metabolic processes. Most oncological and neurological PET imaging involves F-18 glucose. Once the radio ligand is intravenously injected, it redistributes. During the decay process, the isotope releases a positron and an electron. The emitted positron travels a short distance, usually 1 mm, before interacting with an electron. The interaction generates two opposite gamma rays. The gamma rays are located in 3D space and mapped on a CT scan, or an X-ray image acquired simultaneously. The applications of PET include:
- Detection of metastasis
- Tracking glucose and oxygen consumption

- Assessing cerebral blood flow and metabolism.
- Pharmacokinetic research and detecting pathological markers.

Single-photon Emission Computed Tomography

The single-photon emission computed tomography (SPECT) camera uses gamma emitters to image the uptake of molecules. Like the CT scan, multiple images are acquired and integrated. This imaging is unlike PET, where the isotope is a positron emitter and must be produced on-site before use. PET is an expensive process compared to SPECT. Technetium-99 SPECT imaging is used for imaging the brain, myocardial perfusion scans, bone scans, parathyroid scans, tumor, and neutrophil scans for infections.

FURTHER READING

1. Bonatti G et al. Neuromonitoring during general anesthesia in non-neurologic surgery. Best Pract Res Clin Anaesthesiol. 2021;35(2):255-66.
2. Hunfeld M et al. A Systematic Review of Neuromonitoring Modalities in Children Beyond Neonatal Period After Cardiac Arrest. Pediatr Crit Care Med. 2020;21(10):e927-33.
3. Millet A et al. Clinical applications of transcranial Doppler in non-trauma critically ill children: a scoping review. Childs Nerv Syst. 2021;37(9):2759-68.
4. Patchana T et al. Increased Brain Tissue Oxygen Monitoring Threshold to Improve Hospital Course in Traumatic Brain Injury Patients. Cureus. 2020; 12(2):e7115.
5. Yeung MK et al. A Systematic Review of the Application of Functional Near-Infrared Spectroscopy to the Study of Cerebral Hemodynamics in Healthy Aging. Neuropsychol Rev. 2021;31(1):139-66.

Vignette: How the Beetles Helped to Develop the Computerized Tomography Scanner

In the 1950s, Godfrey Hounsfield was a talented inventor at the Electrical and Musical Industries (EMI) in England. He built the first transistor-based computer and pioneered the idea of three-dimensional human body imaging. However, in 1962, the EMI had difficulty supporting its research. It needed around 700,000 pounds to build the scanner. The Department of Health paid EMI about £600,000. Around that time, the company signed on a young pop group, the Beetles. It was not an accident because the company was also a leader in sound-recording technologies. EMI-recording devices were groundbreaking and greatly benefited the Beetles in the success of their records. The success of the Beetles enabled EMI to balance the books for Hounsfield to continue his research. It led to the development of the first CT scanner in 1971.

Chapter 14

Positioning during Neurosurgery

INTRODUCTION

Anesthesia increases the risk of injury during positioning for surgery by annulling pain, suppressing protective reflexes, and abolishing the motor tone.

Positioning patients for neurosurgery has several underlying objectives:
- Provide adequate access to the surgical site.
- To maintain anatomical orientation
- To ensure free drainage of blood and irrigating fluids.
- To provide comfortable access to the site to reduce operator fatigue
- To provide adequate access to IV ports and monitoring interfaces
- To minimize nerve or spine injury
- To reduce the possibility of hemodynamic complications
- To be able to reposition for resuscitation if needed safely.

Safe positioning requires appropriate devices to support the patient, to have adequate staffing available to safely move the patient, to monitor potential hazards due to positioning, and to assess and follow up with the patient in the rare event of iatrogenic injury.

GENERAL POSITIONING CONCERNS

Positioning a patient requires planning and preparation before surgery.
- *Prepositioning concerns include:*
  - *Patient posture:* Severe kyphosis, scoliosis, ankylosing spondylitis, or contractures may restrict adequate movement of limbs and the spine such that the supporting devices have to be modified for a given patient. Allen frame can flex in the mid-section for patients with severe spinal deformity.
  - *Patient-specific anatomic concerns:* Patients may have pacemaker/AICD, implantable ports, and transplanted organs or colostomies that need protection during positioning.
  - *Nature of bed and supporting devices:* The nature of the operating table, the type of the frame, arm boards, suspending weight, and padding devices have to be available and checked before positioning.
  - *Type of the head fixation:* Headrest vs. pin fixation. The latter enables traction and avoids pressure on the eyes.

- *Concerns during positioning:*
  - Ensure planned, controlled, and coordinated movement of the patient.
  - Ensuring adequate depth of anesthesia.
  - Log rolling the patient.
  - Ensure cervical spine care.
  - Careful hemodynamic monitoring: In a high-risk patient, the arterial line can be placed on the side of the turn and, with due care, need not be disconnected to provide a continuous assessment of the blood pressure.
  - Place additional monitors, such as precordial Doppler, after final positioning since the heart's position might change when the patient is moved.
- *Final position concerns:*
  - Reconnecting ventilation.
  - Reconnecting monitors
  - Ensure unrestricted access to IV ports, A-line, and neuromuscular monitoring sites.
  - Check pressure points.
  - Check limb position and padding.
  - Check that the counterweights supporting the head are freely suspended.
  - Place warming blankets
  - Confer baseline electrophysiology assessment after positioning if monitored.
- *Potential complications related to surgical positionings:*
  - *Cardiovascular effects:* Hypotension, vascular graft occlusion, impaired venous drainage, air embolism.
  - *Respiratory effects:* Endotracheal tube dislodgement and endobronchial intubation
  - *Nerve injuries:* Commonest site is the ulnar nerve. Injuries can be due to compression/pressure (blood pressure cuff, tourniquet, unpadded superficial nerve), stretch (unsupported limb/overextended joints), hypotension, and preexisting neuropathy.
  - *Ocular injuries:* Direct compression of the globe, lens displacement, hypotension, emboli
  - *Pressure sores:* Direct pressure on the skin, prolonged surgery, and hypotension.

JACKSON FRAME
Pros
The Jackson Frame is a lightweight carbon fiber frame that permits the virtual suspension of the patient with minimal skin contact and improves

imaging for spine surgery. It can also enable the rotation of the subject when the anterior and posterior approaches are needed. Despite the rotation capability, the patients requiring prone surgeries are induced on a stretcher and then transferred to the table.

Cons

Jackson frame requires personnel training before use, the ability to hand over the patient safely from the delivering to the receiving team, and care in positioning and padding the pressure points. Skin breakdown has been reported with the use of the frame. Intubating patients when on Jackson table can be difficult due to restricted access. Difficulties in positioning pads and protecting pressure points are encountered while rotating the patient during surgery. Staff injuries have occurred during the positioning of the patients. The frame is now routinely used for most spine surgeries.

PIN FIXATION

- It securely positions the head and the cervical spine.
- It avoids pressure on critical structures such as the eyes.
- It provides surgical traction when needed.
- It is ideal for intraoperative X-ray imaging.
- It is essential for imaging-guided navigation devices.

Precautions

- Ensure adequate depth of anesthesia.
- The hypertensive response to pining can be mitigated by local anesthetic infiltration.
- Ensure that the weights supporting the head are freely suspended at all times.

Pros

- It provides secure positioning.
- The face and eyes remain accessible and are protected from pressure during prone spine surgery.

Cons

- Hypertensive response
- Bleeding from pin sites is frequently seen after surgery.
- Scalp lacerations and site infections
- Intracranial bleed

COMMON SURGICAL POSITIONS

Supine

- The standard supine position poses minimal hemodynamic risks or chances of nerve injury. Lumbar support by flexing the knees is desirable to avoid backache during lengthy procedures.
- A contoured (lawn chair) position with slight head elevation and flexion of the hip and the knees is preferable to the horizontal position for prolonged surgeries. It improves venous drainage and reduces the risk of hyperextension of the knees and consequent nerve injuries.
- The arms are usually supported on padded arm boards to access IV ports and arterial lines and enable neuromuscular monitoring. Arms should not be abducted beyond 90° to avoid brachial injuries. They should be secured with straps to avoid being dislodged from the board during surgery.
- Head elevation (anti-Trendelenburg) predisposes to postural hypotension and venous air embolism (VAE). During neurosurgical operations, the head may be turned laterally or flexed. Flexion of the head can result in endobronchial intubation. Extreme head positioning can impede venous return [increase bleeding and intracranial pressure (ICP)] and injure the brachial plexus.
- *Possible nerve injuries in the supine position include:*
  - Brachial plexus injuries due to pressure on nerve roots or turning away the head with the arm fixed to the table.
  - Radial nerve compression in the spiral groove posterior humerus.
  - Ulnar nerve compression behind the medial epicondyle.
  - Median nerve due to extension of the wrist.

Lateral

The lateral position is used mainly for approaching the posterior fossa and the temporoparietal tumors. Often it is briefly used for the placement of a spinal drain. The lateral position is advantageous in awake craniotomies as the tongue falls to one side to open the airway.

The main considerations are:

- To avoid any traction on the neck that could injure the brachial plexus or cervical cord.
- Use a shoulder roll under the chest but beneath the axilla to prevent brachial plexus injury.
- The author's preference is to put the arterial line in the dependent wrist and to zero the transducer at the precordium. It is easy to observe the A-line placed in the dependent radial artery. Two IV lines are usually placed, one in either arm.

- A pillow is placed between the legs so the lower leg extends and the upper flexes.
- The upper arm requires an armrest or pillow support.

Prone
- Requires transfer from the stretcher to the operating table.
  - Injuries possible to patient and staff.
  - Disconnection and reconnection of lines and monitors should be undertaken efficiently with minimal delay.
  - Hazards significantly increase for morbidly obese patients.
- Access to the patient, such as during spine surgery, may be limited.
- Requires protection of face, eyes, and ears
- Padding of nerve pressure points that are likely to be concealed under the drapes.
- *Neck flexion* can impair venous return, increase the risk of bleeding, increase the ICP, and cause tongue swelling. It can also result in endobronchial intubation.

Abdominal compression: Increases airway pressure, decreases venous return (decrease in preload can cause hypotension and increase bleeding during spine surgery), and increases the possibility of VAE because spinal veins have no valves and can entrain air during hypotension.

Special concerns:
- A transplanted kidney in the groin may be injured due to pressure.
- An intraocular prosthesis can be displaced.
- An increase in intraocular pressure could worsen glaucoma.
- Pacemakers need to be padded to prevent skin breakdown.
- Intravenous access ports on the chest need to be protected.
- Hyper-abducted arms may lead to thoracic outlet syndrome.
- Enterostomies have to be adequately padded.
- Recent coronary artery bypass vein grafts can be compressed and lead to myocardial ischemia.

Sitting Position
Due to the risk of venous air embolism, the sitting position is best avoided during neurosurgery. The main advantage of the sitting position is surgical orientation and free drainage of blood and cerebrospinal fluid (CSF) from the operating site.
- *Contraindications to sitting position:*
  - Hemodynamic instability
  - Right to left shunts.
  - Ventriculoatrial shunt

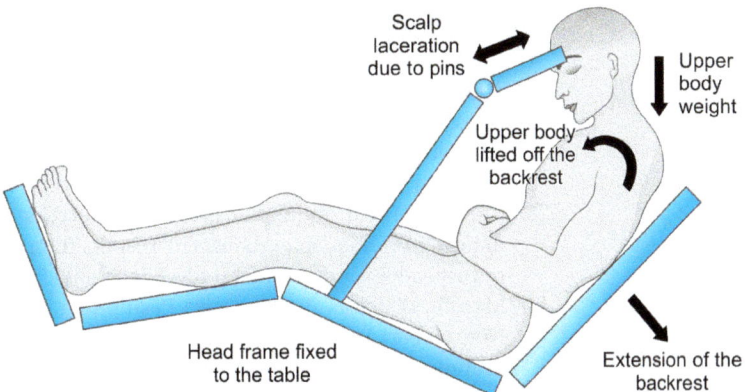

Fig. 1: Sitting position showing mechanism of injury with extension of the back.

- Cervical spondylolisthesis
- Severe atherosclerotic disease
- *Concerns with neck flexion:* At least two finger breadth between the chin and chest.
    - Endobronchial intubation.
    - Impaired venous return decreased cardiac output and hypotension.
    - Swelling of the face and tongue.
    - Mid-cervical tetraplegia can result from extreme head flexion, usually at the C5 level. It may be related to a tethered cord or preexisting spine condition, spondylosis/spondylolisthesis.
    - Brachial injury from improperly supported arms.
- *Circulatory effects:*
    - Postural hypotension
    - The transducer height is raised to ensure adequate cerebral perfusion.
    - Zero the arterial transducers at the external auditory meatus.
    - Precordial Doppler is placed for monitoring VAE after position, but access to precordium may be limited, such as in obese patients.
- Excessive CSF drainage with pneumocephalus can delay recovery.
- *Support of the arms:* Brachial plexus injury is possible if arms hang freely.
- The back of the table cannot be lowered if the head is secured to the mid-table. It is imperative to be familiar with the operating table. Otherwise, serious injury is possible if the back is lowered when the head is still fixed in pins, **(Fig. 1)**. To avoid such an injury, the head pin support is sometimes fixed to the upper portion of the table and not the mid-section.
- Patient exposed—resulting in hypothermia
- The patient may slide during surgery. Flexion of the knees and support below the ankles can minimize the risk. The downward slide can cause spinal injury with the head fixed with pins.

FURTHER READING

1. Chui J et al. Perioperative Peripheral Nerve Injury after General Anesthesia: A Qualitative Systematic Review. Anesth Analg. 2018;127(1):134-43.
2. Himes BT et al. Trelstad-Andrist K, Maloney PR, et al. Outcomes in single-level posterior cervical spine surgeries performed in the sitting and prone positions. J Neurosurg Spine. 2020;p.1-7.
3. Kurihara M et al. Estimation of the head elevation angle that causes clinically important venous air embolism in a semi-sitting position for neurosurgery: a retrospective observational study. Fukushima J Med Sci. 2020;66(2):67-72.
4. Marotta DA et al. Perioperative Positioning in Neurosurgery: A Technical Note on Park Bench Positioning for the Obese Patient Using the "Arrowhead" Technique. Cureus. 2021;13(8): e16932.
5. Sakakura K et al. Intraoperative Head Slippage with the Head Clamp System Can Occur During Epileptic Surgery. World Neurosurg. 2020;142:e453-7.

Vignette: The History of the Operating Table

Until the 19th century, most surgeries were done sitting using wooden chairs. These wooden chairs had several straps to prevent awake patients from moving and falling if rendered unconscious. Wooden surgical chairs were widely used for surgery until the 1890s. Some of the chairs could be flattened to serve as operating tables. Most operating tables, including those during the Civil War, were made of wood and had little flexibility. One of the first surgical tables that could be rotated and raised or lowered to meet surgical needs was developed in 1851 by Carl Emmert. This basic design was used for the next 150 years. Most operating tables consisted of a flat top and a central support with a base that was either fixed or on wheels. The central support and their metal construction restricted X-ray imaging on these tables. Modern carbon fiber-built Jackson frames do not have a central support or a metal plate to hold the patient; thus, they permit virtually unrestricted X-ray imaging from almost any angle.

Chapter 15: Anesthetic Neuroprotection and Neurotoxicity

INTRODUCTION

It was long held that anesthetic drugs, which suppress neuronal excitability and metabolism, can protect against neurological injury. However, evidence supporting anesthetic neuroprotection has failed to emerge from well-controlled clinical trials. In contrast, the neuroprotective effect of hypothermia in improving clinical outcomes is evident when instituted immediately before and sometimes after an ischemic event. Cases of survival after prolonged accidental hypothermia further support these clinical reports. The failure of pharmacological neuroprotection may reflect an actual failure of drugs or the insensitivity of clinical trials, given the complexity of the clinical disease.

PHARMACOLOGIC NEUROPROTECTION VS. HYPOTHERMIA

Barbiturate pre-treatment is the only example of an anesthetic drug that can provide some clinical neuroprotection. Though the evidence to support their its use remains weak. Other anesthetic drugs, including volatile agents, have failed to demonstrate neuroprotective effects in clinical trials. This is in sharp contrast to hypothermia which is beneficial before and sometimes after an ischemic event. Neuroprotective effects of hypothermia are most evident in the setting of preemptive cooling during aortic surgery and intraoperative circulatory arrest. Hypothermia is also beneficial in hypoxic neonatal injury use and to a lesser extent, in post-arrest ischemic injury in adults.

- *Clinical status of hypothermia:*
  - *Benefits established for:*
    - Prevention of neural injury due to planned intraoperative cardiac arrest or vascular occlusion, such as during aortic surgery.
    - Hypoxic/ischemic brain injury in neonates
    - The benefits during postcardiac arrest in adults are contested as they could also be due to the prevention of hyperthermia.
  - *The benefits of hypothermia are unproven in:*
    - Traumatic brain injury
    - Stroke

- *Methods of inducing hypothermia:*
  - Global cooling:
    - Cooling mattresses
    - Ice packs over large arteries
    - Pharmacological hypothermia
      - Drugs directly affect thermoregulation contrast from the use of vasodilators that are used to enhance core cooling.
        - It can cause mild to moderate hypothermia.
        - The mechanism of action is still under investigation.
      - In preclinical stages, the following classes of drugs cause hypothermia:
        - Cannabinoids
        - Narcotics
        - Neurotensin
        - Capsaicin
        - Thyroid hormone derivatives, e.g., 3-iodothyronamine
        - Adenosine and adenine derivatives
        - Gases: Xe and helium
      - *Limitations:*
        - Pharmacological side-effects
        - Poor control of hypothermia
  - Regional Cooling:
    - Local brain cooling with ice packs.
    - Intra-arterial cold saline infusion
  - Combined global and regional.
- *Factors affecting the outcome of hypothermia treatment:*
  - Indication
  - Comorbidities
  - Time lag in the initiation of treatment.
  - Rate of cooling
  - The extent of cooling (mild, moderate, or profound)
  - Rate of rewarming
  - Management of rewarming, e.g., management of shivering.
- *Cellular mechanism of neuroprotection by hypothermia:*
  - Reduction of cerebral metabolic rate by 6%/°C, or more
  - Reduction of ICP
  - Attenuation of blood-brain barrier disruption
  - Delay or interruption of the apoptotic cascade, such as caspase-9.
  - Delay in the increase of intracellular H^+ and Ca^{++} and the activation of the downstream enzymes
  - Attenuation of inflammatory response
  - Attenuated increase in free radical production
- *Neuroprotection by anesthetic drugs can be due to the following:*
  - Decreased cerebral metabolism.

- Free radical scavenging
- Decreased intracranial pressure (ICP)
- Improved cerebral perfusion.
- Flow metabolism coupling can redirect flow to ischemic areas.
- Sedation facilitates ICU care and minimizes secondary insults.
- Facilitates hypothermia—minimizes shivering.
- *Non-anesthetic neuroprotective agents:*
  - Calcium channel blockers
  - Magnesium
  - Free radical scavengers
  - Excitatory amino acid modulators
  - Trophic factors
  - Cytokine inhibitors
  - Statins
  - Erythropoietin
  - Anti-inflammatory drugs.
- *Effective neuroprotective strategies:*
  - Therapeutic hypothermia
  - Prevention of hyperpyrexia
  - Prevention of hyperglycemia
  - Preventing secondary injury:
    - Acidosis
    - Hypercalcemia
    - Hyponatremia
    - Hypomagnesemia
    - Seizures
    - Infections
- *Why has neuroprotective pharmacotherapy failed in clinical trials?*
  - Diverse mechanisms
  - Time dependency
  - The complexity of the clinical injury
  - Failure of drug delivery
  - Problems in translating animal models.
  - Problems with clinical trials.

NEUROPROTECTION IN SPECIFIC CIRCUMSTANCES

Neuroprotection in Neonates

- *Potential applications for neuroprotective interventions:*
  - Premature infants
  - To enhance brain maturation
  - Treatment of ischemic injuries
  - Excitotoxic injuries
  - Hemorrhagic injuries

- *Interventions:*
  - Avoiding prematurity
  - Antenatal steroid treatment
  - Magnesium sulfate
  - Nonsteroidal anti-inflammatory drugs
  - Delayed clamping of the cord
  - Therapeutic hypothermia
  - Avoiding hyperthermia
  - Recombinant human erythropoietin
  - *Others, preclinical:*
    - Melatonin
    - Topiramate
    - Xenon
    - Allopurinol
    - Fetal cell therapy.

Neuroprotection in Stroke

The quest to provide clinical neuroprotection for ischemic stroke with drugs in the last three decades has been frustrating. **Figure 1** shows the complexity of the problem and the futility of single-point interventions. Stroke treatment will probably require not one but several timely pharmacological interventions tailored to evolving tissue injury.

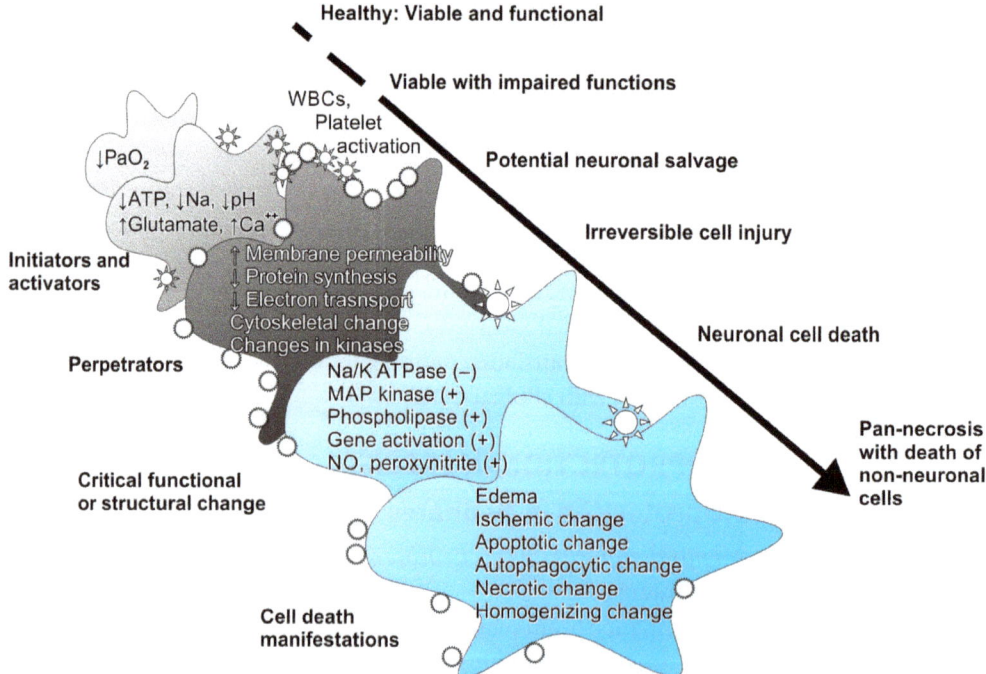

Fig. 1: Pathways of ischemic brain injury are dynamic and crosstalk with each other. Interrupting a single pathway is unlikely to improve clinical outcomes, nor could it be judged reliably by a single time-point assessment.

- *Potential neuroprotection targets:*
  - Oxidative stress
  - Excitotoxicity
  - Inflammation
  - Prevent blood-brain barrier disruption.
  - Apoptosis
  - Autophagy.
- *Potential interventions with examples:* The benefits of pharmacological interventions remain unproven in clinical stroke trials. It is possible that the beneficial effects of these drugs, often in experimental models, only are being overlooked due to the inherent complexity of the clinical disease. Potential interventions for stroke include:
  - Moderate hypothermia
  - *Calcium antagonists:*
    - *Calcium channel blockers:* Nimodipine
    - *Calcium chelators:* DP-b99
  - *Free radical scavengers:* Edaravone
  - *Gamma-aminobutyric acid (GABA) antagonists:* Clomethiazole
  - *Nitric oxide antagonists:* Lubeluzole
  - *Phosphatidylcholine precursor:* CPD-choline
  - *Leukocyte adhesion inhibitors:* anti-intercellular adhesion molecule (ICAM) antibody
  - *Glutamate antagonists:*
    - *AMPA antagonist:* BIIR 561 CL
    - *N-Methyl-d-aspartate (NMDA) antagonist:*
      - Magnesium
      - Memantine
      - Remacemide
- *NMDA channel blocker:* Ketamine
- *Opiate antagonists:* Naloxone
- *Membrane stabilizer:* Piracetam.

Anesthetic Neurotoxicity

Figure 2 shows the diversity of factors that can potentially confound the assessment of the neurotoxicity of anesthetic drugs. Again, in preclinical bench studies, there is emerging evidence of the toxicity of anesthetic drugs, but similar evidence is lacking in clinical trials.
- *Laboratory studies:* Anesthetic exposure can lead to:
  - Apoptosis
  - Impaired neurogenesis
  - Impaired dendritic development
  - *In subhuman primates:*
    - 3-hour anesthetic exposure results in apoptosis
    - Repeat anesthetic exposures alter behavior and increase anxiety.
    - A 5-hour exposure can cause motor deficits.

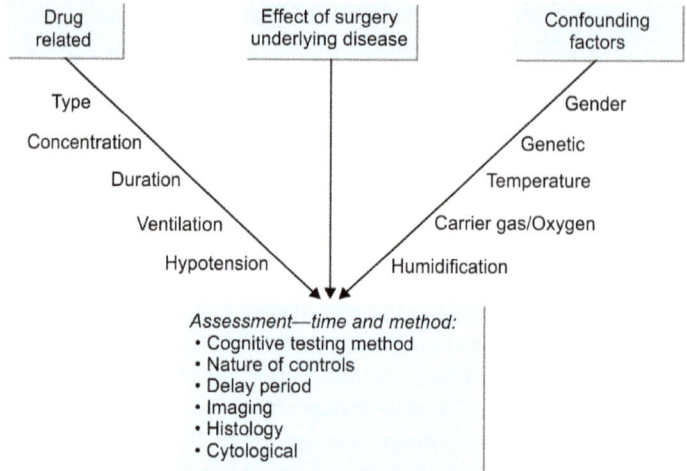

Fig. 2: Factors affecting effects of anesthetic drug neurotoxicity.

- *Potential mechanisms:*
  - *GABA activation:* Unlike adults, GABA is an excitatory neurotransmitter in fetal life. Its activation by anesthetics leads to excitotoxic injury.
  - NMDA inhibition
  - Interference with trophic factors
  - Increased accumulation of post-mitotic cell cycle proteins leading to apoptosis.

VOLATILE ANESTHETICS VERSUS TOTAL INTRAVENOUS ANESTHETICS

Some reports suggest that volatile agents attenuate the increase in S-100B (a marker for brain injury) during cardiopulmonary bypass and result in better neurological scores at 24 hours. However, intraoperatively no significant differences in cerebral oxygenation parameters were evident between the two. Such observations suggest that volatile agents can confer some degree of neuroprotection compared to total intravenous anesthetics (TIVA). However, during neurosurgery, TIVA is preferred for both practical (such as evoked potential monitoring) and theoretical considerations (such as, preserving autoregulation and flow metabolism coupling while decreasing the ICP).

Human studies: MASK, PANDA, and GAS did not provide evidence of neurotoxicity—
- *General Anesthesia or Awake Regional Anesthesia (GAS) trial:* Randomized controlled trial of about an hour of sevoflurane anesthesia vs.

CHAPTER 15 Anesthetic Neuroprotection and Neurotoxicity

awake regional techniques. 722 subjects randomized to the two groups showed no cognitive impairment when assessed at 5 years of age.
- *Mayo Anesthesia Safety in Kids (MASK) Trial:* Compared intelligence quotient of 997 unexposed, single-exposed, and multiple-exposed children <3 years of age were evaluated at 8–12 years and 15-20 years. It found that the IQ scores were unaffected by anesthetic exposure.
- *Pediatric Anesthesia Neurodevelopment (PANDA) Trial:* Prospective trial in children with <3 years of age undergoing inguinal hernia repair with siblings serving as control. 105 sibling pairs compared with retrospective anesthetic exposure (20-240 min) and prospective IQ testing at about 10 years of age. No difference in IQ scores between the anesthesia-exposed and unexposed groups.
- *The limitation of clinical trials:*
  - Exposure to anesthetics is too short.
  - Outcome assessment is too early in development.
  - The outcome assessment lacks sophistication.
  - Better trial designs are needed
  - There may not be any effect of short-term exposure to anesthesia.

Current Status

- FDA recommends that parents should be informed of the potential risk of neurotoxicity.
- Harm also results from inadequate pain relief.
- Thus, the "potential" risk of anesthetic neurotoxicity has to be weighed against the harm from inadequate surgical pain relief.
- There is no scientific basis for delaying necessary surgery.

FURTHER READING

1. Clausen NG et al. Anesthesia Neurotoxicity in the Developing Brain: Basic Studies Relevant for Neonatal or Perinatal Medicine. Clin Perinatol. 2019;46(4):647-56.
2. Lee KH et al. Crosstalk between Neuron and Glial Cells in Oxidative Injury and Neuroprotection. Int J Mol Sci. 2021;22(24):13315.
3. Manzella FM et al. Synthetic neuroactive steroids as new sedatives and anaesthetics: Back to the future. J Neuroendocrinol. 2022;34(2):e13086.
4. Var SR et al. Microglia and Macrophages in Neuroprotection, Neurogenesis, and Emerging Therapies for Stroke. Cells. 2021;10(12):3555.
5. Wu Z et al. Epigenetic Alterations in Anesthesia-Induced Neurotoxicity in the Developing Brain. Front Physiol. 2018;9:1024.

Vignette: Accidental Hypothermia and Prolonged Cardiopulmonary Resuscitation

Accidental hypothermia can be due to exposure to cold air, submersion in cold water, or when people are buried in an avalanche. Among these conditions, immersion in cold water seems to have the best neurological outcome. It is possible that the aspiration of cold water during drowning rapidly cools the brain and provides a greater degree of neuroprotection. There are several reports of hypothermic drowning. Despite the resuscitation lasting for hours, the patients recovered with virtually no neurological deficits. In two extreme examples, the patients were found by the riverside gasping for breath. In one instance, a young man was found an hour after he had gone missing. On the initial examination by the medics, he was found to have a rectal temperature of 27.5°C. He required 7 hours of cardiopulmonary resuscitation (CPR) before cardiac functions recovered. In the second case, a 65-year-old woman who had disappeared by midnight was found gasping on a snow-covered bank several hours later. Her CPR lasted 8 hours and 40 minutes, and she recovered completely. Her core temperature was 28°C initially, but later during resuscitation, it was decreased to 20.8°C. The cases like these show the protective nature of hypothermia. Although it could be argued that the arrest duration in these cases is misleading because some degree of cerebral perfusion was possible during CPR.

Section 2

Neuropathology for Anesthesiologists

- Raised Intracranial Pressure and CSF Drainage Procedures
- Hydrocephalus in Children
- Atherosclerotic Cerebrovascular Disease
- Brain Tumor Pathology
- Brain Edema and Herniation
- Cerebral Aneurysms
- Subarachnoid Hemorrhage and Cerebral Vasospasm
- Pathophysiology of Arteriovenous Malformations
- Surgical Treatment of Chronic Pain
- Developmental Abnormalities of Spine and Scoliosis
- Pathophysiology of Spinal Cord Injury
- Movement Disorders
- Seizure Types and Treatment
- Venous Air Embolism
- Traumatic Brain Injury
- Targeted Temperature Management
- Peripheral Neuropathies
- Brain Death

Chapter 16

Raised Intracranial Pressure and CSF Drainage Procedures

INTRODUCTION

Intracranial pressure (ICP) is the pressure exerted on the cranial vault by the cranial contents: brain tissue, cerebrospinal fluid (CSF), and blood. ICP is usually under 10-15 mm Hg in the supine position. The ICP fluctuates, and the instantaneous waveform reflects the composite changes in cerebrovascular tone, respiration, and blood pressure. An increase in ICP is most frequently due to traumatic brain injury. Other causes include strokes and tumors. Rarely, the increase in ICP can be idiopathic. Commonly used brain imaging methods, such as magnetic resonance imaging (MRI) and computed tomography (CT), can indirectly reveal the increase in ICP by showing compression of the ventricles or displacement of anatomical structures. However, ventricular cannulation and CSF pressure measurements are the most reliable methods of measuring ICP.

PATHOLOGY OF RAISED INTRACRANIAL PRESSURE

The three intracranial components are brain tissue (85%, about 1350 mL), blood (10%, about 130-150 mL), and cerebrospinal fluid (CSF, 5%, about 75 mL). All three components are incompressible.

According to the *Monro-Kellie doctrine*, any increase in the volume of one has to be offset by a decrease in the volume of another. CSF and blood have extracranial drainage that can rapidly adjust to changes in tissue volume. Thus, a slight initial increase in tissue volume does not increase ICP. However, when blood and CSF outflow compensatory mechanisms are exhausted, the ICP rise is rapid. With chronic increases in ICP, adaptive changes occur, such as a decrease in CSF formation, an increase in CSF outflow, or a reduction in the tissue water content that permits the expansion of other intracranial components.

An ICP of 20 mm Hg is the accepted upper physiological limit. The normal ICP varies with age. It is typically 10-20 mm Hg in adults, 7-10 mm Hg in children, and 2-6 mm Hg in infants. In any given patient, absolute ICP might not reflect the risk of brain injury or herniation. Survival with ICP >50 mm Hg has been reported in patients with traumatic brain injuries and with higher ICP with brain tumors.

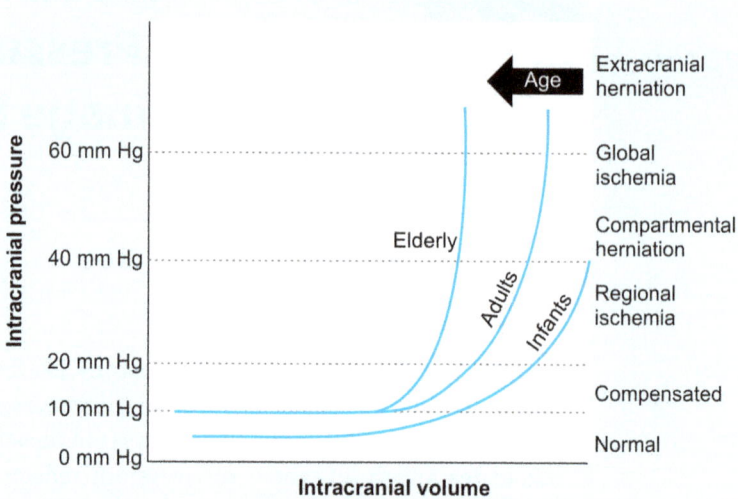

Fig. 1: A representation of the intracranial pressure-volume relationship with age and its impact on tissue perfusion.

Intracranial elastance is the increase in intracranial pressure for a unit increase in volume. Elastance is the inverse of intracranial compliance. However, the term compliance is frequently inaccurately used to describe that relationship. **Figure 1** *shows the intracranial elastance curve or the theoretical intracranial pressure-volume relationships.*

Cerebral elastance curves: Intracranial elastance is a mono-exponential relationship. **Figure 1** shows three cerebral elastance curves. The first ICP curve is from an infant with low intracranial pressure, in whom the rise in pressure is gradual due to open skull sutures and fontanelle. The second and third curves represent a healthy young adult and an elderly. In the elderly, due to cortical atrophy, increased resting CSF and blood volumes, and increased outflow resistance, the rise of ICP is somewhat more rapid compared to young adults. **Figure 2** shows that a decrease in intracranial blood volume by hyperventilation or a reduction of tissue volume by mannitol can also decrease the ICP. Shunt-dependent patients with atrophied collateral CSF drainage pathways, like the elderly, have a steeper rise in ICP. **Figure 3** shows the effect of a progressive increase in ICP on tissue perfusion with an increasing injury volume. Note that some blood in venous sinuses and some CSF in the ventricles cannot drain to compensate for increased tissue volume due to an injury.

Causes of Raised ICP

- *Increased tissue volume:*
  - Edema
  - Hemorrhage/hematoma

CHAPTER 16 Raised Intracranial Pressure and CSF Drainage Procedures

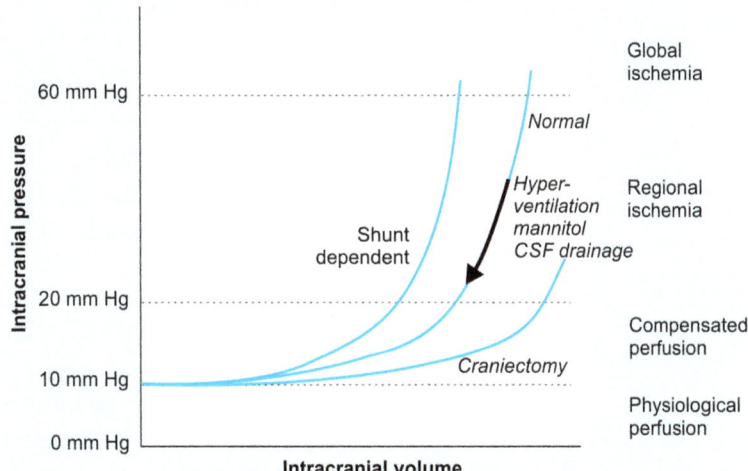

Fig. 2: Conceptual representation of the effect of reduction of blood volume by hyperventilation, of tissue shrinkage with hypertonic mannitol, and of CSF drainage, on the ICP. The increase in elastance by removal of a portion of the skull by craniectomy contrasts with the decrease seen in shunt-dependent patients.

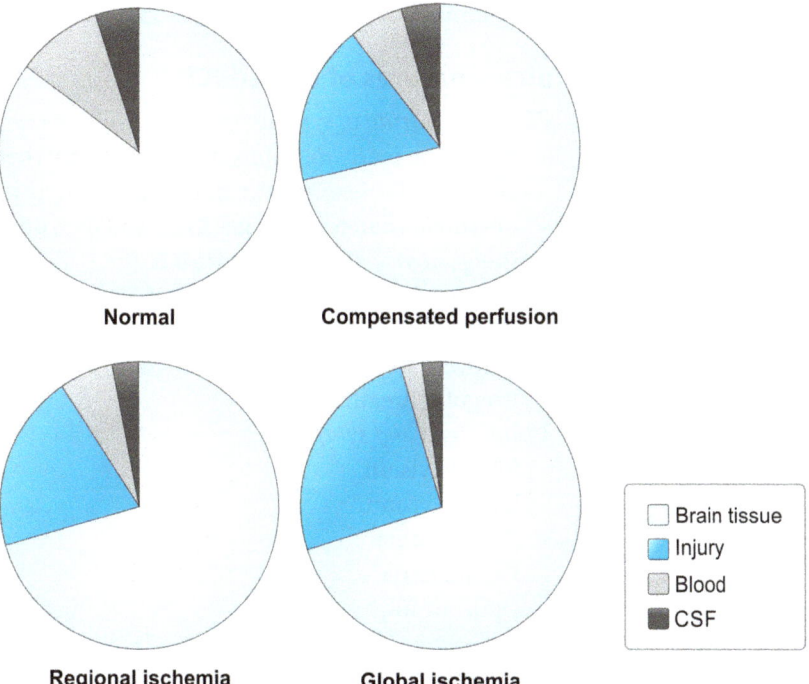

Fig. 3: Conceptual representation of the effects of injury on intracranial compartmental sizes and the failure of tissue perfusion.

- Tumors
- Infections/abscess
- *Increased CSF volume:*
  - *Obstruction to flow:*
    - Communicating hydrocephalus
    - Noncommunicating hydrocephalus
  - *Increased production:* Choroidal tumors
  - *Decreased absorption:* Post meningitis.
- *Increased blood volume:*
  - Hypercapnia
  - Venous sinus thrombosis
  - Congestive heart failure
  - Intravenous vasodilators (nitroprusside/nitroglycerin/hydralazine) increase ICP, while Ca^{++} channel blocker, nimodipine, does not increase ICP.
  - Intraarterial vasodilators used in the treatment of vasospasm can increase the ICP)
- Idiopathic intracranial hypertension
- *Skull deformities:* Single suture synostosis
- *Drugs:*
  - Tetracycline/doxycycline
  - Vitamin A overdose

Clinical Features of Raised ICP

- *The clinical triad of symptoms:*
  - Headache (early morning, postural: worse when supine)
  - *Vomiting:* Projectile, early morning at waking up
  - Cognitive changes/changes in personality/impaired consciousness
- *Cushing's signs—the triad of raised ICP:*
  - Increased pulse pressure (increased systolic and decreased diastolic blood pressure)
  - Bradycardia
  - Irregular breathing
- *Visual signs and symptoms:*
  - Blurred vision
  - Double vision
  - Photophobia
  - Papilledema
  - Optic atrophy

Consequences of Raised ICP

- Decrease in regional, and later global, cerebral blood flow with changes in cognition.

- Throbbing early morning headache due to pressure on the dura mater.
- Cranial nerve compression, such as the III cranial nerve palsy. It results in dilated pupils that are nonreactive to light. It usually indicates an ICP exceeding 30-35 mm Hg.
- Herniation of the brainstem with changes in blood pressure and respiration.

MANAGEMENT OF RAISED INTRACRANIAL PRESSURE

- *Initial measures:*
  - Head elevation, 30–45°, blood pressure permitting.
  - Neutral position to ensure free venous drainage.
  - Avoid systemic hypotension (SBP <90 mm Hg)
  - Avoid hypertension (SBP >160 mm Hg)
  - Avoid hypoxia (PaO_2 <60 mm Hg)
  - Avoid hypercapnia ($PaCO_2$ <35-40 mm Hg)
  - Consider mild sedation.
- *Advanced measures:*
  - *Consider mannitol.*
  - Consider intubation and mechanical ventilation
    - Consider additional sedation.
  - Consider invasive monitoring with an arterial line, possibly central venous line.
  - Treat hyperpyrexia
  - Treat hyperglycemia
  - Consider isotonic fluids such as normal saline; Avoid Ringer's Lactate
  - Mild hyperventilation ($PaCO_2$ 30-35 mm Hg)
  - *Levels of hyperventilation:*
    - *Normocapnia:* $PaCO_2$ 35–40 mm Hg
    - *Hyperventilation:* $PaCO_2$ 30–35 mm Hg
    - *Augmented hyperventilation:* $PaCO_2$ 25–30 mm Hg
    - *Aggressive hyperventilation:* $PaCO_2$ <25 mm Hg
  - Consider hypertonic saline.
  - Consider lumbar CSF drainage
- *Extreme measures:*
  - *Consider deep sedation with IV anesthetic to:*
    - Increase sedation to blunt response to noxious stimuli.
    - Decrease cerebral metabolic rate for oxygen.
    - Decrease ICP
    - Decrease chances of convulsion
    - Reverse cerebral steal.
  - *Consider hypothermia.*
  - *Consider decompressive surgery.*

Ventriculostomy

This is the most common emergency CSF drainage procedure.

Indications

- Acute hydrocephalus:
  - Tumors
  - Subarachnoid hemorrhage (SAH)
  - Meningitis
  - Stroke
- Obstructed or infected ventriculoperitoneal shunt
- *Monitoring ICP:*
  - Traumatic brain injury
  - Subarachnoid hemorrhage
  - Stroke
- Intraoperative relief for tense brain
- *Adjuvant to other treatment procedures:*
  - Intra-arterial (IA) vasodilator treatment for SAH
  - IA thrombolysis
  - Intrathecal therapies for malignancy or infections

Contraindications

- Coagulopathy
- Anticoagulants and antiplatelet drugs
- *Local infections:*
  - Scalp
  - Abscess

Procedure: If non-urgent, the procedure is done with ultrasound, endoscopic, or image navigation. In an emergency, often by the bedside, anatomical landmarks guide the procedure. The classical trephination hole is 1-inch lateral and ½-inch anterior to the coronal plane. The frontal horn of the lateral ventricle is usually 5–6 cm below the site when oriented perpendicular to the skull. The other anatomical approaches are listed in **Table 1**.

Table 1: Ventriculostomy landmarks.

Approach	Landmarks
Kocher's point	1.5 cm anterior to coronal suture in the mid-pupillary plane
Keen's point	3 cm posterior and 3 cm above the pinna
Dandy's point	3 cm above and 1.5 cm lateral to the inion
Frazier's point	6 inches above and 3 cm lateral to the inion
Paine's point	Tip of an isosceles triangle 3.5 cm base and 2.5 cm side resting on the Sylvian vein.
Tubb's point	Through the roof of the orbit in the mid-pupillary plane at 45° to the horizontal and 15° medially.

Care of CSF drain:
- A typical CSF drainage system is shown in **Figure 4**.
- Monitor hourly drainage.
- Observe the ICP waveform:
  - Typically, ICP waves are tri-phasic superimposed on a sinusoidal respiratory wave. Watch for pathological Lundberg's waves with a significant, sustained rise in ICP.
  - The low amplitude or absent waveform could indicate a blockage.
- Observe the height of the drainage.
- Observe for any soakage around the wound site.
- Hourly neuro-examination

Complications of CSF drain:
- Hemorrhage, tissue trauma or vascular injury.
- Infection
- Technical failure
- Over-drainage can lead to aneurysmal hemorrhage.
- Blockage:
  - Kinked drain
  - Blood clots

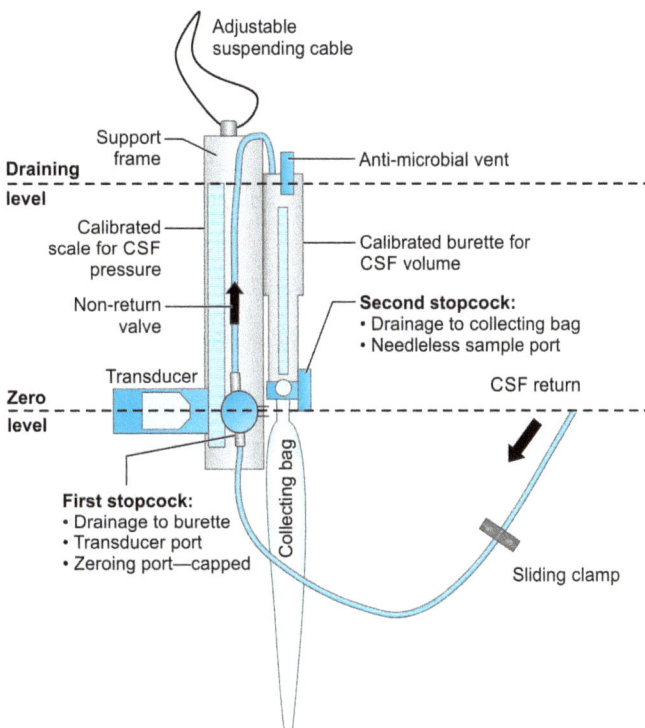

Fig. 4: CSF collecting system—side view.

- Fibrinous plugs
- Less likely with an anterior approach than with the posterior one
- CSF leak
- Pneumocephalus
- Skull fractures

Lumbar Cerebrospinal Fluid Drain

Indications

- Ongoing or expected CSF leak.
- Decreases ICP during trans-sphenoid surgery/craniotomy.
- Evaluation of normal pressure hydrocephalus
- Thoracoabdominal aortic repair and CSF pressure under 10 mm Hg
- Intrathecal drug delivery

Drainage Method

- Continuous with the preset level of drainage carries the risk of over-drainage.
- Intermittent drainage according to ICP/surgical need or volume-limited drainage.

Contraindications

- *Raised ICP:* Tumor and communicating hydrocephalus
- Low platelets (<50 k/mm^3) or coagulopathy
- Drains in SAH can decrease the transmural pressure gradient and increase the risk of bleeding.
- Local infection.

Lumbar CSF pressure: 10 mm Hg (horizontal lateral position)

A routine CSF sample is assessed for cell count, CSF protein and glucose, and Gram stain.

Complications of Lumbar Drain

- Tonsillar herniation during placement
- Overdrainage can result in pneumocephalus.
- Spinal headache
- Vestibulocochlear dysfunction
- Ocular abnormalities
- Infection
- *Hemorrhage:* Subdural or intracerebral hemorrhage
- *Recumbency related:* Deep vein thrombosis.
- Accidental dislodgement

CHAPTER 16 Raised Intracranial Pressure and CSF Drainage Procedures

FURTHER READING

1. Aghayev K et al. Advances in CSF shunt devices and their assessment for the treatment of hydrocephalus. Expert Rev Med Devices. 2021;18(9):865-73.
2. Bakhshi SK et al. Lumbar Drain for Temporary Cerebrospinal Fluid Diversion: Factors Related to the Risks of Complications at a University Hospital. World Neurosurg. 2020;143:e193-8.
3. Ginalis EE et al. A review of external lumbar drainage for the management of intracranial hypertension in traumatic brain injury. Neurochirurgie. 2022; 68(2):206-11.
4. Sunderland GJ et al. Neurosurgical CSF Diversion in Idiopathic Intracranial Hypertension: A narrative review. Life (Basel). 2021;11(5):393.
5. Tan J et al. Intraoperative lumbar drainage can prevent cerebrospinal fluid leakage during transsphenoidal surgery for pituitary adenomas: a systematic review and meta-analysis. BMC Neurol. 2020;20(1):303.

Vignette: Spaceflight Associated Neuro-Ocular Syndrome (SANS)

In the absence of gravity, cerebral hemodynamics are significantly altered. There is mild persistent intracranial hypertension during prolonged space flight. The increase in ICP could be due to cephalad redistribution of arterial blood pressure in weightlessness or an increase in venous pressure. The latter is thought to decrease CSF resorption. Typically, spaceflight-induced hemodynamic changes peak at about three weeks, and adaptation occurs by about the 45th day. The primary adaptive mechanism is cerebral vasoconstriction. Cerebral autoregulation is preserved during space flight and could even be improved in its early stages. The main effect of the sustained increase in ICP is on the perfusion of the optic nerve head. Visual impairment has been noted during and after prolonged space flight. NASA has termed this as Spaceflight Associated Neuro-ocular Syndrome (SANS). Several astronauts have required CSF drainage on return from space.

Chapter 17: Hydrocephalus in Children

INTRODUCTION

Definition: Hydrocephalus is excessive cerebrospinal fluid (CSF) accumulation in cerebral ventricles. It is usually a chronic condition that leads to enlargement of the ventricles and thinning of the cortex.

CLASSIFICATION OF HYDROCEPHALUS

Congenital vs. Acquired Hydrocephalus

- *Congenital:*
  - *Aqueductal stenosis:* Enlargement of lateral ventricles.
  - *Arachnoid cysts:* Often occur in the III ventricle.
  - *Dandy-Walker syndrome:* IV ventricular enlargement with cerebellar atrophy
  - *Neural tube defects, including Arnold Chiari malformation II:* Fourth ventricle outflow obstruction and hydrocephalus.
- *Acquired:*
  - *Intraventricular hemorrhage:*
    - Typically, in premature neonates
    - Blocks arachnoid villi.
  - Meningitis
  - Head injury
  - Brain tumors.

Communicating vs. Noncommunicating

- *Communicating hydrocephalus:* Ventricles communicate with each other without any obstruction to CSF flow. It is primarily due to a failure of reabsorption of CSF, excessive formation, or normal pressure hydrocephalus. Imaging reveals the absence of an obstructing lesion. Communicating hydrocephalus is seen with meningitis due to arachnoid villi damage.
- *Noncommunicating hydrocephalus:* It is due to CSF flow obstruction that prevents flow between ventricles. It can lead to asymmetric ventricular dilation. It can be due to congenital abnormalities, arteriovenous malformations, or tumors.

Differential Diagnosis
- Cortical atrophy
- Developmental anomalies of periventricular structures such as corpus callosum agenesis and septo-optic dysplasia.

CLINICAL SIGNS
- *Infants (Figure 1)*:
  - Failure to thrive.
  - Irritability
  - Nausea, vomiting, and lethargy
  - Cranial growth (diameter) exceeds face growth.
  - Increased head circumference
  - Poor head lift and control
  - Suture separation with increased fontanelle size and bulging
  - Delayed fontanelle closure
  - *Macewen's crackpot sign:* Percussing the skull at the junction of frontal, temporal, and parietal bones results in resonant sound due to suture dehiscence.
  - *Trans-illumination:* Bight light illuminates the head of the infants with hydrocephalus due to excessive cerebrospinal fluid.
  - Prominent scalp veins due to reverse intracranial flow
  - VI cranial nerve (CN) paralysis with a medial deviation of the eyes.
  - *Sunset sign:* Seen in 40% of cases with hydrocephalus. It is an early sign of the disease before the enlargement of the head. Sunset is appearance due to the sclera that can be seen between the iris and the upper lid. The sign is due to the distension of the aqueduct and the compression of the peri-aqueductal structures.

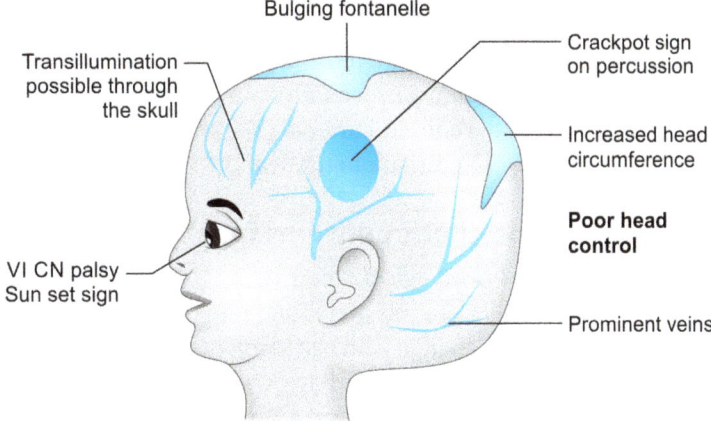

Fig. 1: Clinical features of hydrocephalus in infants.

- The reflexes are hyperactive.
- The respiration is irregular with apneic spells.
- *Children:*
  - Headache
  - Nausea and vomiting
  - Gait changes
  - Paralysis of upward gaze
  - VI CN paralysis
  - Papilledema
  - Impaired development
  - Impaired cognition

INVESTIGATIONS

- A plain X-ray of the skull shows a copper-beaten appearance due to excessive cortical convolutional markings.
- CT/MRI:
  - Enlarged head circumference.
  - Ventricular dilation without cortical shrinkage in contrast to other causes of cognitive impairment.
  - III ventricle herniation into sella turcica
  - Erosion of sella turcica resulting in empty sella syndrome
  - Corpus callosum atrophy
  - Attenuation of the temporal horns.

MANAGEMENT

Medical management: In neonates, medical treatment with acetazolamide with furosemide may be indicated. Such treatment could lead to electrolyte imbalances and metabolic acidosis.

Surgical intervention: Possible surgical treatments in children includes:
- Choroid plexectomy
- Third ventriculostomy
- Shunting procedures
  - Ventriculoarterial (VA) and
  - Ventriculoperitoneal (VP) shunts.

Anesthetic Concerns for Shunt Surgery in Children

- *Physiological concerns:*
  - Cerebral metabolic rate ($CMRO_2$) and cerebral blood flow (CBF) change with age in infants.
    - Neonates have low $CMRO_2$ and CBF compared to adults.
    - $CMRO_2$ and CBF increase in infancy and by early childhood exceed adults.

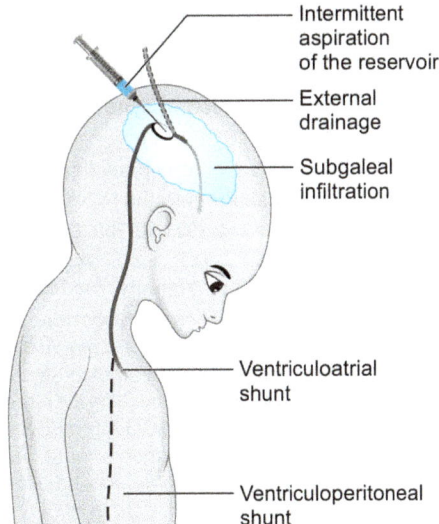

Fig. 2: CSF drainage options in neonates and infants.

- Cerebral autoregulation develops in-utero. In the pre-term infants, pressure autoregulation improves with 23 to 33 weeks of gestational age. The low cerebral blood flow at birth (20 mL/100g/min) rapidly increases to peak at 5 years of age. The lower limit of cerebral autoregulation in infancy corresponds to the lower mean arterial pressure. Beyond infancy, the difference between the mean arterial pressure/cerebral perfusion pressure and the lower limit of autoregulation remains relatively constant.
- *The effects of raised ICP,* such as nausea, vomiting, poor feeding, and obtunded sensorium, predispose to dehydration and hypovolemia.
- *Difficulty in intubation due to an enlarged head*
- *Effects of acute ICP decompression:* Reverse herniation with bradycardia/arrest. The risk is greater in children due to high vagal tone.
- *Shunt surgery in neonates:*
  - Neonates ≤1.5 kg are at risk of germinal matrix hemorrhages present with hydrocephalus.
  - In newborns and ill infants, CSF can be drained into the subgaleal tissue or tapped from a subcutaneous Ommaya reservoir without requiring a formal shunt early in life **(Fig. 2)**.

FURTHER READING

1. Carlstrom LP et al. A clinical primer for the glymphatic system. Brain. 2022; 145(3):843-57.

2. Koutsouras GW et al. Pathophysiologic mechanisms and strategies for the treatment of post-hemorrhagic hydrocephalus of prematurity. Childs Nerv Syst; 2022;38(3):511-20.
3. Varagur K et al. Syndromic Hydrocephalus. Neurosurg Clin N Am. 2022;33(1):67-9.
4. Yamada S. Cerebrospinal fluid dynamics. Croat Med J. 2021;62(4):399-410.
5. Yin R et al. Progression in Neuroimaging of Normal Pressure Hydrocephalus. Front Neurol. 2021;12:700269.

Vignette: The Treatment of Hydrocephalus

Hydrocephalus was known to Hippocrates and later to Galen. The condition was considered to be excess water around the brain. Abu al Qasim Al Zahrawi, in the 10th century, first reported the drainage of subcutaneously collected CSF in an infant with hydrocephalus. Al Zahrawi is widely considered to be the father of surgery. A French anatomist and surgeon, Claude Nicholas LeCat (1700–1768) described ventricular puncture in 1744. However, these methods had little application without antisepsis. Wernicke described sterile ventricular puncture in 1881. Quinke introduced the sterile lumbar puncture method in 1891. The first ventriculogaleal shunt was done in 1893 by Mikulicz. The development of shunt technology faced many hurdles, such as infection, surgical complications and occlusion. By the 1950s, techniques for ventriculoperitoneal, lumboperitoneal, ventriculocaval, and other shunts had been developed, but none were successful. Shunt surgery became practical with the development of silicone tubes and better valve designs in the 1960s.

Chapter 18: Atherosclerotic Cerebrovascular Disease

INTRODUCTION
Atherosclerotic cerebrovascular disease is the narrowing the vascular lumen by atheromatous plaques, calcium deposits, and muscular hypertrophy.

RISK FACTORS FOR ATHEROSCLEROTIC DISEASE
- *Gender:* 9% of men and 7% of women have atherosclerotic carotid arterial disease
- *Age:*
  - Cellular senescence with age predisposes to atherosclerosis.
  - There is a three-fold increase in the incidence of the disease over 70 years of age than under that age.
- *Concurrent diseases:*
  - Peripheral vascular disease
  - Hypertension
  - Diabetes
  - Dyslipidemias
  - Obesity
- *Lifestyle:*
  - Smoking
  - Sedentary lifestyle
- *Genetics:* Genes for advanced glycation end-products and RAGE (receptor for advanced glycation end-products) play a significant role in the progress of the disease.

PATHOLOGY
- Formation of atheromatous plaque typically occurs in the proximal 1–2 cm of the carotid bifurcation
- Plaque ulceration, rupture, bleeding, thrombosis, and embolism lead to acute or chronic cerebral vascular insufficiency, transient ischemic attacks, or strokes.
- *Embolism:* More Likely in the MCA than the ACA
- *Stenosis: Grades:* Mild <49%, moderate 50–69%, severe 70–99%, and complete 100%
- *Syndromes:* Ipsilateral stroke, ipsilateral transient ischemic attack (TIA), and amaurosis fugax (transient unilateral blindness)

Table 1: Society of Radiologists in Ultrasound: Criteria for the assessment of carotid stenosis.

Severity	Primary		Additional	
	Peak systolic velocity (PSV)	Duplex ultrasound	ICA/CCA PSV	ICA EDV
Normal	<125 cm/s	No plaque No thickening	<2.0	<40 cm/s
Mild<50%	<125 cm/s	Plaque or Thickening	<2.0	<40 cm/s
Moderate 50–69%	125–230 cm/s	Plaque	2.0–4.0	40–100 cm/s
Severe ≥70%	>230 cm/s	Plaque narrow lumen	>4.0	>100 cm/s
Near occlusion	Not applicable	Very narrow lumen	Not applicable	Not applicable
Total occlusion	Not applicable	No lumen	Not applicable	Not applicable

(ICA: internal carotid artery; CCA: common carotid artery; EDV: end-diastolic velocity; PSV: peak systolic velocity)

INVESTIGATIONS

- Carotid bruit poorly predicts stenosis.
- Duplex ultrasound assessment of the severity of stenosis **(Table 1)**
- MR angiography
- CT angiography
- Interventional angiography (gold standard).

DIFFERENTIAL DIAGNOSIS

- Brain tumors
- Intracranial hemorrhage
- Stroke in evolution, a poorly characterized entity with progressive neurological deficits
- Ictal and postictal states
- Raised intracranial pressure, tissue edema, and hydrocephalus
- Drug overdose
- Infection
- *Metabolic:* Glucose, electrolytes, acidosis, and organ failure.

ETIOLOGY OF STROKE

Table 2 shows the etiology of stroke. Most strokes are due to thromboembolic disease.

Table 2: Types and clinical features of ischemic and hemorrhagic strokes.

	Thrombotic stroke	Embolic stroke	Watershed infarction	Parenchymal hemorrhage	Subarachnoid hemorrhage
Etiology	Clot develops In situ	Usually thrombi; rarely vegetations, valvular calcifications; infective debris	Shock; heart failure; postural hypotension	• Hypertension • AVMs and cavernous malformations	• Usually aneurysmal • Rarely AVM or traumatic
Incidence	Increases with age; males	Slight female bias, later presentation, more atrial fibrillation	Underestimated	Increases with ages; males; more frequent in Afro-American/Hispanic	Bimodal in young and elderly, female bias; more frequent in Asian population
%-of all stroke	70%	15%	<5%	10–15%	<5%
Onset	H/o Transient ischemic attacks, gradual	Abrupt and catastrophic	Proportional to the severity of hypotension	A focal deficit that progresses over minutes to hours	Abrupt and catastrophic
Risk factors	Atherosclerosis, hypertension, diabetes, smoking alcohol, drugs	Atrial fibrillation, atherosclerosis, hypertension, diabetes, smoking	• Cardiopulmonary bypass with MAP <60 mm Hg • Hypotension	80% hypertension 80% no pathology, such as cavernous and AV malformations	• Family history • Hypertension • Polycystic kidneys
Treatment	• Anticoagulation • Antiplatelets thrombolysis	• Anticoagulation • Antiplatelets thrombolysis • Rx of the cause	Correction of hypotension and anemia	Surgical intervention	Surgical intervention
Outcome	20% early mortality	30% early mortality; increases dramatically with repeat episodes	Worse prognosis if deep and bilateral	35% fatal; 20% full recovery	Significant pre-hospital mortality; 33% early deaths; 33% good outcome outcome

Flowchart 1: Multiple pathways of ischemic brain and reperfusion injury.

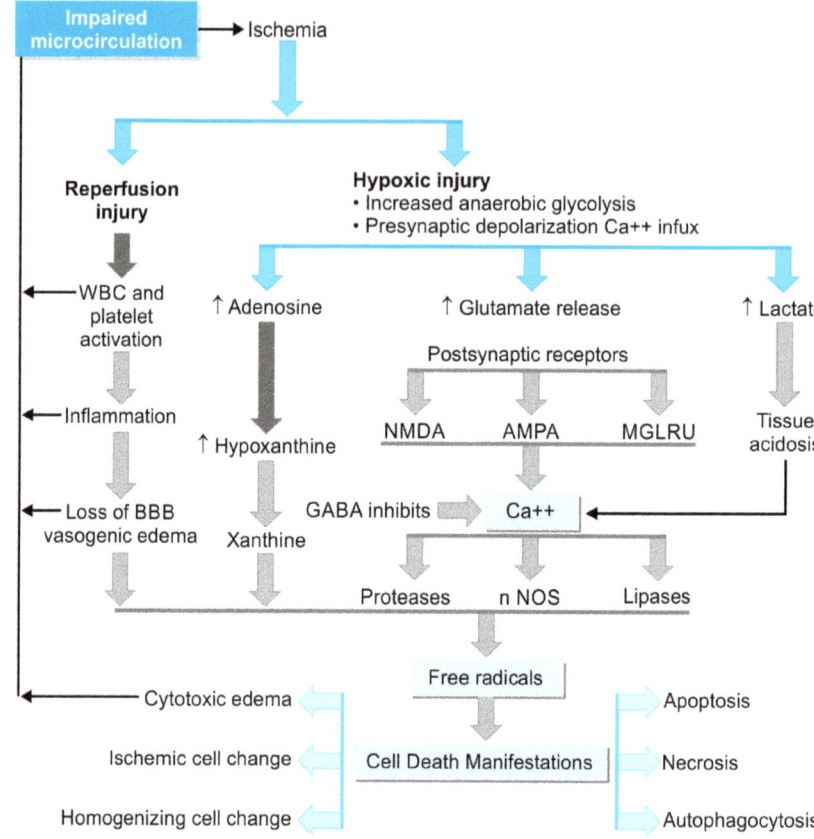

(GABA: gamma-aminobutyric acid; NMDA: N-methyl-D-aspartate; AMPA: α-amino-3-hydroxy-5-methyl-4-isoxazolepropionic acid; MGLRU: metabolic glutamate receptors; nNOS: neuronal nitric oxide synthetase)

BIOCHEMICAL EVENTS IN STROKE

The complex pathogenic cascades of stroke are shown in **Flowchart 1**. These injury pathways are constantly evolving and cross-talk with each other. Some of the critical pathological events are as follows:
- Critical reduction in blood flow
- Depletion of ATP
- Failure of the ATP-dependent Na^+ pump
- An intracellular surge of Ca^{++}
- Activation of intracellular necrotic and apoptotic cascades
- *Necrotic or apoptotic cell death:*
  - *Necrotic death:* Mediated primarily by the intracellular Ca^{++} surge that activates phospholipases. Damage to the mitochondrial cell membrane worsens energy failure and lactic acidosis. Release of free radicals/fatty acids/arachidonic acid occurs. The latter activates

platelets to result in microcirculatory failure due to thrombogenesis, vasospasm, and edema.
Subsequent neutrophil activation leads to the formation of hydrogen peroxides and free radicals, leading to tissue necrosis.
- *Apoptotic cell death:* Also known as programmed cell death. It is primarily due to the activation of caspases and other genetic pathways. It is characterized by cell shrinking and nuclear condensation, which ultimately leads to phagocytosis of the cells without triggering an inflammatory response.

STROKE TREATMENT

Early Diagnosis and Treatment

- *Early diagnosis:*
  - *Quick test:* "Smile, Talk, and Raise arms" = STRoke rule out
  - *Or FAST:* Facial drooping, Arm weakness, Speech difficulties, Time to call emergency services
- *Clinical signs: Hemiplegia, hemineglect, and aphasia: Suspected stroke*
- *Immediate transfer to the stroke center*
- *IV tPA if criteria met:*
  - *Inclusion criteria:*
    - Stroke (<4.5 hours) with measurable neurological deficits
  - *Exclusion criteria (0-3 hours):*
    - *Evidence of active bleeding:* ICH or SAH
    - Internal hemorrhage
    - Coagulopathy
    - Severe uncontrolled hypertension
    - Increased chances of bleeding
    - Intracranial aneurysms and malformations
    - Recent traumatic brain injury and brain or spine surgery
  - *Additional exclusion criteria between 3 and 4.5 hours:*
    - Age >80 years
    - Severe stroke
    - On anticoagulants
    - History of diabetes or prior stroke

Stroke Assessment

- *Clinical status based on the National Institute of Health Stroke Status Scale (NIHSS)* **(Table 3):** It scores sensory and motor functions, neglect, language, vision, gaze, and ataxia. The total score is 42. The individual scores are aggregated:
  - *0:* No stroke
  - *1-4:* Minor
  - *5-20:* Moderate
  - *20:* Severe

Table 3: National Institute of Health Stroke Scale

1a	LOC overall	0: Alert; 1: Drowsy; 2: Stuporous; 3: Coma
1b	LOC 2 questions	0: Both correct; 1: One correct; 2: None correct
1c	LOC to 2 commands	0: Obeys both; 1: Obeys one; 2: Obeys none
2	Gaze	0: normal; 1: Partial gaze palsy; 2: Persistent deviation
3	Hemianopia	0: None; 1: Partial; 2: Complete; 3: Bilateral
4	Facial paresis	0: None; 1: Minor; 2: Partial; 3: Complete
5a	Left arm	0: No drift; 1: Drift; 2: Insufficient elevation of the limb; 3: No elevation; 4: No movement; X: Untestable
5b	Right arm	
6a	Left lower limb	0: No drift; 1: Drift; 2: Insufficient elevation of the limb; 3: No elevation; 4: No movement; X: Untestable
6b	Right lower limb	
7	Limb ataxia	0: None; 1: In one limb; 2: In two limbs
8	Sensory	0: Normal; 1: Partial loss; 2: Severe loss
9	Language	0: Normal; 1: Mild/moderate aphasia; 2: Severe aphasia; 3: Mute
10	Dysarthria	0: Normal speech; 1: Mild; 2: Unintelligible; X: intubated
11	Extinction or inattention	0: No neglect; 1: Partial neglect; 2: Complete neglect

(LOC: Level of consciousness)

Stroke Investigations

- Non-contrast CT:
  - Rule out hemorrhage.
  - See the extent of the infarction.
  - ASPECT: Alberta Stroke Program Early CT score gives 1 point for differentiating gray and white matter in 10 regions: Caudate, putamen, internal capsule, insular cortex, and six defined areas of the cortex in the middle cerebral artery (MCA) distribution.
- CT angiogram for the site of occlusion
- MRI DWI MR angiogram or perfusion CT is useful at or beyond 6 hours to determine the value of mechanical clot extraction.

Clot Retrieval

- *Indications:*
  - Age >18 years
  - A pre-stroke Modified Rankin's Score of 0 or 1 (*see* **Table 4**)
  - NIHSS score ≥6
  - ASPECTS ≥6
  - Occlusion in the internal carotid artery (ICA) or proximal MCA
- For treatment after 6 hours and sometimes up to 24 hours, consider age <80 years, site of occlusion ICA/proximal MCA, or M1 portion of MCA. NIH injury severity score is <20, core volume is 20–50 mL, and perfusion imaging to infarct volume is >1.8.

Table 4: Clinical status by modified Rankin's scale.

0	Asymptomatic
1	Fully functional despite symptoms
2	Self-sufficient, some limitations of previous activities, and independent
3	Needs some assistance and can walk independently
4	Needs assistance for self-care and is unable to walk without assistance
5	Bedridden, incontinent, and needs nursing care

Studies Supporting Clot Retrieval

- *1980–1999:* Evidence was gathered that recanalization of arteries was possible in stroke. These studies (IV-tPA, PROACT I, and PROACT II) focused on tPA and prourokinase to lyse the clot and showed that such treatments could be effective.
- In 2004 MERCI device trial involving 114 patients showed that safe recanalization was possible in 53% of the cases with mechanical clot extraction and improved stroke outcomes.
- In 2013, three clinical trials (IMS III, MR-RESCUE, and SYNTHESIS) using MERCI and IA tPA failed to show the benefits of endovascular. Still, the limitations of these trials regarding treatment selection, randomization, and controls paved the way for follow-up studies.
- These results were superseded by five trials (MR CLEAN, EXTEND-1A, ESCAPE, REVASCAT, and SWIFT PRIME) in 2015 showed an almost two-fold improvement in the quality of survival after clot extraction with newer devices compared to medical management.

CONCERNS WITH RADIOLOGICAL INTERVENTIONS

- Clot aspiration is more straightforward than using a clot retriever.
- *Stent retriever:* A wire cage device traps and retrieves the clot.
- Intra-arterial (IA) thrombolysis is less frequently used due to the risk of hemorrhagic conversion.

OUTCOME OF STROKE

- Hemorrhagic stroke is worse than ischemic stroke.
- *Ischemic stroke:*
  - Complete recovery = 25%
  - Minor disability = 15%
  - Moderate disability = 15%
  - Major disability = 30%
  - Death = 15%

FURTHER READING

1. El Hadri K et al. Inflammation, oxidative stress, senescence in atherosclerosis: thioredoxine-1 as an emerging therapeutic target. Int J Mol Sci. 2021;23(1):77.

2. Ghelani DP et al. Ischemic stroke and infection: A brief update on mechanisms and potential therapies. Biochem Pharmacol. 2021;193:114768.
3. Ni D et al. Recent insights into atherosclerotic plaque cell autophagy. Exp Biol Med (Maywood). 2021;246(24):2553-8.
4. Tekle WG et al. Intracranial atherosclerotic disease: current concepts in medical and surgical management. Neurology. 2021;97(20 Suppl 2): S145-57.
5. Tomerak S et al. Systemic inflammation in COVID-19 patients may induce various types of venous and arterial thrombosis: a systematic review. Scand J Immunol. 2021; 94(5):e13097.

Vignette: Rudolf Virchow and his follies.

Rudolf Virchow (1821–1902) is the Father of Modern Pathology. He made innumerable contributions to medicine, with over 2000 invaluable publications. Virchow described that stasis and coagulation led to venous thrombosis and pulmonary embolism but not the third component of the triangle, endothelial injury. The term "Virchow Triad" is often invoked to explain the occurrence of strokes or pulmonary emboli. Beyond pathology, Virchow's contributions extended to public health and politics. However, this man of great talent opposed two major scientific concepts of his time: Charles Darwin's theory of evolution and Ignaz Semmelweis's idea of hand washing for preventing infection during surgery. Though Darwin was successful, Semmelweis was ridiculed by his peers. Semmelweis had a nervous breakdown and died in an asylum. Semmelweis and Henry Hill Hickman, who first brought the concept of anesthesia, are tragic illustrations of how corrupt, incompetent, and savage scientific peer review process can be!

Chapter 19: Brain Tumor Pathology

INTRODUCTION

A brain tumor is an abnormal growth of cells that can be benign or malignant. Primary tumors arise locally in the brain (**Fig. 1**). A secondary tumor metastasizes to the brain from an extraneous site. Brain tumors become symptomatic when they infiltrate a vital brain region, press on a critical structure, obstruct the flow of cerebrospinal fluid (CSF), increase intracranial pressure, or cause a hemorrhage. Brain tumors are therapeutically challenging because of the vulnerability of the host organ to injury. They are often diagnosed late in the course of the disease and respond poorly to chemo- and radiotherapy. The survival rate of patients with aggressive brain tumors remains exceedingly poor.

PRIMARY BRAIN TUMORS

- *Gliomas:* Glioblastoma multiforme (GBM) is an aggressive brain tumor with a doubling time of about 19 days. Its survival time is limited to 10–14 months. The prognosis with GBM is better in younger and higher functioning people and those with methylated O6-methylguanine-DNA-methyltransferase (MGMT) promoter gene. GBMs progress over time from lower to higher, more invasive grades.

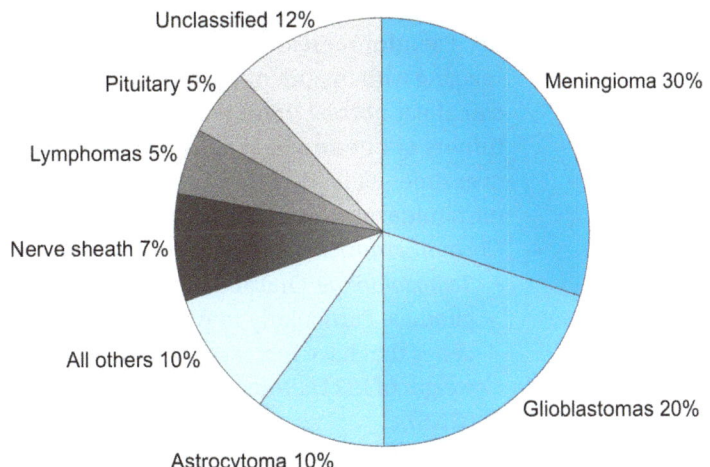

Fig. 1: Distribution of primary brain tumors.

- Grades of GBM:
  - *Grade I:* Slow-growing, non-infiltrative tumors with normal cells.
  - *Grade II:* Mixture of malignant and healthy cells
  - *Grade III:* Anaplastic tumors
  - *Grade IV:* Anaplastic tumors with necrosis
- *Meningiomas:* Benign, atypical, or malignant (rare)
- Primitive neuroectodermal tumors from cell remnants of fetal development, usually in pediatric patients
- *Pituitary tumors:* Adenoma, carcinoma, craniopharyngioma, and cysts
- Pineal tumors
- *Choroid plexus tumors:* Papillomas and carcinomas
- Skull-base tumors
- Nerve sheath tumors
- *Cysts:* Epidermoid, dermoid, arachnoid, colloid, pineal, and cleft cyst
- Mixed cell types malignancies.

SECONDARY BRAIN TUMORS

About 25% of all malignancies are due to brain metastasis. They could be solitary or multiple metastatic lesions or result in diffuse carcinomatosis.

TUMOR TREATMENT MODALITIES AND ANESTHETIC IMPLICATIONS

- *Surgery:* While surgery is indicated as a treatment for many brain tumors, it is usually contraindicated when tumors are bilateral, such as most butterfly wing tumors, inaccessible tumors, or tumors involving vital centers.
- *Radiation:* Most brain tumors are treated with radiation. Radionecrosis of tumors can lead to an increase in size, new deficits, or seizures. Effects of radionecrosis do not reverse over time, while those of pseudoprogression do. Pseudoprogression is an apparent increase in tumor size on imaging with treatment. Radiation exposure in the pediatric age group can affect normal brain development. Radiosensitivity of most brain tumors is intermediate, and resistance to treatment often develops over time. Radiosensitizers can enhance treatment response, such as nitroimidazoles, hyperbaric oxygen, and induced hyperthermia.
- *Chemotherapy:*
  - *Temozolomide:* Oral alkylating agent, first-line treatment of grade 2–4 gliomas. Particularly in patients with methylated MGMT promoter genes that have increased sensitivity to the drug. It has a molecular weight of 192 Daltons. It freely penetrates the central nervous system (CNS).
  - *Lomustine:* An oral alkylating agent that can cause bone marrow suppression and hepatic and renal toxicity.

- *Procarbazine:* Oral alkylating agent can cause bone marrow suppression, CNS toxicity, and hypersensitivity reaction.
- *Vincristine:* Given IV, it can cause a severe local reaction, bone marrow suppression, gastrointestinal (GI) side effects, peripheral neuropathy, and hepatic and renal toxicities.
- *Cisplatin:* Given IV, bone marrow suppression and GI side effects are common, CNS side effects in the elderly, peripheral neuropathy, and cardiotoxicity.
- *Other tumor treatments in clinical trials:*
  - *Anti-vascular endothelial growth factor (VEGF) treatment:* Bevacizumab is a potent anti-VEGF drug and has been used with conventional chemotherapy.
  - Tyrosine kinase inhibitors.
  - Oncolytic viruses
  - Immunotherapy

ANESTHETIC CONCERNS
- Increased ICP
- Neurological deficits
- Seizures and anticonvulsant treatment
- *Perioperative steroid:* Dependence, withdrawal, weight gain, replacement, worsening diabetes, hypertension
- Vascular access
- *Infections:*
  - *Increased infection/sepsis risk*
  - *Oral fungal infections*
- Nausea and vomiting
- If δ-amino levulinic acid (δ-ALA) is used for tumor imaging, the patient will be photosensitive and needs to be protected from light. The operating room lights have to be appropriately dimmed.
- *Side effects of chemotherapy:*
  - *Bone marrow suppression:*
    - *Decreased Hb:* Anemia
    - *Decreased platelets:* Increased bruising
    - *Decreased WBCs:* Infection risk
  - Deafness
  - Nephrotoxicity
  - Hepatotoxicity
  - Pulmonary fibrosis
  - Cardiotoxicity.

Nausea and Vomiting in Patients on Chemotherapy

- *Clinical types of nausea and vomiting with chemotherapy:*
  - *Anticipatory:* Psychogenic vomiting triggered by past experiences
  - *Acute:* Within minutes of the start of the chemotherapy infusion
  - *Delayed:* Within 24 hours after treatment and lasts for a week
  - *Breakthrough:* Occurs despite antiemetic treatment
  - *Refractory:* Resistant to treatment
- *Pharmacological management:*
  - *D2 receptor in CTZ:* Metoclopramide
  - *Central sedative:* Lorazepam
  - *$5\text{-}HT_3$ blockers:* Ondansetron, dolasetron, and palonosetron
  - *NK1 receptor antagonists:* Aprepitant and netupitant
  - *H_2 blockers:* Ranitidine, famotidine, and cimetidine
  - *First-generation H_1 blockers:* Promethazine, prochlorperazine, meclizine, and doxylamine
  - *Second-generation H_1 blockers:* Loratadine and desloratadine
  - *Steroidal anti-inflammatory drugs:* Dexamethasone.
- *Perioperative care:*
  - With chemotherapy, maintain regular antiemetic cover starting 24 hours before to 7 days after
  - Do not discontinue if asymptomatic.
  - Fasting appropriately
  - Move the patient slowly to avoid motion sickness.
  - Avoid strong smells.
  - *Pretreatment:* Ondansetron, ranitidine, and dexamethasone
  - Gastric decompression
  - Total intravenous anesthesia is superior to volatile agents.

Anesthetic Choice in Patients with Systemic Malignancy

The effect of anesthesia on the clinical course of malignancy is unproven in clinical trials. The concerns include the following:
- Manipulation of the tumor during surgery, surgical stress, and immunosuppression may predispose to metastatic disease.
- Narcotics may suppress immune functions.
- Regional techniques with better perioperative pain control may be superior to general anesthesia.

Changing Profile of Central Nervous System Tumors

Advances in genomic cancer treatment that uses receptor-specific monoclonal antibodies have increased the survival of cancer patients. However, the inability to deliver the same compounds effectively across the blood–brain barrier (BBB) has led to increased metastatic cancers in

CHAPTER 19 Brain Tumor Pathology

the brain and the spine. Unlike primary brain tumors, the metastatic tumors are likely to be multifocal within the brain/spine. Many of these patients are in frail health.

Tumor Blood Flow

- The brain tumor blood flow is highly variable within a given tumor, over time, across tumor types, and from one patient to another.
- Tumors often have specific regions of very high blood flow mimicking AV fistulae like shunts, but other regions of the same tumor can be relatively ischemic.
- On average, the tumor blood flow is less than the cerebral blood flow. For GBMs, the tumor blood flow correlates with the virulence of the tumor.
- However, due to widespread cystic and necrotic changes in virulent tumors, the blood flow in these tumors does not always linearly increase as the disease progresses.
- Meningiomas with excessive blood flow may require preoperative embolization to reduce blood loss.

Tumor Blood Flow Autoregulation

- Tumor tissue lacks autoregulation. In contrast to the tumor, the surrounding brain can react to physiological factors that modulate the blood flow. Regional differences in blood flow regulation can affect the blood flow distribution to brain tumors.
- Hypoventilation or hypercapnia vasodilates the healthy brain tissue. It has a minimal effect on brain regions with impaired autoregulation, thus diverting blood from tumors or ischemic areas to healthy tissue. This redistribution of the blood flow from regions with impaired autoregulation to healthy ones is called "*cerebral steal*". Hyperventilation or hypocapnia results in vasoconstriction in the healthy areas of the brain. Thus, blood is redistributed from the healthy brain to the tumor or ischemic regions where vascular regulation is impaired. This phenomenon is known as "*inverse steal*".
- The factors that affect tumor blood flow could affect bleeding during resection. During the excision of large brain tumors, conventional interventions such as head elevation, modest hypocapnia, low-pressure ventilation, total intravenous anesthesia (TIVA), osmotic diuretics, and steroids might help reduce blood loss.

Intracranial Pressure Concerns with Large Brain Tumors

Large brain tumors with mid-line shifts obliterated ventricles are at risk of herniation. These patients are often hypertensive. Thus, the induction strategy should include smooth intubation with minimal hypertensive response.

Furthermore, the skull's interior is compartmentalized by dura into supratentorial and infratentorial compartments. The former is further divided into the left and the right side. Brain tissue herniation through the dural openings can block CSF drainage, increasing compartmental pressure, causing brain bulging, and worsening operating conditions. CSF drainage can help reduce pressure and facilitate surgery. CSF drainage and rapid tumor debulking might be necessary to decrease intracompartmental pressure and restore cerebral perfusion to healthy brain tissue in the compartment.

Intraoperative Brain Tumor Imaging

Most malignant brain tumors recur due to residue at the edges of tumor resection. Incomplete glioma resection directly affects patient survival. Dyes, such as fluorescein and 5-aminolevulinic acid, are used to identify the tumor margins during surgery guided by tissue fluorescence **(Table 1)**.

Blood Loss during Tumor Resection

In most brain or spine surgeries, it is impossible to compress the tissue to prevent blood loss. Strategies to contain blood loss and minimize blood transfusions include:
- Avoidance of antiplatelet and anticoagulant drugs before surgery
- Test for and correct any coagulopathies before surgery.
- Preoperative embolization when possible
- Consideration for preoperative erythropoietin and blood harvest with primary brain tumors.
- *Intraoperative:*
  - *Surgery:*
    - Proper positioning:
      - Safe head elevation
      - Unobstructed venous return

Table 1: Comparison for fluorescein and 5-ALA for intraoperative tumor imaging.

	Fluorescein	5-Aminolevulinic acid
Source	Synthetic	Hemoglobin metabolite
FDA approved	2006	2017
Dose	3 mg/kg IV during surgery	20 mg/kg oral 4 hours before surgery
Peak excitation	490 nm	405 nm
Peak emission	525 nm	Green–red complex pattern
Adverse effects	Allergic reactions	Allergic reaction, photosensitivity for 24 hours, mild leukocytosis, thrombocytopenia, anemia, and increased liver enzymes
Human clinical use	Extensive	Very limited

CHAPTER 19 Brain Tumor Pathology

- Good surgical technique
- Diathermy, gel foam, cellulose
- The topical coagulant, human gelatin-thrombin matrix (Floseal™), is effective in most situations.
- Use of antifibrinolytics (TXA) carries the risk of seizures, risk-benefits unproven therefore avoided.
- Cell savers cannot be used in cases of malignancy or infections
- *Anesthesia:*
  - Intraoperative volume expansion and blood harvest
  - Good regional venous return
  - Low-pressure ventilation
  - Mild hypotension
  - Antifibrinolytics (potential side-effects: Seizures, delirium, transient ischemic attacks)
  - Monitoring coagulation thromboelastography
  - Replacement of platelets and coagulation factors.

Effect on Perioperative Cognition and Delayed Awakening

Anesthesia can unmask neurological deficits. Large brain tumors (>3.5 cm), independent of their location, can delay awakening. Furthermore, neurological symptoms might worsen in the immediate postoperative period compared to preoperative examination. Care must be taken in dosing long-acting narcotics (hydromorphone boluses/sufentanil infusion) and avoiding hypothermia. Delayed emergence can result in unnecessary CT scans. See **Appendix 18**.

FURTHER READING

1. Baliga S et al. Brain tumors: Medulloblastoma, ATRT, ependymoma. Pediatr Blood Cancer. 2021;68(Suppl 2):e28395.
2. Galbraith K et al. Molecular pathology of gliomas. Surg Pathol Clin. 2021;14(3):379-86.
3. Papic V et al. Primary intraparenchymal meningiomas: a case report and a systematic review. World Neurosurg. 2021;153:52-62.
4. Plant-Fox AS et al. Pediatric brain tumors: the era of molecular diagnostics, targeted and immune-based therapeutics, and a focus on long-term neurologic sequelae. Curr Probl Cancer. 2021;45(4):100777.
5. Tadros S et al. Pathological Features of Brain Metastases. Neurosurg Clin N Am. 2020;31(4):549-64.

Vignette: Longest Glioblastoma Multiforme Survivor

After glioblastoma multiforme (GBM) diagnosis, survival seldom exceeds 12–18 months. However, in 2017, a report from Rome, Italy, described the 22-year-long survival of a male patient with frontal GBM. The patient was 44 year old at the time of diagnosis. He underwent complete resection with follow-up radiotherapy. After surgery, his weakness in the contralateral arm resolved over the next few weeks. The biopsy confirmed GBM, and samples obtained during surgery were repeatedly analyzed afterward. Serial MR and CT follow-ups and clinical examinations remained negative until the age of 66 years when the report was published.

Chapter 20: Brain Edema and Herniation

INTRODUCTION

According to the Monro Kellie doctrine, the sum of brain tissue, cerebrospinal fluid, and blood volume is constant. Should one of these intracranial components increase in volume, it is at the expense of another. Brain edema is a common feature of neurological injuries, leading to the expansion of tissue volume. The increase in tissue volume leads to increased intracranial pressure and, in-extremis, brain herniation. Brain herniation is the displacement of the brain tissue either extracranially or across a dural compartment due to increased intracranial pressure.

CEREBRAL EDEMA

Definition: Cerebral edema is the excessive fluid accumulation in the brain tissue. In the gray matter, a 2% increase in water content (from 80 to 82%) leads to edema. In the white matter, a 9% increase in water content (from 68 to 77%) leads to tissue edema.

Types of Cerebral Edema

Cerebral edema, as previously defined, is an increased tissue water content. However, the clinical picture is often more complex. For example, in the early stages of cytotoxic edema, there may be a shift of water into the cell from the interstitial space without a net increase in tissue water content. When the blood-brain barrier (BBB) is compromised, the water content is further increased in later stages.

Based on the underlying pathology, cerebral edema is classified as:
- *Vasogenic edema:*
  - It is due to the disruption of the BBB.
  - Seen with tumors, trauma, infections, contusions, and hemorrhages.
  - The disruption results in the leakage of proteins across the BBB, resulting in increased fluid in the interstitial space.
  - It mainly affects the white matter.
  - On CT scans:
    - Gray and white matter remain distinct.

CHAPTER 20 Brain Edema and Herniation

- Edema affects the white matter primarily
- Extends in a finger-like fashion
  - On MRI scan:
    - Hyperintense T2 signal
    - Fluid-attenuated inversion recovery (FLAIR) signal
    - No diffusion restriction
- *Cytotoxic edema:*
  - Cytotoxic edema is due to cell energy failure, secondary to anoxia.
  - Failure of ATPase-dependent Na^+/K^+ pump with the accumulation of water in the cells.
  - Consequently, cells swell, and extracellular volume is reduced.
  - It mainly affects gray matter and white matter astrocytes.
  - BBB remains intact, with capillary permeability unaltered.
  - On CT scans:
    - Difficult to detect.
    - Changes seen are due to ionic edema.
  - On MRI scans:
    - No changes in T1 and T2 images
    - High diffusion-weighted imaging (DWI) signal
    - Low apparent diffusion coefficient (ADC) signal
    - Both DWI and ADC track the movement of water molecules, and changes last for days after injury.
    - Diffusion restricted.
- *Ionic edema:*
  - Often conflated with cytotoxic edema
  - It is a later stage of cytotoxic injury due to replenishment of the depleted interstitial Na^+ concentration from the capillaries.
  - The Na^+ gradient leads to an influx of Cl^- and water.
  - Results in interstitial tissue edema that follows cytotoxic edema.
  - Ionic requires some degree of reperfusion. It is thus seen mainly in the periphery of ischemic strokes.
  - On CT scans:
    - Area of low attenuation of signal due to water influx
    - The distribution of edema follows vascular territories.
    - Loss of gray and white matter differentiation
    - Cortical swelling
  - On MRI scans:
    - High T2 signal in gray and white matter
    - Strong FLAIR signal in gray and white matter
    - Some restrictions in diffusion on DWI
- *Combined cerebral edema:*
  - A mixed picture of both vasogenic and cytotoxic edema

- Includes edema due to:
  - Acute hypertension
  - Traumatic brain injury
  - Intoxications
    - Water intoxication/acute hyponatremia
  - Systemic infections:
    - Sepsis
    - Severe inflammation
  - Local infections:
    - Encephalitis
    - Parasitic infections
    - Abscesses
  - Metabolic conditions like
    - Liver failure
    - Reye's syndrome
    - Diabetic ketoacidosis
    - Hyponatremia
    - Carbon monoxide poisoning
    - Lead poisoning
- *CT and MRI:* Mixed cytotoxic and vasogenic features
- *Interstitial cerebral edema:*
  - Increased CSF pressure leads to periventricular edema.
  - Interstitial edema can be due to
    - Acute hydrocephalus
    - Meningitis
  - CSF ventricular outflow is obstructed, and the flow is reversed.
  - Fluid accumulates in the extracellular compartment.
  - Astrocytes swell and are necrosed
  - Radiological shows as a halo around the ventricle
    - Is an early diagnostic feature of hydrocephalus.
- *High altitude cerebral edema (HACE):*
  - Typically seen at 13,000 ft, but can occur at lower altitudes.
  - Usually occurs after 48 hours.
  - Etiology complex: Hypoxia leads to:
    - Impairment of Na^+/K^+ ATPase pump
    - Vasodilation
    - Release of vascular endothelial growth factor (VEGF), cytokines, nitric oxide, and free radicals
  - It can be associated with high-altitude pulmonary edema.
  - Symptoms include headache, nausea, fatigue, anorexia, insomnia, lightheadedness, confusion, and ataxia.
  - Edema can be rapid.
  - Brain herniation can occur in 24 hours.

Management of Cerebral Edema

- Cerebral ischemia can create a vicious cycle of edema, leading to increased intracranial pressure (ICP), decreased cerebral perfusion, worsening ischemia, and edema.
- Three-pronged strategy:
  1. Prevention of cerebral edema:
     - Ensure adequate tissue oxygenation.
     - Ensure adequate tissue perfusion.
     - Safe treatment of hypertension.
     - Improve venous return.
     - Prevent coughing or straining.
     - Anticonvulsants
  2. Treatment of cerebral edema and increased ICP:
     - Steroids are helpful in vasogenic edema but can worsen outcomes in other situations, like traumatic brain injury.
     - Decrease ICP:
       - Hyperventilation
       - Hypertonic agents
       - CSF drainage
       - Decompressive craniectomy
  3. Treating underlying cause:
     - Tumor excision
     - Correction of hyponatremia and other metabolic anomalies
     - Removal of the underlying cause, e.g., lead or carbon monoxide
     - *HACE:* Return to a lower altitude, hyperbaric chamber.

BRAIN HERNIATION (FIG. 1)

- *Clinical features:*
  - Impaired cognition, seizures, or unconsciousness
  - Asymmetric pupils, anisocoria, pupillary dilation
  - Motor weakness, posturing
  - Respiratory irregularities
  - Heart rate and blood pressure changes
  - Hypothalamic insufficiency
  - Respiratory arrest
- *Specific herniation syndrome* (**Table 1**)
- *ICP tracing: See the chapter on ICP monitoring.*
  - Presence of a dicrotic wave with P2 higher than P1 and P3
  - Pathological waves:
    - *A wave or plateau of waves:* Giant (to 50–100 mm Hg) increase in ICP for 5–20 minutes, possibly due to autoregulatory vasodilation

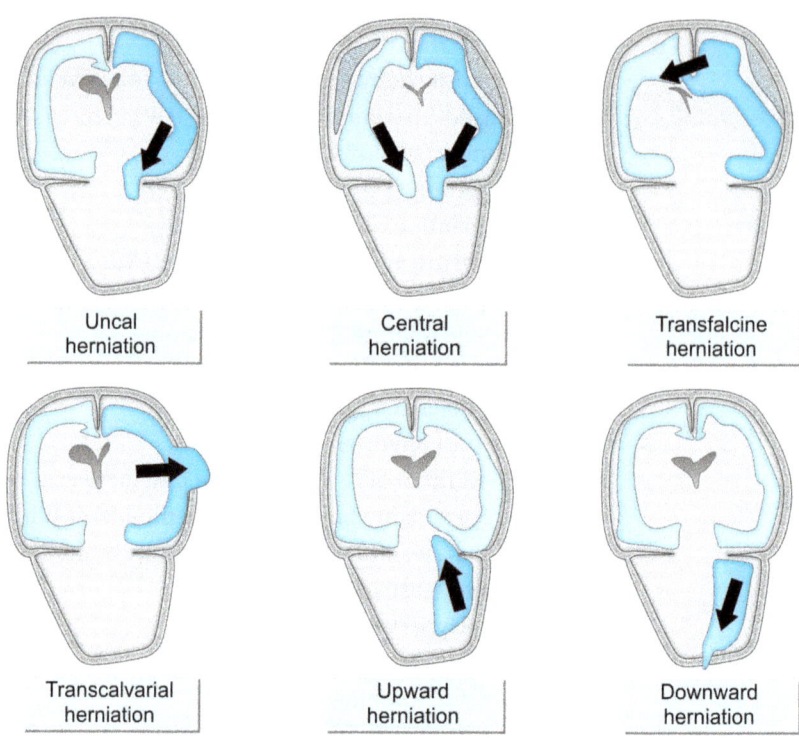

Fig. 1: Types of brain herniation.

in response to tissue ischemia, poor prognosis, and indicates impending brain herniation or irreversible ischemia.
- *B waves:* Spontaneous moderate increase in ICP (to 20–30 mm Hg) at a frequency of 0.5 to 2/min and possibly due to an autoregulatory response to decreased cerebral perfusion pressure (CPP).
- Investigations:
  - Imaging—MRI/CT: Characteristic findings—
    - Tissue displacement
    - Ventricular compression and dilation
    - Tissue infarction
- *Differential diagnosis of brain herniation:* Acute and profound change in consciousness in the setting of known brain injury. These include:
  - Seizures
  - Acute hydrocephalus
  - Tension pneumocephalus
  - CSF over-drainage
  - Meningitis
  - Electrolyte imbalance

CHAPTER 20 Brain Edema and Herniation

Table 1: Types of cerebral herniation.

Types	Site	Clinical features
Supratentorial		
Uncal	Temporal lobe under tentorium cerebelli	*Cushing's triad*: Hypertension, bradycardia, abnormal respiration; evidence of increased ICP: headache, nausea, vomiting, and impaired cognition; eyes: III CN palsy, blurred vision, field cuts, and dilated pupils; motor: contralateral hemiparesis, Babinski's sign +ve, and decorticate posture
Central	Both temporal lobes through tentorium cerebelli	Bilateral non-reacting pinpoint pupil and loss of consciousness
Sub-falcine	Under falx cerebri	The most common type, the ACA is compressed by the cingulate gyrus; contralateral motor weakness; if on dominant site, receptive or sensory aphasia; and ipsilateral weakness
Transcalvarial	Breeched skull	Depends on site
Infratentorial		
"Ascending" transtentorial	Through tentorium cerebelli	Due to the upward displacement of the cerebellum, compression of the brainstem, and occlusion of PCA: Nausea, vomiting with impaired consciousness; can be due to decompression of the lateral ventricles with raised ICP
"Downward" transtentorial	Foramen magnum (central)	Brainstem and upper spinal cord compression with PCA and VA occlusion. Presents with posturing (decorticate, decerebrate, and loss of brainstem reflexes); respiratory changes (Cheyne–Stokes, Biot's, or ataxic and apnea); ultimately leads to fixed dilated pupils and respiratory arrest

(ACA: anterior cerebral artery; CN: cranial nerve; ICP: intracranial pressure; PCA: posterior cerebral artery; VA: ventriculoatrial)

Intraoperative Brain Herniation

Management of a Tight Brain

- The intraoperative tight brain is an example of calvaria herniation.
- A tight brain prevents surgeons from safely accessing the cranial vault contents during surgery.
- A tight brain pushes at the dural edge and does not pulsate with the heartbeat.
- A relaxed brain is covered with a relaxed dura; the dura is easy to separate from the underlying brain tissue, and when the brain is exposed, it is not congested; it does not push on the dural edge and is pulsatile with each heartbeat.
- Rule out light anesthesia, pain, inadequate muscle relaxation, and high peak airway pressures.
- Check head position for impaired venous return.

- Elevate the head (5–10°) to improve venous return.
- Ensure adequate cerebral perfusion pressure.
- Increase minute ventilation (MV) using the following formula:
  - MV desired = (ETCO$_2$ × current MV)/desired ETCO$_2$
  - Send a blood gas to check arterial to end-tidal CO$_2$ gradient.
  - Target PaCO$_2$ 25–35 mm Hg.
  - Check ABG 10–15 minutes after adjusting ventilation.
- *Consider:* (i) Mannitol with a total dose usually not exceeding 1 g/kg; or (ii) 3% saline, usually in 2 mL/kg doses.
- Check the depth of anesthesia if using >1 MAC of volatile anesthetic, give a bolus of propofol 1 mg/kg, and support BP if needed.
- Decrease volatile agents to ≤1 MAC by supplementing total intravenous anesthesia (TIVA). Preferable to shift to TIVA altogether when possible. Ensure adequate paralysis while adjusting anesthetic doses.
- Drain cerebrospinal fluid through the pre-existing spinal drain or via the operating site.
- *Rule out rare causes:* Hypoglycemia, seizures, and remote bleeding from the pin site.
- Discuss the need to extend craniotomy with the surgical team.
- Surgical decompression and removal of herniating brain tissue.

FURTHER READING

1. Deng YY et al. Progress in drug treatment of cerebral edema. Mini Rev Med Chem. 2016;16(11):917-25.
2. Iftikhar S et al. The association of posterior reversible encephalopathy syndrome with COVID-19: a systematic review. Ann Med Surg (Lond). 2021;72:103080.
3. Liotta EM et al. Cerebral edema and liver disease: classic perspectives and contemporary hypotheses on mechanism. Neurosci Lett. 2020;721:134818.
4. Zheng H et al. Mechanism and therapy of brain edema after intracerebral hemorrhage. Cerebrovasc Dis. 2016;42(3-4):155-69.
5. Zusman BE et al. Cerebral edema in traumatic brain injury: a historical framework for current therapy. Curr Treat Options Neurol. 2020;22(3):9

Vignette: Cranial Trephination

Worldwide, some 1,500 skulls have been found that show cranial trephination. Specimens have been found in Europe, Mesoamerica, China, Africa, and Polynesia. The earliest specimens have been found in Gobekli Tepe in Tukey, that date back to 9000 BCE. However, most other trephinations date to 5000–3000 BCE. Many skulls show healing along the edges, suggesting the person survived the surgery. Others show cracking of the skull or an incomplete procedure, which suggests an early adverse outcome. Trephination is mentioned in the Hippocratic treatises. Galen warned that the procedure could lead to unconsciousness. Why did the Neolithic populations undertake such a dangerous operation? Recent excavations in Russia revealed a large group of related individuals, most of whom showed trephination. The finding suggests that trephination was partly a cult practice or had religious significance. Although there could also be medical reasons for such a procedure, such as pain, head injury, epilepsy, or psychiatric disorders.

Chapter 21: Cerebral Aneurysms

INTRODUCTION

Cerebral aneurysms are abnormal focal dilations of intracranial arteries. The patient often presents with an acute onset hemorrhage with neurological deficits due to the disruption of the lesion. Unruptured aneurysms might be diagnosed during an unrelated workup. They may present with headaches, visual deficits, facial paralysis, or hemiparesis.

PATHOLOGY

Incidence: About 2 to 5% of the general population has brain aneurysms, while the incidence of subarachnoid hemorrhage (SAH) is 10 per 100,000.

Location: The anterior communicating and the internal carotid arteries account for two-thirds of all aneurysms, while the middle cerebral artery accounts for another fifth (**Fig. 1**).

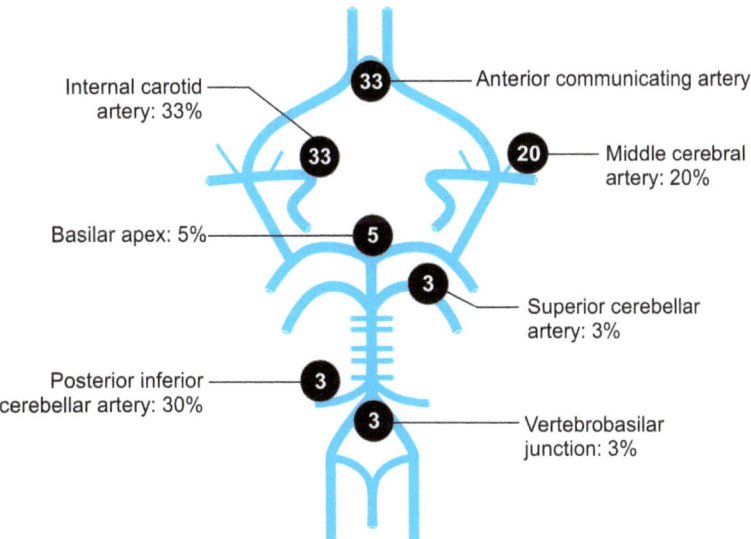

Fig. 1: Location of brain aneurysms.

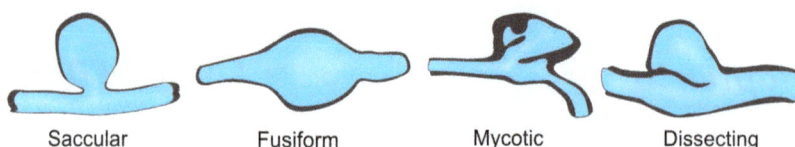

Fig. 2: Types of intracranial aneurysms.

Types: Saccular, fusiform, mycotic, and dissecting **(Fig. 2)**.
- *Saccular aneurysms:* It is the most common type of intracranial aneurysm. Saccular aneurysms are connected to the parent artery with a definable neck. The apex is the weakest part, called the dome, while the body is called the sack. A narrow neck of an aneurysm is favorable to both coiling and clipping.
- *Fusiform aneurysms:* Concentric dilation of the artery with no neck. They are, therefore, challenging to treat and carry a poor prognosis.
- *Mycotic aneurysms:* Mycotic aneurysms occur when infection damages the vessel wall. The infection is usually bacterial and not fungal, as the name suggests.
- *Dissecting aneurysms:* Intimal tears lead to blood collecting in the vessel wall. Over time, progressive weakness leads to aneurysm formation. Dissection of the vessel wall could also lead to the complete occlusion of the artery. Usually, they are amenable to stent treatment.

RISK FACTORS FOR ANEURYSM FORMATION

Flowchart 1 shows the factors that influence the formation and development of cerebral aneurysms.
- *Congenital:*
  - Seen with polycystic kidney disease, connective tissue disorders (Ehlers–Danlos syndrome, Marfan's syndrome, and fibromuscular

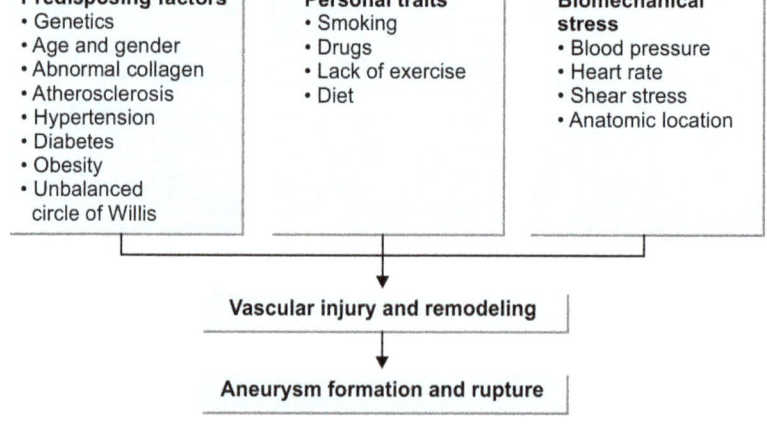

Flowchart 1: Risk factors for aneurysm formation.

Table 1: Approximate % cumulative risk of aneurysm rupture based on size and location.

Location	<7 mm	<7 mm separate aneurysm rupture	7–12 mm	13–25 mm	>25 mm
Cavernous ICA	0%	0%	0%	3%	6%
ACAs, MCA, Non-cavernous ICA	0%	2%	3%	15%	40%
PCA	3%	4%	15%	20%	50%

(ACAs: anterior cerebral or anterior communicating arteries; ICA: internal carotid artery; MCA: middle cerebral artery; PCA: posterior cerebral artery)

dysplasia), Moyamoya disease, and familial clusters of intracranial aneurysms.
- Patients with polycystic kidneys have a 12% chance of intracranial aneurysms that increase to 22% if there is a positive family history of aneurysms or hemorrhagic stroke.
- *Familial cluster:* If there is one affected first-degree relative, then there is a 4% chance for an aneurysm to develop. If there are two affected first-degree relatives, there is a 10% chance of having an aneurysm.
- A previous history of SAH suggests a 15% chance of having other aneurysms.
- *Acquired:*
  - Hypertension
  - Cigarette smoking
  - Cocaine abuse
  - Alcohol abuse.
- *The risk of aneurysm rupture increases with the following* **(Table 1)**:
  - Posterior circulation
  - Anterior communicating artery aneurysm
  - Large aneurysm
  - History of hypertension
  - Cigarette smoking.
- Biomechanical factors showing formation, growth and rupture of aneurysms are shown in **Figure 3**.

CLINICAL PRESENTATION

- *Unruptured aneurysm:*
  - It can be an incidental finding during workups for other complaints, like headaches, cranial nerve palsies, and seizures.
- *Ruptured aneurysms:*
  - *Sentinel hemorrhage:* About 40% of patients have a history of recent severe headaches during the previous month.
  - *Thunderclap headache* is severe, crescendo headache peaking in a minute with nausea, vomiting, obtunded sensorium or coma. May be accompanied by fever and convulsions.

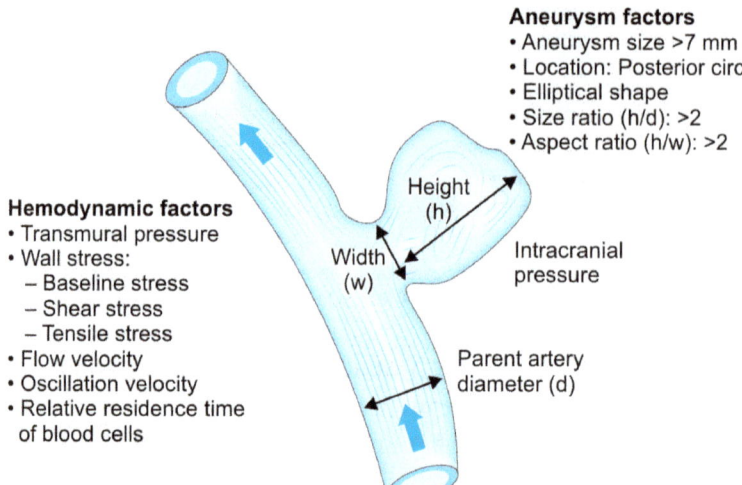

Fig. 3: Mechanical factors affecting aneurysm formation, growth, and rupture.

INVESTIGATIONS

- *Non-contrast CT scan:* Such a scan has 90–100% sensitivity under 6 hours after rupture but decreases afterward.
- MRI T2 FLAIR is highly sensitive for detecting blood.
- *LP:* High opening pressure, blood in cerebrospinal fluid that does not clear in the fourth tube, xanthochromia (most sensitive indicator), and crenated RBCs.
- *CT and LP:* If CT and LP are negative, no workup is recommended.
- CTA may be negative for aneurysms <3 mm
- If the DSA is negative, repeat at 10–14 days; 20% might reveal an aneurysm at this stage.

Indications to Treat an Aneurysm

- Symptomatic aneurysm irrespective of size
- Unruptured aneurysm >7 mm
- Aneurysms in the posterior circulation
- Aneurysm with a secondary lobe
- Increasing size over time
- Life expectancy >5 years

Clipping versus Coiling of Unruptured Aneurysms

- Clipping carries higher earlier morbidity and mortality, but coiling has a greater recanalization rate, delayed rupture, and a higher likelihood of retreatment.
- Neurological complications are marginally more significant with coiling than clipping.

FURTHER READING

1. Chung BJ et al. Identification of hostile hemodynamics and geometries of cerebral aneurysms: a case-control study. AJNR Am J Neuroradiol. 2018;39(10):1860-66.
2. Etminan N et al. Unruptured intracranial aneurysms-pathogenesis and individualized management. Dtsch Arztebl Int. 2020;117(14):235-42.
3. Rousseau O et al. Location of intracranial aneurysms is the main factor associated with rupture in the ICAN population. J Neurol Neurosurg Psychiatry. 2021;92(2):122-8.
4. Texakalidis P et al. Aneurysm formation, growth, and rupture: the biology and physics of cerebral aneurysms. World Neurosurg. 2019;130:277-84.
5. van Kammen MS et al. Heritability of territory of ruptured and unruptured intracranial aneurysms in families. PLoS One, 2020;15(8):e0236714.

Vignette: A Brief History of Brain Aneurysms

Imhotep (2725 BCE), in the Edwin Smit papyri, described the treatment of "vessel swelling" with heated knives, which might be the first surgical treatment of the disease. In the 4th century BC, Hippocrates described "apoplexy" as severe headaches leading to death. E. Flaenius Rufus described the dilation of arteries due to trauma in 117 BCE. Around that time, Galen coined the term "aneurysm" to describe abnormal arterial dilation. "Carotid aneurysm" was first reported in an autopsy by Morgagni in 1761. Francisci Biumi reported the first rupture of an aneurysm, described in an autopsy in 1765. John Blackall described the rupture of a basilar apex aneurysm and fatal subarachnoid hemorrhage in 1810. However, without any imaging methods, the diagnosis of aneurysms remained challenging. Surgeons like Harvey Cushing would insert needles in tumors to determine if they were cysts or aneurysms, often with disastrous consequences. The breakthrough came in 1927 when Egas Moniz injected strontium bromide into a surgically exposed carotid artery to visualize the cerebral vessels of a patient using X-rays. The birth of cerebral angiography permitted an effective treatment of the disease using clipping, trapping, or coiling.

Chapter 22: Subarachnoid Hemorrhage and Cerebral Vasospasm

INTRODUCTION

Subarachnoid hemorrhage (SAH) is blood collected between the pia mater and the arachnoid.

PATHOLOGY

- *Nontraumatic SAH:*
  - *Berry aneurysms:* 80%
  - *Arteriovenous malformations:* 10%
  - *Others 10%:*
    - Mycotic aneurysms
    - Angiomas
    - Neoplasms
    - Cortical vein thrombosis
- *Traumatic SAH:*
  - The most frequent cause of SAH.
  - *Associated with:*
    - Blood over cerebral convexity
    - Other local injuries to the scalp, skull, or brain (contusion) are evident.
    - *A source of bleeding is evident:* Brain contusion, arterial or venous disruption.

PRESENTATION

Prodromal symptoms may herald aneurysmal SAH.
- *Prodromal symptoms:*
  - *Sentinel hemorrhage:* Mild headache and fever-mimicking viral fever
  - *Mass effects:* Isolated cranial nerve palsy, such as with III nerve resulting in ptosis (2%)
  - *Emboli:* History suggestive of TIA or embolic strokes with
    - Sensory or motor disturbances (5%)
    - Seizures (5%)

- *The classic presentation of SAH:*
  - *Thunderclap headache:*
    - Seen in 50% of SAH
    - Conversely, only 10% of thunderclap headaches are due to SAH.
  - Dizziness (10%)
  - Nausea and vomiting
  - Neck rigidity and pain
  - *Visual changes:*
    - Visual disturbances
    - Photophobia
    - Diplopia (2%)
    - Orbital pain (5%)
  - Loss of consciousness
  - Seizures

EXAMINATION

- Hypertension and tachycardia
- Fever
- *Meningeal signs:*
  - *Neck rigidity:* Resistance felt on flexing the neck.
  - *Kernig's sign:* With the patient lying flat and the hip and knees flexed to 90°, patients experience pain and spasms extending the knee beyond 135°.
  - *Brudzinski's sign:* With the patient lying flat and palm restraining the chest, the flexion of the neck causes involuntary flexion of the hips.
- Retinal hemorrhage
- Papilledema
- Focal and global neurological signs

INVESTIGATION

- *Routine:*
  - Complete blood count
  - Basic metabolic profile
  - Coagulation studies
  - Arterial blood gas
  - EKG and cardiac enzymes
  - Chest X-ray
- *Neurological:*
  - Lumbar puncture
  - **Table 1** distinguishes between traumatic tap and SAH.
- *Imaging studies:*
  - CT scan

Table 1: Features of blood in the CSF sample due to traumatic tap vs. SAH.

	Traumatic tap	SAH
Clinical syndrome	It depends on the underlying disease	Headache, nuchal rigidity, and fever features suggestive of irritation due to SAH
Appearance	Bloody but clears over time	Blood tinged does not change
RBCs	Decline	Persist >100,000/mm^3
RBC morphology	Normal RBCs	Crenated RBCs
WBC: RBC ratio	Same as blood	Greater than blood
Spun supernatant	Clear	Xanthochromic
Clotting	Possible	Unlikely
Protein content	<serum proteins	> serum proteins
LP at a higher level	Usually normal	Xanthochromic

(LP: lumbar puncture)

- CT angiography
- If CT negative:
    - MRI
    - MRA may not rule out aneurysms.
- Digital subtraction angiography is the gold standard.

HUNT AND HESS GRADE: CLINICAL ASSESSMENT

I. Mild headache or asymptomatic
II. Moderate-to-severe headache, neck rigidity, and cranial nerve deficits only
III. Drowsiness, confusion, and mild (usually motor) deficits
IV. Stupor with severe deficits
V. Moribund

MODIFIED FISHER'S GRADE ON COMPUTED TOMOGRAPHY

- *Grade 0:* No SAH or intraventricular hemorrhage evident, Clinical vasospasm risk 0%
- *Grade 1:* Focal or diffuse thin SAH with no intraventricular hemorrhage. Clinical vasospasm risk 24%
- *Grade 2:* Focal or diffuse SAH with intraventricular hemorrhage. Clinical vasospasm risk 33%
- *Grade 3:* Thick SAH without intraventricular hemorrhage. Clinical vasospasm risk 33%
- *Grade 4:* Thick SAH with Intraventricular hemorrhage. Clinical vasospasm risk 40%

RISK OF INTRACRANIAL HEMORRHAGE IN NEUROSURGICAL DISEASES

- *With brain aneurysms:*
  - *Chances of rebleed: Day 1:* 4%; *Day 2:* 2%; and *Day 3-14 days:* 0.2% each day
  - *The risk of rebleeding:* 20% in the first two weeks and 50% in 6 months.
  - Hence, the urgency to treat early.
- *With traumatic brain injury (TBI) have:*
  - Approximately 30% of patients TBI coagulopathy
  - Factors that increase the risk of bleeding after TBI:
    - Glasgow coma score <8
    - Systolic blood pressure <90
    - Pre-hospital fluid infusion of more than 2L
    - Age >75
- *With AVM bleed:*
  - An AVM bleed is usually parenchymal and intraventricular, rarely subarachnoid bleed.
  - The overall risk of AVM hemorrhage ranges from 2-8% annually.

COMPLICATIONS OF SUBARACHNOID HEMORRHAGE

- *Cerebral effects of SAH:*
  - *Direct and indirect effects of blood over time:*
    - Mass effect and increased intracranial pressure (ICP)
    - Abnormal vascular reactivity, even in the absence of cerebral vasospasm
    - Focal neurological symptoms
- *Cerebral vasospasm:*
  - *Angiographic spasm* is seen in 30% of patients after SAH. Half of those patients have clinical symptoms. The usual symptoms are changes in cognition, pronator drift, impaired speech, or motor weakness. With the occurrence of the symptoms, vasospasm is described as *"symptomatic vasospasm".*
  - *Delayed ischemic neurological deficit (DIND)* is the occurrence of new neurological deficits, typically in the second week after SAH. Vasospasm is often diagnosed at the bedside using a transcranial Doppler that reveals an increase in the flow velocity.
  - On angiography, cerebral vasospasm can be *proximal* (seen as a local narrowing of the major arteries) or *distal* (increased contrast transit time). About 50% of all patients with SAH develop vasospasm as diagnosed by TCD. About 30% demonstrate narrowing on an angiogram. 20-40% of patients with demonstrable SAH develop neurological symptoms depending on the severity of the bleeding.

- The incidence of vasospasm after SAH depends on the following:
  - Amount of blood in the basal cisterns
  - History of hypertension
  - History of smoking
  - Left ventricular hypertrophy on EKG
  - Other risk factors for vasospasm include a history of rebleed, poor glycemic control, excessive alcohol intake, leukocytosis, and in patients with prolonged QTc.

Ultrasonic Diagnosis of Cerebral Vasospasm

- Middle cerebral artery (MCA) velocity measurements through the temporal window are possible in 90% of the cases.
- Normal MCA systolic flow velocity = 60 cm/s
- Mild spasm MCA systolic flow velocity >120 cm/s
- Moderate spasm MCA systolic flow velocity >160 cm/s
- Severe spasm MCA systolic flow velocity >200 cm/s

Lindegaard's Ratio

Lindegaard's ratio: The ratio between blood flow velocity in the MCA to the ipsilateral internal carotid artery (ICA). An increase in flow velocity could be due to either vasospasm or a net increase in cerebral blood flow. The two are differentiated by calculating Lindegaard's ratio. The significant values are:

- *<3:* No vasospasm and possible hyperemia
- *3–4.5:* Mild vasospasm
- *4.5–6:* Moderate vasospasm
- *>6:* Severe vasospasm

Management of Cerebral Vasospasm

- The therapeutic goals are to maintain perfusion pressure, correct hypovolemia, and avoid anemia.
- The classical triple H therapy (hypervolemia, hypertension, and hemodilution) has not proven beneficial.
- *Blood pressure targets:*
  - If the aneurysm is clipped, systolic BP can be increased to 180–200 mm Hg to increase cerebral perfusion.
  - If untreated, systolic BP is limited to 140–150 mm Hg.
- IV nimodipine is preferred to treat vasospasm. Nicardipine can cause systemic hypotension and is primarily used as an antihypertensive.

- Intra-arterial verapamil is used to treat vasospasm when medical management fails. It can cause bradycardia, hypotension, and an increase in ICP.
- *Others:* Magnesium sulfate, statins, and endothelin antagonists.

Cardiac Injury

Massive catecholamine surge adversely affects the myocardium (Takotsubo syndrome), especially in the elderly. Microinfarcts can be seen on autopsy.

- *Arrhythmias:*
  - Seen in most patients, are usually transient, lasting three days.
  - ST segment changes and conduction defects
  - Atrial and ventricular ectopy
- *Myocardial injuries:*
  - Elevated BNP
  - Elevated troponins
  - Wall motion abnormalities
  - Cardiogenic shock
  - *Takotsubo syndrome:* Echocardiogram shows hypokinesia unrelated to vascular distribution. Four types of syndromes are described based on the region of the left ventricle that is hypokinetic:
    - *Apical type:* Most common
    - *Global type:* Worst outcome
    - Mid-ventricular type
    - Basal type

Pulmonary Injury

Etiology: Pulmonary injury after SAH can be due to the following:
- Aspiration
- Acute respiratory distress syndrome (ARDS)
- Transfusion-related acute lung injury (TRALI) in TBI cases
- *Neurogenic pulmonary edema (NPE):*
  - Acute respiratory distress due to central nervous system injury is usually due to hypothalamic or brainstem disturbances. It is characterized by extravascular accumulation of interstitial fluid within 30–60 minutes but usually <4 hours after neural injury.
  - *Clinical features:* Pulmonary edema with dyspnea, tachypnea, rales, and crackles
  - *Diagnostic findings:* Hypoxemia, $P_{(A-a)}O_2$ >200 mm Hg; leukocytosis; CXR bilateral alveolar infiltrates and cardiomegaly.
  - *The trigger for NPE:* Intracranial hemorrhage, traumatic brain injury, stroke, epilepsy, intracranial infections; *postoperative:* posterior fossa surgery and carotid endarterectomy, ECT, and drugs, e.g., amphetamines

- *Etiology:* Catecholamine storm: systemic hypertension, systemic vasoconstriction, pulmonary volume load, increased pulmonary capillary permeability, fluid exudation, and pulmonary edema combined with cardiogenic shock.
- *Differential diagnosis of NPE:*
  - Cardiogenic pulmonary edema
  - Aspiration pneumonia
  - Pneumonitis
  - Transfusion-related acute lung injury (TRALI)
  - Negative pressure pulmonary edema
  - Sepsis
- *Treatment:*
  - *Supportive:* Ventilation, oxygenation, fluids, vasoactive drugs, and diuretics
  - Positive end-expiratory pressure (PEEP) with inotropic support using norepinephrine and dobutamine.
  - Steroid use remains controversial unless NPE is related to brain tumors.
  - Milrinone is effective in NPE when due to brainstem encephalitis.
  - *In refractory cases:* ECMO is needed but carries a high risk of intracranial hemorrhages.
- *The outcome of NPE:*
  - Resolves within 72 hours in 50%
  - *If unresolved, it carries high mortality:* 60–100%
  - Worse with Takotsubo syndrome
- Pituitary dysfunction:
  - Decreased cortisol.
  - Diabetes Insipidus
- Metabolic dysfunction:
  - Hyperglycemia
  - Hyponatremia
  - Hypocalcemia
  - Hypomagnesemia

OUTCOME OF SUBARACHNOID HEMORRHAGE

- The risk of poor outcome after aneurysmal SAH include:
  - Age >70
  - Poor Fisher grade
  - Poor World federation of Neurosurgeons' grade IV and V
  - Aneurysms >20 mm
- Death after SAH is likely due to cerebral infarction.

CHAPTER 22 Subarachnoid Hemorrhage and Cerebral Vasospasm

- Despite treatment, 20% of the patients with SAH die in a hospital, 40% have a good neurological outcome, and 40% have severe neurological deficits.
- Perhaps the most reliable way of predicting outcome of SAH is the neurological assessment after initial resuscitation using the World Federation of Neurosurgical Societies Scale. The WFNS Scale that ranks SAH from Grades I to V based on Glasgow Coma scale (GCS) values.
  - Grade I: GCS 15, 70% survival.
  - Grade II: GCS 14, 60% survival.
  - Grade III: GCS 13, 50% survival.
  - Grade IV: GCS 7–12, 30% survival.
  - Grade V: GCS 3–6, 10% survival.

FURTHER READING

1. Alotaibi AS et al. Central nervous system causes of sudden unexpected death: a comprehensive review. Cureus. 2022;14(1):e20944.
2. Goertz L et al. Impact of aneurysm morphology on aneurysmal subarachnoid hemorrhage severity, cerebral infarction and functional outcome. J Clin Neurosci. 2021;89:343-8.
3. Muhammad S et al. Inflammation and anti-inflammatory targets after aneurysmal subarachnoid hemorrhage. Int J Mol Sci. 2021;22(14):7355.
4. Stokum JA et al. When the blood hits your brain: the neurotoxicity of extravasated blood. Int J Mol Sci. 2021;22(10):5132.
5. Xu Z et al. Intracranial aneurysms: pathology, genetics, and molecular mechanisms. Neuromolecular Med. 2019;21(4):325-43.

Vignette: Understanding "Apoplexy"

In the 5th Century BCE, Hippocrates believed that apoplexy was due to the bile collection in the brain. The obstruction blocked the flow of animal spirits contained in the ventricles. Galen thought apoplexy was due to the blockage of humor by phlegm. However, the cause of apoplexy remained confusing for the next 2000 years. A Swiss physician, Johann Jakob Wepfer, first described the anatomy of cerebral circulation, including the Circle of Willis. Wepfer, in 1658, provided correlations between clinical features and autopsy findings in cases of apoplexy. Wepfer distinguished between hemorrhagic and embolic strokes. One year later, William Cole, an English physician, coined the term "stroke" to modernize the ancient concept of apoplexy.

Chapter 23
Pathophysiology of Arteriovenous Malformations

INTRODUCTION
Arteriovenous malformations (AVM) are developmental abnormalities in which arteries, through a network of dysmorphic vessels, directly drain into veins without the intervening capillaries. The pathological lesion appears to be a tangled mass of blood vessels that causes symptoms due to its bulk, location, changes in cerebral and systemic hemodynamics, or due to rupture.

PATHOLOGY
- *Arteriovenous malformations:* Although considered congenital, brain AVMs present in the third or fourth decade of life, which on imaging, appear as a tangle of abnormal vessels.
- They are the most common vascular malformations of the brain. Venous malformation and cavernous malformations are less frequent abnormalities.
- About 1% of the general population is diagnosed with AVMs. However, they are found in 2% of autopsies suggesting that the disease often remains asymptomatic.
- They account for about 1% of all intracranial bleeds.

CEREBROVASCULAR EFFECTS OF AVMs
- AVMs are usually divided into a high-flow region called the "*nidus*" and a surrounding region of dysplastic vessels. There is usually one or more feeding arteries supplying the lesion. The hemodynamic effects of the AVM can extend beyond the lesion and create a hypotensive zone **(Fig. 1)**.
- AVM vessels do not demonstrate vascular reactivity. As a result, the increased flow through the lesion rapidly increases the shear on the vessel wall. AVM vessels are dysplastic and structurally deficient. The breach of walls can lead to bleeding with minimal hemodynamic stress. Hemosiderin deposits are often seen in AVMs and are suggestive of past rupture. Thrombosis is frequently seen within the AVM vessels and, in some instances, can lead to spontaneous regression of the lesion.

CHAPTER 23 Pathophysiology of Arteriovenous Malformations

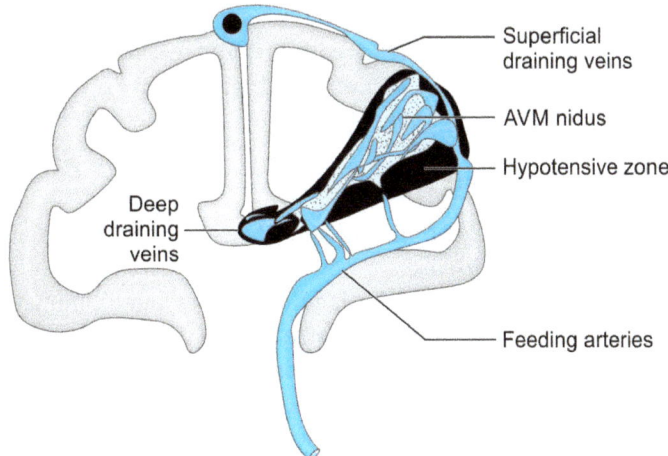

Fig. 1: AVM with hypotensive zone shown in solid black.
(AVM: arteriovenous malformation)

- AVMs have been characterized based on their size as small (<3 cm), medium (3-6 cm), or large (>6 cm) or their blood flow of low (200-500 mL/min), medium (500-1,000 mL/min), or high (>1,000 mL/min).
- Blood flow through the AVM can result in shunting blood from around the lesion and decrease the regional perfusion pressure, thus creating a hypotensive zone. The region around the AVM adapts to such chronic hypotension and preserves neurological functions.
- Ablation of the AV fistula can result in a sudden increase in the perfusion of the hypotensive zone surrounding the AVM, potentially leading to postoperative bleeding.
- About 10% of the AVMs are associated with aneurysms.

CLINICAL PRESENTATION
- Usually present in young individuals.
- *Symptoms:*
  - *Intracranial hemorrhage:* 50%: Headache, nausea, vomiting, change in consciousness.
  - *New onset seizures:* 25%
  - *Asymptomatic, incidentally diagnosed:* 15%
  - *Progressive neurological deficits:* 10%
- *Bleeding from AVMs:*
  - Usually, parenchymal or intraventricular
  - The overall risk of AVM hemorrhage for a patient is 2-8% per year.
  - AVMs at greater risk of bleeding include:
    - Those presenting as hemorrhage.

- Small AVMs <3 cm diameter
- High feeding artery pressure
- Deep venous drainage
- Intranidal aneurysms

INVESTIGATIONS

- *Cerebral angiography* is the gold standard for the diagnosis of the disease.
  - Identifies feeding arteries and draining veins.
  - Reveals the structure of the nidus.
  - Provides an estimate of the volume of flow through the lesion.
- *Magnetic resonance imaging:*
  - Reveals the location and size of the lesion.
  - Can identify high-flow areas
  - Can reveal complications, such as:
    - hemorrhage
    - edema
    - atrophy
- *Computed tomography:*
  - Reveals the location and size of the lesion.
  - Unruptured AVMs have no edema and no mass effect.
  - Due to hyperdense signals from blood in the normal brain, AVM hemorrhage is difficult to detect on CT scans.
  - CT angiogram can show the flow dynamics of the lesion.
  - In contrast-CT, the lesion appears as a "bag of worms".

ANESTHETIC IMPLICATIONS

- Unlike aneurysms, bleeding from the AVM is not directly related to the arterial or transmural pressure gradient.
- Rebleed rates are much lower for AVMs than aneurysms.
- Hypertensive episodes are better tolerated as the AV fistula decompresses the increase in pressure.
- Surgical resection of the AVM is complicated because extensive dissection may be required to gain access to the arterial feeders. These are first ligated, while the draining veins are last to resect.
- Postoperative bleeding can occur from the AVM residue or dysplastic arteries in the AVM bed.
- High-resolution imaging is often done to ensure complete resection after surgery.

ANEURYSM VS AVM SURGERY

Aneurysm versus AVM surgery is shown in **Table 1**.

Table 1: Aneurysm versus AVM surgery.

	Aneurysms	AVMs
Clinical picture		
Incidence	20% of all strokes	Rare
Age at presentation	75% incidence 45–65 years	Peak incidence 10–30 years
Risk of bleeding	2% per day post bleed	2% per year
Hemodynamic factors affecting bleed	BP management critical	BP is one of the several factors affecting bleed
Consequences of bleed	Catastrophic	Relatively mild
Anesthetic management		
Arterial line	Awake	Can be placed after induction
Hyperventilation	Decreasing ICP can increase transmural pressure prior to bone flap removal	To decrease the mass effect
Hypothermia	Indicated to protect the brain	Avoided to minimize coagulopathy
Temporary occlusion	Often may require an increase in CO_2 and BP	Not needed; AVM surgery arterial feeders occluded before draining veins
Post-treatment management	BP near normal	Mild hypertension to test surgical hemostasis after resection
Postoperative angiogram	In the ORs	In angiographic suite

(AVM: arteriovenous malformation)

MOYAMOYA DISEASE

Moyamoya disease: Moyamoya in Japanese means "*puff of tobacco smoke*". The term describes its angiographic characteristic. The disease presents ischemic stroke in children (juvenile form) or, in adults, intracerebral hemorrhage (ICH). The underlying pathology is a result of stenosis of the carotid artery or its major branches. Consequently, hypoperfusion results in distal reactive capillary, AVM, or aneurysm formation. Moyamoya disease (MMD) has to be ruled out in any child with a stroke.

Pathology

- The pathological feature of MMD is the progressive stenosis of the cerebral arteries with the development of basal collateral channels that yield the characteristic angiographic picture.
- The primary pathology seems to be intimal proliferation and inflammation leading to progressive stenosis, but the typical picture may not always be evident:
  - In classical MMD, stenosis is bilateral but can be unilateral.
  - Reactive blood vessel formation might not be seen in the early stages.

- *Incidence in Japan:* 4/100,000 population; the incidence is less in the United States.
- There is a 2:1 female preponderance and a familial predisposition.
- The etiology of primary MMD is unknown. Genetic predisposition, abnormal stem cells, aberrant cytokine response, and abnormal vascular proliferation all seem to play some role.
- Almost 95% of patients with familial MMD in the East Asian population have the Ring finger (RNF213) gene. The gene is also found in 80% of the sporadic MMD but less than 2% of the general population.
- Secondary MMD is associated with inflammatory diseases of the head and neck, such as Graves' Disease, systemic lupus erythematosus (SLE), meningitis, traumatic brain injury (TBI), and radiation treatment.
- *Clinical course:*
  - Progressive disease major stroke or death in 75% within two years.
  - *Juvenile disease:* Transient ischemic attack (TIA) in 41%, stroke in 40%, and neurological symptoms with crying (hyperventilation).
  - *Adult disease:* Hemorrhages are seen in 60% of the patients. The location can be thalamic, intraventricular, or subarachnoid.
- *Diagnosis:*
  - CT, MRI or MRA, and angiography can reveal the lesion.
  - *Rete mirabile:* Abnormal communication between an internal carotid artery (ICA) and the external carotid artery (ECA).
  - Blood flow studies, PET or Xe CT, show a decrease in cerebral blood flow (CBF) in children while being relatively normal in adults.
- *Angiographic Suzuki grades:*
  - *Stage 1:* Narrowing of ICA apex
  - *Stage 2:* Initiation of Moyamoya collateral; anterior cerebral artery (ACA), middle cerebral artery (MCA), and posterior cerebral artery (PCA) are dilated.
  - *Stage 3:* Progressive collateral development with ICA narrowing
  - *Stage 4:* Circle of Willis occluded, extracranial-to-intracranial collateral develop, and Moyamoya vessels regress
  - *Stage 5:* Disease advances
  - *Stage 6:* Complete absence of cerebral arteries and Moyamoya vessels.

Treatment

Medical Management

Conservative management is unproven. Strategies to prevent stroke (such as antiplatelet drugs, anticoagulants, and steroids), measures to augment blood flow (such as calcium-channel blockers, mannitol, and hemodilution), or those to prevent infection (antibiotics) have been ineffective.

Surgery

- Decompression of hematoma
- *MCA revascularization:*
  - Superior temporal artery–middle cerebral artery (STA–MCA) bypass
  - *Encephalo-myo-synangiosis (EMS):* Temporalis muscle graft put on the cortex
  - *Encephalo-duro-arterio-synangiosis (EDAS):* STA stitched to dura
  - Omental graft with vascular pedicle
- *ACA revascularization:* Burr holes and glial ribbon
- Stellate ganglion block

Anesthesia Management

Concerns in Children

- High cerebral metabolic rate for oxygen in children
- Critical reduction in blood flow at the baseline
- Cerebral blood flow (CBF) may decrease with crying-induced hyperventilation.
- Hypoventilation due to excessive sedation may lead to cerebral steal, i.e., diversion of blood flow from ischemic regions.
- Preoperative hydration.
- Consider pre-medication with midazolam.
- Consider preoperative EEG monitoring, if possible.
- Inhalation or IV induction as clinically needed.
- Invasive arterial blood pressure monitoring
- Essential to maintain hemodynamic stability:
  - Avoid hypertension that can disrupt fragile vessels.
  - Avoid hypotension that may decrease cerebral perfusion pressure.
- Mild hypercapnia with a $PaCO_2$ of about 40-45 mm Hg is desirable to augment collateral blood flow.

Adult Moyamoya Disease

- Hemorrhage risk is significant due to the fragility of vessels, yet the tissue is ischemic; therefore, rigorous BP control is needed.
- Patients are often obese; OSA risk assessed.
- Awake arterial line and close hemodynamic and $PaCO_2$ monitoring essential.
- EEG/SSEP might be used; therefore, consider total intravenous anesthesia (TIVA).
- Avoid hypo- or excessive hypercapnia; target $PaCO_2$ of 40–45 mm Hg.
- Avoid hyper- or hypotension.

Postoperative Concerns

- No immediate benefits from indirect bypass procedures; tissue takes months to revascularize.
- Extubation is desired to permit neurological examination after surgery.
- Smooth hemodynamic control during extubation
- Hypotension can lead to graft occlusion.
- Stroke, TIA, and ICH are possible.
- Delayed awakening may need a CT scan to rule out bleeding.
- Aspirin may be started on the second postoperative day to prevent graft occlusion.
- A cerebrospinal fluid leak is possible under skin closure.

FURTHER READING

1. Chen CJ et al. Brain arteriovenous malformations: a review of natural history, pathobiology, and interventions. Neurology. 2020;95(20):917-27.
2. Florian IA et al. An insight into the microRNAs associated with arteriovenous and cavernous malformations of the brain. Cells. 2021;10(6):1373.
3. Florian IA et al. 'De Novo' Brain AVMs-hypotheses for development and a systematic review of reported cases. Medicina (Kaunas). 2021;57(3):201.
4. Koch MJ et al. Dynamic changes in arteriovenous malformations (AVMs): spontaneous growth and resolution of AVM-associated aneurysms in two pediatric patients. Pediatr Neurosurg. 2019;54(6):394-8.
5. Sakata A et al. Evaluation of cerebral arteriovenous shunts: a comparison of parallel imaging time-of-flight magnetic resonance angiography (TOF-MRA) and compressed sensing TOF-MRA to digital subtraction angiography. Neuroradiology. 2021;63(6):879-87.

Vignette: Brain Arteriovenous Malformation

The Egyptians, in 1500 BCE, were probably aware of brain AVMs. However, the history of the disease is relatively recent. Luschka and Virchow, in the mid-19th century, described brain AVMs as vascular hamartomas or tumors. Steinheil provided the first clinical description of the disease in 1895. The development of angiography by Egaz Moniz in 1927 paved the way for the in-vivo detection of the disease. Bergstrand first angiographically diagnosed the condition in 1936. The first AVM was resected in 1932 by Herbert Olivecrona, a Swedish neurosurgeon. Much of the recent research in cerebral AVMs was pioneered by the late William L. Young, a neuroanesthesiologist.

Chapter 24: Surgical Treatment of Chronic Pain

INTRODUCTION

Pain that persists beyond its beneficial purpose of alerting that a tissue injury has occurred that lasts for more than three months is called chronic pain. Chronic pain is a complex entity that has mixed characteristics of two extremes: (1) neuropathic pain and (2) nociceptive pain **(Table 1)**.

PATHOLOGY OF CHRONIC PAIN (FIG. 1)

Abnormal pain perception can arise due to disorders of:
- *Transduction:* Abnormal transduction of pain triggers.
- *Transmission:* Abnormal transmission to the spinal cord.
- *Modulation:* Abnormal modulation in the peripheral and central nervous systems.
- *Perception:* Abnormal psychogenic response.

Abnormal Transduction

- Transduction is the process through which receptors convert mechanical, chemical, and thermal stimuli into electrical impulses.
- There are three types of pain receptors: (1) nociceptive mechanoreceptors, (2) nociceptive mechanothermal receptors, and (3) polymodal receptors.

Table 1: Neuropathic and nociceptive pain.

	Neuropathic pain	Nociceptive pain
Source	Neural injury, may have sensory/motor deficits	Tissue injury, may have evidence of inflammation
Nature	Sharp shooting well-localized; spontaneous, random	Dull, aching, throbbing; triggered by activity
Pain hypersensitivity	Allodynia (nonpainful stimuli cause pain), hyperalgesia	Local hyperalgesia possible
Skin changes	Altered color or temperature, swelling, and sudomotor changes	Rare
Radiation	Distal along the dermatome	Proximal diffuse

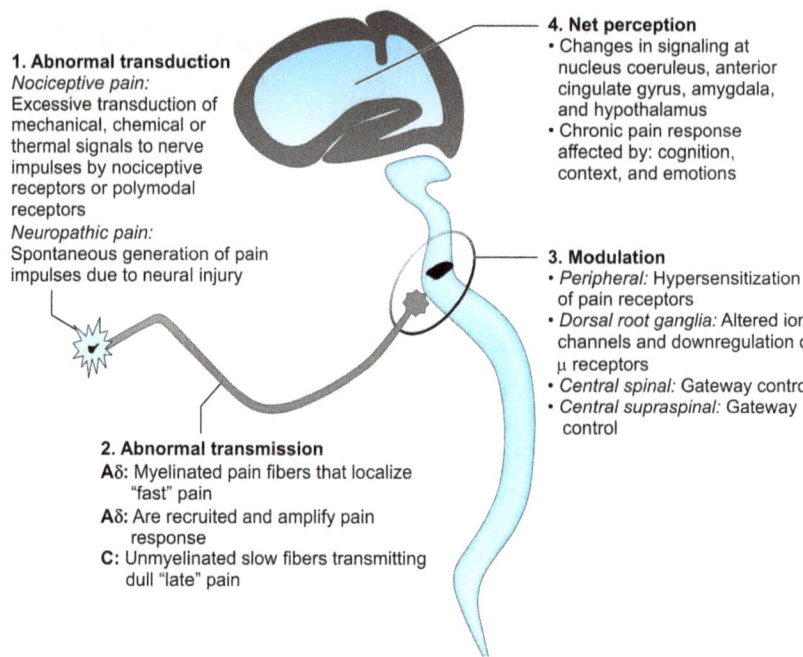

Fig. 1: Pathogenesis of chronic pain.

- *Nociceptive receptors:*
    - They are naked nerve endings of Aδ- and C-fibers
    - The Aδ mechanoreceptor and mechanothermal receptors sharply localize the pain
    - Polymodal pain receptors respond to chemical, mechanical, and thermal stimuli. They transmit through unmyelinated C-fibers.
    - These receptors have voltage- or ligand-gated ion channels:
        - Voltage-gated channels, such as Na^+ channels, play a significant role in neuropathic pain.
        - Ligand-gated channels respond to inflammatory cytokines and play a substantial role in nociceptive pain.

Abnormal Transmission
- *Two types of fibers usually transmit pain:*
    1. *Aδ-fibers:*
        - The Aδ fibers are linked to nociceptive mechano- or thermal receptors.
        - Are myelinated.
        - Sharply localize the pain.
        - The conduction velocity is about 5–30 m/s.
        - Generate the fast response to pain known as "fast pain".

2. *C-fibers:*
   - C-fibers are linked to the polymodal naked nerve endings.
   - They are small unmyelinated fibers.
   - Diffuse pain localization.
   - The conduction velocity is 0.5–2.3 m/s.
   - Generate a slow response to pain known as "late pain."
- *Additionally, Aβ-fibers are recruited in chronic pain:*
  - These fibers usually innervate:
    - *Pacinian corpuscles:* Sense deep pressure and high-frequency vibrations.
    - *Meissner's corpuscles:* Low-frequency vibration and fine touch.
  - *Are heavily myelinated:*
    - Transmit impulses at 30–70 m/s.
    - However, in chronic pain, these nerve fibers can increase the excitability of spinal cord neurons.

Abnormal Modulation

Abnormal modulation of pain in chronic pain state occurs at several levels:
- *Modulation of pain receptors:*
  - Sensitization of pain receptors is due to the peripheral release of tissue metabolites. These include:
    - Fatty acids and prostaglandins increase cGMP and lower the action potential threshold.
    - Release of other mediators:
      - Calcitonin G-related peptide
      - Substance P
      - *Others:* Bradykinins, growth factors, and cytokines.
    - *Sensitization* of pain receptors results in excessive pain signals relative to injury.
- *Modulation at the dorsal root ganglion:*
  - Enhanced pain response can be due to several changes in the signal pathway at the dorsal ganglion level. These include:
    - Abnormal Na channels lead to excessive or spontaneous discharge by dorsal root ganglion cells.
    - Excessive discharge by voltage-gated Ca^{++} channels in the dorsal root ganglia and spinal cord.
    - Increased sensitization to glutamate causes persistent pain.
    - Downregulation of μ opioid receptors.
- *Spinal pain modulation:*
  - Gateway control theory **(Fig. 2)**:
    - Injury activates pain C-fibers; however, the simultaneous activation of large Aδ-fibers (touch/vibration) inhibit pain transmission.

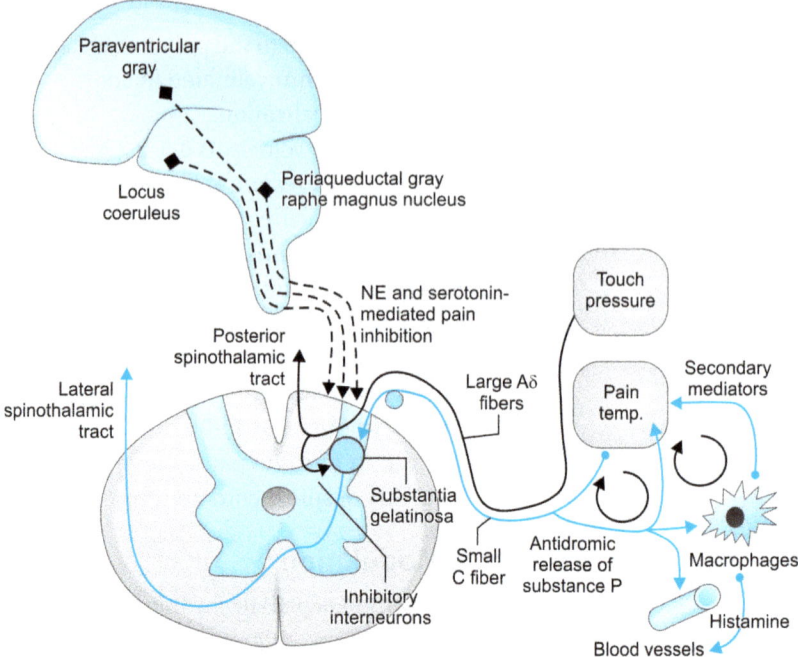

Fig. 2: Modulating chronic pain by gateway control theory and descending tracts. (NE: norepinephrine)

- Pain and temperature activate the small C-fibers. The C-fibers relay to the Rexed lamina II synapse. They release excitatory neurotransmitters and substance P. Through the interneurons, they activate forward pain transmission through the anterior and lateral spinothalamic tracts. In addition, the antidromic release of substance P also enhances peripheral pain sensitization.
- The Aβ and Aδ- fibers are activated by gently rubbing the injury site. These fibers ascend in the posterior spinothalamic tracts. From there, interneurons converge on the substantia gelatinosa and release glutamate that inhibits pain transmission.

- *Supraspinal pain modulation:* Several nuclei in the mid-brain can inhibit pain transmission at the spinal level. Descending fibers can be norepinephrinergic (e.g., periventricular gray matter) or serotonergic fibers (e.g., locus coeruleus) that descend on substantia gelatinosa and inhibit pain transmission.

Abnormal Perception

- The state of cognition, the context of pain, and the emotional state modulate pain perception.
- Many regions of the brain that modulate sleep, anxiety, and depression play a role in chronic pain perception. They also have some degree of

neurotransmitter overlap. These brain centers provide targets for surgical interventions for ablative or stimulatory treatments. Potential anatomical targets for treating chronic pain and its affective manifestations are shown in **Figure 3**.

- Anormal pain perception can be due to the following:
  - The imbalances in neurotransmitters such as dopamine, GABA, norepinephrine, opioids, and serotonin
  - Abnormal signal modulation in the medulla and the periaqueductal gray.
  - *Abnormal central processing:* The locus coeruleus, anterior cingulate gyrus, amygdala, and hypothalamus play a role in pain perception and emotional response.

SURGICAL INTERVENTIONS FOR CHRONIC PAIN

- *Although surgery (Fig. 3) offers several sites for intervention in patients with chronic pain, the overall strategy is to use multimodality narcotic-sparing treatments (Fig. 4). These surgical interventions include:*
- *Decompressive procedures:*
  - *Nerve decompression:*
    - *Peripheral nerves:* For example, median nerve decompression for carpal tunnel syndrome.
    - *Cranial nerves:* For example, microscopic decompression of the trigeminal nerve

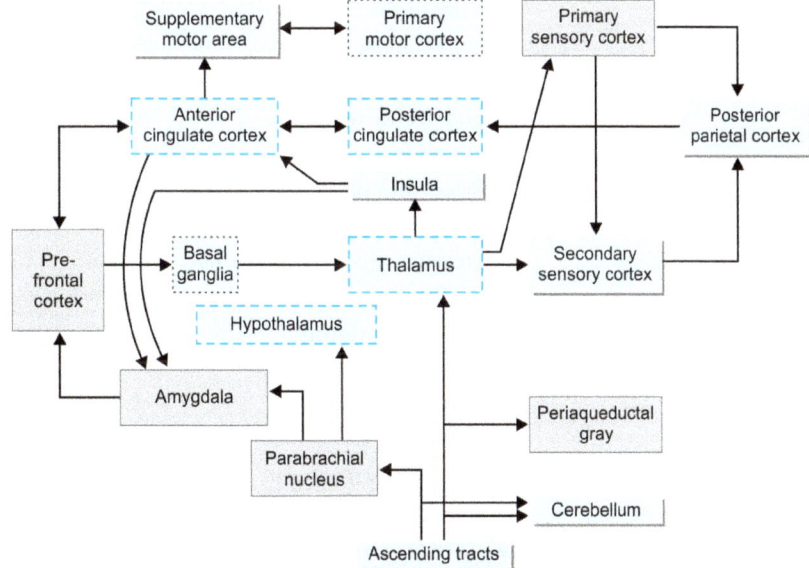

Fig. 3: Chronic pain treatment by ablation (dashed) or stimulation (dotted) of specific structures in the afferent pain pathways.

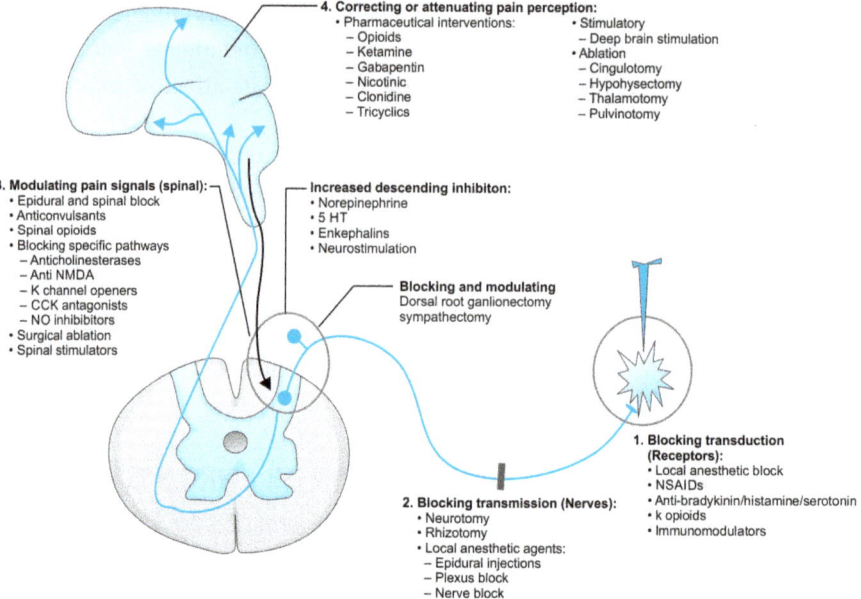

Fig. 4: Strategy to treat chronic pain. (CCK: cholecystokinin; NMDA: N-methyl-d-aspartate; NSAIDs: nonsteroidal anti-inflammatory drugs)

- *Nerve roots:* Decompressive surgery
- *Cord compression:* Decompressive spine surgery.
- Ablative procedures:
    - *Peripheral nerve:*
        - Neurotomy
        - Neuroma excision
    - Sympathectomy
    - Ganglionectomy
    - *Spinal cord:*
        - Dorsal root entry zone lesion
        - Anterolateral cordotomy
        - Extra-lemniscal myelotomy
    - *Brainstem:*
        - Mesencephalotomy
    - *Brain:*
        - Hypophysectomy
        - Pulvinotomy
        - Medial thalamotomy
        - Cingulotomy
- *Stimulatory procedures:*
    - Peripheral nerve stimulation
    - Spinal cord stimulation

CHAPTER 24 Surgical Treatment of Chronic Pain

- Motor cortex stimulation
- Deep brain stimulation.
- *Implantation of infusion pumps for:*
  - Chronic non-cancer pain control with opioids
  - Muscle spasms and spasticity treatment with baclofen.

CHRONIC PAIN SYNDROMES DUE TO NERVE INJURIES

- *Carpal tunnel syndrome:*
  - Most common peripheral neuropathy
  - Median nerve compression under the flexor retinaculum
  - Affects lateral 3-1/2 fingers.
  - Worse at night.
  - Hypothenar and thenar muscle wasting
- *Cubital tunnel syndrome:* Second most frequent peripheral neuropathy due to ulnar nerve compression in the postcondylar canal.
- *Other nerve compression:*
  - *Suprascapular nerve* under the supraspinatus ligament causes shoulder pain.
  - *Sciatic nerve* under the pyriformis muscle mimics lumbar radiculopathy.
  - *Brachial plexus* due to compression at the thoracic outlet due to the first rib
  - *Lateral cutaneous nerve* compression under the inguinal ligament or *Meralgia paresthetica*
  - *Digital nerve compression* in the foot or *Morton's neuroma.*
- *Trigeminal neuralgia:* Severe hemifacial pain may be triggered by contact with specific trigger points. It may be due to the compression of the nerve by an artery.
  - *Medical treatment:*
    - Nonsteroidal anti-inflammatory drugs (NSAIDs)
    - Antidepressants
    - Anticonvulsants.
    - Opioids
  - *Surgical treatment:*
    - Trigger point block
    - Chemical neurolysis with glycerol or alcohol
    - Radiofrequency ablation
    - Craniotomy and microvascular decompression.
- *Neuropathic pain syndromes* are due to partial nerve injuries. Neuropathic pain can be postoperative due to iatrogenic nerve injuries; intercostal neuralgia due to herpes virus infection; coeliac plexopathy due to malignant infiltration; or after limb amputations:
  - Neuropathic pain is difficult to treat.
  - A multidisciplinary approach is necessary.

- The goal of treatment has to be defined:
  - Palliation of pain
  - Restoration of sleep
  - Return to functionality.
  - Improved quality-of-life.
- The treatment modalities include:
  - *Over-the-counter analgesics:* Aspirin, ibuprofen, and acetaminophen are usually ineffective but often used.
  - *Anticonvulsants:* Carbamazepine, gabapentin, and lamotrigine
  - *Antidepressants:* Amitriptyline and desipramine
  - *Local anesthetic agents:* Topical lidocaine
  - Topical capsaicin
  - Narcotics
  - Surgical interventions.

FURTHER READING

1. Goebel A et al. The autoimmune aetiology of unexplained chronic pain. Autoimmun Rev. 2021;21(3):103015.
2. Kandić M et al. Brain circuits involved in the development of chronic musculoskeletal pain: evidence from non-invasive brain stimulation. Front Neurol. 2021;12:732034.
3. Pahng AR et al. The convergent neuroscience of affective pain and substance use disorder. Alcohol Res. 2021;41(1):14.
4. Patel R et al. Neuropharmacological basis for multimodal analgesia in chronic pain. Postgrad Med. 2022;134(3):245-59.
5. Ye D et al. Painful diabetic peripheral neuro- pathy: role of oxidative stress and central sensitisation. Diabet Med. 2022; 39(1):e14729.

Vignette: Algea—The Personification of Pain

Algea was the personification of spirits of pain and suffering in Greek mythology. They were the three daughters of Eris, the goddess of strife. The three Algea were: (1) Lupe: the personification of pain, grief, and distress; (2) Ania: the personification of distress, sorrow, trouble, and boredom; and (3) Achus: the personification of ache and anguish. What has been described by the Algean mythology are the essential components of chronic pain: pain, depression, withdrawal, and anxiety! Perhaps the most severe chronic pain in Greek mythology was dealt to Prometheus. Prometheus stole the fire from Mount Olympus, which angered Zuses. Prometheus was chained to the rock. Each night an eagle attacked him and nibbled his liver. The next day the liver regrew, and the punishment was repeated. The question is not about the pain, but how did the Greeks know about liver regeneration?

Chapter 25

Developmental Abnormalities of Spine and Scoliosis

INTRODUCTION

Surgery on the spine is one of the most extensive and invasive neurosurgical procedures. It is estimated that 2–3% of the US population have scoliosis, and a tenth of these patients need treatment. An estimated 1.5 million spinal instrumentations are undertaken in the US each year. Developmental abnormalities of the spine may be diagnosed in utero or soon after birth and may require urgent correction in some cases.

SPINAL DEFORMITIES

- Spina bifida is the incomplete fusion of the spinal canal of a varying degree of closure.
- Closure of the neural tube occurs in the first month of gestation.
- Incidence in the US is 0.7/1,000 live births.
- Familial clusters are seen.
- There is a 4% incidence in the sibling of an affected child.
- It is associated with folate deficiency during pregnancy, maternal obesity, diabetes, and the use of the anticonvulsant drug (carbamazepine/valproic acid).
- It is confirmed in utero by high alpha-fetoproteins in amniotic fluid.
- *Clinical presentation ranges from:*
  - *Spina bifida occulta* is the most benign form of the disease. It is asymptomatic or presents with low backache. On examination, a tuft of hair or a dimple over a lumbar spine is frequently seen at the L5 level. It is often an incidental radiological finding. X-rays show the incomplete fusion of the spinous process and spinal process cleft.
  - *Meningocele:* Cerebrospinal fluid (CSF) filled sac formed by herniating meninges through a vertebral defect. Besides the lumbar and thoracic spine, meningoceles can occur due to the failure of the fusion of skull plates. Cranial defects are seen in the occipital, frontal-ethmoid, or nasal region. Neurological deficits are not seen.
  - *Syringomyelia:* During development, the central canal of the neural tube closes at the fourth ventricle floor. When the closure is incomplete, cystic lesions (syrinx) develop in the spinal cord that

may be isolated or communicate with the spinal CSF. Syringomyelia presents as headache, pain, weakness, numbness of arms or legs; stiffness of the back, shoulder, arms, and neck; loss of sensitivity pain and temperature in hands; later incontinence and loss of balance.
- *Myelomeningocele:* Herniating meningeal sac contains the spinal cord or nerves. It is the most common defect. If the defect is at the thoracic level or higher, it can have severe neurological impairment with sensory, motor, and bladder dysfunction.
- *Myelocele:* Spinal cord exposed with no overlying meningeal coverings. There can be associated Arnold Chiari malformation with hydrocephalus. Weakness of the lower limbs, incontinence, and deformities of the leg and feet are other abnormalities in the central nervous system. Chiari malformation can be associated with hydrocephalus in the first year of life.
- *Tethered cord:* A thickened filum terminale bridges the conus and the lumbar or sacral vertebrae. Consequently, flexion and extension of the spine cause traction on the spinal cord resulting in neurological symptoms. The treatment consists of transecting the filum terminale.
- *Diastematomyelia:* A defect in the fusion of the neural tube leads to the spinal cord's division. Typically affects the lumbar vertebrae and is associated with structural deformities of the spine, kyphosis, scoliosis, and myelomeningocele.

Management
- *In-utero surgery:* Reconstructive surgery for major neural tube defects can be undertaken in-utero and has improved survival. It is usually undertaken in carefully selected patients during the 23rd to 26th week of gestation. The surgery is performed on the mother under general anesthesia. The fetus is optimally positioned under laparoscopic guidance. The uterine and amniotic cavities are carefully incised, and the defect is repaired. The outcome of fetal surgery is considered to be better than postnatal repair.
- *Pediatric spine surgery:*
  - *Preoperative concerns:*
    - It may require urgent surgery due to potential CSF leak and infection in neonates and preterm infants.
    - It is associated with other spinal malformations (Chiari), hydrocephalus, and other neurological syndromes.
    - Co-morbidities involve other organs (kidneys) and cardiovascular and respiratory systems.
    - May have a history of past surgery.
    - Latex sensitivity is seen in about 66% of the patients.
    - Potential blood loss requires coagulation screening.

- *Intraoperative care:*
  - Intubation in unusual positions, e.g., lateral
  - Positioning while protecting the defect
  - Possible migration and dislodgement of the tube
  - Adequate vascular access and invasive monitoring as needed
  - *Avoid hypothermia:* Operating room temperature, forced air warming fluids, and blood
  - Evoked potential (EP) monitoring in children may be improved with ketamine infusion.
- *Postoperative care:*
  - Postoperative ventilation
  - Optimum fluid resuscitation
  - Multi-modality pain management.

ARNOLD CHIARI MALFORMATION

- *Type 1:* Descent of cerebellar tonsil results in CSF collection and syrinx formation. Typical symptoms include suboccipital headache with coughing; visual symptoms (blurred vision, flashing lights, diplopia, and nystagmus); impaired ocular movement; brainstem symptoms (apnea and bradycardia); hydrocephalus symptoms (headache, nausea, vomiting, and lethargy); and spasticity due to cord compression.
- *Type 2:* Meningomyelocele leads to the downward displacement of cerebral tonsils; hydrocephalus is common; ocular symptoms are less marked.
- *Surgical risks:*
  - Residual neck pain and stiffness
  - Neurological injuries
  - *Vascular complications include:*
    - *Vertebral artery injury:* Net effect depends on collateral blood flow.
    - *Posterior inferior cerebellar artery injury:* Wallenberg syndrome: Dysphagia, stridor, nausea, vomiting, vertigo, nystagmus, and abnormal gait and balance.

SCOLIOSIS

- Scoliosis is the *lateral* bending of the spine in contrast to kyphosis, which is the *anterior-posterior* (AP) curvature.
- It occurs in 2–3% of the population.
- Onset is usually 10–15 years; it may be seen in infancy and childhood.
- There is no gender bias.
- 38,000 spinal fusions per year in the US.
- 30,000 treated with braces per year in the US.

Etiology of Scoliosis

- Idiopathic (80%), usually diagnosed at puberty. In children, scoliosis is classified as infantile <3 years, juvenile 3–10 years, and adolescent >11 years.

- *Congenital:* Due to the developmental abnormality of the vertebrae, seen in early childhood.
- *Neuromuscular:* Progressive disease usually due to cerebral palsy, spinal muscular atrophy, muscular dystrophy, degenerative diseases, or trauma.

Clinical Features
- Postural tilt, asymmetric shoulders, waist, head not centered.
- Less than a quarter of scoliosis patients have pain.
- Pain in a patient with scoliosis requires ruling out other spinal pathologies.

Preoperative Assessment
Cobb's Angle
- The angle is considered the gold standard for assessing the severity of scoliosis.
- Cobb's angle **(Fig. 1, Angle A)** is the angle between the planes of the top of the most tilted upper and the bottom of the most tilted lower vertebra of the scoliotic curve.
- An AP chest X-ray identifies the most displaced vertebrae on the top and bottom of the spinal curve. Lines on the curve are drawn on the top of the uppermost vertebrae and the lowermost vertebrae. Perpendiculars are drawn from these lines toward each other. If the spine were perfectly aligned, these perpendiculars would be parallel. Cobb's angle is the intersection of these perpendiculars **(Fig. 1, angle B)**.

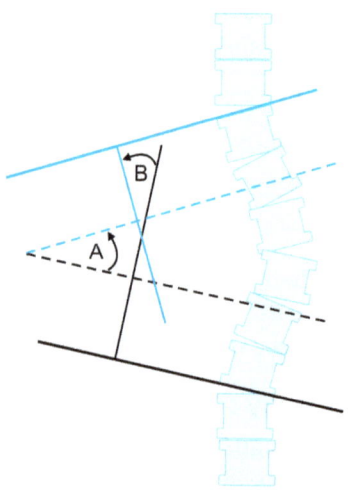

Fig. 1: Determination of Cobb's angle.

- *Significance of Cobb's angle:*
  - *>10°:* Diagnostic threshold for scoliosis
  - *10–30°:* Significant scoliosis
  - *40°:* Surgical correction
  - *65°:* Restrictive lung disease
  - *>100°:* Exertional dyspnea
  - *>120°:* Chronic alveolar hypoventilation.

Adam's Test
- It is a screening tool used in schools.
- With the feet together, the patient bends 90 degrees at the waist. The observer standing behind the patient, looks for the asymmetry of the trunk.
- The test is a good screening test but does not determine the type and severity of the spinal deformity.

Radiological investigations such as X-rays, CTs, and MRIs are required to assess the severity of scoliosis and rule out other pathologies.

Impaired Pulmonary Functions
Scoliosis can affect pulmonary functions in several ways:
- Reduction in lung volumes results in restrictive lung disease and hypoplastic lung.
- Inefficient functioning of the respiratory muscles, intercostals, and diaphragm.
- Underlying neuromuscular disease
- Decreased diffusion capacity.
- V/Q mismatch
- Increased work of breathing
- Alveolar hypoventilation
- Pulmonary hypertension
- Secondary changes such as chronic infection and atelectasis.
- Respiratory failure.

Cardiovascular Effects
- Pulmonary artery hypertension
- Right heart failure
- Congestive heart failure

Anesthetic Concerns
- *Severity of scoliosis:*
  - Extent of deformity
  - Respiratory and cardiovascular functions

- Pain
- Neurological deficits
- General physical condition.
- *Preoperative optimization:*
  - Pulmonary functions
  - Treatment of chest infections
  - Correction of anemia
  - Correction of right heart failure
  - *Pain pretreatment strategy:* For neuropathic and inflammatory pain.
- *Induction:*
  - Airway and intubation:
    - Positioning for intubation
    - Temperature probe
    - Bite block
  - Total intravenous anesthesia (TIVA) setup
  - *Vascular access:* Central venous access for significant blood loss
  - Antibiotics and antifibrinolytics
  - *Monitoring:*
    - *Hemodynamic:* A-line, central venous pressure (CVP), EKG.
    - *Respiratory:* Capnography and airway pressure.
    - Temperature
    - *Neurological:*
      - Processed EEG as a bispectral index (BIS) or power spectrum
      - Raw EEG
      - Sensory evoked responses
      - Motor evoked responses
      - Possibility of awake testing
      - *Muscle relaxation:* Twitch monitor
  - *ABG:* Oxygenation, hematocrit, base deficits, and lactic acidosis
  - *Coagulation:* Clinical, Laboratory coagulation tests, Rotational thromboelastometry/ thromboelastography (ROTEM/TEG)
  - *I/O:* Input, urine output, blood loss, and coagulation.
- *Anesthetic choice:* TIVA and TIVA drug selection: Propofol/ narcotic
- *Positioning:*
  - Pinning
  - Prone positioning
  - Modification and padding
  - Eye protection.

Intraoperative Care

- *Blood conservation:*
  - Preoperative blood harvest
  - Intraoperative blood harvest

CHAPTER 25 Developmental Abnormalities of Spine and Scoliosis

- Cell saver
- Induced hypotension
- Antifibrinolytics.
- *Possible intraoperative events:*
  - Prolonged surgery
  - Blood loss
  - Excessive volume resuscitation
  - Hypotension
  - Decreased urine output.
  - Loss of evoked responses
  - Venous air embolism.

Emergence Concerns

- Edema of the face and airway
- Tongue swelling and injury
- Leak test
- Delayed emergence
- Inadequate ventilation.

Postoperative Care

- Postoperative ventilation
- Postoperative pain management
- New neurological deficit
- Visual loss and corneal abrasion.

Complications and Outcomes of Spine Surgery

- Overall, the complication rate in spine surgery is around 15%.
- Complication rates are sometimes linked to the underlying pathology.
  - Scoliosis correction in patients with underlying neuromuscular disease has the highest incidence of complications, about 35% average aggregated rate).
  - Another high-risk group is patients with congenital cardiac morbidities.
- *Complications include:*
  - *Post-surgery pain:*
    - 50% have reduced pain after surgery.
    - 40% of patients have no change in the amount of pain.
    - 25% may be dissatisfied with the outcome of surgery.
  - Blood loss and transfusion
  - *Infection:* 3–10% incidence
    - *Wound site:* May occur years later.
    - Urinary infection.

- Postoperative neurological deficits
- Progression of the curve
- Impaired spinal cord flexibility
- Repeat operations.
- *Death:* Post-surgical mortality is rare after spine surgery, but in patients with underlying neuromuscular disease can be about 5%.

FURTHER READING

1. Forster JG et al. Anaesthetic considerations in posterior instrumentation of scoliosis due to spinal muscular atrophy: case series of 56 operated patients. Acta Anaesthesiol Scand. 2022;66(3):345-53.
2. Jug M et al. 3D model-assisted instrumentation of the pediatric spine: a technical note. J Orthop Surg Res. 2021;16(1):586.
3. Lin Y et al. Influences of thoracic spinal deformity on exercise performance and pulmonary function: a prospective study of 168 patients with adolescent idiopathic scoliosis. Spine (Phila Pa 1976). 2022;47(3):E107-15.
4. Martin BD, et al. Factors affecting length of stay after posterior spinal fusion for adolescent idiopathic scoliosis. Spine Deform. 2020;8(1):51-6.
5. Tsirikos AI et al. Cyanotic congenital cardiac disease and scoliosis: preoperative assessment, surgical treatment, and outcomes. Med Princ Pract. 2020;29(1):46-53.

Vignette: Evolution of the Spine

In the furthest recesses of evolution, perhaps for the first one and half a billion years, life evolved as individual cells. Over time, those cells aggregated, and primitive organisms evolved. Most early animals had soft bodies. Some developed hard encrustations, while others developed shells. Nature experimented with diverse body plans. By the time the Cambrian explosion occurred some half a billion years ago, a race was on. It was driven by a simple principle: "Eat or be eaten". Thus, there was an evolutionary need for animals to move, hunt and escape effectively. Around that time, some animals developed a primitive spine, the notochord, to control their movements. A handful of animals retain a notochord in their adult life. These include amphioxus, coelacanth, lamprey, and lungfish. These animals are considered to be living fossils. Due to their ability to locomote effectively, vertebrates have dominated evolution ever since, underwater, on land, or in the air.

Vignette: Talking of Evolution, Just How Smart Were the Dinosaurs?

In 2004, a fossil hunter in England found an odd-shaped pebble on the beach. The pebble turned out to be a 133-million-year-old endocast of the dinosaur brain. Though endocasts of dinosaur brains are exceedingly rare, those of modern hominids have been extensively studied. The hominid casts reveal the evolution of various regions of the hominid brain, such as the development of speech areas. The hominid casts show the rapid growth of the human brain compared to higher apes. The dinosaur brain endocast belonged to a relative of the Iguanodon, an herbivore. Most endocasts do not preserve tissue details, but the mineralization preserved some of those structures in this case. The endocast showed surface vessels, meninges, and some layers of the cortex. Scanning electron microscopy and CT images of the cast revealed similarities with avian and crocodilian specimens. Based on this specimen, it was summarized that the brain size and intelligence of the dinosaurs could match those of present-day reptiles and birds.

Chapter 26: Pathophysiology of Spinal Cord Injury

INTRODUCTION

A spinal cord injury (SCI) is an injury to the spinal cord or its terminal nerves that constitute cauda equina. SCI results in the impairment or loss of sensory, motor, and autonomic functions at and below the level of injury. An estimated 20,000 people sustain spinal cord injuries each year. An estimated quarter of a million or more people live with these injuries.

Patients may present for surgical spine injury management or complications requiring surgical interventions.

PATHOLOGY OF SPINAL CORD INJURY

- *Incidence:*
  - 70% are traffic related.
  - 2× more in men than in women.
  - Peak age 20–40 years.
- *Determinants of outcome:*
  - Age and comorbidities
  - Level of injury
  - *The severity of injury:* Partial or complete
  - Prevention of secondary injury
- *Primary and secondary injury:*
  - *Primary injury:* Primary injury is immediate at the time of impact. *Types of primary injuries:*
    - A contusion is the bruising of the cord due to disruption of the blood capillaries and venules, which triggers an inflammatory response.
    - A laceration is an injury with physical disruption of the tissue.
    - A hematoma is the collection of blood in extravascular space.
  - *Secondary injury:* Secondary injuries evolve over the next several hours and are due to:
    - Cord hypoperfusion/ischemia
    - Edema
    - Inflammation
    - Activation of neutrophils
    - Oxygen and free radical-induced injuries

- Excitotoxic injury, e.g., due to glutamate release
- Apoptosis
- Glial scarring.

CLINICAL CONSEQUENCES

- *Neurological effects:*
  - *Spinal shock* is the complete transient loss of sensory, motor, and autonomic responses at any level of spine injury. Resulting in the loss of flaccid paralysis, loss of reflexes, hypothermia, ileus, bradycardia, and hypotension.
  - *Neurogenic shock:* Sudden loss of autonomic tone with spinal injuries (above T6) redistributes blood volume, and results in hypotension and bradycardia.
  - *Autonomic hyper-reflexia:*
    - Seen with SCI at or above the T6 level.
    - Pain below the level of injury results in vasoconstriction.
    - Intense vasoconstriction causes hypertension, bradycardia, and arrhythmias.
    - However, above the injury level, there is vasodilation resulting in headaches, flushing, and nasal stuffiness.
    - In severe cases, autonomic hyperreflexia can cause seizures and intracranial hemorrhages.
- *Neurologic syndromes:*
  - *Cervicomedullary syndrome* is due to the compression of the lower brainstem and upper spinal cord. It presents with occipital headache, neck pains, numbness, motor weakness, lower cranial nerve paralysis, dizziness, and gait instability.
  - *Central cord syndrome:* Motor and sensory losses of the upper extremity with partial loss below; due to the injury to corticospinal pathways and extreme extension of the cervical spine.
  - *Anterior cord syndrome:* Usually due to ischemic injury to the anterior two-thirds of the spine in the spinal artery distribution; affects corticospinal (motor weakness) and spinothalamic (loss pain and temperature sensation) and autonomic reflexes (hypotension) below the level of injury.
  - *Posterior cord syndrome* is the least frequent spine injury and is typically due to hyperflexion of the spine. The posterior cord syndrome presents with the loss of proprioception, fine touch, pressure and vibration sensations, and deep tendon reflexes.
  - *Brown-Sequard syndrome* is due to hemisection of the spinal cord. It presents with ipsilateral loss of motor function, vibration, position, and deep touch with the contralateral loss of pain, temperature, and light touch sensations.

- *Conus medullaris syndrome:* It is the terminal part of the spinal cord located in an adult between L1 and L2. Injuries to conus medullaris affect the sacral segments. The conus medullaris syndrome affects bowel and bladder functions early. The lower limb sensation, motor power, and reflexes are relatively spared.
- *Cauda equina syndrome* is due to an injury to the bundle of nerves extending L2 to the sacrum. It impacts lumbosacral nerve roots with the corresponding loss of motor and sensory sensations affecting the saddle area and a loss of perineal reflexes.

- *Respiratory complications:*
  - Airway obstruction
  - *Associated trauma:* Hypoxia (thoracic injury) and hypoventilation (C spine)
  - Aspiration
  - Pulmonary edema
  - Hypoventilation
  - Pulmonary embolism.
- *Cardiovascular:*
  - *Bradycardia:* Loss of cardio accelerator fibers (T1-5)
  - Ventricular arrhythmias
  - Postural hypotension
  - Neurogenic shock
  - *Autonomic hyperreflexia*
- *Gastrointestinal system:*
  - Stress ulcers
  - Gastroparesis
  - Ileus
  - Occult peritonitis
  - Fecal impaction.
- *Genitourinary system:*
  - Neurogenic bladder
  - Atonic bladder
  - Stones
  - Infection
- Impaired thermoregulation
- *Skin:* Decubitus ulcers
- *Musculoskeletal:*
  - Muscle spasms
  - Spasticity and contractures
  - Osteoporosis
- *Thrombogenesis:*
  - Deep venous thrombosis
  - Pulmonary embolism

Investigations

- *Radiological studies:*
  - X-ray spine
  - Computed tomography
  - MRI
- *Electrophysiological studies:*
  - *Somatosensory evoked potential (SSEP):* Loss of SSEP carries a poor prognosis in settings of traumatic SCI, although some patients with initial loss of SSEPs might still recover cord function.
  - Motor evoked potentials (MEP) Like the SSEPs, the loss of MEPs predicts poor recovery after SCI. Both SSEP and MEPs can be used to monitor SCI over time. A possible alternative to conventional MEPs is transcranial magnetic stimulation which can be done with minimal sedation but is challenging to undertake in clinical settings.
  - Brainstem auditory evoked responses: SCI leads to deafferentation and displacement of cortical function over time. Consequently, it alters the amplitude and latency of brainstem auditory evoked responses.
  - EEG and Processed EEG to monitor sedation/depth of anesthesia.
  - Electromyography.
- *Effect of anesthetics on evoked potentials (EPs):*
  - A significant change is defined as a 50% decrease in amplitude and a 10% increase in latency **(Table 1)**.
  - Avoid volatile agents.
  - Ketamine, methohexital, and etomidate may be better for recording EPs but lack the quality of propofol anesthesia.
  - *Signal attenuated by:* Deep anesthesia, hypothermia, anemia, hyperventilation, and hypotension.

Table 1: Effect of anesthetics on somatosensory evoked potentials.

	Latency	Amplitude
Narcotics	+	–
Benzodiazepines	0	–
Propofol	++	– – –
Etomidate	– –	++
Dexmedetomidine	0	–
Ketamine	– –	++
Barbiturate	++	– – –
Volatile agents	++++	– – – –
Nitrous oxide	++	– –

Notes: +: Increases; –: Decreases; 0: no effect

- *Ultrasonography* for intraoperative imaging and blood flow monitoring
- *Lumbar puncture* and dural pressure monitoring for ensuring cord perfusion.

MANAGEMENT GOALS
- Spinal cord stabilization
- Maintenance of spinal cord perfusion
- Airway and oxygenation
- Metabolic correction
- Pain relief
- Traction
- *Spinal cord protection:*
    - Hypothermia unproven
    - High-dose steroids carry the potential risk of infection with no proven benefits.
    - Several novel treatments, from proteins to stem cells, remain unproven.
- Surgical decompression and stabilization are effective.

DELAYED COMPLICATIONS OF SPINAL CORD INJURY
- *Cardiovascular:*
    - Persistent orthostatic hypotension
    - Autonomic hyper-reflexia
- *Respiratory:* With high cervical injuries:
    - Persistent respiratory insufficiency
    - Ventilator dependency
    - Chest infections
- *Neurological:*
    - Persistent neurological deficits
    - Muscle spasticity
    - Neuropathic pain
- *Urinary tract:*
    - Infection
    - Calciuria
    - Atonic bladder
    - Incontinence
- *Gastrointestinal tract:*
    - Stress ulcers
    - Constipation
    - Bowel dysfunction
- Heterotopic ossifications of joints such as hips, knees, and elbow
- Bedsores
- Immunodeficiency.

FURTHER READING

1. Gong L et al. Changes in transcriptome profiling during the acute/subacute phases of contusional spinal cord injury in rats. Ann Transl Med. 2020;8(24):1682.
2. Pinchi E et al. Acute spinal cord injury: a systematic review investigating miRNA families involved. Int J Mol Sci. 2019;20(8):1841.
3. Yang LY et al. Exerting the appropriate application of methylprednisolone in acute spinal cord injury based on time course transcriptomics analysis. Int J Mol Sci. 2021; 22(23):13024.
4. Zhang Y et al. Acute spinal cord injury: pathophysiology and pharmacological intervention (Review). Mol Med Rep. 2021;23(6):417.
5. Zrzavy T et al. Acute and non-resolving inflammation associated with oxidative injury after human spinal cord injury. Brain. 2021;144(1):144-61.

Vignette: Spinal Injuries

The Edwin Smith Papyrus (c1550–1650 BCE) reveals that the ancient Egyptians knew about the spinal cord. They described the vertebrae. They knew the motor fibers crossed over, so that the brain injuries would affect the opposite side. Neck stiffness was routinely tested for during head and spine injury assessment. Hippocrates described spine traction in the 5th century BCE to treat such injuries. Around 600AD, Paul of Aegina provided a detailed description of the types of spinal dislocations, the careful use of traction, and the surgical repair of spinal injuries. He was the first to perform laminectomy and corpectomy. He described the devastating effects of cervical spine injuries and the hazards of treating them recklessly. A thousand years later, Ambroise Pare' recommended similar treatment for spine injuries. Modern spine surgery with an intense multidisciplinary approach came towards the end of the second world war and was pioneered by Ludwig Guttmann (1899-1980). Guttmann's spine surgery unit at the Stoke Mandeville Hospital set the standards of spine surgery care in the latter half of the twentieth century. However, there is a new era in spinal surgery with minimally invasive techniques and image-guided neurosurgery that make yesterday's advances look relatively modest.

Chapter 27: Movement Disorders

INTRODUCTION

Movement disorders syndromes are characterized by abnormal (excessive or insufficient) movements that are not due to weakness or spasticity. These typically arise from pathologies in the extrapyramidal system or basal ganglia. The common syndromes seen are:
- Parkinson's disease (PD)
- Essential tremors
- Restless leg syndrome
- Involuntary movements
- Huntington's chorea
- Wilson's disease
- Drug-induced movement disorders.

PARKINSON'S DISEASE

Pathology

Idiopathic Parkinson's disease (IPD) is a progressive neurodegenerative disorder. IPD affects 1% of people >60 years of age. It has a male predominance (1.5:1). It is characterized by resting tremors (70%), rigidity (90%), and bradykinesia (100%). It is initially due to the loss of dopaminergic neurons and later by the loss of other neurotransmitters **(Fig. 1)**. It gradually progresses to dementia.

Etiology

- Histologically, IPD shows degenerative changes in the neuromelanin-containing dopaminergic neurons in the substantia nigra.
- The presence of hyaline eosinophilic "Lewy bodies" is pathognomonic of the disease.
- Genetic factors predispose to neuronal damage by environmental toxins that lead to a familial form of the disease.
- Secondary PDs are seen due to many neuronal injuries; however, they do not manifest with all the clinical features of IPD. Encephalitis, trauma, toxins (CO and Mn), stroke, and drugs can cause PD-like syndromes.

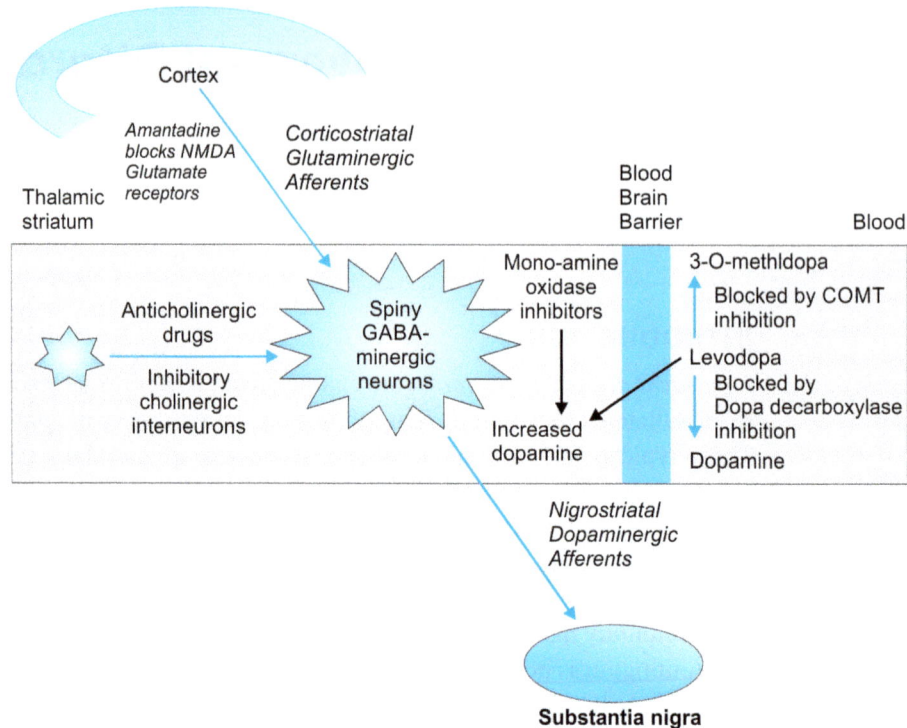

Fig. 1: Site of action of drugs for Parkinson's Disease treatment. (NMDA: N-methyl-D-aspartate, COMT: catecholamine methyl transferase; GABA: Gamma-aminobutyric acid).

- Some drugs used in the peri-operative period can cause PD-like symptoms. These include:
  - *Antipsychotics:* Haloperidol
  - *Antiemetic:* Prochlorperazine and metoclopramide
  - *Antihypertensive:* Reserpine
  - Neurotoxic compounds such as 1-methyl-4-phenyl-1,2,3,6-tetra-hydro-pyridine (MPTP) can cause PD-like syndrome in illicit drug users.

Clinical Features

- *Early Symptoms often preceding diagnosis:*
  - Hyposmia
  - Fatigue
  - Depression
  - Constipation
  - Sleep disorders of the rapid eye movement phase
- *Classic symptoms at diagnosis*
  - *Tremors:* Intention tremors, 4–7/s; relieved by rest
  - *Rigidity:* Mask-like facies, micrographia, and cogwheel rigidity
  - *Bradykinesia:* Festinating gait; postural instability

- *Late symptoms—several years after diagnosis:*
  - Drug-resistant rigidity, freezing, postural instability, and falls
  - Dysphagia
  - Sialorrhea
  - Nocturia and urinary urgency
  - Postural hypotension
  - Anxiety and depression
  - Cognitive decline and dementia

Treatment

Figure 1 and **Table 1** provide a summary of Parkinson's disease treatments.

ESSENTIAL TREMORS (ET)

- Tremors worsen with emotional stress and purposeful movements. It is the most common movement disorder in the United States, affecting 10 million patients. It typically presents in the young and worsens with age.
- *Pathology:* Abnormalities in electrical signal processing by the thalamus.
- *Etiology:* It is a familial disorder with 5× greater incidences in families.

There is a 50% chance of inheriting the disease from an affected parent. ET can also be sporadic with no familial history. ET increases the risk of Alzheimer's disease and is associated with a 4× increase in the likelihood of Parkinson's disease.

Table 1: Treatment of Parkinson's disease.

	Mechanism of action	Drug	Indication	Side-effects
First line	DA precursors, Dopa decarboxylase inhibitors	Levodopa/ Carbidopa	Monotherapy	Nausea, orthostatic hypotension, hallucination, and dyskinesia
		Levodopa/ Benserazide	Monotherapy	Anorexia, nausea, vomiting, dizziness, insomnia, headaches
Second line	DA agonists	Pramipexole	Monotherapy	Nausea, orthostatic hypotension, sleep disturbances, psychosis, edema, impulse control disorder
		Ropinirole	Monotherapy	
		Bromo-criptine	Failed pharmacotherapy	Avoid with h/o hypertension and migraine; side-effects: dizziness, hypoglycemia, impaired sleep, hallucinations, rhinitis, and pulmonary fibrosis

Contd...

Contd...

Mechanism of action	Drug	Indication	Side-effects
Monoamine oxidase B inhibitor (MAO-BI)	Selegiline	Adjunctive therapy	Dizziness, headache, stimulant effect, increased levodopa side-effects
	Rasagiline	Monotherapy or Adjunct therapy	Flu-like symptoms: headache, arthralgia, nausea, rash, constipation, and increased levodopa side-effects.
MAO-BI + Anti-glutaminergic	Safinamide	Adjunct to decrease off time	Orthostatic hypotension, fall risk, increased liver enzyme
COMT inhibitor	Entacapone	Adjunct therapy	Dizziness, drowsiness, diarrhea, hallucination, fever, muscle stiffness, confusion
	Tolcapone	Adjunct therapy	
Anti-cholinergic	Trihexy-phenidyl	Adjunct therapy	Dizziness, blurred vision, dry mouth, constipation, urinary retention, impaired sweating, behavioral changes
	Biperiden	Adjunct therapy	
Third line Mixed (dopamine release/anti-cholinergic/NMDA antagonist)	Amantadine	Adjunctive therapy to decrease dyskinesia	Orthostatic hypotension, syncope, edema. Avoid 14 days before and after the flu vaccine

Surgical treatment: Drug refractory disease

DBS site	Thalamus	Decreases tremor only	Intracranial hemorrhage, infection (4%), stroke (2%); periodic battery change
	Subthalamic	Overall improvement	
	Globus Pallidus	Overall improvement	
Ablative	Thalamus	Decreases tremor only	Bleeding, infection, stroke. Unilateral treatment only
	Subthalamic	Unproven	
	Globus Pallidus	Overall improvement	

(DA: dopamine; MAO-B I: monoamine oxidase B inhibitor; COMT: catecholamine methyl-transferase; DBS: deep brain stimulation)

Table 2: Treatment of essential tremors.

Beta-blockers	Propranolol, metoprolol	Fatigue, bradycardia, depression, dizziness, erectile dysfunction, 505 respond to treatment, but tolerance develops in 10–15%
Anticonvulsants	Primidone, gabapentin	Are the second line of treatment. Side-effects include nausea, vomiting, confusion, sedation, irritability, ataxia weight gain
Na$^+$ channel blockers	Topiramate Zonisamide	Sedation, fatigue, ataxia, paresthesia
Tranquilizers	Benzodiazepines: Lorazepam Clonazepam	Drowsiness, fatigue, dependence, abuse risk
Botox injections	Effect time-limited, Persistent weakness	
Surgery	Deep brain stimulation/unilateral thalamotomy	

- *Clinical features:* These tremors affect the hands and arms, head, neck, and vocal cords but rarely affect the lower extremities, so disturbances in balance are rare.
- *A cluster of movement disorders:* ET may mimic Parkinson's disease and dystonia. Hyperthyroidism, antidepressant drugs, and toxins may also cause tremors.
- *Other causes of tremors include* psychogenic tremors, physiologic tremors, orthostatic tremors, and task-specific (writing) tremors.

Treatment

- *Medical treatment:* Propranolol (50–70% respond), primidone, other anticonvulsants, and anxiolytics **(Table 2)**.
- *Surgical treatment:*
  - Deep brain stimulators are used for resistant cases and have replaced thalamotomy.
  - *Focused ultrasound for movement disorders:* Using MRI guided focused ultrasound, it is now possible to ablate specific brain regions, such as the thalamus, to treat movement disorders. The procedure is usually done under sedation. The main side-effect of such treatment are headache, nausea, and sensory changes during the procedure. Ataxia and sensory changes may persist long term.

RESTLESS LEG SYNDROME

- Willis–Ekbom disease, or restless leg syndrome, is an unpleasant sensation resulting in an irresistible urge to move, typically in the evenings or at night.

- It is a familial disorder that manifests in middle-aged people. It is due to the disruption of dopamine pathways in the basal ganglia.
- It is also associated with end-stage renal disease, iron deficiency anemia (IDA), and drugs with extrapyramidal side-effects, such as metoclopramide, haloperidol, and antidepressants.
- *Treatment:* Treat any underlying causes such as IDA. Pharmacological therapies include anti-epileptics, such as gabapentin, and dopaminergic agents, such as ropinirole, rotigotine, and pramipexole.
- Opioids and benzodiazepines are also helpful.

OTHER MOVEMENT DISORDERS

- *Tourette's syndrome:* Neurological syndrome with involuntary repetitive tics, blinking, and shrugging of shoulders with offensive vocalizations. Its treatment usually requires psychotherapy, alpha-2 adrenergic agonists such as clonidine, or antipsychotic drugs.
- *Huntington chorea:* It is an autosomal dominant progressive degenerative disorder. It is characterized by progressive impairment of gait, movement, and dementia. It requires symptomatic treatment.
- *Wilson's disease:* Hepatolenticular degeneration: It is a genetic disorder of copper metabolism with liver and brain damage. Tremors, muscle stiffness, impaired sight, deafness, anxiety, and personality changes are evident in the later stages. It is treated with dietary changes and chelating agents.

FURTHER READING

1. Church FC. Treatment options for motor and non-motor symptoms of Parkinson's disease. Biomolecules. 2021;11(4):612.
2. Jellinger KA. Neuropathology and pathogenesis of extrapyramidal movement disorders: a critical update. II. Hyperkinetic disorders. J Neural Transm (Vienna). 2019;126(8):997-1027.
3. Raza C et al. Shakeel, Parkinson's disease: Mechanisms, translational models and management strategies. Life Sci. 2019;226:77-90.
4. Stoker TB et al. Emerging treatment approaches for Parkinson's disease. Front Neurosci. 2018;12:693.
5. Yim RLH et al. Peri-operative management of patients with Parkinson's disease. Anaesthesia. 2022;77(Suppl 1):123-33.

Vignette: How Animal Motor Systems Outclass Human Capabilities

Power: *An African dung beetle can lift 1100× its body weight, the human equivalent of lifting 68,000 kg.*
Speed: *The fastest reflexes: Trap-jaw ants: 0.15 milliseconds; humans: around 80 milliseconds and some 500× slower.*
Jumps: *Flea jumps 220× body length and 150× height. The equivalent human jump would be 400 m long and 220 m high. The Olympic triple jump pit would be a kilometer long if human athletes were as good as the fleas.*

Chapter 28: Seizure Types and Treatment

INTRODUCTION

Epilepsy is characterized by the repeated occurrence of sudden transient episodes of motor, sensory, autonomic, or psychic dysfunction due to abnormal cortical discharges observable by electrocorticography. Epilepsy can be primary, idiopathic, or secondary to developmental abnormalities, infection, trauma, tumors, metabolic, or vascular disease. Convulsions associated with acute metabolic disorders, such as hypoglycemia, are not considered epileptic. Clinical diagnosis of epilepsy requires two unprovoked seizures at least 24 hours apart or a single seizure episode with a likelihood of recurrence.

PATHOLOGY

- *Incidence and etiology:*
  - *Bimodal:* Seventy-five percent of the patients are <5 years of age, while elderly (>60 years) also present with new onset seizures, often with status epilepticus (SE).
  - *In neonates:* Developmental abnormalities, hypoxic injury, hypoglycemia, electrolyte imbalance, intracranial hemorrhage, errors of metabolism, and maternal drug abuse.
  - *In infants and children:* Febrile seizure, the onset of idiopathic seizures, central nervous system infections such as *Haemophilus influenzae* or *Staphylococcal pneumonia* and brain tumors.
  - *In young adults:* Onset of idiopathic seizures, substance abuse, and trauma.
  - *Adults:* Idiopathic, progressive brain disease, trauma, and congenital diseases, such as tuberous sclerosis or neurofibromatosis.
- *Underlying pathology:*
  - *In elderly:* Tumor, trauma, and cerebrovascular accident.
  - Clinical features of epilepsy are enumerated in **Tables 1** and **2**.
  - Epilepsy could be convulsive or non-convulsive.
  - Generalized tonic-clonic status epilepticus (GTCSE) is a seizure lasting at least 5 minutes or two convulsions without intervening recovery.
  - *Absence status epilepticus:* Prolonged absence seizure with characteristic 3/s spike and wave pattern on electroencephalogram (EEG).

Table 1: Classification, clinical, and electroencephalographic features of seizures.

Type	Clinical	EEG
Partial seizures (focal/local) seizures		
Simple partial seizures	Focal seizure sensory or motor; consciousness remains intact	Localized seizure activity
Complex partial seizures	Confused behavior, with impairment of consciousness	Generalized abnormal EEG activity persisting in the anterior temporal lobe
Partial seizure with secondary generalization	A focal seizure that spreads to the other hemisphere	Variable findings with spread to the other side.
Generalized seizures		
Absence seizures	Transient loss of consciousness with varying degrees of clonic motor activities ranging from blinking of eyelids to jerking of the body	Bilateral synchronous 3/s spike and wave pattern
Myoclonic seizures	Localized clonic jerks	A brief burst of multiple spikes
Clonic seizures	Seen in children; generalized clonic contractions with unconsciousness and autonomic dysfunction	Fast 10 Hz activity with slow waves and an occasional spike and wave pattern
Tonic seizures	Opisthotonus, unconsciousness, and autonomic dysfunction	Fast rhythmic activity at 9–10 Hz, sometimes increasing in amplitudes though decreasing in frequency
Tonic-clonic seizures	Major generalized tonic-clonic activity	Fast spike and wave activity at 4–5 Hz
Atonic seizures	Sudden loss of postural tone, falling on one side	Spike and wave complexes at 1–2 Hz but increasing in frequency

(EEG: electroencephalogram)

- *Simple partial status epilepticus:* Persistent focal seizures often due to metabolic disorders.
- *Complex partial status epilepticus:* Persistent confusion state without clearing of consciousness.

DIFFERENTIAL DIAGNOSIS
- Shivering
- Syncope
- Transient ischemic attack
- Migraine
- Hypoglycemic convulsions
- Pseudoseizures.

Table 2: Clinical features of epilepsy.

Type	Clinical characteristic
Focal seizures	Limited to one hemisphere, 60% of all seizures usually present with aura, generally of short duration, with motor, sensory, behavioral, and psychological manifestations
Generalized seizures	They are associated with loss of consciousness with motor manifestations; they can be tonic, clonic, tonic-clonic, atonic, and myoclonic; focal manifestations can precede these symptoms
Nonepileptic seizures	Epileptic seizures without typical electroconvulsive features
Absence seizure	Aura is rare, typically without motor manifestations, and postictal confusion
Uncinate seizure	Olfactory hallucination
Juvenile myoclonic epilepsy	Strong family history, GTCS, myoclonus, or absence seizure manifestations, and EEG multiple spikes
West syndrome	Neonates, complex manifestation, progressive disease, mental retardation, EEG: spikes and slow waves; Rx: ACTH and steroids
Lennox–Gastaut syndrome	Drop attacks (up to 50/day); may progress to GTCS with mental retardation
Todd's paralysis	Persistent postictal motor or sensory deficits last up to 60 minutes

(EEG: electroencephalogram; GTCS: generalized tonic–clonic status)

STATUS EPILEPTICUS

Seizures that last>5 minutes or short seizures lasting <5 minutes without return of consciousness or seizures resistant to front-line anticonvulsants (benzodiazepines and phenytoin in adequate doses). Consider inadequate doses of anticonvulsant drugs if a patient on treatment has SE.

Management of Status Epilepticus

- Protect the patient from injury, assess and secure the airway and ensure adequate breathing and ventilation.
- Obtain brief history while securing the IV line:
  - Past seizure
  - Diabetes
  - Major medical issues
  - Drug or alcohol withdrawal.
- Consider the possibility of nonseizure.
- Check vitals (pulse oximetry, blood pressure, temperature, and EKG).
- Finger stick glucose.

- Obtain blood sample if needed, start second IV line:
  - *Samples for:*
    - Hemogram
    - Basic metabolic profile
    - Liver function test
    - Blood sugar
    - Drug screen
    - Anticonvulsant drug levels
  - CT scan.
- Start normal saline. Give:
  - 50 mL of 50% dextrose IV
  - 100 mg thiamine IV or IM.
- *Stop seizures:* Benzodiazepines (midazolam/diazepam/lorazepam) IV stat.
- *If seizures persist after 20 minutes, despite benzodiazepines (first line drugs), consider a second-line drug* **(Table 3)**:
  - Phenytoin/fosphenytoin may take time to load (contraindications include allergy, heart block, and bradycardia). Then consider valproic acid or phenobarbital.

Table 3: Drugs for the treatment of status epilepticus.

Drug	Dose	Comment
First-line drugs: Safely terminate seizures		
Lorazepam	0.2 mg/kg	Less hypotension than diazepam, the anticonvulsant effect lasts 6–12 hours; 0.3–9 mg/h used as an infusion as an alternative to phenobarbital
Midazolam	0.05 mg/kg	Higher doses of 0.2 mg/kg are used; IV midazolam can also be given by the IM, buccal, or intranasal route
Diazepam	0.1 mg/kg	If higher doses are used (0.3 mg/kg), respiratory depression is likely and ventilatory support might be necessary
Second-line drugs: If no response in 20 minutes		
Phenytoin/fosphenytoin	20 mg/kg	Fosphenytoin, unlike phenytoin, is water soluble and can be given IM; phenytoin can cause purple glove syndrome, which is a severe tissue drug reaction that can occur even without extravasation; a maintenance dose of 5–7 mg/kg/day TID
Sodium valproate	40 mg/kg	6 mg/kg/min; maintenance dose 30–60 mg/kg/day BID
Levetiracetam	20 mg/kg	100 mg/min; maintenance dose 2–4 g/day
Phenobarbital	20 mg/kg	50–75 mg/min; maintenance dose 1–4 mg/kg/day BID
Lacosamide	400 mg IV 5 minutes	Pre- and post-Rx EKG needed; maintenance dose 400–600 mg/day BID
Third-line drugs: Anesthetic doses for intractable seizures		
Propofol	2 mg/kg	Repeat to a max dose of 10 m/kg; it may require ventilation and cardiovascular support
Midazolam	0.2 mg/kg	Repeat to a max dose of 2 mg/kg; it may require ventilation and cardiovascular support

CHAPTER 28 Seizure Types and Treatment

- Intubate with propofol and muscle relaxants (succinylcholine, if K within normal limits)
- Alert EEG lab for emergency recording
- If seizures persist after propofol induction, consider phenobarbiturate 20 mg/kg at 100 mg/min.
- *Seizures persist at 40 minutes:* Consider continuous infusions of midazolam or propofol.

Antiepileptic drug side-effects: Patients on anticonvulsant drugs are at risk of sedation, cognitive impairment, ataxia/impaired coordination, withdrawal syndrome, depression with suicidal ideation; bone marrow, liver, or renal impairment; and weight gain or loss. Anticonvulsant drugs induce hepatic enzymes, compete with protein binding, and have significant drug interactions.

Anticonvulsant - neuromuscular blocking drugs interaction:
- Effect of anticonvulsants:
  - Minimal potentiation of neuromuscular block with acute use.
  - Resistance to neuromuscular block with prolonged use
  - Resistance due to pre- and post-receptor effects
- Long-term anticonvulsant use:
  - Significant tolerance can result with steroidal relaxants.
  - Increased protein binding
  - Increased hepatic clearance.
  - Upregulation of acetylcholine receptors.

FURTHER READING

1. Khateb M et al. The effect of anti-seizure medications on the propagation of epileptic activity: A review. Front Neurol. 2021;12:674182.
2. Kim H et al. Antiepileptic drug selection according to seizure type in adult patients with epilepsy. J Clin Neurol. 2020;16(4):547-55.
3. Siddiqui MK et al. A review of epileptic seizure detection using machine learning classifiers. Brain Inform. 2020;7(1):5.
4. Turek G et al. Seizure semiology, localization, and the 2017 ILAE seizure classification. Epilepsy Behav. 2022;126:108455.
5. Varatharajah Y et al. Electrophysiological correlates of brain health help diagnose epilepsy and lateralize seizure focus. Annu Int Conf IEEE Eng Med Biol Soc. 2020;2020: 3460-64.

Vignette: A Brief History of Epilepsy

Akkadian, a Babylonian tablet dated from 2000 BCE, describes epilepsy and its features. Epilepsy was documented in the Edwin Smith Papyrus 3500 years ago. It is also documented in Chinese texts dating to 770 BCE. In the 5th century BCE, Hippocrates considered it a sacred disease due to its inexplicable nature. He described its clinical manifestations. Hippocrates described it as a treatable brain disorder. The disease ran in families, and its prognosis was worse if it occurred at a young age. However, little progress was made in treating the disease until 1857, when Sir Charles Locock introduced potassium bromide. Locock realized that potassium bromide did not cure the disease but suppressed convulsions. The bromide treatment was used until the early 20th century when barbiturates were first used to treat convulsions.

Chapter 29

Venous Air Embolism

INTRODUCTION

Venous air embolism (VAE) is the entrainment of air into the veins from an operating field.

PATHOLOGY

- *Predisposing factors:*
    - Air entrainment requires a pressure gradient of >5 cm H_2O between the venous entrainment site and the right atrium. A 14 G (1.8 mm internal diameter) needle with a 5 cm H_2O pressure gradient can entrain 100 mL of air/s.
    - *Risk of VAE during neurosurgery:*
        - *High risk:* Sitting position and posterior fossa surgery.
        - *Medium risk:* Spine fusion, cervical laminectomy, and craniosynostosis
        - *Low risk:* Burr holes, deep brain stimulator, and arterial and central venous line placements
        - It can occur at any time during posterior fossa surgery, even postoperatively.
        - With transesophageal echocardiogram (TEE), VAE is detected in 100% of sitting position surgeries.
- *Incidence:*
    - Posterior fossa (50%) > cervical laminectomies (25%) in sitting position; both surgeries in sitting position have a greater incidence of air embolism compared to lateral approach to posterior fossa surgery (12.5%).
    - Increased incidence during posterior fossa surgery due to:
        - Presence of large venous sinuses in the posterior fossa
        - Presence of emissary veins (non-retractile) in the squamous part of the occipital bone
        - Dry operating field condition
        - Systemic hypotension and reduced cardiac output.
- *Other possible sites of air entrainment:*
    - Around central venous lines, if placed in the neck

- During rapid resuscitation through the peripheral IV line
- Pin fixation sites.
- *Other neurosurgeries associated with VAE:*
  - Stereotactic surgery in a sitting position, sometimes in awake patients
  - Spine surgery
  - VA shunt placement
- *Other surgeries with VAE:*
  - Laparoscopic cholecystectomy
  - Central venous line placements
  - Endoscopic procedures
  - Hip surgery
  - Accidental injections during radiological procedures.

HEMODYNAMIC EFFECTS

- The clinical syndrome depends on the rate of air entrainment. Any surgery in which the operating site is above the heart carries the risk of air embolism:
  - *Slow entrainment of air* partially obstructs the right ventricular outflow. Air enters the pulmonary vascular bed. There is a release of cytokines and neurogenic vasoconstriction [Bezold–Jarisch reflex (BZR]. BZR, during PE, stimulates the J-receptors, causing apnea, bradycardia, and hypotension. Turbulent flow activates platelets. Pulmonary vascular constriction and bronchoconstriction decreased $ETCO_2$ and increased ETN_2, decreased cardiac output, and shunt resulting in hypoxia.
  - *Rapid air entrainment:* Right ventricular outflow obstruction and cardiac arrest
- *The hemodynamic effects of venous air embolism depend on the following:*
  - Volume and rate of air entrainment
    - Usually said to be 1 mL/kg/min
    - Bolus of 3 mL/kg fatal
  - Presence of a right-to-left shunt
  - Underlying cardiac function
  - Concurrent use of nitrous oxide
- *Acute VAE:* Signs and symptoms based on air volume in the right ventricle:
  - *Small Volume (<0.5 mL/kg):*
    - Gasp, wheezing, altered mental state, decreased $ETCO_2$, increased ETN_2, increased airway pressures, decreased SaO_2, sinus tachycardia, and ventricular ectopy.
  - *Medium Volume (0.5–1.5 mL/kg):*
    - *Respiratory:* Bronchoconstriction: Dyspnea, wheezing, increased airway pressures; pulmonary vasoconstriction

- *Cardiac:* Right ventricular outflow obstruction, right heart strain, tall peaked P waves, ST segment depression, increased jugular venous pressure (JVP), and hypotension
- *Cerebral:* Ischemia due to hypotension and altered mental status
- Large volume (>1.5 mL/kg):
  - Precordial pain and cardiovascular collapse.

GIRARD'S SCALE

- *Grade I:* Precordial Doppler detection only
- *Grade II:* Grade I + decreased ETCO$_2$
- *Grade III:* Grade II + 20% change in heart rate and blood pressure
- *Grade IV:* Grade II + 40% change in heart rate and blood pressure
- *Grade V:* Circulatory collapse
- Venous air embolism in awake patients:
  - Can occur during:
    - Stereotactic surgery in a sitting position
    - Placement and removal of central venous lines
  - Clinical signs and symptoms of venous air embolism:
    - Coughing
    - Gasp with air entrained at 0.4 mL/kg/min
    - Tachyarrhythmias
    - Shortness of breath
    - Anxiety
    - Confusion
    - Chest pain
    - *Change in S$_1$ intensity:* 1.7 mL/kg/min
    - *Classical mill-wheel murmur:* 2 mL/kg/min
    - Cardiovascular collapse
- *Venous air embolism in anesthetized patients:* The detection thresholds for VAE under general anesthesia are listed in **Table 1**.

TRANSESOPHAGEAL DOPPLER (TEE)

- TEE was not used extensively in the past as bulky probes pressed the tongue to impede venous return.
- Compact TEE probes are now available and therefore are more useful.
- TEE has a high sensitivity for VAE. It can detect right to left shunt, assess cardiac functions, and help in resuscitation.
- It requires time for placement and technical expertise.
- *Grading of VAE* based on imaging of the bubble volume relative to the right ventricular outflow tract (RVOT) volume:
  - *Grade 1:* Single bubble
  - *Grade 2:* <50% RVOT volume

Table 1: Detection of venous air embolism.

Modality	Threshold (mL/kg/min)	Comment
TEE	0.02	Expertise is needed; placement can put pressure on the tongue; highly sensitive and helpful to assess cardiac function and help in guiding treatment
PC Doppler	0.2	Highly sensitive, constant noise, diathermy artifacts
PA catheter	0.25	Invasive, seldom used clinically, but it can aspirate air
ETN_2	0.4	ETN_2 sampling is not available in most centers
CVP	0.4	Earlier than the increase in pulmonary vascular resistance
$ETCO_2$	0.4	Most useful for a 3 mm Hg sudden decrease without change in ventilation diagnostic; gradual $ETCO_2$ decline can be due to hypothermia, hyperventilation, and reduction of cardiac output; sudden drop can also be due to PE from a thrombus
SaO_2	–	Due to bronchospasm, pulmonary vascular spasm, right ventricular dysfunction and outlet obstruction, and V/Q mismatch
EKG	0.6	Sinus tachycardia, right ventricular strain, and ST segment depression
MAP	0.7–1.5	Late depends on the rate and volume of air entrained and myocardial functions

(EKG: electrocardiogram; MAP: mean arterial pressure; PA: pulmonary artery; PC: precordial; TEE: transesophageal echocardiogram)

- *Grade 3:* 50–99% RVOT volume
- *Grade 4:* 100% RVOT volume

PRECORDIAL DOPPLER

- *Precordial Doppler probe for the detection of VAE:*
    - It has an emitting and receiving frequency of 2–3 MHz.
    - It has a diameter of 1 inch.
    - It has two piezoelectric sensors for continuous signal processing: one for generating sound, while the other receives the reflected signal.
- The 2–3 MHz ultrasound can penetrate tissues to 10 cm.
- Doppler is highly sensitive, and sound analysis of the mill-wheel murmur reveals an increase in amplitude with a shift toward higher frequencies with the increasing volume of entrained air.
- The device is usually put slightly to the right of the sternum and tilted towards the right atrium.
- In the sitting position, the heart might be recumbent, and the probe might need to be placed to the left of the sternum.
- The probe is tested by listening to changes in heart sound by rapid injection of 10 mL of agitated saline of albumin. The dissolved air is sufficient to test the placement of the probe.

PREVENTION OF VENOUS AIR EMBOLISM

- *Positioning:*
  - Minimize the use of a sitting position.
  - If a central venous catheter has been placed: Zero CVP to RA (V intercostal space), watch changes in pressure by raising the transducer to the operating height before moving the patient. The test helps to anticipate the venous pressure changes with positioning and the need for supplemental fluids.
- *Avoid hypovolemia:*
  - Gradually position.
  - Consider a judicious IV fluid supplement.
  - RA pressure of 10–15 cm H_2O
- *Use of antishock trousers*
- *Avoid N_2O that can diffuse into and expand the entrained air.*
- *Positive end-expiratory pressure (PEEP):*
  - *Advantages:* Increases regional venous pressure.
  - *Disadvantages:* Increases risk of paradoxical embolism; the release of PEEP can lead to VAE.
  - PEEP use for VAE prevention is questionable.
  - Low levels (<5 mm Hg) are cautiously used for improving oxygenation.
- *RA catheter:*
  - Pros:
    - A multi-orifice catheter is ideally positioned 2 cm below the superior vena cava and right atrium (SVC/RA) junction, preferably at an angle of 80°, can help aspirate air and prevent it from reaching the RV.
    - It helps to detect VAE due to the increase in CVP.
    - Aspiration offers a means of removing air from the RA and confirming the diagnosis.
    - Enables delivery of potent vasoconstrictors.
    - Assists in determining the level of safe head elevation.
  - Cons:
    - Placement of long-arm catheter takes time.
    - It takes expertise to place a long-arm catheter in the correct location guided by a biphasic P wave on the EKG.
    - Air aspiration during VAE is relatively ineffective.
    - Corrective measures instituted at early detection, by monitoring precordial Doppler, decrease the chances of successful aspiration.
    - Placement of the line via the internal jugular vein creates a route for air embolism. When access to the SVC/RA is obtained through the internal jugular vein, a purse string suture should be placed

around the catheter to prevent air from entraining along the central venous catheter.
- The benefits of placing the catheter remain unproven. Within seconds of entrainment, air reaches the RV, rendering aspiration ineffective.

Thus, the routine use of a multi-orifice catheter has declined in recent years. Emphasis is now placed on alerting the surgeons, flooding the field, and other measures guided by precordial Doppler.

MANAGEMENT OF VAE

- *Be vigilant:* Any procedure in which the operating site is 5 cm above the level of the heart or any operation requiring gas insufflation carries the risk of VAE. The severity of VAE and the corresponding clinical features are listed in **Table 2**.
- An acute 3 mm Hg drop of $ETCO_2$ indicates VAE.
- Prevent further entrainment.
  - Alert the surgeons
  - A dry operating field carries a greater risk of VAE.
  - Entrainment of air can sometimes be seen in veins egressing the surgical site.
  - Flood the field with saline, pack it with wet swabs, and apply wax to bone edges.
  - Identify and seal the source when possible.
- Switch to 100% oxygen and shut off nitrous oxide. Changing the net fresh gas flow or ventilator rate is to be avoided, as it makes assessing the recovery from VAE ($ETCO_2$) challenging.
- If a CV catheter has been placed, aspirate to confirm and treat VAE.

Table 2: Clinical severity of air embolism.

Severity	Detected by	Trigger	Pathophysiology	Symptoms
Subclinical	TEE, precordial Doppler, ETN_2	Minimal air entrainment	Trace air in RA	None
Mild	Decreased $ETCO_2$ and SaO_2	Mechanical, platelet activation	Impaired gas diffusion	Gasp, cyanosis
Moderate	Increased CVP; Increased HR; Decreased MAP	Increased RV strain, decreased CO, decreased RV and LV functions	Decreased cardiovascular function	Tachycardia, arrhythmias, and hypotension
Severe	Abnormal S1, mill-wheel murmur	RV and LV failure	Myocardial ischemia, collapse	Hypotension, arrest

(CVP: central venous pressure; LV: left ventricle; MAP: mean arterial pressure; RA: right atrium; RV: right ventricle; TEE: transesophageal echocardiogram)

- Support the blood pressure with fluids and pressor agents.
  - Maintain adequate CVP.
  - Institute inotropic support as needed with dobutamine and ephedrine.
  - Despite pulmonary arterial hypertension (PAH), small doses of norepinephrine are safe.
  - Treat arrhythmias
- Consider compressing the jugular vein if $ETCO_2$ continues to decrease.
- The use of PEEP in preventing VAE is controversial. In theory, PEEP increases CVP; however, it can also decrease the preload and cause a paradoxical air embolism.
- Coordinate with the surgical team to place the patient in the Trendelenburg position and not lower the back unless pins fixed to the upper section of the table.
  - Increases venous return.
  - Increases operative site venous pressure.
  - May decrease right ventricle outflow obstruction.
  - The classical left lateral decubitus position (Durant's maneuver) is not universally considered to be effective.
- In extremis, take the patient out of pins, cover the operating site, and place in the Trendelenburg position with or without left lateral tilt.
- *Hyperbaric oxygenation:*
  - Decreases bubble size.
  - Increases N_2 reabsorption.
  - Improves oxygenation.
- In extremis, perfluorocarbon infusion may be considered. Perfluorocarbon has $10^5 \times$ greater affinity to CO_2, N_2, and O_2 than blood and may help absorb entrained air.

FURTHER READING

1. Al-Afif S et al. Analysis of risk factors for venous air embolism in the semisitting position and its impact on outcome in a consecutive series of 740 patients. J Neurosurg. 2021:1-8.
2. Elouardi Y et al. Fatal venous air embolism during lumbar spondylolisthesis surgery. Indian J Anaesth. 2021;65(2):171-3.
3. Gey L et al. Cerebral venous sinus air embolism following removal of intracranial pressure monitoring device: About an exceptional and fatal complication. Neurochirurgie. 2022;68(2):249-51.
4. Günther F et al. Venous air embolism in the sitting position in cranial neurosurgery: incidence and severity according to the used monitoring. Acta Neurochir (Wien). 2017;159(2):339-46.
5. Kurihara M et al. Estimation of the head elevation angle that causes clinically important venous air embolism in a semi-sitting position neurosurgery: a retrospective observational study. Fukushima J Med Sci. 2020;66(2):67-72.

CHAPTER 29 Venous Air Embolism

Vignette: Cerebral Air Embolism in Commercial Flights

Based on control tower communications, about 15,000 emergencies occur during commercial flights in the US each year. About one in 600 commercial flights have a medical emergency. The most common emergencies are seizures, gastrointestinal complaints, respiratory difficulties, chest pain, and cardiac arrest. Some of these emergencies are easy to explain and are linked to the low cabin pressure and partial pressure of oxygen. Therefore, worsening respiratory and cardiac problems are expected.

Inflight seizures are rare and constitute less than a tenth of a percent of all inflight emergencies. Usually, in-flight seizures are triggered by sleep deprivation during travel in epileptic patients. However, cerebral air embolism can cause seizures as well. These patients usually are middle-aged with a history of respiratory disease, in whom seizures can be due to bullae in the lungs. Bullae can be the source of air entrainment leading to air embolism. There may be a history of inflight seizures in these patients. In severe cases, unconsciousness and in-flight death can occur. Prevention includes vigilance and avoiding flying if there is a history of significant lung disease or unexplained seizures. If an episode occurs during flight, oxygen supplementation, return to a lower altitude, and as soon as possible hyperbaric oxygen treatment might be necessary.

Chapter 30

Traumatic Brain Injury

INTRODUCTION

Traumatic brain injury (TBI) is the impairment of brain functions due to the abrupt movement of the head resulting from a fall, blow or jolt. TBI is characterized by changes in consciousness, memory loss, disorientation, or focal neurological symptoms. These manifest varyingly, from exceedingly transient disturbances to fatal outcomes. Annually in the United States, approximately 2.5 million traumatic brain injuries result in 50,000 deaths. A third of injuries are in the pediatric age group. About 13 million people live with disabilities due to TBIs.

PATHOLOGY

- *Primary brain injury:*
  - *Acceleration and deceleration injuries:* The brain, suspended in the CSF, can move within the cranial vault as the neural tissue is relatively elastic. A sudden linear or rotational movement can push the tissue against the bony confines of the skull to cause injury.
  - *Concussion:* Altered consciousness without structural damage.
  - *Contusion:* Disruption of capillaries and venules with increased edema (low attenuating lesions on CT scans) or extravasation of blood (high attenuating regions on CT scans).
  - *Laceration:* Tear of the pia-arachnoid membrane with tissue disruption.
  - *Diffuse axonal injuries:* Rotational acceleration/deceleration injuries cause microscopic axonal injuries in the corpus callosum and rostral brainstem with immediate unconsciousness without evidence of injury on CT. They are classified as mild (coma <6 hours), moderate (coma 6–24 hours), or severe (coma for months).
  - *Hematoma:*
    - *Subgaleal:* Extracranial bleed between the pericranium and the galeal aponeurosis seen in neonates. It usually happens after a difficult delivery or suction extraction. It can lead to hemorrhagic shock in neonates.
    - *Epidural:* Arterial bleed between dura and skull.
    - *Subdural:* Between dura and arachnoid, typically due to venous-tears, can be acute or chronic to cause a rise in intracranial

pressure (ICP), and can be fatal; seen in extremes of age; with anticoagulation; and with minimal trauma.
    - *Intraparenchymal bleeding* is usually due to vascular and microvascular pathologies or trauma.
    - *Subarachnoid hemorrhage* is not restricted to a region; hence, it is not considered a hematoma.
  - *Countercoup injuries* are on the opposite side of impact.
  - *Penetrating brain injuries* can be low (knives) or high velocity (bullets) or due to skull fragments.
- Secondary brain injury: Multiple mechanisms that include:
  - Hypoxia/ischemia
  - Edema
  - *Metabolic:* Hyperglycemia/acidosis/hypercalcemia
  - *Children at greater risk:*
    - $CMRO_2$ is higher in children versus adults, 6.0 versus 3.5 mL/100 g/min.
    - Cerebral blood flow (CBF) is higher in children versus adults, 100 versus 50 mL/100 g/min.
    - ICP (2-4 mm Hg) is lower in children vs. 10-15 mm Hg in adults
    - However, cranial compliance is better in children.

CLINICAL FEATURES

- TBI associated with cervical spine injuries in 6% of patients.
- With severe head injury or Glasgow Coma Scale (GCS) <8: Other injuries that require surgery are likely to occur in 25% of the patients, while overall, 50% of patients have other injuries.
- Closed head injury unlikely to cause shock in adults.
- *Scalp:* Highly vascular and can result in significant bleeding.
- *Skull fractures:*
  - Simple
  - Comminuted
  - Depressed
  - Basilar
  - *Skull base fractures:*
    - *Bleeding from the nose, nasopharynx, and ears*
    - *Battle sign:* Mastoid ecchymosis
    - *Raccoon eyes:* Periocular hematoma
    - *CSF rhinorrhea and otorrhea*
    - *Double-ring sign:* Halo around blood stain with CSF leak
  - *Increased ICP:* Headache (occipital), nausea/vomiting (projectile), impaired mentation, altered consciousness, bradycardia, hypertension, unilateral pupillary dilation, and abnormal breathing and seizures.

Score	Adult	Children	Infant
Best eye opening			
4	Spontaneous	Spontaneous	Spontaneous
3	Verbal	Verbal	Verbal
2	Pain	Pain	Pain
1	None	None	None
Best verbal response			
5	Oriented converses	Appropriate speech	Appropriate interaction
4	Disoriented converses	Inappropriate speech	Inappropriate
3	Inappropriate speech	Moaning	Cries to pain
2	Incomprehensible	Irritable/inconsolable	Moans
1	None	None	None
Best motor response			
6	Normal response	Normal response	Normal response
5	Localizes pain	Localizes pain	Withdraws to touch
4	Withdraws to pain	Withdraws to pain	Withdraws to pain
3	Abnormal flexion	Abnormal flexion	Abnormal flexion
2	Abnormal extension	Abnormal extension	Abnormal extension
1	None	None	None

Table 1: Glasgow Coma Scale for adults, children, and infants.

Assessment of Traumatic Brain Injury

- *Traumatic brain injury severity based on GCS **(Table 1)**:*
    - *Minimal:* GCS 15, no amnesia or unconsciousness.
    - *Mild:* GCS 14, unconsciousness <5 minutes, impaired alertness, and memory
    - *Moderate:* GCS 9–13, unconsciousness >5 minutes, and focal deficits
    - *Severe:* GCS 5–8
    - *Critical:* GCS 3–4.

Pitfalls of the Glasgow Coma Scale

- Other factors could affect cognition:
    - Concurrent alcohol intake
    - Metabolic factors
- Compounding effects of other neurological influences, such as seizures
- Questionable weightages of parameters that are skewed toward motor assessment.
- The verbal response cannot be evaluated in intubated patients.
- Does not assess brainstem responses.

Table 2: Marshall's CT based classification of TBI.

Class	Injury	Finding	Mortality
I	Diffuse injury	Normal CT	<1%
II	Diffuse injury	• Cisterns seen; mid-line shift <5 mm • Foreign bodies seen • No high/mixed density lesion >25 cm^3	10%
III	Diffuse injury with edema	• Cisterns decreased or absent • Mid-line shift <5 mm • No high/mixed density lesion >25 cm^3	15%
IV	Diffuse injury with shift	• Mid-line shift >5 mm • No high/mixed density lesion >25 cm^3	25%
V	Evacuated mass lesion	Any surgically treated lesion	50%
VI	Nonevacuated mass lesion	Unevacuated high/mixed density lesion >25 cm^3	60%

Other Coma Scales

- *Pediatric Coma Scale* is a modification of GCS for infants and children.
- *Modified Glasgow Coma Scale:* Assesses motor activity, brainstem reflexes, and consciousness, each on a 1-6 point scale.
- *The four scale:* Full outline of unresponsiveness (FOUR) was developed to assess unconsciousness in patients with or without an endotracheal tube. It assesses eye opening, motor response, brain stem reflexes, and respiration on a 0–4 scale.

Marshall's CT class: Marshall's CT scan-based classification of traumatic brain injury is in **Table 2**.

Serum Markers of Traumatic Brain Injury

Role of biochemical markers: Biochemical markers are needed to determine prognosis, determine treatment response, and detect secondary brain injury, but they are still investigational:
- *s-100 B:*
  - Initial released after TBI. S100b is not specific to cerebral injury as it occurs in non-neuronal cells like adipocytes.
  - Cerebral s100B peaks at 12–24 hours after injury.
  - Half-life 30-90 min
  - CSF concentrations are 100× serum
  - An increase in serum s100B may predict outcome of TBI:
    - 100B as a predictor of the Glasgow Outcome Scale (GOS) score:
      - s100B <0.3 µg/mL, GOS = 5
      - s100B 0.3–0.5 µg/mL, GOS = 4

- s100B 0.5–0.75 µg/mL, GOS = 3
- s100B 0.75–1.0 µg/mL, GOS = 2
- s100B >1 µg/mL, GOS = 1.
- *Other markers* include Glial fibrillary protein (GFP), neuronal-specific enolase (NSE), and *plasma-free DNA*.

Magnetic Resonance Imaging Assessment of Traumatic Brain Injury

- MRI imaging is superior to a CT scan for imaging posterior fossa injuries.
- T2 image is better for intraparenchymal lesions.
- FLAIR (fluid-attenuated inversion recovery) for detecting edema.
- The location of injuries can have prognostic values, such as in the brainstem, the hypothalamus, and the basal ganglia.
- Magnetic resonance spectroscopy can detect lactic acidosis which predicts a poor outcome.

Electroencephalography

Percent alpha variability (PAV) on EEG represents the changes in the rhythm in response to stimulation. The loss of PAV in TBI is a predictor of a poor prognosis of 6-month survival and as is the silence in this frequency band. High PAV was usually associated with a better outcome. Due to background sedation in critically ill patients, the usefulness of electroencephalography (EEG) in TBI is somewhat limited.

Evoked Potentials

- Bilateral loss of evoked potential (EP) beyond a week carries a very poor prognosis.
- Conversely, the preservation of evoked response carries a better prognosis.

High-Risk Traumatic Brain Injury

Glasgow outcome scale:
- *Score 1:* Death
- *Score 2:* Persistent vegetative state
- *Score 3:* Severely disabled.
- *Score 4:* Moderately disabled.
- *Score 5:* Minor residual deficits.

Predictors of poor outcome:
- GCS <8
- Prolonged hypotension (SBP <90 mm hg)
- Fixed dilated pupils.
- Diffuse axonal injury.

CHAPTER 30 Traumatic Brain Injury

- Post-traumatic amnesia >7 days
- Altered mental state/unconsciousness >24 hours

Predictors of poor prognosis in children:
- <4 years
- Cardiopulmonary resuscitation (CPR);
- Hypoxia (PaO_2 <60 mm Hg),
- Hypotension (SBP <70 + 2 × age),
- Hyperthermia (>38°C)
- Hyperglycemia (glucose >250 mg/dL)
- Other injuries.

FURTHER READING

1. Böhm JK et al. Extended coagulation profiling in isolated traumatic brain injury: a CENTER-TBI analysis. Neurocrit Care. 2022;36(3):927-41.
2. Faden AI et al. Bidirectional brain-systemic interactions and outcomes after TBI. Trends Neurosci. 2021;44(5):406-18.
3. Przekwas A et al. Biomechanics of blast TBI with time-resolved consecutive primary, secondary, and tertiary loads. Mil Med. 2019;184(Suppl 1):195-205.
4. Sekar S et al. Concussion/mild traumatic brain injury (TBI) induces brain insulin resistance: a positron emission tomography (PET) scanning study. Int J Mol Sci. 2021;22(16).
5. Toro C et al. Association of brain injury biomarkers and circulatory shock following moderate-severe traumatic brain injury: a TRACK-TBI study. J Neurosurg Anesthesiol, 2021.

Vignette: Phineas Gage: How His Head Injury Impacted Neuroscience?

Phineas P. Gage was a young, literate, energetic, enterprising railroad worker. At 4:30 PM on September 13, 1848, Gage was preparing a gunpowder explosion. As he momentarily turned his head, the gunpowder ignited. It launched an iron bar at his face. The bar was an inch thick, 3 feet long, and weighed about 6 kg. The iron bar pierced his left cheek and traversed through his brain, exited the skull, and landed 100 yards away. Gage bled profusely from the injury but remained conscious throughout his ordeal. Before his injury, Gage had been assessed by a physician, John Harlow. Harlow also followed him after the injury. He observed that Gage had changed from a restrained, responsible man to a disinhibited, unemployable person. His dysfunction was initially severe but gradually improved. Gage died during a seizure twelve years later, at 36 years of age. John Harlow believed that the change was due to the frontal lobe injury. In the 1850s, phrenology was the prevailing pseudoscience that attributed personality traits to the shape of the skull. Gage's case revealed that there could be an organic basis to behavior and that different parts of the brain probably work together to influence it.

Chapter 31: Targeted Temperature Management

INTRODUCTION

Manipulation of brain temperature is an essential part of modern neuroanesthetic practice. Mild to moderate hypothermia can mitigate ischemic neurological injury but can impair cognition, and profound hypothermia causes systemic complications. Hypothermia, however, remains the most reliable neuroprotective tool in clinical practice. Conversely, hyperthermia can potentiate neurological injury, and malignant hyperthermia requires early recognition and prompt specific treatment.

BRAIN TEMPERATURE

- Brain tissue accounts for 20% of total body metabolism; it is an imported source of heat generated in the body.
- Brain temperature is dynamically linked to neuronal activity.
- Brain temperature can differ by as much as 2–3 °C compared to core temperature.
- When measured directly, brain tissue temperature exceeds the arterial blood temperature.
- Regions of the brain that are constantly active, like the hippocampus, have a higher temperature than regions like the cortex that are intermittently active.
- Drugs (e.g., cocaine), motivation, and sensory stimuli affect regional brain temperature.
- Neuronal activation, such as painful stimuli, causes an immediate and sustained increase in brain temperature.
- *Brain temperature effects:*
  - *Neuronal functions:* Cognition, clinical and electrophysiological monitoring
  - Brain metabolism
  - Regional blood flow
  - Blood-brain barrier permeability
  - Permeability of cell membranes to ions and water
  - Glial cell metabolism
  - Neuronal injury
  - Metabolic monitoring, such as microdialysis

Targeted Temperature Management

Targeted temperature management (TTM) provides a target temperature and specifies the duration of hypothermia.

- *Indications:*
  - *In adults:* Cardiac arrest after the return of spontaneous circulation.
  - *Neonatal:* Perinatal hypoxia-ischemia and birth asphyxia.
  - Role in stroke and traumatic brain injury
- *Hypothermia can be classified as:*
  - *Normothermia:* Up to 36–38.0 °C
  - *Mild hypothermia:* 32–36 °C
  - *Moderate:* Up to 28–32 °C
  - *Profound/severe:* <32 °C
- The techniques for inducing hypothermia are listed in **Table 1**
- *Rationale:*
  - Decreases $CMRO_2$ 5–7%/°C
  - Decreases excitotoxic neurotransmitter (glutamate) release.
  - Decreases blood-brain barrier breakdown.
  - Decreases edema.
  - Decreases intracranial pressure (ICP).
  - Reduces the likelihood of hemorrhagic transformation.
  - Mitigates hyperthermic injury.
- *Concerns and side-effects:*
  - Delays in the institution of hypothermia decrease the potential benefits
  - Impairs cognitive assessment

Table 1: Methods to induce hypothermia.

Technique	Cooling rate	Advantages	Disadvantages
Ice packs over large superficial arteries	1.5°C/h	It readily instituted and could be applied to the whole body	Poor control, and frostbites, limit patient care and may prevent effective defibrillation
Cooling helmet	1.5°C/h	Effective in neonates	Scalp injury possible
Cold fluid circulating pads	3°C/h	Effective and can also be used for rewarming with warm water	Skin injury is possible and difficult in obese
Cold IV fluids	Up to 4°C/h	Rapid, helpful in obese, but volume limited to 30 mL/kg	Ineffective over time and fluid overload
Intravascular cooling catheters	Up to 4.5°C/h	Rapid onset	Invasive and can cause DVT
Antipyretics	Up to 0.4°C/h	Readily instituted	Oral administration needed

(DVT: deep venous thrombosis)

- Slows enzymatic reaction decreases drug clearance and prolongs drug effects.
- It impairs coagulation and platelet functions to cause disseminated intravascular coagulation.
- Causes a leftward shift of the oxygen-hemoglobin dissociation curve.
- Increases infection rates.
- *Fluid and electrolyte imbalances:*
  - Hypovolemia
  - Hyperglycemia
  - Hypokalemia
  - Hypomagnesemia.
- *Arrhythmias:* Bradycardia, heart blocks, ventricular ectopy, cardiac arrest
- Organ dysfunction such as kidney, liver, and pancreatic dysfunction
- Tissue injuries such as frost bites of fingers and toes, rhabdomyolysis
- Shivering during and after hypothermia
- Delays determination of brain death.

Shivering

- Shivering is an involuntary motor response to hypothermia.
- Cooling the pre-optic region of the hypothalamus leads to shivering.
- The descending neural pathways traverse the medial forebrain bundle, the spinal cord, to end in the anterior horn cells.
- Shivering is characterized by grouped discharges on electromyography. There are two patterns:
  - A phasic pattern that waxes and wanes due to postoperative hypothermia (defined as a core temperature of 33–35 °C)
  - A clonic pattern that is seen after recovery from volatile general anesthetics
- *Shivering scale:*
  - *Grade 0:* No shivering
  - *Grade 1:* Mild fasciculation of face and neck
  - *Grade 2:* Visible tremors
  - *Grade 3:* Gross generalized muscular activity.
- *Side-effects:* Distressing for the patient. It can increase metabolic rate by 500%, increase heart rate and blood pressure, increase myocardial oxygen consumption, increase intracranial pressure, decreases cerebral perfusion pressure, brain tissue oxygen tension and augments pain.
- *Treatment:*
  - Forced warm air blanket.
  - Warm blankets
  - Meperidine in 15-25 mg increments
  - *Other treatments:* Physostigmine and clonidine

CHAPTER 31 Targeted Temperature Management

- May require sedation with midazolam, fentanyl, dexmedetomidine, or propofol.
- If febrile, consider acetaminophen.

Hyperthermia

Core temperature >99.7–100.9 °F or 37.5–38.3 °C
Dangerous if core temperature >104 °F or 40 °C.

- ***Etiology in neurological ICU:***
  - Infection
  - Transfusion reaction
  - *Central fever:*
    - Etiology often unknown
    - Intraventricular hemorrhage (IVH)
    - Subarachnoid hemorrhage (SAH)
    - External ventricular drain
    - Prolonged ICU stay.
  - Deep venous thrombosis
  - *Drugs:* Include phenytoin, carbamazepine, sulfa drugs, and penicillin
- ***Malignant hyperthermia (MH):***
  - *Etiology:*
    - Autosomal dominant disorder of calcium metabolism.
    - MH is largely due to an error in encoding ryanodine receptor 1 (RyR-1) on chromosome 19.
  - *Clinical presentation:*
    - Fever in 66% of the patients
    - Tachycardia in 50% of the patients
    - Trismus or masseter rigidity in 33% of the patients
    - Muscle rigidity in 20% of the patients
    - High-end tidal CO_2
    - *Subsequently:* Hyperventilation, rhabdomyolysis, severe acidosis, electrolyte imbalance (hyperkalemia), tachyarrhythmia and cardiovascular collapse, renal failure, and disseminated intravascular coagulation (DIC).
  - *Triggering agents:*
    - Succinylcholine
    - Volatile agents
    - Stress
    - Reaction to drugs may be delayed for 24 hours.
  - *Drugs considered safe to use:*
    - *Intravenous anesthetics:* Propofol, ketamine, etomidate
    - Sedatives like midazolam and other benzodiazepines
    - Local anesthetic agents

- Opiates
- Non-depolarizing neuromuscular blockers
- Nitrous oxide unlike volatile agents
- *Treatment:*
  - Early recognition essential
  - Aggressive supportive treatment
  - Large bore IV and cold fluids
  - Surface cooling
  - Arterial line essential
  - *Dantrolene dose:* 2.5 mg/kg rapid IV
  - Consider higher doses (10 mg/kg) if rigidity persists
  - *Dantrolene side effects:*
    - Drowsiness
    - Dizziness
    - Weakness
    - Tiredness
    - Nausea
    - Vomiting
    - Diarrhea.
- **Serotonin syndrome:**
  - The syndrome is triggered by psychoactive drugs such as monoamine oxidase inhibitors (MAOIs), selective serotonin reuptake inhibitors (SSRIs), tricyclic antidepressants, LSD, and cocaine.
  - *Clinical syndrome:* Presents 6–24 hours after drug exposure
    - Agitation, tremors, seizures
    - Autonomic disturbances
    - Hyperreflexia myoclonus
    - Hyperthermia
  - *Treatment:*
    - Drug discontinuation
    - *Serotonin antagonists:* Bromocriptine
    - *Supportive treatment:* Sedation, paralysis, intubation, ventilation, cardiovascular support, and fluids
    - Target temperature management
- **Neuroleptic malignant syndrome:**
  - *Etiology:*
    - Altered dopamine neurotransmission
    - Neuroleptic drugs (Haldol)
    - Antiemetics (phenothiazine, metoclopramide, droperidol, and prochlorperazine).
  - *Clinical features:*
    - Hyperpyrexia, rigidity, autonomic disturbances including fever, and altered mental status.

CHAPTER 31 Targeted Temperature Management

- *Treatment:* Discontinue Rx, symptomatic, dantrolene, bromocriptine, and sedatives.
- **Delirium tremens (DT):**
  - *Etiology:* 24–48 hours after alcohol withdrawal
  - *Clinical features:*
    - Anxiety, confusion, restlessness, and agitation
    - Tremors
    - Tachycardia and hypertension
    - Fever, sweating, and dehydration
    - Seizures
  - *Treatment:*
    - Benzodiazepines and adequate sedation.
    - Thiamine does not affect symptoms but helps prevent Wernicke's encephalopathy.

FURTHER READING

1. Evald L et al. Prolonged targeted temperature management reduces memory retrieval deficits six months post-cardiac arrest: A randomised controlled trial. Resuscitation. 2019;134:1-9.
2. Kim JG et al. Efficacy of the cooling method for targeted temperature management in postcardiac arrest patients: A systematic review and meta-analysis. Resuscitation. 2020;148:14-24.
3. Litman RS et al. Consensus Statement of the Malignant Hyperthermia Association of the United States on Unresolved Clinical Questions Concerning the Management of Patients with Malignant Hyperthermia. Anesth Analg. 2019;128(4):652-9.
4. Rüffert H et al. Consensus guidelines on perioperative management of malignant hyperthermia suspected or susceptible patients from the European Malignant Hyperthermia Group. Br J Anaesth. 2021;126(1):120-30.
5. Sawyer KN et al. Relationship between duration of targeted temperature management, ischemic interval, and good functional outcome from out-of-hospital cardiac arrest. Crit Care Med. 2020;48(3):370-77.

Vignette: An Early Report of a Familial Cluster of Malignant Hyperthermia Patients
Although malignant hyperthermia (MH) was first reported in pigs in 1900, the first clinical report was provided by E Penny in 1919. During surgery for a ruptured kidney, the patient became rigid, stopped breathing, and died. It was later found that the patient's mother had similarly passed away four years ago while undergoing a uterine operation. Two other family members died in the following years after exposure to chloroform. The condition was described as "hereditary susceptibility to chloroform", but features suggest an MH reaction to the anesthetic. The classic MH syndrome was not described until 1960 by Denborough and Lovell, some 40 years later.

Chapter 32: Peripheral Neuropathies

INTRODUCTION

Peripheral neuropathy is an injury to a peripheral nerve that impairs sensory, motor, or autonomic functions in a given dermatomal distribution. The disease can affect a single nerve (mononeuropathy) or several nerves (polyneuropathy). Sensory neuropathy presents with tingling, numbness, or pain. The pain can feel like pinpricks, throbbing, or burning. Motor neuropathies present as muscle weakness. Autonomic neuropathies, for example, can affect regional vasomotor responses, cardiovascular responses, or bowel functions.

ETIOLOGY

- *Traumatic:*
  - Direct nerve injuries
  - Positioning-related nerve injuries
  - Compression injuries, such as during tourniquet use.
- *Hereditary:* Charcot Marie–Tooth disease.
- *Entrapment syndromes* may be due to repetitive injuries, myxedema, rheumatoid arthritis, amyloidosis, and acromegaly.
  - The common sites are:
    - Median (carpal tunnel)
    - Ulnar (cubital tunnel)
    - Lateral cutaneous (meralgia paresthetica)
    - *Other common nerve injuries:* Radial nerve, Femoral nerve, Peroneal nerve
- *Metabolic:*
  - Diabetes mellitus
  - Uremia
  - Hypothyroid
  - Alcohol
  - Vitamin B_{12} deficiency
  - Porphyria.
- *Ischemic lesions:*
  - Diabetes mellitus
  - *Vasculitis:* Polyarteritis nodosa and systemic lupus erythematosus.

- *Systemic:*
  - Guillain–Barré syndrome
  - Cancers
  - Sarcoid
  - Syphilis
  - Collagen disorders.
- *Toxins:*
  - Insecticides
  - Heavy metals.
- *Drugs:*
  - Cisplatin
  - Doxorubicin
  - Isonicotinic acid hydrazide
  - Phenytoin
  - Hydralazine
  - Amiodarone.

CLINICAL FEATURES

- *Type of onset:* Sudden (trauma and compression), rapid (infective, diabetes, rheumatoid arthritis, and polyarteritis nodosa), slow, intermittent, and progressive as with autoimmune diseases, e.g., SLE.
- *Type of distribution:* Mono- or polyneuropathy; Pattern of distribution (characteristic nerve compression sites; proximal (rare, e.g., porphyria), or distal (Guillain–Barré syndrome)
- Associated comorbidities include diabetes or uremia, drug treatment, environmental exposure, and functional conversion reactions.
- *Clinical Assessment of motor power:*
  - 0/5 No contraction or movement
  - 1/5 Contraction visible/palpable but no movement
  - 2/5 Movement seen but not antigravity
  - 3–/5 Limited active movement against gravity.
  - 3+/5 Active movement against gravity that ceases when minimal resistance is applied.
  - 4/5 Active movement against gravity and mild resistance
  - 4+/5 Active movement against gravity and moderate resistance
  - 5–/5 Subnormal power
  - 5/5 Normal power

INVESTIGATIONS

- Electromyography.
- *Nerve conduction studies:* The loss of myelin slows nerve conduction and increases latency, conduction block, and temporal dispersion.

- *Autonomic response assessment,* such as heart rate variation with respiration or posture.
- *High-resolution MR imaging.*
- *High-frequency ultrasound imaging.*
- *Nerve or nerve-muscle biopsy:* Vasculitis, leprosy, amyloid, sarcoid, and leukodystrophies.
- *Diagnostic metabolic screen:*
  - *Blood:* Glucose, urea/creatinine, B_{12} deficiency, blood cell count, erythrocyte sedimentation rate (ESR), and thyroid screen.
  - *Cerebrospinal fluid (CSF):* Cytological studies to rule out infection and malignancy. Lyme polymerase and cytomegalovirus-branched chain DNA arrive at a specific diagnosis.

ANESTHETIC IMPLICATIONS

- Etiology and distribution.
- *Regional versus general anesthesia:*
  - Regional preferred, when possible.
- *Regional concerns:* A greater sensitivity to local anesthetic drugs:
  - Documentation of preexisting neurological deficits is essential if a regional technique is considered.
    - Spinal blocks
    - Regional blocks.
- *General anesthetic concerns:*
  - *Muscle weakness and atrophy:*
    - *Competitive blockers:* Prolonged effects
    - *Depolarizing muscle relaxants:*
      - Contraindicated.
      - Result in severe hyperkalemia
  - *Pharmacological concerns:* Narcotics are safe when care is taken not to depress respiration
  - *Cardiovascular effects:*
    - Postural hypotension
    - Bradycardia

FURTHER READING

1. Kollmer J et al. Magnetic resonance neurography: Improved diagnosis of peripheral neuropathies. Neurotherapeutics. 2021;18(4):2368-83.
2. Merheb D et al. Drug-induced peripheral neuropathy: Diagnosis and Management. Curr Cancer Drug Targets. 2022;22(1):49-76.
3. Patel K et al. Electrodiagnosis of common mononeuropathies: median, ulnar, and fibular (peroneal) neuropathies. Neurol Clin. 2021;39(4):939-55.
4. Vaz A et al. Complex regional pain syndrome after severe COVID-19 - A case report. Heliyon. 2021; 7(11):e08462.
5. Yakoby J et al. Guillain-Barré syndrome after novel coronavirus disease 2019. J Emerg Med. 2021;61(4):e67-70.

CHAPTER 32 Peripheral Neuropathies

Vignette: Role of Electricity in Nerve Transmission

The word "nerve" can be traced to the ancient Greeks, which means tendon, fiber, band, or sinew. In ancient Greece, it was believed that animal spirits transmitted information through the nerves. It was not until the second century that Galen described the brain as the vital organ of cognition, with the nerves playing a role in transmitting information. Rene Descartes, in 1664, published a figure that showed nerves transmitting pain impulses from the toes to the brain. Sir Isaac Newton (1717) believed nerves transmitted information through vibrations in an electric aether that permeated the nerves. Luigi Galvani, in the 1780s, demonstrated the role of electricity in transmitting impulses through nerves and provoking muscle contraction.

Chapter 33

Brain Death

INTRODUCTION

Brain death implies the irreversible cessation of all brain functions, including the brain stem. Irreversible means a failure to recover function, regardless of any therapeutic intervention.
- Diagnosis of brain death requires:
  - Meet the prerequisite requirements for severe brain injury by ruling out drugs, hypothermia, hypotension, or any metabolic/endocrine cause.
  - *Clinical exam:*
    - No response to pain
    - No cranial nerve reflexes.
    - No pupillary response to light
    - No oculocephalic response
    - No corneal reflex
  - *Apnea test:* No spontaneous respiratory effort in response to increasing CO_2.
  - Ancillary tests to support the diagnosis.

DIFFERENTIAL DIAGNOSIS

- *A persistent vegetative state* is the state of complete unawareness of self or the environment, although there may be some preservation of hypothalamic and brain stem functions. It lasts more than a month in severe traumatic and nontraumatic brain injury settings. The patient may exhibit preservation of some responses to noxious, auditory, tactile, or visual stimuli. Prolonged survival is possible, but the life expectancy is 2–5 years with supportive care. Recovery after 12 months is rare.
- *Locked-in syndrome* is characterized by a complete lack of motor functions, other than the movement of the eyes and the eyelids. The vision, hearing, and cognition are intact. The patients cannot talk, swallow, speak, or demonstrate any motor activity other than eye movements and blinking. The syndrome can be complete or incomplete, with no motor control or some motor control, respectively. The typical syndrome is due to pontine infarction due to basilar artery occlusion. Other causes include severe muscular diseases and meningitis.

- *Other differential diagnoses:*
  - Neurological diseases resulting in coma.
  - Profound hypothermia
  - Sedative/paralytic drug overdose

Prerequisites for Diagnosing Brain Death
- Establish the diagnosis of coma.
- The core temperature should be at least 36°C.
- Systolic blood pressure of 100 mm Hg; if needed, use vasopressin and other pressors.
- *Rule out:*
  - Metabolic abnormalities
  - Endocrine abnormalities
  - Acid-base imbalances
  - *Drugs:* Five half-lives of sedative-hypnotics should have elapsed.

Clinical Examination
- *Pain response:*
  - Assessment of cranial nerves may be challenging with facial trauma.
  - *Typical sites for eliciting pain response:*
    - Pressure on the supra-orbital ridge, sternum, angle of the mandible,
    - Pinching of the trapezius, anterior axillary fold
  - Pain response is usually a grimace or motor movement.
- *Spinal reflexes:* Dermatomal nociceptors or muscle stretch receptors can trigger a motor response. These spinal reflex responses can persist after brain death. They do not exclude the diagnosis of brain death.
  - *Examples of spinal reflexes seen after brain death include:*
    - Muscle fasciculation in the limbs in response to pain
    - Myoclonic jerks of the limbs
    - Twitching of facial muscles
    - Plantar flexion, or repetitive flexion and extension of the toes
    - Pronator extension response with the turning of the head.
    - Flexion of the quadriceps muscles in response to pain
    - *Lazarus sign:* Flexion of one or both arms towards the chin, as if reaching for the endotracheal tube and then relaxing them to the side.
- *Cranial nerve testing:*
  - *Light reflex (CN II):* Pupils 4-9 mm, non-reactive to light
  - *Doll's eyes (CN III, IV, and VIII):* The eye is fixed despite the sudden movement of the head.

- *Corneal reflex (CN V and VII):* No blinking in response to corneal stimulation.
- *Caloric test (CN VIII):* Failure of eyes to move towards the ear canal being irrigated with cold fluid.
- *Gag reflex (CN IX):* Absence of palatal movements in response to pharyngeal stimulation.
- *Cough reflex (CN X):* Absence of coughing in response to tracheal stimulation.

Primary Apnea Test

- Baseline $PaCO_2$ of 35–45 mm Hg, and PaO_2 of 200 mm Hg, continue with continuous positive airway pressure and positive end-expiratory pressure while discontinuing ventilation. Supplement oxygen during apnea testing.
- *The anticipated rise in $PaCO_2$:*
  - *0–2 min:* 5 mm Hg/min
  - *2–10 min:* 2 mm Hg/min
  - A 20 mm Hg increase without respiratory effort is consistent with brain death.
  - A net increase in 60 mm Hg in 8–10 minutes suggests brain death.
- Test terminated if systolic blood pressure decreases below 100 mm Hg or arrhythmias occur.

Secondary Tests

- *Electroencephalogram (EEG):* Amplitude <2 microvolts at maximum gain (2 microvolt/mm) for 2 minutes 24 hours apart.
- No somatosensory evoked responses
- *Transcranial Doppler (TCD):* Absence of flow or flow reversal in late diastole probably best observed via the trans-orbital window.
- Angiography, computed tomography, and magnetic resonance imaging: Absence of cerebral blood flow.
- *Radionucleotide scan:* Absence of perfusion but can yield false-positive results.

PROBLEMS IN DIAGNOSING BRAIN DEATH

- *Clinical examination:* May be difficult due to facial trauma.
- *Apnea test:* Affected by hypothermia, hypoxia, and hypotension; unreliable in chronic CO_2 retaining patient.
- *TCD:* Sonication sites may be difficult to access.
- *Metabolic testing:* Pharmacodynamic sensitivity to drugs affected by liver or kidney disease.
- *Electroencephalogram (EEG):* Affected by electrical interference, hypothermia, and drugs.

FURTHER READING

1. Busl KM et al. Apnea testing for the determination of brain death: A systematic scoping review. Neurocrit Care. 2021;34(2):608-20.
2. Kirschen MP et al. New perspectives on brain death. J Neurol Neurosurg Psychiatry. 2021;92(3):255-62.
3. Lerner DP et al. Metabolic values precluding clinical death by neurologic Criteria/Brain death: Survey of neurocritical care society physicians. J Clin Neurosci. 2021;88:16-21.
4. Murphy L et al. Toxicologic confounders of brain death determination: A narrative review. Neurocrit Care. 2021;34(3): 1072-89.
5. O'Keeffe FJ et al. Diagnosing death 50 years after the Harvard brain death report. New Bioeth. 2021;27(1):46-64.

Vignette: The First Description of Locked-in Syndrome

Alexandre Dumas (1802-1870) wrote his classic work, The Count of Monte Cristo, in 1844-45. Contained in the book is the description of Monsieur Noirtier de Villeforte. Monsieur Villeforte was an older man who could hear and see but could not move. Dumas described him as "a corpse with living eyes" or "a soul trapped in a body that no longer obeys its commands".

The more detailed description precisely describes the clinical features of locked-in syndrome. "Sight and hearing were the only senses remaining. It was only, however, by means of one of these senses that he could reveal the thoughts and feelings that still occupied his mind, and the look by which he gave expression to his inner life was like the distant gleam of a candle which a traveler sees by night across some desert place, and knows that a living being dwells beyond the silence and obscurity. In his eyes, shaded by thick black lashes, was concentrated, as it often happens with an organ which is used to the exclusion of the others, all the activity, address, force, and intelligence which were formerly diffused over his whole body; and so although the movement of the arm, the sound of the voice, and the agility of the body, were wanting, the speaking eye sufficed for all".

Dumas did not have any medical training. The vivid description of stroke patients in his writings was primarily due to his friendship with a physician, Dr. Thibaut, with whom he rounded at Charite' Hospital Paris. Also, he had a fear of apoplexy or stroke. The disease affected his paternal lineage, leading to his mother's death. Dumas himself succumbed to a stroke on December 5, 1870.

Section 3

Neuroanesthesia Case Management

- Preoperative Assessment of Neurosurgical Case
- Routine Craniotomy under General Anesthesia
- Awake Craniotomy for Seizure Disorders
- Carotid Endarterectomy
- Carotid Artery Stenting
- Cerebral Arteriovenous Malformation Resection
- Clipping of Cerebral Aneurysms
- Treatment of Cerebral Vasospasm
- Deep Hypothermic Circulatory Arrest
- Management of Traumatic Brain Injury
- Brain Herniation
- Decompressive Craniectomy
- Cerebrospinal Fluid Leak
- Cervical Decompression
- Acute Spinal Injury
- Intraoperative Evoked Potential Changes
- Posterior Fossa Surgery
- Transsphenoid Hypophysectomy
- Endoscopic Third Ventriculostomy and Shunt Procedures
- Anesthesia for Electroconvulsive Therapy
- Pregnant Patient for Neurosurgery
- Pediatric Neurosurgery Patient
- Biopsy for Creutzfeldt–Jakob Disease
- Postoperative Vision Loss
- Robot-assisted Surgery and Laser Interstitial Thermal Therapy
- Patient with Ventricular Assist Device
- Post-craniotomy Pain Management
- Massive Blood Transfusion
- Brain Death and Organ Harvest

Chapter 34: Preoperative Assessment of Neurosurgical Case

INTRODUCTION

Seven hundred thousand patients undergo neurosurgery in the US and Canada each year, and 14 million are treated globally. Neurosurgical interventions are required for traumatic brain injury, stroke, epilepsy, and brain tumors. Other frequent indications of neurosurgery are hydrocephalus, infections, vascular malformation, neural tube defects, spine injuries, and spine tumors. The distribution of neurosurgical procedures is bound to change with technological advances. These include advances in spine surgery, endovascular surgery, minimally invasive brain surgery, neural implants, and stroke treatments. Preoperative evaluation for neurosurgical patients has to be comprehensive. Neuropathology may affect the central nervous system in isolation, such as in the case of a primary brain tumor. However, most neurosurgical patients also have systemic complaints. These complaints can be due to the systemic manifestations of neurological diseases, underlying pathogenic mechanisms affecting other organs, systemic effects of drugs, or concurrent illnesses. Therefore, preoperative assessment of neurosurgical cases requires thorough neurological and systemic evaluation.

GOALS OF PREOPERATIVE ASSESSMENT

- Establish rapport.
- Assess medical fitness for the planned surgery.
- Review and update investigations as needed.
- Document baseline condition before surgery.
- Plan the safest course of surgery.
- Inform the patient about the anesthetic plan.
- Inform of anticipated complications.
- Premedicate if necessary.

SPECIAL CONSIDERATIONS FOR NEUROSURGICAL PATIENTS

- *Pre-existing cognitive impairments:*
  - History may be limited or unreliable.

- Difficult to undertake preoperative assessment.
- Explaining risks and concerns may be difficult.
- Problems in obtaining consent.
- *Neurological diseases may have systemic effects, such as:*
  - *Cardiovascular:*
    - *Increased intracranial pressure (ICP) can cause* hypertension and bradycardia.
    - *Subarachnoid hemorrhage (SAH) can cause* neurogenic pulmonary edema or Takotsubo cardiomyopathy.
    - *Brain tumor patients may have* steroid-induced hypertension or diabetes.
  - *Respiratory:* Increased incidence of aspiration pneumonia in comatose, neurogenic pulmonary edema, impaired cough and decreased respiratory effort, and central respiratory dysregulation.
  - *Gastrointestinal:* Stress ulcers and gastric stasis
  - *Metabolic:* Steroid-induced diabetes; syndrome of antidiuretic hormone (SIADH)/diabetes insipidus (DI): Electrolyte imbalances.
  - *Urinary:* Urinary tract infection (UTI).
- *Often urgent or semi-urgent procedures:* May not have time to optimize the patient:
  - Herniating brain, stroke, or cord compression emergency in minutes.
  - Aneurysmal SAH, subdural hematoma (SDH), or vasospasm treatment in hours.
  - Tumor or unruptured aneurysm treatment in days.
- At risk for neurological complications. Even without complications, symptoms might worsen due to residual anesthetics. These deficits clear over the first 24 hours.
- *Cardiovascular Assessment:* Tight hemodynamic control is needed during surgery.
  - Baseline BP determines intraoperative BP control.
  - Tight BP control is needed for most procedures.
  - Mild hypotension is used to decrease blood loss during tumor and spine surgery.
  - Steroids may cause hypertension and fluid retention.
- *Respiratory concerns*:
  - Central respiratory depression.
  - *Impaired respiratory function:* Restrictive lung disease in spine cases and neurogenic pulmonary edema with severe neurological injuries.
  - Judicious narcotic use.
  - Obstructive sleep apnea (OSA).
  - Smoking
- Drugs that affect anesthetic management
  - *Steroid:* Withdrawal and increased blood sugar.
  - *Anticonvulsants:* Tolerance to competitive muscle relaxants.
  - *Diuretics:* Hypovolemia and electrolyte imbalance.

- *The potential risk for major bleeding:*
  - Major spine surgery
  - Large brain and vascular spine tumors.
  - Aneurysms and arteriovenous malformations of the brain
  - Patients on anticoagulants or with impaired coagulation
- *Position-related considerations:*
  - The prone position is potentially hazardous for patients with ocular implants, renal transplants, and recent coronary venous grafts.
  - Sitting position not ideal with patent foramen ovale or poor cardiovascular status
- *Increased risk for sore throat:*
  - Usually prolonged surgical procedures.
  - Friction between the tube and the vocal cords during positioning.
  - Pressure on the tube during surgery, such as anterior cervical decompression.

Perioperative Anxiety

- *Perioperative anxiety has many components:*
  - Underlying diagnosis
  - Surgery and surgical outcome
  - *Anesthesia:* Pain, loss of control, and physical exposure.
  - *Recovery:* Location, duration, treatment for pain and vomiting
  - Underlying anxieties can be challenging to discuss in cases with poor outcomes, such as advanced malignant tumors and high-risk vascular surgeries. However, there can be non-medical anxieties as well:
    - *Financial:* Cost of procedure, its impact on life and livelihood
    - Quality of life after the procedure, rehabilitation
    - The personal impact of neurological disease and treatment
- *Communication:*
  - It has to be empathetic.
  - Communication is both verbal and nonverbal.
  - Communication has to be precise with well-rehearsed questions
  - The tone of voice and content of the conversation matter.
  - Past surgical experience may influence patient behavior.
  - Provide the details of the anesthetic and postoperative care.
  - Inform cautiously about any anticipated anesthetic problems.
  - Facts must be clearly stated without provoking anxiety.

Suggested Approach

Chart Review

- Read the notes carefully before talking to the patient.
- Discuss the case with the surgical team and identify specific concerns they might have beforehand.

- Due to the COVID epidemic, contact is limited, and social distancing rules must be followed appropriately.
- Scrub your hand with sanitizer before approaching the patient.
- *Preoperative discussion, the author's approach:*
  - Identify the patient (salutation and full name), surgeon, and operation without looking at the chart and then cross-check identifiers.
  - Contrary to medical history-taking, do not begin by asking what the presentation of the disease was but summarize the salient points of their medical history. By doing so, you are indicating that you are familiar with their medical concerns, and you can win their trust and put them at ease.
  - Confirm the medical history systematically and then ask for any additional information they would like to provide.
  - Examine the patient.
  - Effective time management is necessary during the preoperative review.
- *Informing about surgery:*
  - Focus on issues related to anesthesia for a given surgery.
  - Discuss potential anesthetic complications and mitigating steps for each.
  - Recognize the need to do so without increasing preoperative anxiety.
  - Present a coherent anesthesia plan.
  - Necessary to elaborate on "postoperative" care, such as pain management, nausea, vomiting, respiratory care, sedation, and intensive care unit (ICU) care. It reassures the patients that they will safely get through the surgery.
  - *Have a positive tone:* Talk about the day after surgery, when possible, "the pain will be much less, "we will have the diagnosis that has been worrying you," "you will not have to worry about the aneurysm once the surgery is over today".

Systemic Review

The American Society of Anesthesiologists (ASA) grades are given in **Table 1**. The risk factors for systemic complications are listed below:

Risk Factors for Cardiovascular Complications

- *Moderate risk factors:*
  - History of coronary artery disease.
  - Chronic stable heart failure.
  - History of stroke and transient ischemic attack (TIA).
  - Insulin-dependent diabetes mellitus (IDDM).
  - End-stage renal disease (ESRD) with sCr >2 mg/dL

CHAPTER 34 Preoperative Assessment of Neurosurgical Case

Table 1: ASA grades with the corresponding examples.

Classification: Definition	ASA examples, although not limited to
ASA I: Normal healthy	*Healthy,* nonsmoking, and minimal alcohol
ASA II: Mild systemic disease	*No functional limitations:* Active smoker, social alcohol, pregnant, mild obesity BMI 30–40 kg/m^2, well-controlled DM, HT, or mild lung disease
ASA III: Severe systemic disease	*Substantial functional limitations:* Poorly controlled DM, HT < lung disease, significant obesity BMI >40 kg/m^2, alcohol abuse, ESRD regular dialysis, pacemaker, moderately reduced EF, MI >3 months, PCA <60 weeks, CAD stents, CVA, and TIA
ASA IV: Severe systemic disease, a constant threat to life	*A constant threat to life:* Recent MI <3 months, CVA, TIA, CAD/stents, unstable angina, severe valvular dysfunction, severely reduced EF, sepsis, DIC, and ERDS with erratic dialysis
ASA V: Moribund, not expected to survive	*In extremis:* Massive trauma, intracranial bleed with mass effect, ruptured aortic aneurysm, ischemic bowel, significant cardiac pathology, multiorgan failure
ASA VI: Brain death	Organ harvest

(ASA: American Society of Anesthesiologists; BMI: body mass index; CAD: coronary artery disease; CVA: cerebrovascular accident; DIC: disseminated intravascular coagulation; DM: diabetes mellitus; EF: ejection fraction; ESRD: end-stage renal disease; HT: hypertension; MI: myocardial infarction; PCA: percutaneous coronary artery; TIA: transient ischemic attack)

- *Severe risk factors:*
  - Unstable angina.
  - Recent myocardial infarction (MI).
  - Decompensated congestive heart failure (CHF).
  - Severe valvular heart disease.

Risk Factors for Respiratory Complications

- The risk factors for postoperative respiratory complications:
  - *Moderate risk factors:*
    - FEV1 30–70%.
    - Moderate pulmonary artery hypertension.
    - OSA
    - Smoking 20-pack years or more
  - *Severe risk factors:*
    - FEV1 <30%.
    - Severe pulmonary artery hypertension.
    - Home oxygen therapy
- *Obstructive Sleep Apnea (OSA):*
  - OSA is a risk factor for hypertension, coronary artery disease, and stroke
  - Diagnosis requires sleep studies that may sometimes be conducted at home.

Table 2: OSA risk assessment: STOP–BANG parameters.

Element	Question
Snoring	Do you snore louder than talking or can be heard next door? Yes/No
Tired	Do you often feel tired, fatigued, and sleepy during the day? Yes/No
Observed	Has anyone observed you stopped breathing? Yes/No
Pressure	Hypertension? Yes/No
BMI	BMI >35 kg/m^2? Yes/No
Age	Greater than 50 years? Yes/No
Neck circumference	Greater than 40 cm or 16 inches? Yes/No
Gender	Male? Yes/No

Table 3: Differential diagnosis of upper respiratory infection (URI).

	Allergy	URI (rhinovirus)	URI (influenza)
History	Allergens known	Seasonal	Seasonal
Conjunctiva: Itching, redness, and watery discharge	Common	Rare	Conjunctivitis possible
Nasal congestion/sneezing	Common	Common	Common
Sore throat	Possible	Common	Common
Cough	Rare	Rare	Common
Headache/fever/malaise/fatigue	Rare	Rare	Common
Muscle pains	Never	Rare	Common
Anesthesia	Proceed	Delay	Delay

- A set of eight questions (STOP-BANG, **Table 2**) with yes/no answers can be used to detect the OSA risk in undiagnosed patients. Four positive responses suggest a high risk of OSA.
- Counterintuitively, recent reports have suggested that periodic hypoxia and hypercarbia in patients with OSA can improve neurological outcomes after subarachnoid hemorrhage.

Diagnosis of Recent Upper Respiratory Infection

Recent URI may increase the chances of intraoperative bronchospasm, may result in severe coughing and bucking at extubation, and could lead to postoperative pulmonary complications. Abnormal airway reactivity can persist for 6 weeks after URI. However, it is often not advisable to postpone neurosurgery for so long. If URI is associated with infection, it is treated for two weeks. The symptoms should resolve at that time to proceed with surgery. URI has to be differentiated from allergic reactions **(Table 3)**.

COVID-19 is a highly contagious coronavirus infection with significant mortality in elderly patients >65 years of age. Symptoms occur 2–14 days after exposure. If suspected on clinical examination, postpone surgery unless it

CHAPTER 34 Preoperative Assessment of Neurosurgical Case

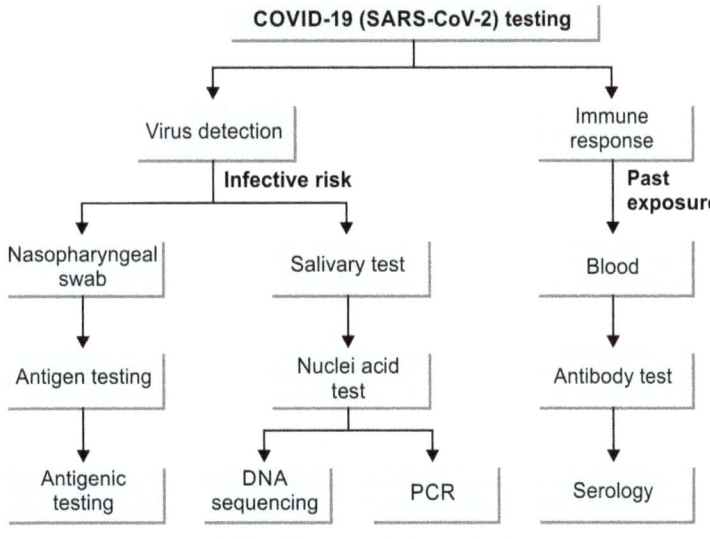

Flowchart 1: Testing for SARS-CoV-2 or COVID-19.

(PCR: polymerase chain reaction)

is a life-threatening emergency, quarantine, and treat with remdesivir. Wait for 7 days or until the nasal swabs are negative for the virus on two exams **(Flowchart 1)**. The guidelines for management are constantly changing with increased immunization, anti-viral drugs, and change in the dominant strain of the virus. Follow the recommended guidelines. The emergence of more infective COVID-19 strains in early 2021, with greater virulence (delta variant) and another more infective and less virulent strain (omicron variant) later in 2021 required health personnel to continue with barrier precautions despite complete immunization. The clinical symptoms of the disease include:

- Fever with chills
- Breathing difficulty or shortness of breath
- Cough
- Fatigue
- Muscle or body aches
- *Loss of taste or smell*
- Sore throat
- Runny nose
- Nausea, vomiting, and diarrhea.

Airway Examination: At-risk Airway

- Mallampati grade III or IV **(Fig. 1)**. It is helpful to add an extra grade if the movement of the cervical spine or the temporomandibular joint is limited.

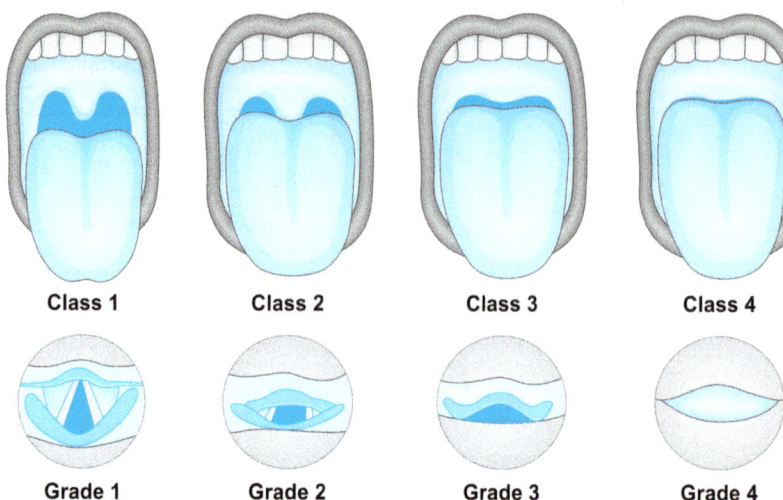

Fig. 1: Mallampati classification and grading of laryngeal view.

- Inability to protract the jaw.
- Thyromental distance (TMD) <4 cm
- Limited neck extension.
- The atlantooccipital joint extension is tested by extending the head with the examiner bracing the lower neck in full flexion.
- The ability to say "E" tests vocal cord adduction.
- *Additional airway risk factors:*
  - Body mass index (BMI) is more important than weight.
  - Weight >100 kg.
  - The beard may conceal a hypoplastic mandible.
  - Hair tied on the top of the head might restrict neck extension.

Routine Investigations

- *Complete blood count (CBC) and hemogram:*
  - *Hemoglobin/hematocrit (Hb/Hct):* Rule out anemia before major surgery and in patients with renal disease or chemotherapy.
  - *Total leukocyte count (TLC):* Rule out an active infection, particularly when the surgery requires the insertion of foreign objects such as shunt placement and spine instrumentation.
  - *Platelets:* Rule out thrombocytopenia.
- *Basic metabolic panel (BMP):*
  - *Blood glucose:* >200 mg/dL increased morbidity. Target 100–150 mg/dL
  - *Blood urea nitrogen (BUN)/serum creatinine (sCr):* Rule out renal disease. Glomerular filtration rate (GFR) <60 mL/min and sCr >2 mg/dL increase perioperative mortality.
  - *Serum Na^+:* Hyponatremia can lead to cognitive decline, and rapid correction can lead to central pontine myelinolysis.

- *Serum K⁺:* It is essential in patients with ESRD or for the use of succinylcholine.
- *Serum Ca⁺⁺:* Its increase might explain behavioral changes.
- Coagulation screen:
  - *International normalized ratio (INR):* Reflects the overall state of coagulation.
  - *Partial thromboplastin time (PTT):* Liver-dependent coagulating factors.
  - *Activated clotting time (ACT):* Monitoring heparin.
- *EKG:* For perioperative comparison, the diagnostic value remains poor.
- *Echo:* Significant changes in myocardial contractility are seen with a severe neurological injury such as aneurysmal hemorrhage or traumatic brain injury (TBI). It is also necessary to manage cases requiring induced hypertension, such as carotid endarterectomy.
- *Stress test:* With history of significant cardiac disease, recent change in symptoms or functional impairment with minimal effort.
- *Chest X-ray (CXR):* Evaluate any infection, possibly tracheal deviation or compression.
- *CT/MRI:* Evaluation of neurological disease severity and airway assessment in patients undergoing c-spine surgery.

Preoperative Medications

- *Continue with:*
  - Antiepileptic drugs
  - Steroids
  - Antibiotics
  - Anti-hypertensives except for Angiotensin Converting Enzyme (ACE) Inhibitors
  - Beta-blockers and clonidine.
  - Anxiolytics
  - Sedative hypnotics, pain medications
  - Parkinson's treatment drugs.
  - Alzheimer's Disease treatment drugs (Donepezil).
- *Discontinue:*
  - Oral hypoglycemic on the day of surgery; if needed, use sliding insulin.
  - ACE inhibitors and angiotensin receptor-blocking drugs can be withheld for 24 hours.
  - Warfarin is discontinued for at least four days and replaced by low molecular-weight heparin if needed.
  - Aspirin clopidogrel (Plavix) is stopped for one week. It can be started within 24 hours of surgery if indicated.

Table 4: Potential neurosurgical complications and their risk factors.

Anesthesia risk	Incidence	Risk factors
Headache	70%	Moderate-to-severe pain after craniotomy
PONV	50%	Female gender, decreased with steroid use
Sore throat	30–50%	Female gender, smoking, and cuff pressure
Shivering	30%	
Postoperative ventilation	5–50%	Heavily biased by intuitional preferences
Postoperative pulmonary complication	4%	4% for supratentorial craniotomies, 1% for spine surgery. Enrollment criteria may exclude prolonged ventilation.
	12%	Infratentorial surgery risk factors include: BT, lower cranial nerve palsies, prolonged intubation, and tracheostomy
	10–30%	After aneurysm surgery, it depends on age, duration of surgery, BT, duration of ventilation, coma grade after wakeup, and tracheostomy
Postoperative seizures	15%	
Anemia (Hct <30%) and blood transfusion	5%	Most neurosurgical patients are not transfused, but postoperative anemia is common, and severity increases perioperative recovery
Postoperative ventilation >48 hours	8%	
Coma	0.3%	
Mortality	4%	Tumor surgery
	4%	Unruptured aneurysm
	2%	Posterior fossa surgery
	1%	Trans-sphenoid surgery

(BT: Blood transfusion; PONV: postoperative nausea and vomiting)

Instructions to the Patient

- Expected procedures in the OR before induction.
- A list of anesthesia-related complications is provided in **Table 4**.
- Wake up in the OR or the ICU.
    - Sore throat
    - Oxygen supplementation
    - Additional lines and monitors
    - Pain management
    - Antiemesis protocol.
- Neurological symptoms can transiently worsen immediately after surgery.
- Describe transfer to post-surgery care unit or ICU.
- Obtain family contact information.
- Inform the family when and who will contact them during the day if surgery is prolonged.

Table 5: Incidence of neurosurgical complications.

	Craniotomies	Spine surgery
Frequent transient complications		
Pain >24 hours	66%	40%
Sore throat/difficulty in swallowing	50%	50%
Nausea	30%	40%
Significant possible complications or 5–20%		
Post-op ventilation	5%	2%
Blood transfusion	6%	5%
Reoperation	5%	2%
Infrequent complications or 1–5%		
Infections: • UTI • Pneumonia • Sepsis	4%	2%
Intracranial hemorrhage	2%	N/A
Reintubation	3%	1%
Wound infection: • Superficial • Deep • Dehiscence • Compartmental	2%	2%
Vascular: • Pulmonary embolus • Stroke	1%	<1%
Rare complications or <1%		
Renal failure/dialysis	0.3%	0.3%
MI	0.3%	0.2%
Nerve injury	0.1%	0.1%
Coma	<1%	0%
Overall Complications	25%	10%

(BT: Blood transfusion; DVT: deep vein thrombosis; CPR: cardiopulmonary resuscitation; MI: myocardial infarction; PE: pulmonary embolism; UTI: urinary tract infection)

Outcome

Cranial cases have 3× complication rates as compared to spinal cases. Overall complication rates are about 15%. However, the data is strongly biased by sicker patients with pre-existing risk factors, particularly neurological morbidities **(Table 5)**.

CASE REPORTS FOR FURTHER DISCUSSION

Case 1: A 52-year-old patient presented with a 3-week history of episodic headache, nausea, vertigo, and ataxia. History was significant for smoking (15 pack- years). He was diagnosed with Holmes–Ades pupils on the left side five years ago. On examination, he was severely hypertensive in the range of 230–250/140–150 mm Hg. The Fundus examination was positive for bilateral papilledema and arteriovenous nipping with exudates. Other than the pupillary abnormalities, the cranial nerve functions were normal. The cerebellar signs were positive, including lack of finger-nose coordination, wide-based gait, and an impaired tandem gait. There was a flexor plantar response, and lower limb reflexes were absent. MRI revealed cerebellar edema with moderate obstructive hydrocephalus. There were minor white matter lesions in the cerebellum. Laboratory investigations revealed mild kidney failure.

Echocardiography revealed left ventricular hypertrophy. There was no other cause of hypertension. A diagnosis of hypertensive encephalopathy with cerebellar edema was made, and a ventriculoperitoneal (VP) shunt placement was planned. *How will you optimize the patient before surgery? When will you operate on him? What blood pressure values do you consider safe for neurosurgical patients? Will suspected white-coat hypertension affect your decision? If so, how will you differentiate acute versus chronic hypertension?*

Case 2: A middle-aged female patient presented with recent-onset confusion and memory loss. She was treated with 4 mg dexamethasone six hourly for five days before admission. She is due for the excision of frontal meningioma. She started antibiotics for UTI treatment since diagnosis. Her preoperative investigations revealed blood sugar of 272 mg%, blood urea of 25 mg/dL, and serum creatinine of 0.9 mg/dL. MRI showed a frontal tumor with extensive edema and mid-line shift. She arrived for afternoon surgery complaining of severe thirst. General anesthesia was induced. Arterial and central venous lines were placed along with a urinary catheter. The baseline sample was sent with a pH of 7.14, PaO_2 of 278 mm Hg, $PaCO_2$ of 27 mm Hg, HCO_3 of 11.1, base excess –17.7, lactate 23.8 mg/dL (2.64 mmol/L), and glucose 719 mg/dL. *How will you proceed? Would you do additional testing before surgery in such a case? What are your goals for blood sugar management before surgery? What if sudden bleeding into the tumors led to an impending herniation, and surgery could not be postponed? What additional problems will diabetic ketoacidosis (DKA) pose in an emergency?*

Case 3: A 59-year-old female achondroplastic dwarf with a long history of morbid obesity with recent weight gain was admitted for spinal correction. Her body mass index (BMI) was 67 kg/m^2, and she had a history of severe sleep apnea. Examination revealed a morbidly obese patient with a class III airway and normal neck extension. There was a history of past surgery with difficult intubations, but the details were unavailable. Routine labs and EKG were unremarkable. Transthoracic echo was advised due to a history of sleep apnea with possible pulmonary artery hypertension but was deemed to be of poor quality for any reliable inference. *How will you proceed with the case? How do you plan to intubate? Is sleep apnea a concern? If so, what additional precautions will you take?*

Case 4: A 60-year-old female with ischemic cardiomyopathy presented with a worsening headache, confusion, and balance problems. MRI revealed multiple intracranial brain tumors and she is posted for craniotomy for tumor resection. Her history was significant for hypertension, MI, coronary artery disease, CHF managed with a left ventricular assist device (LVAD; Heartmate II) for two years, and COPD. Due to repeated past episodes of GI bleeding, her INR goal was set at 1.3–1.8. Medications included carvedilol, furosemide, K supplements, albuterol-ipratropium inhaler, warfarin, omeprazole, trazodone, fluticasone- salmeterol, aspirin low dose, and sildenafil. A preoperative exam revealed a 42 kg 155 cm female with a pulse of 83 bpm and a BP of 102/69 mm Hg. Her LVAD was set at 8,200 rpm, with a power of 4.7 and a pulse index of 6.7. The laboratory results on the day of surgery had a Hb of 8.8 gm/dL, a platelet count of 9.7×10^9/L, INR of 1.6, PTT of 27 seconds, and PT of 19.4 seconds. *What are the problems in such a patient? How will you manage anticoagulation in a case with LVAD for neurosurgery? What preoperative corrections will you undertake before surgery?*

Case 5: A 57-year-old man with a 3-day history of unconsciousness was due for a decompressive craniotomy. His history was significant for severe aortic stenosis, aortic insufficiency, and coronary artery disease. He was admitted for bypass surgery and valve replacement when he sustained the intracranial bleed. The patient was intubated and mechanically ventilated. His laboratory reports revealed an increased white cell count of 26,000/µL; other reports were unremarkable. Doppler ultrasound revealed a valve area of 0.9 cm^2, aortic valve pressure gradient of 86 mm Hg, and concentric ventricular hypertrophy with 54% ejection fraction. Computed tomography revealed coronary atherosclerosis and 10%, 85%, and 70% stenosis of anterior descending, left circumflex, and right coronary arteries, respectively. CT scan of the brain revealed cerebral infarction with hydrocephalus. *How will you proceed in this case? Will you correct aortic valve stenosis before craniotomy? What risk do you anticipate in the case of severe aortic stenosis (AS) with raised ICP?*

CASE REPORT REFERENCES

Case 1: O'Riordan S et al. Reversible hypertensive cerebellar encephalopathy and hydrocephalus: J Neurol Neurosurg Psychiatry. 2007;78(9): 1008-9.

Case 2: Ramessur S et al. Hyperglycaemia and cerebral edema in a patient with a meningioma receiving dexamethasone: Anaesthesia. 2011; 66(2):127-31.

Case 3: Veevaete L et al. Three anesthetic challenges for spinal surgery in a morbidly obese achondroplastic dwarf. Acta Anaesth Belg. 2017;68:95-8.

Case 4: Vandse R et al. Successful perioperative management of a patient with the left ventricular assist device for brain tumor resection: case report and review of the literature. Case Rep Anesthesiol. 2015;2015:839854.

Case 5: Xu AJ et al. Anesthetic management for craniotomy in a patient with massive cerebellar infarction and severe aortic stenosis: a case report. Int J Clin Exp Med. 2015;8(7):11534-8.

FURTHER READING

1. Dong W et al. Deep brain stimulation for the treatment of dopa-responsive dystonia: a case report and literature review. World Neurosurg. 2020;136: 394-8 e5.
2. Goodhart IM et al. Patient-completed, preoperative web-based anesthetic assessment questionnaire (electronic personal assessment questionnaire preoperative): development and validation. Eur J Anaesthesiol. 2017;34(4): 221-8.
3. Hadanny A et al. Preoperative evaluation of coagulation status in neuromodulation patients. J Neurosurg. 2021;1-7.
4. Harland TA et al. Frailty as a predictor of neurosurgical outcomes in brain tumor patients. World Neurosurg. 2020;133:e813-8.
5. Kurosu K et al. Preoperative prognostic nutritional index as a predictive factor for medical complication after cervical posterior decompression surgery: a multicenter study. J Orthop Surg (Hong Kong). 2021;29(1):23094990 211006869.
6. Padevit L et al. Smoking status and perioperative adverse events in patients undergoing cranial tumor surgery. J Neurooncol. 2019;144(1):97-105.
7. Stumpo V et al. Enhanced recovery after surgery strategies for elective craniotomy: a systematic review. J Neurosurg. 2021;1-25.
8. Tulloch I et al. Assessment and management of preoperative anxiety. J Voice, 2019;33(5):691-6.

Vignette: Why the Russians Failed to Reach the Moon First?

In the 1960s, the Russian space program was well ahead of the Americans at the height of the space race. Russia had launched the first satellite, put the first man in space, and soft-landed Luna 9 on the moon. Soviets were ready to put a man on the moon. However, on January 14, 1966, tragedy struck. The architect of the Russian space program, Sergei Pavlovich Korolev, responsible for all these successes, was to undergo routine surgery. Korolev's jaw had been broken when he was incarcerated in Siberia by Stalin. The injury limited his mouth opening, and it made intubation difficult. During the removal of a rectal polyp, he started bleeding. As the bleeding continued, they had to open the abdomen to control it. Eight hours later, Sergei Pavlovich Korolev—the world's most talented rocket designer-lay dead on the operating table without an endotracheal tube. His death, in part, was undoubtedly due to a failed intubation. The Russian space program never recovered from Korolev's death.

CHAPTER 34 Preoperative Assessment of Neurosurgical Case

Vignette: History of Endotracheal Intubations

Ancient Indian and Egyptian texts describing intubation have been dated to the second millennium BCE. Hippocrates described endotracheal intubation around 400 BCE. Avicenna, father of early modern medicine in 10th century Persia, described intubation to treat dyspnea. In the 16th century, Vesalius described using a reed placed in the trachea to enable ventilation in animals. Modern intubation technique was discovered to overcome upper airway obstruction for diphtheria in the 19th century. William Macewen did the first intubation for anesthetic needs in 1879. Franz Kuhn developed the first metal endotracheal tubes in the early 1900s. Benjamin Babington developed the first glottis scope in 1929. Magill in England and Lundy in the US developed the modern intubation technique.

Chapter 35: Routine Craniotomy under General Anesthesia

INTRODUCTION

A craniotomy is the breech of skull integrity needed to access the underlying tissue, and the bone removed is replaced afterward. Craniectomy, in contrast to craniotomy, removes a part of the skull. Craniotomies are frequently indicated for the treatment of:
- Head injury and intracranial hemorrhages
- *Tumors:* biopsy, excision, or local chemotherapy
- *Vascular lesions:* Aneurysms and vascular malformations
- Hydrocephalus, CSF drainage, and ICP monitoring.
- Epilepsy, Parkinson's Disease, and movement disorders
- Abscesses and infections

The common craniotomies include:
- Conventional approaches such as supraorbital, frontal, bifrontal, orbito-zygomatic, temporal, pterional or frontal temporal, retro-sigmoid, trans-labyrinthine, or sub-occipital.
- Stereotactic CT or MRI-guided craniotomies.
- Endoscopic guided craniotomies that permit direct visualization.

A craniotomy can be minimally invasive such as for a needle biopsy or the placement of a shunt. Conversely, it could be extensive with significant blood loss, such as with a bi-frontal approach for vascular meningioma.

NEUROANESTHETIC CONCERNS

- *Specific neurosurgical concerns and preoperative planning:*
  - The severity of neurological disease
  - Raised intracranial pressure (ICP)
  - Desired hemodynamic goals
  - Neurological monitoring
  - Possible blood loss
- Smooth induction and safe intubation
- *Monitoring:*
  - Hemodynamic and critical body functions
  - Depth of anesthesia
  - Metabolic
  - Neurological

CHAPTER 35 Routine Craniotomy under General Anesthesia

- *Intraoperative*:
  - Ensuring depth of anesthesia
  - Desired hemodynamic and respiratory goals
  - Neuromuscular blockade
  - Core temperature management
  - Blood loss and fluid balance
  - Strategies to decrease blood loss.
  - Care of bulging brain tissue
  - Neuroprotective strategies
- *Emergence*:
  - Extubation strategy
  - Antiemesis
  - Hemodynamic control
  - Neurological assessment
- Postoperative care
  - Pain management

Preoperative Assessment

History

- *Neurological:*
  - Specific neurological deficits
  - Seizures and seizure control
  - Muscular disease, weakness, or wasting.
  - *Symptoms of raised ICP* include impaired cognition, headache, and photophobia.
- *Respiratory:* A history of COPD, bronchial asthma, recent upper respiratory infection (URI), and smoking is significant not only for optimizing intra- operative ventilation but also for planning extubation.
- *Cardiovascular system:* Brain tumors have the highest incidence between the fifth and seventh decades, coinciding with increased age-related cardiovascular disease.
  - *Hypertension:* Age, steroid use, and perioperative anxiety increase BP. Hypertension can shift autoregulatory control, affect blood loss, and increase the risk of intracranial hemorrhage. Antihypertensive drugs can cause intraoperative hypotension. Hypertension can be a sign of raised ICP.
  - *Congestive heart failure:* Neurological disease can restrict exercise assessment. Echocardiography is indicated for high-risk cases.
  - *Cardiac arrhythmias:* Bradycardia with escaped beat possible due to the raised ICP.

- History of deep vein thrombosis (DVT,) calf pains, and tenderness as tumors and antiepileptic drugs may affect activity, increasing chances of DVT and pulmonary embolism (PE).
- *Airway*:
  - A history of difficult intubation
  - Past craniotomy may limit mouth opening.
    - If recent, swelling and edema make mouth opening difficult and restrict the temporomandibular joint (TMJ).
    - If remote, fibrosis of the temporalis muscle can lead to atrophy and limit mouth opening due to pseudoankylosis of the TMJ.
- History of postoperative nausea and vomiting (PONV)
- *Current medical treatment:*
  - *Anticonvulsant consideration:* Last dose, any side effects, and withdrawal syndrome; hepatic enzyme induction and drug interactions; tolerance to competitive muscle relaxants
  - Steroid dose dependency and possible withdrawal
  - Current antihypertensive and angiotensin-converting enzyme ACE inhibitors
  - Appropriate discontinuation of anticoagulant and antiplatelet drugs
- Allergy to antibiotics (cephalosporin), and anticonvulsants.
- Allergy to soy and eggs no longer precludes the use of propofol. Should an allergic reaction occur with propofol it should be investigated to identify the cause.
- Allergic reactions (urticaria, hypotension, and wheezing) are often confused with side effects (such as sedation, nausea, and vomiting).

Examination

- *Cognitive status:*
  - Preexisting deficits might worsen immediately after surgery.
  - History might not be available from the patient.
  - The ability to follow simple commands is necessary for extubation.
- *Vital signs*:
  - *Blood pressure (BP):* Baseline BP provides pressure targets for neurosurgical procedures. For example, BP is kept 20–30% above baseline during carotid occlusion and 10% below baseline after endarterectomy. However, in other surgeries, there are widely accepted preset BP limits. For example, during extubation for tumor resections, the systolic BP is kept at ≤140 mm Hg, and with an unruptured aneurysm, it is ≤150 mm Hg.
  - Bradycardia/hypertension are indicative of the raised ICP
  - *Respiratory:* Smoking and a recent respiratory infection may make extubation challenging. Elective surgery is avoided in the settings of ongoing URI; however, a delay might not be possible in urgent cases (tumors, aneurysms, and many emergencies).

- *Airway examination*:
  - Helpful to add a point to the Mallampati score if any of the elements from b to e listed below are positive.
    a. Mallampati score
    b. Thyromental distance (TMD) <4 cm
    c. Neck flexion
    d. The atlantooccipital joint extension (extension of the head with the examiner bracing the neck in full flexion)
    e. Jaw protraction
    f. Ability to say "E" for adduction of the vocal cords.

Main Risks to Inform Patients
- The neurological function takes time to recover after surgery.
- Headache is likely and will be promptly treated.
- PONV, especially in patients with a history of PONV
- Sore throat that is usually transient
- Possibility of blood transfusion
- Bruises for IV, a line, or needles for electrophysiological monitoring.
- Possibility of awareness during extubation
- Surgical risks best left to surgeons: In general:
  - Risk of postoperative intracranial hemorrhage (ICH): 1%
  - Risk of infection: 2%
  - Postoperative (0–24 hours) transient neurological deficits: 10%

Setup of the Operating Room
- Machine check, circuit check, suction check, ensure vaporizers are adequately filled, adequate pumps available, and drugs prepared.
- *Airway equipment:*
  - Plan for three airway management strategies: For example, (i) direct laryngoscopy, (ii) bougie-assisted intubation, and (iii) laryngeal mask airway (LMA)
- *Direct laryngoscopy:*
  - *Laryngoscopes:* Operator preference—usually two blades, Mac 3 and 4, are opened and tested.
  - Consider a shoulder ramp for the obese or a shoulder roll positioned under the scapula to extend the neck.
  - Ability to lower the head of the table to extend the neck.
  - *The goal of positioning:* To the extent possible, draw a straight line from the upper incisor to the upper end of the thyroid cartilage in your sightline.
- Bougie-assisted intubation
- Glidescope or fiber-optic assisted intubation

- *Accessories:* Optimum-sized oral airway and nasal trumpet and LMAs
- *Bite blocks* necessary for electrophysiological (EP) monitoring.
- *Other equipment:* Esophageal temperature probe, nasogastric (NG) tube, condenser humidifier, eye lubricant, and sealing tape.
- *Neuromuscular monitor*

Monitoring

Routine Anesthesia Monitors

- *EKG:* Three channels—II (for rhythm), V (for ischemia), and CM-5 (combined rhythm and ischemia)
- *Respiratory rate from EKG* by thoracic impedance
- *Pulse oximeter* for pulse pleth (volume) and oxygen saturation
- *An esophageal temperature probe* is avoided in trans-sphenoid and cervical spine surgery. *Alternate sites:* axilla, urinary catheter, and, where appropriate, nasopharynx.
- *Noninvasive blood pressure (NIBP)* can be unreliable in the following situations:
  - in extremes of BP
  - morbidly obese patients
  - severe bradycardia
  - atrial fibrillation
- *Arterial line:* Pre-induction A-line is indicated when NIBP is unreliable; hemodynamically unstable patients or instability is expected, as with cardiac disease. *Certain surgeries:* Carotid endarterectomy, aneurysm surgery, cerebral vasospasm, Moyamoya disease, and critical spinal cord perfusion.
- *Information provided by the A-line:*
  - Heart rate
  - Electromechanical functioning of the heart: rhythm
  - Systolic, diastolic, and mean BPs
  - Site-specific perfusion pressure
  - Preload (volume) status by pulse pressure variation
  - *Myocardial contractility:* Upstroke of the arterial pulse
  - Cardiac output: Area under pressure–time curve
  - Detection of pulseless electrical activity
  - Effectiveness of CPR
  - Samples for hemogram, biochemical, and coagulation studies
- *Urinary output:*
  - *Parameters:* Volume, color, specific gravity, and electrolyte content. Informs about:
    - *Volume resuscitation:* Concentrated scant urine indicates hypovolemia.
    - Observing mannitol response is important while treating ICP.

CHAPTER 35 Routine Craniotomy under General Anesthesia

- Diabetes insipidus during pituitary surgery and rarely with propofol infusion
- Renal perfusion or injury with high-dose pressor drug use
- Neuromuscular monitoring
- *Processed EEG* for total intravenous anesthesia (TIVA) cases
- *Respiratory monitoring:*
  - Rate, volume, and minute ventilation to achieve the desired $ETCO_2$.
  - Optimizing minute ventilation guided by repeat blood gases.
  - Airway pressure, if excessive, can impede venous return and increase ICP.
  - *$ETCO_2$ monitoring:*
    - Acute decrease with the venous air embolism (VAE)
    - A rapid increase occurs with malignant hyperpyrexia (MH)
    - A gradual decrease occurs with hyperventilation or hypothermia.
    - Low $ETCO_2$ occurs with pulmonary emboli.
    - A sudden absence – a disconnection of the breathing system
    - A sloping expiratory curve suggests bronchospasm.
    - Irregular tracing or curare cleft with inadequate muscle relaxation
    - Stable $ETCO_2$ provides a measure of cardiac output.
  - Volatile anesthetic concentrations

Induction

The goal of induction is to achieve pleasant and hemodynamically stable intubation with a combination of the drugs listed in **Table 1**.

Table 1: Standard anesthesia drugs used in neurosurgery cases.

Drug	Typical dose	Comment
Fentanyl	50–100 mg	Apnea and hypotension are possible with higher doses
Midazolam	1–2 mg	Avoid in elderly and with dementia
Lidocaine	1 mg/kg	Treatment of pain with propofol and hypertension with intubation
Propofol	1–2 mg/kg	The usual induction agent that can cause hypotension
Rocuronium	0.6 mg/kg	Rapid reversal is possible with sugammadex if needed
Succinylcholine	1.5 mg/kg	Rapid and profound relaxation
Phenylephrine	40–80 µg boluses	Often given with propofol to avoid hypotension
Ephedrine	5–10 mg boluses	Treat hypotension with bradycardia
Labetalol	10–20 mg boluses	Prevent or treat hypertension
Esmolol	10–30 mg boluses	For rate control
Nicardipine	100–250 µg boluses	For increased BP with bradycardia
Sugammadex	1 mg/kg with TOF = 4	4 mg/kg with TOF <2 and 16 mg/kg for immediate recovery of NM blockade

(NM: neuromuscular; TOF: train-of-four)

Strategies to Decrease Response to Intubation
- Ensuring adequate depth of anesthesia before intubation
- Limit laryngoscopy to 20 seconds.
- Do a test laryngoscopy.
- Supplemental intravenous anesthetics if needed after test laryngoscopy.
- *Supplemental narcotics:* Fentanyl or remifentanil bolus
- Supplemental lidocaine (1 mg/kg)
- Topical intratracheal lidocaine via a catheter
- Bolus of esmolol 10–30 mg
- *Minor points:*
  - If the laryngeal view is good, avoid using stylet for intubation; it achieves better tube placement under vision.
  - Observe the response to endotracheal tube (ETT) placement before inflating the cuff slowly unless there is risk of aspiration.

Preoperative Interventions At/Immediately after Induction
- *Steroids:* Dexamethasone 10 mg at induction for most tumors.
  - Avoid in an awake patient as it causes perineal itching.
- *Antiepileptic drugs (AEDs):* Fosphenytoin or levetiracetam at induction.
- *Antibiotics:* Within 60 minutes before incision
- *Compression stockings* for DVT prophylaxis
- *Mannitol* (0.25–1 g/kg, IV) at skin incision, due to rebound increase in ICP, there is a trend to avoid its use or decrease the dose.
- *Fluorescein* (3 mg/kg, IV), as requested.

Steroid Replacement
- *Minor surgical stress:* 25 mg hydrocortisone or 5 mg methylprednisolone
- *Moderate surgical stress:* 25 mg IV hydrocortisone q 6/8 hours or 5 mg IV prednisolone q 8 hours; taper over two days.
- *Major surgery:* 25–50 mg IV hydrocortisone q 6/8 hours or 5 mg IV prednisolone q 8 hours; taper over two days.
- *Critical illness:* 50–100 mg IV hydrocortisone every 6/8 hours with fludrocortisone 50 µg/day; gradual taper over days.

Positioning
Before positioning, pin fixation is usually necessary. Ensure adequate depth of anesthesia and muscle relaxation before pin fixation. Supplemental propofol (20–50 mg) or narcotic (fentanyl 50–100 µg) is given along with IV saline flush. If the patient is hemodynamically unstable, topical local anesthetics can be injected at the pin site. In the final position, ensure that the venous return is not compromised, the limbs are well supported, all pressure points are adequately padded, IVs flow freely, and monitoring is functioning.

Table 2: Drug infusions used during maintenance of anesthesia.

Drug	Infusion dose	Comment
Propofol	50–100 µg/kg/min	If used as a sole agent at <50 µg/kg/min, recall is possible
Lidocaine	1–3 mg/kg/h	For analgesia, better emergence and avoid with renal failure
Remifentanil	0.1–0.3 µg/kg/min	Short acting and consider supplemental narcotics at the end
Sufentanil	0.5–3 µg/kg/h	Reduce infusion rates with skin closure
Rocuronium	0.01 mg/kg/min	Titrated to the level of paralysis
Phenylephrine	10–100 µg/min	As needed to maintain BP

Maintenance of Anesthesia

- Ensure depth of anesthesia while avoiding excessive [>1 minimum alveolar concentration (MAC)] volatile agents.
- TIVA with drugs listed in **Table 2** is a viable alternative to volatile agents and has the advantage of more favorable cerebral hemodynamic effects.
- Use processed EEG to ensure adequate depth of anesthesia.
- Most tumor surgeries require mild hyperventilation (ETCO$_2$ of 28–32 mm Hg). However, hypercapnia may be indicated to increase the collateral blood flow in Moyamoya disease or during temporary arterial occlusion. Hyperventilation is avoided in the initial phase of aneurysm surgery.
- Adequate muscle relaxation.
- Mild 5° anti-Trendelenburg position to ensure adequate venous return.
- During neurosurgery, there may be a preference for normal saline instead of Ringer's Lactate, which is slightly hypotonic.
- Avoid fluid runoff with large bore IVs.
- Check for the crystallization of 20% mannitol in the bag before infusion over 20–30 minutes via a 0.2-µm filter; rapid mannitol infusion can increase ICP, cause hyperkalemia and acidosis, and precipitate congestive heart failure. Mannitol is usually started at the skin incision, and the infusion should end when the bone flap is lifted.
- Avoid hypothermia, as it can inhibit coagulation and lead to post-operative shivering. Mild hypothermia is beneficial during vascular occlusion when indicated.
- Monitor urine output (volume and color).
- *Monitor blood loss:* Blood loss assessment becomes difficult as blood is collected in a plastic cone below the incision site or may flow onto the floor and is usually mixed with irrigation fluids. Blood is also mopped up in cotton towels. In the case of suspected excessive bleeding, the

best measure for adequate blood replacement is serial hemoglobin and hematocrit measurements.
- Repeat antibiotics and steroids as needed.

Preparation for the End of the Case

The author's approach to fast-track wake-up is listed in **Appendix 18 a–c**. Typical preparatory steps for wake-up are:
- Antiemetic drugs
- Narcotics for smooth emergence and postoperative pain.
- Timely tapering of volatile anesthetic use.
- Taper muscle relaxants
- Have a backup of IV propofol should any abrupt movement is observed.
- Avoid airway manipulation or reversal of muscle paralysis when the head is secured in pins.
- Reverse paralysis when headpins are removed to avoid scalp injury.
- Inspect the pin site for any bleeding; treatment may require pressure and injection of FlosealTM or a stitch.
- Ensure the bite block is in place and perform oral suctioning.
- The verbal response might be challenging for patients who are neurologically compromised.
- *For aphasic patients, extubation can be done if:*
  - The airway was safely maintained at induction.
  - There was no difficulty in intubation.
  - No change in airway since
  - Adequate spontaneous tidal volume and minute ventilation
  - Protective cough reflex present
  - End-tidal vapor concentration stable at "0" for a few minutes
  - Suctioning of the pharynx yields no secretions.

Emergence from Anesthesia

Emergence Problems

- Coughing and bucking
- Emergence hypertension
- Emergence hypotension
- Delayed emergence
- Postoperative agitation and delirium
- Nausea and vomiting

Coughing and Bucking

At-risk Patients

- History of smoking
- History of asthma and COPD

CHAPTER 35 Routine Craniotomy under General Anesthesia

- Recent cough and cold
- Robust young individuals
- OSA

Management

- *At induction:*
  - 5% lidocaine viscous gel on ETT before intubation
  - Intracuff lidocaine
- *During surgery:*
  - TIVA with propofol and remifentanil
  - TIVA with propofol sufentanil
  - Lidocaine infusion intraoperative
- *At the time of extubation:*
  - Suctioning the patients (oral/ETT) prior to the reversal of paralysis
  - Low-dose remifentanil infusion at wake up
  - Intravenous lidocaine infusion
  - Dexmedetomidine infusion
  - Low-dose fentanyl bolus (25-50 µg)
  - IV lidocaine bolus
  - Endotracheal lidocaine sprayed slowly with a small bore needle.
  - *After ventilation is established:* Low-dose hydromorphone 0.2 mg boluses may be used, typically requiring 1-3 doses.
- Deep extubation is possible for peripheral neurological surgery but not craniotomies. A new onset deficit would require reintubation; deep extubation is routinely avoided.
- *Complications of coughing and bucking:*
  - Raised ICP
  - Raised BP
  - Desaturation
  - Increased bleeding
  - Negative-pressure pulmonary edema

Emergence Hypertension

Target Blood Pressure Management

- Confer with the surgeons to decide on hemodynamic targets.
- *Typical targets:*
  - *At/not exceeding baseline SBP:* Tumor surgery (SBP often arbitrarily requested at 120-140 mm Hg).
  - *<20% baseline SBP:* Arteriovenous malformation (AVM) resection
  - *>20% baseline SBP:* Carotid endarterectomy (CEA) during occlusion but at or below SBP after endarterectomy
  - *Unprotected aneurysms:* Not to exceed SBP of 150 mm Hg.
  - *Protected aneurysms in settings of vasospasm SBP:* 180 mm Hg.
  - Ischemic stroke SBP of 150-200 mm Hg

- *Emergence hypertension:*
  - Almost 90% of neurosurgical patients need anti-hypertensive treatment.
  - TIVA is less likely to cause emergence hypertension compared to volatile anesthetics.
  - Complications due to the emergence hypertension:
    - Risk of bleeding
      - *Intracerebral hemorrhage:* Tumor or AVM bed
      - *Subdural hemorrhage:* Craniotomy/Pin sites
      - *Subarachnoid hemorrhage:* Aneurysms

Emergence Hypotension
- *Etiology:*
  - Anesthetic overdose
  - Antihypertensive drugs
  - Hypovolemia
  - Neurological injury
- *Complications:*
  - Delayed emergence
  - Watershed infarcts
- *Treatment:* Fluids and pressors as needed

Management of postoperative neurological dysfunction: New neurological deficit, delayed emergence, or delirium.

Neurological Deterioration after Craniotomy
- *Residual anesthetics:* Prolonged surgery with drug cumulation and long-acting narcotics can delay emergence and unmask preexisting neurological deficits.
- *Hematoma:* The risk of bleeding is about 1% and can occur remote from the operating site
- Infarction
- Seizures
- *Pneumocephalus:* Benign or tension
- *Tension pneumocephalus:* Ball valve obstruction to airflow, lets air in but cannot get out. Expansion of the trapped air due to nitrous oxide diffusion or the warming of trapped air from room to body temperature. The risk increases with the excessive drainage of cerebrospinal fluid (CSF) or extensive tissue resection.
- Acute hydrocephalus
- Edema
- Vasospasm
- *Neurological findings are often seen on emergence:*
  - Impaired cognition

- *Hyperreflexia:* Due to lack of cortical inhibition, spinal reflexes may be accentuated and manifest as:
  - Bilateral clonus
  - Bilateral Babinski
  - Hyperactive tendon reflexes
  - Opisthotonus
- Shivering
- Sluggish or absent pupillary response
- Unmasking of neurological deficits
- Hallucination
- Delirium

Delayed Emergence (Table 3)

- Delayed emergence is wakeup exceeding 30 minutes.
  - Can result in respiratory depression.
  - Overall risk 3%
  - Intracranial tumors >3 cm with mass effects
  - High-risk cases:
    - ASA (American Society of Anesthesiologists) III or greater.
    - Age >70 years

History

- Review anesthetic drugs and doses.
- Review immediate vital sign trends, core temperature, $ETCO_2$, and respiratory effort, if any.
- Review of medical, neurological, and pharmacological history
- History of substance abuse and self-medication

Examination

- *Vital signs:*
  - Core temperature

Table 3: Causes of delayed emergence.

Anesthetic or pharmacological causes	Neurologic causes	Metabolic causes
Overdose	Unmasked deficit	Hypothermia
Long-acting narcotics	New stroke	Hypo/hypercarbia
Residual volatile agents	Pneumocephalus	Hypo/hyperglycemia
Residual paralysis	Intracranial hemorrhage	Electrolyte imbalance (Na/Ca/Mg)
Steroid psychosis	Cerebral edema	Hyperosmolar state
Central cholinergic syndrome	Seizures	Hypothyroidism
Drug withdrawal	Catatonia	Thiamine deficiency
	Extrapyramidal syndrome	

- Heart rate, BP (bradycardia and hypertension, with decreased consciousness suggestive of raised ICP)
    - $ETCO_2$, respiratory rate, and tidal volume
    - Neuromuscular functions
- *Laboratory investigations:*
    - *Arterial blood gas (ABG):* $pH/PaCO_2/PaO_2$
    - *Metabolic screen:* $Na/Ca/Mg/PO_4$/glucose/lactate
    - EEG
    - CT
- *Treatment:*
    - Correct hypothermia.
    - Correct electrolyte and metabolic errors.
    - *Carefully consider reversing agents, which may cause pain and agitation:*
        - *Muscle relaxant:* Extra dose of sugammadex
        - Naloxone for narcotics
        - Flumazenil for benzodiazepines
        - Doxapram for sedative drugs
        - Atipamezole for dexmedetomidine (experimental)
    - Reversal of anesthesia with analeptics, such as doxapram, carries the risk of agitation, confusion, and seizures.
    - Consider anticonvulsive drugs (ACDs) for seizures.

POSTOPERATIVE DELIRIUM

Definition: Acute change in consciousness is characterized by inattention and disorganized thinking. Delirium is associated with decreased survival, extended ICU stays, and poor prognosis. The overall incidence of delirium after neurosurgery is about 10%.

Risk Factors

- Age
- Anemia
- Prior psychiatric history
- Poor functional status
- Low educational levels
- Respiratory disease
- Bilateral tumors
- Large tumors

Management

- Rule out and correct hypoxia, pain, discomfort (catheter), electrolyte imbalance, sepsis, and drug withdrawal.
- *Pharmacotherapy:* Use the lowest effective dose for the shortest time.
- Drugs are usually reserved for agitation in patients at risk of self-harm.

CHAPTER 35 Routine Craniotomy under General Anesthesia

- For immediate control of the situation, a bolus of propofol might be necessary while ensuring adequate breathing.
- Lorazepam can be used with caution; benzodiazepines can aggravate delirium.
- *Drugs used for treatment:*
  - Haloperidol
  - Droperidol
  - Chlorpromazine
  - Thioridazine

Postoperative Nausea and Vomiting (PONV)

PONV usually occurs within 24–48 hours of surgery. It can manifest as:
- *Nausea:* Sensation of the urge to vomit
- *Retching:* Sensation of vomiting without expelling gastric content
- *Vomiting:* Expulsion of gastric content

Incidence

- Can be exceedingly high (80%) with a history of risk factors.
- The overall risk of nausea is 50%
- The overall risk of vomiting is 50%
- Without any risk factors: 10%

Adult Risk Factors

- Female gender
- History of PONV
- History of motion sickness
- Age <30 years
- Use of narcotics
- Use of volatile agents, nitrous oxide
- Nonsmokers

Risk Factors for PONV in Children

- Surgery >30 min
- Family history of PONV
- Age >3 years

Pathology

- *Mechanism of PONV:*
  - Chemoreceptors triggering PONV are located throughout the medulla and brain stem
  - These receptors are sensitive to toxins, metabolites, and drugs
  - *The vomiting center is a loose cluster of neurons that includes:*
    - Chemoreceptor trigger zone in caudal IV ventricle

- Area postrema
- Nucleus tractus solitarius (NTS)
- *The vomiting center receives afferent from:*
  - Vagus from the gastrointestinal tract mediated by $5HT_3$ receptors.
  - From vestibular system (motion sickness)
  - The limbic system (Psychogenic vomiting)
- CTZ senses chemo-triggers in blood and cerebrospinal fluid
- *Vomiting center afferent relay to:*
  - CTZ communicates with NTS via dopamine-2 receptors.
  - NTS stimulates:
    - Rostral nucleus
    - Nucleus Ambiguous
    - Ventral respiratory group
    - Dorsal motor nucleus of the vagus
- The $5HT_3$ and Dopamine (D-2) receptor blockers prevent vomiting.

Management:
- Antiemetic drugs are the mainstay of treatment **(Table 4)**.

Table 4: Antiemetic drugs.

	Ondansetron	Dolasetron	Metoclopramide	Droperidol
Mechanism of action	$5HT_3$ antagonist	$5HT_3$ antagonist, more efficacious than ondansetron	Dopamine antagonist	• Dopamine antagonist • Antipsychotic
Dose	0.15 mg/kg (max 8 mg) q 4 hrs	0.35 mg/kg to a maximum of 12.5 mg	0.1 mg/kg	2.5 mg max, observe for 30 min, repeat 1.25 mg
Half life	6 hrs	8 hrs	6 hrs	2 hrs
24 hrs dose	16 mg	12.5 mg	0.5 mg/kg 24 hrs	7.5 mg
Side-effects	• Prolonged QTc • Others rare	Prolonged QTc	• Tardive dyskinesia • Prolonged QTc	• Prolonged QTc • Arrhythmia • Extra-pyramidal effects • Neuroleptic malignant syndrome
Contraindications	• Patient on apomorphine • Allergy to the drug	• Prolonged QTc • Sick sinus syndrome • Chemotherapy induced vomiting • Hypokalemia • Hypomagnesemia	• Avoid in epilepsy • Parkinson's disease • Prolactinomas • Pheochromocytoma	• Inc. QTc • Serious arrhythmias • Allergy to the drug • Hypokalemia/hypomagnesemia

CHAPTER 35 Routine Craniotomy under General Anesthesia

- *Other measures include:*
  - Propofol, decadron, scopolamine (patch), and anxiolytics
  - Acupressure at Neiguan point, on the inside of the wrist.
  - Avoiding fast, abrupt movements during the transportation of the patient that can trigger motion sickness.
- *Ondansetron:*
  - It is the front-line drug for PONV treatment.
  - It is ineffective for motion sickness.
  - Its use with apomorphine can lead to excessive sedation and hypotension.
  - It is metabolized by the liver; the dose is limited to 8 mg/24 hrs in liver failure.
  - Dose-dependent QTc prolongation. Caution with heart failure, severe bradycardia, and electrolyte imbalances. Prescreening EKG is not recommended, although EKG monitoring is desirable with the potential for QTc prolongation.
  - Side effects are rare, including headache, fatigue, chills, dry mouth, and constipation.

CASE REPORTS FOR FURTHER DISCUSSION

Case 1: A 59-year-old male presented to the hospital with dysarthria and lower limb weakness for a month. A CT scan revealed hemangioblastoma of the right cerebellum. History was significant for well-controlled diabetes and hypertension. Prone position craniotomy for the excision of the tumor was planned. Preoperative laboratory reports and tests were unremarkable, including CXR and pulmonary function tests. The patient underwent 4-hour surgery under general anesthesia with endotracheal intubation. The induction was with glycopyrrolate, propofol, remifentanil, and rocuronium. The single attempt ETT placement was atraumatic.

Anesthesia was maintained with target-controlled propofol infusion aimed at a Bispectral index score (BIS) of 40 (total dose 3 g), remifentanil (total dose 4 mg), and rocuronium (total dose 105 mg). The total blood loss was 500 mL, and the urine output the 1,250 mL. The fluid input, including mannitol, was 1,750 mL. On completion of the surgery, he was alert and spontaneously breathing oxygen via a face mask. Postoperative blood gases revealed PaO_2 of 147 mm Hg and $PaCO_2$ of 31 mm Hg. Four hours after the surgery, the patient developed stridor and swelling of the neck, but SaO_2 remained at 100%. By hour 6, the SaO_2 decreased to 90% on 10-L oxygen flow. *What is the differential diagnosis of postoperative respiratory distress in a patient who underwent prone posterior fossa surgery? How will you conservatively manage this case? What devices can you use to give positive pressure support with spontaneous breathing? What is the role of racemic epinephrine? Will you consider heliox? How will you intubate this patient?*

Case 2: A 36-year-old man presented for a suboccipital craniotomy for acoustic neuroma resection. He had a 7-month history of bilateral tinnitus, unstable gait, and impaired balance. Medical history was significant for hypertension and hyperlipidemia. There was a history of dysphagia that had resolved spontaneously. He had a history of mitral valve repair and closure of patent foramen ovale. His medications included aspirin (stopped seven days previously), rosuvastatin, lisinopril, and propranolol. Preoperative clinical exam and investigations were non-contributory. CT scan showed a left cerebellopontine angle tumor (4 × 4 × 3 cm) inferior to VII and VIII cranial nerve origin with compression of the cerebellum, brainstem, aqueduct, and the IV ventricle. After the induction of anesthesia, the head was turned to the right. Anesthesia was maintained with the infusion of propofol 120–140 μg/kg/min and remifentanil 0.15–0.2 μg/kg/min. During surgery, the patient's brainstem auditory evoked potentials declined and did not recover. The surgery lasted 8 hours. The net positive fluid balance was 695 mL. Thirty minutes before waking up, propofol and remifentanil infusions were stopped. At the wake-up time, the patient remained unresponsive. The temperature was 37°C, and heart rate was 67 bpm, BP was 119/52 mm Hg, and the spontaneous respiratory rate was 12 bpm. Both pupils were reactive and equal in size. There was no evidence of any neuromuscular paralysis. His glucose was 162 mg/dL. Blood gases and electrolytes were in the normal range. The BIS values remained low in the sixties.

There was no response to 0.2 mg flumazenil or 80 μg naloxone. A CT scan done at 3 hours was negative for bleed, infarct, or hydrocephalus. The patient responded to verbal commands 6 hours after surgery when extubated. He was oriented in time and place and had no gross neuro deficits. *What potential neurological/neurosurgical factors could have contributed to delayed awakening? What is context-sensitive half-life? Describe the management of infusions of propofol and remifentanil over prolonged anesthesia.*

Case 3: A 61-year-old man underwent several operations to treat glioblastoma multiforme (GBM), along with radiation to the tumor site and treatment with Avastin that can inhibit wound healing. During these treatments, he developed a pseudoaneurysm that also required a craniotomy. He developed a CSF leak that required an additional craniotomy. The leak persisted, and a ventriculoperitoneal shunt was planned for CSF diversion. The patient developed left-sided weakness and decreased sensations five days after the shunt. The CT scan revealed significant tension pneumocephalus beneath the craniotomy site. An urgent craniotomy relieved the pneumocephalus, and the skull was closed with a new titanium graft. However, the CSF leak recurred soon after discharge. Again, the patient developed a tension pneumocephalus with left-sided weakness and gait instability. This time, a rotational skin flap with superior temporal artery was planned to encourage wound healing. During surgery, it was noted that the brain was very tense and that his heart rate had decreased to the mid-40s with a significant elevation of BP. It was noted that nitrous oxide was being used. The gas flow was immediately stopped, and a needle was introduced into the tumor cavity. A gush of air was released, and BP and heart rate normalized soon after that. *What was the cause of pneumocephalus in this case? What are the pros and cons of using nitrous oxide in neurosurgery? What are other surgeries that carry the risk of pneumocephalus?*

Case 4: An 11-year-old girl presented with a 2-month-long history of headache, vomiting (1–2/week), dizziness, dysmetria, and abnormal gait. MRI was consistent with a large medulloblastoma with obstructive hydrocephalus. She underwent a successful suboccipital craniotomy with CSF drainage. Postoperatively, the patient developed severe nausea and vomiting, with ten or more daily episodes lasting several days. It responded better to intravenous than oral metoclopramide. A month later, radiotherapy was started. The radiation treatment lasted 30 sessions over six weeks. However, nausea and vomiting persisted throughout this time. *What are the risk factors for PONV? Why are patients with brainstem lesions at a greater risk for PONV? What are the perioperative precautions that prevent PONV? What are the major antiemetic drugs, and what is the effect of anticonvulsants in such cases?*

Case 5: A 45-year-old woman presented with headache, neck stiffness, and altered sensorium. A cerebral angiogram revealed a ruptured anterior communicating artery aneurysm clipped via the pterional approach. After the clipping, the patient was slow to recover from anesthesia. Neurological examination revealed signs consistent with cerebellar dysfunction. A postoperative CT scan showed a right cerebellar hemorrhage. The patient was investigated for the potential cause of remote cerebellar bleeding, such as BP spikes or coagulopathy, but none was found. *What are the causes of delayed emergence after anesthesia? What investigations will you do to rule them out? How does excessive CSF drainage lead to postoperative bleeding?*

CASE REPORT REFERENCES

Case 1: Shin HW et al. Post-operative respiratory difficulty due to asymptomatic anterior cervical osteophyte after brain tumor surgery: a case report. Korean J Anesthesiol. 2016;69(6):640-3.

Case 2: Munis JR et al. Delayed emergence from anesthesia associated with absent brainstem reflexes following sub-occipital craniotomy. Neurocrit Care. 2006;5(3):206-9.

Case 3: Singh M et al. Intraoperative development of tension pneumocephalus in a patient undergoing repair of a cranial-dural defect under nitrous oxide anesthesia. J Surg Tech Case Rep. 2015;7(1):20-2.

Case 4: Tsai KC et al. Gabapentin for postoperative vomiting in children requiring posterior fossa tumor resection. Pediatr Neonatol. 2015; 56(5):351-4.

Case 5: Landeiro JA et al. Remote hemorrhage from the site of craniotomy. Arq Neuropsiquiatr. 2004;62(3B):832-4.

FURTHER READING

1. Aurilio C et al. Multimodal analgesia in neurosurgery: a narrative review. Postgrad Med. 2022;134(3):267-76.
2. Ibrahim IM et al. Efficacy of dexmedetomidine infusion without loading dose on hemodynamic variables and recovery time during craniotomy: a randomized double-blinded controlled study. Anesth Pain Med. 2021. 11(2):e113410.
3. Mallari RJ et al. Streamlining brain tumor surgery care during the COVID-19 pandemic: a case-control study. PLoS One. 2021;16(7):e0254958.
4. McCullough IL et al. Opioid-free anesthesia for craniotomy. J Neurosurg Anesthesiol. 2021; PMID: 34469414.
5. Sato T et al. Comparison of remimazolam and propofol in anesthetic management for awake craniotomy: a retrospective study. J Anesth. 2022; 36(1):152-5.

Vignette: The First Neurosurgeon

Harvey Cushing is widely recognized as the father of modern neurosurgery. However, the first surgeon ever appointed exclusively for treating brain diseases was Victor Horsley. In 1886, Horsley was appointed to the National Hospital for the Paralyzed and Epileptics at Queen's Square in London. Cushing toured Europe and trained under Victor Horsley. Thus Victor Horsley gets the credit for being the first neurosurgeon.

Vignette: Surgery by Neanderthals?

"Shanidar-1" is a designated Neanderthal skeleton dating to 60,000 to 30,000 BCE. It was found in Shanidar cave in northern Iraq. The skeleton is of a man aged between 35 and 40 years who suffered a significant head injury in his youth. The analysis of the bones has revealed extensive arthritis. There is considerable wear and tear on the teeth, suggesting he ate a softer diet. Ossicles in the ear indicate that he was probably deaf. However, the most stunning feature of the skeleton is a clean amputation at the lower humerus with the healing of the stump. Such an injury is unlikely to be accidental, suggesting a possible surgical intervention. If this injury represents a surgical intervention, it would be a stunning achievement. When it comes to intelligence assessment, there is an overwhelming bias against the Neanderthals.

Most bone art and cave paintings from around 30,000 to 40,000 years found in Europe have been attributed to modern humans, although the Neanderthals lived in the same places around the same time. Evidence suggests that Neanderthals were dexterous with tools, as evidenced by their perforated shell beads. They were cognitively advanced, as evidenced by cave paintings, which antedate modern humans. Thus, the cognitive and social behavior of the Neanderthals was comparable to early humans. Could Shanidar-1 be the evidence of surgery by the Neanderthals? Perhaps! At the very least, surgery aside, the skeleton suggests that the Neanderthals were not the brutes as they have been portrayed in popular culture but took care of the old and the infirm members of their groups.

Chapter 36

Awake Craniotomy for Seizure Disorders

INTRODUCTION

Awake craniotomy is a craniotomy under dynamic sedation. Dynamic sedation implies that the level of sedation is titrated continuously to meet the surgical needs of the moment. The level of sedation ensures adequate patient comfort and temporary affective dissociation during most of the operation. However, sedation is reduced to enable testing of cortical functions by verbal commands. Awake craniotomy is indicated for surgery near the speech and motor cortex, excision of epileptic foci, stereotactic brain surgery for movement disorders, and ablation of deep brain structures for pain treatment. Its relative simplicity and rapid postoperative recovery have expanded the application to excision biopsies, stereotactic biopsies, and ventriculostomies. Awake craniotomy carries the risk of significant intraoperative complications. It requires careful assessment of the patient's airway and the ability to cooperate during the procedure. There are several approaches to ensure the safety of the procedure. The patient's characteristics primarily determine the approach used in a given case.

NEUROANESTHETIC CONCERNS

- Epileptic seizure
- Clinical classification
- Pathogenesis and perioperative triggers
- Preoperative work up
- *Awake craniotomy:*
  - Indications/contraindications
  - Preoperative preparation
  - Techniques
  - Cortical mapping
  - Complications
- Ambulatory neurosurgery.

Epileptic Seizure

An epileptic seizure is a spontaneous, abnormal, and paroxysmal discharge of neurons that affects sensory, motor, or behavioral functions or alters consciousness. For the diagnosis of epilepsy, there must be two seizure episodes 24 hours apart, a seizure episode with the likelihood of another seizure, or a diagnosis of known seizure syndrome but no longer seizing.

Epilepsy is classified based on the presentation, although the underlying pathology is often age-dependent. In children, seizures are often precipitated by febrile episodes or may be idiopathic. In juveniles, seizures are usually idiopathic. In middle-aged patients, epilepsy is usually due to trauma and tumors. In the elderly, epilepsy is often due to tumors or cerebrovascular accidents.

Clinical Classification

Incidence: Partial (55%), generalized (40%), unclassified (5%).
- *Partial seizures:* These are usually due to focal hemispheric pathology. They are simple when there is no alteration in consciousness but with motor (Jacksonian seizures), sensory, autonomic, or psychic symptoms. They are complex when there is a change in consciousness, often with an aura preceding the seizure. Both simple and complex partial seizures can progress to generalized seizures.
- *Generalized tonic–clonic seizures (GTCS):* These present with bilateral symmetrical motor activity and unconsciousness.
- *Myoclonic seizures* present as jerky movements during which the patient is usually conscious.
- *Atonic seizures* are due to the sudden loss of motor tone and present as drop attacks or inexplicable falls.
- *Absence seizures* arise from the temporal lobes; when generalized, they impair consciousness without motor involvement.
- *Mesial temporal sclerosis:* Often presents with an aura that warns of an impending seizure. Seizures are associated with sensory disturbances, absence seizures, behavioral changes, muscle spasms, or convulsions. These seizures are associated with amnesia and postictal confusion. The onset of these seizures is in the late first decade. Seizures increase in complexity and duration. The effect on speech may suggest pathology localized to the dominant hemisphere. Mesial temporal sclerosis presents a history of febrile seizures, often with a family history of seizures.

  On investigation:
  - MRI shows hippocampal atrophy.
  - EEG shows spikes over the temporal lobes.
  - Fluorodeoxyglucose-PET imaging shows temporal lobe hypometabolism.
  - *Wada test:* Amnesia after intracarotid anesthetic injection in the side of the lesion can predict post-surgical deficit.

- *Mixed seizures:* Share the characteristics of two or more seizure disorders.
- *Unclassified seizures:* Complex seizures that do not fit any defined pattern.
- *Nonepileptic seizures:* About 20% of seizures are without electrical discharges, called nonepileptic or pseudo-seizures. They present with convulsions or jerky movements, falls, rigidity, staring, or loss of attention. These are usually due to psychological stress.

Pathogenesis

- *Structural abnormalities:* Developmental defects, hypoxic injuries, stroke, traumatic brain injury (TBI), tumors, and infective mass lesions (cysticercosis or toxoplasmosis)
- *Genetic and familial:* Juvenile myoclonic epilepsy, tuberous sclerosis, or neurofibromatosis
- Drug or drug withdrawal
- *Metabolic:* Inborn errors in metabolism, acquired metabolic abnormalities such as hypoglycemia, hyponatremia, hypocalcemia, or hypomagnesemia
- *Infectious:* Encephalitis, meningitis
- *Immune disorders:* Lupus or Hashimoto's thyroiditis
- *Idiopathic:* Epilepsy without apparent pathology manifests as childhood and juvenile absence seizures, myoclonic seizures, or generalized tonic-clonic seizures.

Perioperative Triggers

- Preoperative fasting (hypoglycemia)
- Drug or alcohol withdrawal
- Sleep deprivation
- Hyperventilation
- Photostimulation
- Metabolic alkalosis/electrolyte imbalance
- Hyperthermia
- Proconvulsive anesthetics/drugs
- Anesthetic and surgery-related changes in drug concentrations
- Neurosurgical complications
- Motor-evoked responses.

Differential Diagnosis

- Cerebrovascular accident (CVA)
- Migraine
- Sleep disorders
- Drugs or substance abuse
- Vestibular disease

- Movement disorders
- Psychological.

Preoperative Assessment

Investigations

- *Complete blood count:*
  - *Anemia/thrombocytopenia:* Valproic acid may induce bone marrow suppression.
- *Electrolytes:* Abnormalities may cause or aggravate seizures
- *Serum concentrations of anticonvulsant drugs:*
  - Determine the adequacy of treatment.
  - Anesthesia and or surgery can alter concentrations of anticonvulsant drugs.
- *Liver function test (LFT):* Valproic acid, felbamate, and phenytoin can affect LFT.
- Coagulation screen
- *EEG:* Diagnostic workup for seizures
- *EKG:* Antiepileptic drugs (AEDs) such as carbamazepine can affect heart rate and QT interval.
- *Imaging for localizing the lesion:*
  - CT scan
  - *MRI:* Non-contrast and contrast-enhanced
  - Functional brain imaging MRI/PET
  - *Angiography:* To rule out suspected vascular disease
  - *Wada testing:* Intra-arterial injection of anesthetic drugs has been used to localize brain functions such as speech and memory and to determine hemispheric dominance before surgical interventions.

Awake Craniotomy

Indications

- Tumor excisions close to eloquent regions of the brain, such as the speech, sensory, or motor cortex.
- Need for the stimulation of deep brain nuclei.
- Epilepsy surgery requiring careful tissue excision in eloquent regions of the brain.
- *Ambulatory neurosurgery:* In selected patients, an early discharge is possible 4–6 hours after awake neurosurgery.

Absolute Contraindications

- Patients who are neurologically impaired, unable to communicate or cooperate or comprehend commands.
- Prolonged surgery
- Large tumor with significant midline shift
- Frequent breakthrough seizures, refractory to medical management.

Relative Contraindications
- Exceedingly anxious patients
- Significant comorbidities such as chronic obstructive pulmonary disease (COPD) or obstructive sleep apnea (OSA)
- Morbid obesity
- Esophageal reflex
- Anticipated difficult airway.

Preoperative Preparation
- Evaluate the patient's ability to cooperate during the procedure.
- Assess their level of anxiety. Claustrophobic patients with anxiety disorders or panic attacks may not be suitable for awake craniotomy.
- Determine their response to pain, such as during the IV placement.
- Assess the airway, including the history of OSA and snoring.
- The airway is better maintained in a lateral than in a supine position.
- Explain the procedure in a simple stepwise manner.

Approaches to Awake Craniotomy
- Awake craniotomy with regional block and minimal sedation: This approach is appropriate for patients with compromised airways, morbid obesity, and severe OSA.
- Awake craniotomy under sedation with minimal airway instrumentation.
- Asleep-awake-asleep craniotomy with laryngeal mask airway (LMA) with the patient breathing spontaneously.
- Asleep-awake-asleep craniotomy with LMA and controlled ventilation.

Scalp Block for Awake Craniotomy
- The seven nerves that need to be blocked to anesthetize the scalp are listed in **Table 1**.

Table 1: Front to back circumferentially, 7 nerves.

Nerves	Injection site	Volume
Supratrochlear	1.5 cm above supraorbital foramen, medial third of the orbit	2 mL
Supraorbital		
Zygomatic-temporal	1.5 cm anterior to tragus, deep subcutaneous injection	5 mL
Auricular-temporal		
Lesser occipital	1.5 cm posterior to antitragus	2 mL
Greater occipital	At mastoid along the nuchal ridge	5 mL
Third occipital		

- Supplemental injections may be needed at the pin sites.
- The block lasts 6–8 hours when performed with a mixture of 0.5% bupivacaine and epinephrine (1:200,000).

Anesthetic Techniques
- *Minimal sedation technique:*
  - Judicious doses of fentanyl and midazolam for background sedation.
  - Anti-emetics are prophylactically given along with steroids, anticonvulsants, and antibiotics.
  - Sedation is maintained by an infusion of either propofol or dexmedetomidine.
  - An arterial line may be placed to monitor the blood pressure to avoid the need to inflate the cuff repeatedly.
  - End-tidal carbon dioxide ($EtCO_2$) monitoring is quantitatively unreliable with a nasal cannula, though it assesses the respiratory rate and can reveal airway obstruction.
  - Anticipating the need for rescue ventilation with little warning, a backup airway management plan (facemask/nasal trumpets/LMA) should always be available. Ensuring that the breathing circuit can extend to the airway in an emergency is prudent.
- *Minimal airway instrumentation:*
  - It provides a deeper level of anesthesia compared to sedation alone.
  - Nasal trumpets may be used.
    - Nasal passages are tested for airflow, and the one with the better flow is selected. The test is not reliable as the posterior passage may be dilated in case of anterior obstruction.
    - Intranasal 2% lidocaine jelly with phenylephrine is used and applied to the trumpet before insertion.
    - Trumpets are placed under sedation with minimal force.
- *Asleep–awake–asleep technique:*
  - Involves placement of an LMA to ensure a deeper level of sedation.
  - The LMA is removed during the brain tissue resection to enable the patient to communicate.
  - Drug selection is similar to conventional deep sedation with propofol. However, greater doses of propofol may be used.
  - $EtCO_2$ can be reliably monitored.
  - The patient breathes spontaneously to decrease the risk of air leaks.
- *Asleep–awake–asleep technique with ventilation:*
  - Mechanical ventilation is used during more profound levels of sedation after LMA placement to permit adequate gas exchange.

CHAPTER 36 Awake Craniotomy for Seizure Disorders

- With this method, hypercapnia and hypoxia can both be avoided.
- LMA is removed during neurological testing.
- Given that the head is secured in pins, a flexible stem LMA might be more useful than the more rigid ones.

Cortical Mapping

- *Cortical mapping:* It is used for localizing sensory, motor cortex, and speech centers in relation to the pathology.
- The sensory cortex is identified by placing a six-electrode strip across the post-central sulci and then observing the phase reversal of the N20 to P20 waves during stimulation on the electrocorticogram.
- Speech function location relative to the seizure focus:
  - The cortex is stimulated using a 2mA that is increased to 10 mA while the surface electrodes monitor the after-discharge.
  - If a seizure is seen, the stimulation current is decreased by 1mA to verify the focus location.
  - The objective is to test speech function while stimulating the seizure focus.
  - The effect can range from no change to complete speech arrest.

Complications of Awake Craniotomy

- Hypotension (50%)
- Tachycardia and hypertension (15%)
- Seizures, on EEG (15%), more likely during epilepsy surgery
- Conversion to general anesthesia (5%)
- Clinical seizures (2%)
- Airway obstruction (2%)
- Hypoxemia (2%)
- Disinhibition (2%)
- Brain swelling (1%)
- Nausea (1%)
- Bradycardia (rare)
- Dysphoric reactions
- Vomiting and aspiration

Ambulatory Neurosurgery

Ambulatory neurosurgery has been proposed for some select neurosurgical procedures in relatively healthy patients, using regional anesthesia and minimal sedation. Careful patient selection is necessary for ambulatory neurosurgery. During the procedure, invasive monitoring and airway instrumentation are kept to a minimum. Patients scheduled for ambulatory neurosurgery should live near the hospital and have a reliable caregiver. The operation should end by early afternoon, typically around 1:00 pm, to enable postoperative monitoring for at least 4 hours. A CT scan is often required before discharge.

CASE REPORTS FOR FURTHER DISCUSSION

Case 1: A 39-year-old patient with uncorrected complex cyanotic congenital heart disease presented with acute right frontal headache, fever, and sensory disturbances on the left side of his body. A week prior, he had undergone laser surgery for hypertrophic nasal turbinate. His cardiac abnormalities included a single ventricle, tricuspid atresia, transposition of great vessels, and bilateral Blalock–Taussig shunts. His history included endocarditis, pulmonary hemorrhage, renal and splenic infarctions, transient ischemic attacks (TIAs), and recurrent supraventricular arrhythmias. Echo revealed a ventricular ejection fraction (LVEF) of 46%. EKG revealed NSR. His room air saturation was 80%, with a hematocrit of 62% and mild leukocytosis. CT scan revealed a ring-enhancing lesion in the right superior temporal gyrus. Contrast-enhanced MRI revealed a lesion consistent with an acute abscess. The patient was scheduled for an awake craniotomy for the abscess excision. *What special precautions will you take given his single ventricle? What medications will you use for sedation? Will you use invasive monitoring?*

Case 2: A 42-year-old female was diagnosed with a frontal glioma and was scheduled for an awake craniotomy with language mapping. Her medical history was significant for ongoing depression. She is reluctant to undergo awake surgery, raising concerns about her cooperation during the procedure. *Would you proceed with the awake craniotomy in a potentially uncooperative patient? How will you plan for such a procedure? If her cortical EEG shows excessive activity, what steps can you take to decrease the chances of intraoperative seizures?*

Case 3: An 11-year-old female with treatment-resistant epilepsy is scheduled for the excision of a neuroepithelial tumor on her motor strip. MRI revealed a 3.5 × 3.5 × 5 cm tumor in the right prefrontal cortex. Despite treatment, the patient has about one seizure each week. She is easily distracted and has difficulty following simple commands. *Is she a candidate for an awake craniotomy? What additional precautions will you take in this case? What would be your anesthesia plan for the procedure? A plan is made to minimize awake time by initial general anesthesia using LMA and inhaled anesthetics. On placing the LMA, there is a notable air leak. What will you do?*

Case 4: A 51-year-old male presented with dysarthria and right hemiparesis and was diagnosed with a stroke two years ago. He was subsequently diagnosed with parietal lobe glioblastoma. His medical history was significant for diabetes, hypertension, and OSA. About two weeks before surgery, he had increased focal seizures involving the upper extremities, and carbamazepine and levetiracetam were increased. After treatment, his serum Na⁺ level decreased from 140 to 130 mEq/L. He was scheduled for tumor resection with an asleep–awake–asleep protocol. After anesthesia was induced, repeat point-of-care tests were done. Serum Na⁺ was 124.5 mEq/L and serum K⁺ was at 4.3 mEq/L. After 200 mL of 20% mannitol, serum Na⁺ further decreased to 117.8 mEq/L, while K+ increased to 5.6 mEq/L. *What are the possible causes of hyponatremia in this case? What are the hazards of rapid mannitol infusion? What risk will hyponatremia pose if the patient is woken up?*

CASE REPORT REFERENCES

Case 1: D'antico C et al. Case Report: Emergency awake craniotomy for cerebral abscess in a patient with unrepaired cyanotic congenital heart disease. F1000Research. 2017;5:2521.

Case 2: Al Shuaibi KM. Awake craniotomy in a depressed and agitated patient. Anesth Essay Res. 2010;4(1):41-3.

Case 3: Labuschagne J et al. Awake craniotomy in a child: assessment of eligibility with a simulated theatre experience. Case Rep Anesthesiol. 2020;6902075.

Case 4: Yamamoto S et al. A case of failed awake craniotomy due to progressive intraoperative hyponatremia. JA Clin Rep. 2018;4:40.

FURTHER READING

1. Korkar GH, et al. Awake craniotomy for epilepsy surgery on eloquent speech areas: a single-centre experience. Epileptic Disord. 2021;23(2):347-56.
2. Lee CZ, et al. An update of neuroanesthesia for intraoperative brain mapping craniotomy. Neurosurgery. 2022;90(1):1-6.
3. Rossi M, et al. Asleep or awake motor mapping for resection of perirolandic glioma in the nondominant hemisphere? Development and validation of a multimodal score to tailor the surgical strategy. J Neurosurg. 2022;136(1): 16-29.
4. Singh K, et al. Anesthesia for Awake Craniotomy, in StatPearls. 2022: Treasure Island (FL)
5. Takami, et al. Perioperative Factors Affecting Readmission after Awake Craniotomy: Analysis of 609 Consecutive Cases. World Neurosurg, 2021.

Vignette: Primitive Techniques of Skull Trephination

In 1865, the first Peruvian skull with trephination was presented to the Western world, and it stunned scholars on either side of the Atlantic. There was great skepticism that someone in a remote South American jungle could undertake such a surgery. Paul Broca in Paris investigated the specimen, and after 11 years of examination, he concluded that the person had survived the surgery. It was a stunning conclusion that was met with universal skepticism. It was not until 1873, after a Neolithic skull with evidence of a similar surgery was found in France, that the possibility of such surgery by relatively primitive cultures was accepted. Soon, other specimens emerged from elsewhere in the world.

These specimens revealed that different techniques were used for trephining the skulls, such as scraping the skull with a piece of glass, using intersecting linear cuts with glass chards or metal blades, cutting a circular groove using a trephine that could be rotated by hand or with a bow, or drilling several close holes and then chiseling the intervening bone bridges.

Primitive trephinations could be ritualistic acts that were sometimes found in several members of a group. However, Hippocrates recommended trephination for treating head injuries. His rationale was to prevent blood stagnation, which he deemed harmful to the patient.

Chapter 37 Carotid Endarterectomy

INTRODUCTION

The first carotid endarterectomy (CEA) was performed in 1953. By 1976, 34,000 CEA procedures were done in the US annually; by 1999, that number had increased to over 81,000. However, the US and European trend has been declining ever since. In 2014, for example, 36,000 CEA procedures were done in the US, while another 10,000 patients were treated by carotid stenting (CAS). It reflects a significant decrease in surgical interventions for treating carotid arterial disease.

Regarding anesthetic care, the surgeon's preference determines whether CEA is undertaken under general or regional anesthesia. Both require close neurological and hemodynamic monitoring. Evidence shows that the prevalence of specific risk factors has increased, yet the morbidity and mortality from both CEA and CAS have declined in the last two decades. The improved outcome could partly be due to better perioperative care of these patients.

NEUROANESTHETIC CONCERNS

- *Pathology of carotid arterial disease:* Carotid artery pathology is usually a part of systemic atheromatous disease. *It is associated with a cluster of diseases that include* hypertension, coronary artery disease, congestive heart failure (CHF), peripheral vascular disease, smoking, obesity, diabetes, and hyperlipidemia.
- High risk CEA
- *Treatment options for carotid arterial disease*
- *Assessment of stenosis*
- *The surgical approach*
- *Three key concerns:*
  - Anticoagulation,
  - Neuromonitoring
  - Controlling hemodynamics
- *Setup of the OR*
- *Preoperative assessment*
- Regional versus general anesthesia (GA).

- Regional techniques
  - Superficial cervical plexus block
  - Deep cervical plexus block
  - Cervical epidural
- General anesthesia
- Postoperative management
- Postoperative complications

Pathology of Carotid Arterial Disease

- Risk factors:
  - Age
  - Diabetes
  - Hyperlipidemia
  - Hypertension
  - Smoking
- Atherosclerotic changes:
  - Formation of a soft plaque:
    - Degenerative changes in the vessel wall
    - Deposition of cholesterol, lipids, and calcium
  - Maturation of the plaque:
    - Fibrous changes
    - Infiltration of macrophages
    - Formation of fatty streaks
  - Degenerative plaques:
    - Necrosis
    - Hemorrhage
    - Thrombosis
- Stroke precipitating factors:
  - *Embolic debris:* Fibrin and platelet, and thromboemboli
  - Thrombosis
  - Stenosis >80% decreases the flow.
  - Complete occlusion.
- Clinical syndromes:
  - Asymptomatic
  - Transient ischemic attacks (TIAs) resolve in 72 hours.
  - *Crescendo TIA:* Increasing frequency of TIAs
  - *Amaurosis Fugax:* Transient blindness
  - *Stroke:* Symptoms lasting >72 hours.

High-Risk CEA Cases

- High-risk cases are often excluded from clinical trials; therefore, risk factors are hard to identify:
  - Age >80 years
  - Previous ipsilateral or contralateral CEA
  - Severe hypertension

- Diabetes
- Poor cardiac status [atrial fibrillation (AF), CHF, coronary artery disease (CAD)/abnormal stress test, and need for heart surgery].
- Renal failure
- Severe pulmonary disease
- Previous neck surgery, radiation treatment, or tracheostomy.

Treatment Options for Carotid Arterial Disease

In general:
- Medical management is indicated for:
    - Complete occlusion
    - Short life expectancy
    - Asymptomatic patients with significant (90%) stenosis
    - Medical management consists of the following:
        - Antiplatelet drugs
        - Statins and lipid-lowering drugs
        - Anticoagulants
        - Treatment for hypertension and diabetes
- CEA has higher earlier mortality compared to CAS.
- CAS may have higher earlier stroke complications.
- Long-term outcomes with both similar
- **Table 1** lists some recent studies assessing carotid artery disease treatments.

Table 1: Treatment of carotid arterial disease.

Trial	Enrollment	Major results
1991: North American Symptomatic Carotid Endarterectomy Trial (NASCET)	659 patients with 70–99% narrowing by angiography	Two-year follow up: Stroke incidence decreased from 26% with medical Rx vs. 9% after CEA. Serious stroke/death were 2.1 and 0.9%, respectively
2004: Asymptomatic Carotid Atherosclerotic Study (ACAS)	1,662 asymptomatic patients with >60% stenosis	Median follow-up 2.7 years; Stroke risk decreased from 11% with medical Rx to 5.1% after CEA
2004: Stenting and Angioplasty with Protection in Patients at High Risk for Endarterectomy (SAPPHIRE)	334 symptomatic and asymptomatic patients	2 × more stroke/MI/death with CEA vs. stenting at 30 days but no difference by 3 years
2009: Carotid Revascularization Endarterectomy vs. Stenting Trial (CREST)	2522 patients randomized to CAS and CEA 2.5 year follow up	Stroke rates acceptable with both Rx. Early stroke CAS 2× CEA. CEA 2 × CAS for MI. CEA better for younger subjects. No long-term difference
2016: Randomized Trial of Stent vs. Surgery for Asymptomatic CEA (ACT I)	1453 with severe asymptomatic stenosis, <79 years, 3: 1: CAS: CEA allocation. 30 days to 5 years follow-up	Early stroke/MI/ death is more in CAS than CEA, but long-term survival is comparable
2021: Second Asymptomatic Carotid Surgery Trial (ACST-2)	3625 asymptomatic patients randomized to CAS (1811) or CEA (1814) 30 days to 5 year follow-up	Similar impact on stroke rate after both treatment on long term follow-up
2022: ACT-I and CREST trials combined data	Total of 2544 asymptomatic patients with >70% stenosis <80 years of age followed up for 4 years	No significant difference between CEA and CAS stroke and survival after the two treatments

(CEA: carotid endarterectomy; CAS: carotid artery stenting ; MI: myocardial infarction)

Indication for Surgery
- *Surgery is indicated for:*
  - Symptomatic carotid disease (TIA, blindness, or transient strokes) with 50–99% stenosis.
  - Asymptomatic patients with >60% stenosis but not >90%.
  - A 70% occlusion corresponds to a lumen of 1.5 mm.
  - TIA risk with asymptomatic patient 1–2%/year.
- *Surgery is contraindicated if there is:*
  - Complete internal carotid artery (ICA) occlusion.
  - Previous stroke with significant deficits on the ipsilateral side.
  - Significant comorbidities.
  - *The carotid artery cannot be accessed safely:*
    - Tracheotomy
    - Radiation to the neck
    - Restricted surgical access.

Assessment of Carotid Stenosis
- *Auscultation:* Bruit.
- *Ultrasound:*
  - *Simple blood flow velocity measurements*
  - Duplex scan—B mode, which permits anatomical measurements.
  - Spectral analysis, which gives a more detailed blood flow velocity profile.
- CT angiography.
- Magnetic resonance angiography.
- *Carotid angiogram:* The gold standard.

CEA Operative Steps
Key surgical steps are common to regional and GA.
- *Positioning:* Neck slightly extended using a shoulder roll and turned to the left or right side at a 30° angle.
- The vertical incision on the anterior border of the sternocleidomastoid muscle
- Alternatively, a transverse incision at the carotid bifurcation can yield better cosmetic results.
- Retractors are placed superficially under platysma to avoid nerve injury.
- *Possible nerve injuries include:*
  - The marginal mandibular branch of the facial nerve (motor supply to the angle of the mouth)
  - Recurrent laryngeal nerve injury (innervates vocal cords)
  - Ansa hypoglossi and hypoglossal nerve (innervation of the tongue).
- The facial vein is ligated and divided where it crosses the carotid sheath.

- *Carotid sheath contents identified:* Common carotid artery (CCA), ICA, internal jugular vein, and vagus nerve.
- Carotid bulb manipulation causes bradycardia and can be anesthetized with lidocaine.
- The upper and lower limits of the plaque are identified by gentle palpation.
- For temporary occlusion the loops are placed as follows:
  - *Loop around CCA:* 2-3 cm below the bifurcation
  - *Loop around external carotid artery (ECA):* 2-3 cm above the bifurcation
  - Vascular clip occludes the superior thyroid artery.
  - *Loop around ICA:* 2-3 cm above the bifurcation.
- Heparin (70-100 units/kg, IV) is given 3 minutes before clamping, and the effect is confirmed by a 2X increase in activated clotting time (ACT).
- *Occlusion sequence:* CCA, ECA, and last ICA
- Arteriotomy and plaque removal.
- Rule out any intimal flap that can lead to dissection. Intima sutured from outside.
- Closure of suture edges with Prolene or with patch graft as needed.
- *Guarded release of vascular clamps in sequence:* ECA followed by CCA and then ICA.

Three Key Concerns during CEA

Three key elements to monitor during surgery are (1) anticoagulation, (2) neurological monitoring, and (3) hemodynamic management.

Anticoagulation

Due to the risk of thrombosis and thromboembolism as a part of the disease process or arterial occlusion, it is required that a certain degree of anticoagulation is maintained during surgery. To do so:
- Antiplatelet drugs are usually continued until surgery.
- During surgery, heparin is given to prolong the ACT time two-fold. The effects of heparin are not reversed at the end of surgery.

Neurological Monitoring

- *Awake* CEA can be performed under superficial and deep cervical plexus block with minimal background sedation. Awake CEA permits gross neurological monitoring and minimizes hemodynamic stress due to intubation or hypotension associated with anesthetic drugs. However, it requires the cooperation of the patient, the ability to understand and express verbal commands, and the ability to perform basic tasks such as squeezing a squeaky toy. In addition, hemodynamic control might be difficult in an awake patient. Furthermore, a gross neurological examination might not detect focal embolic injury. Awake CEA is usually an institutional or individual preference, and there is no clear benefit of regional versus GA on the neurological outcome.

- *Mean arterial and stump pressure monitoring:* In most CEA, patients have normal intracranial pressure (ICP); hence monitoring the mean arterial pressure (MAP) can provide a measure of cerebral perfusion pressure (CPP). The goal during ICA occlusion is to maintain the MAP 20% above the resting blood pressure. The target blood pressure is based on the extent of collateral perfusion on the angiogram in consultation with the surgeon.

  Stump pressure: Pressure distal to the occluded ICA, if <25 mm Hg from the proximal pressure indicates the need for shunt placement.

- *Transcranial Doppler (TCD) monitoring:* TCD provides:
  - TCD provides a reliable way to assess carotid artery flow changes during CEA.
  - It can help detect the release of embolic materials at the clamping and unclamping of the ICA,
  - Predict the risk of stroke, e.g., when there is a ≥90% decrease in the middle cerebral artery (MCA) flow velocity on clamping and a ≥100% increase in pulsatility index on the release of the clamp.
  - The risk of neurological injury increases when these changes are seen in symptomatic patients and those with ≥70% occlusion.
  - A >175% increase in the flow velocity after CEA is suggestive of cerebral hyperperfusion syndrome.
  - However, TCD monitoring is not always possible due to the absence of a suitable window, which is generally limited to the MCA territory.

- *Near-infrared spectroscopy (NIRS):* NIRS compares cerebral tissue oxygen saturation ($rSaO_2$) on the ipsilateral and contralateral cerebral hemispheres. However, NIRS provides a relative change from baseline values; it has a high negative but a low positive predictive value. A 20% reduction in $rSaO_2$ indicates cerebral ischemia, and a 17% reduction indicates a need for shunt placement.

- *EEG, processed EEG, and evoked responses:* Bi-hemispheric two-channel EEG monitoring montage provides a good assessment of cortical perfusion. However, EEG monitoring, even with an eight-channel montage, can easily miss focal neurological injury. EEG monitoring could be challenging when there is baseline asymmetry between the two hemispheres. Processed EEG parameters, such as total power, power spectrum analysis, and spectral edge frequency, can result in the loss of information during signal processing and are best interpreted alongside the raw EEG data. Bispectral index devices only monitor the activity of the frontal cortex and thus have limited value during CEA. Unlike somatosensory evoked responses, the motor-evoked potential seems to be a better predictor in detecting ischemia and the need for shunt placement.

Hemodynamic Management

- *Preoperative plan:* Before the induction of anesthesia based on baseline resting blood pressure and heart rate, the severity of the carotid arterial disease, the extent of collateral circulation, and the cardiovascular reserve of the patient, a clear plan for hemodynamic management has to be planned in consultation with the surgical team. Hypotension is avoided at induction, and hypertension at about 20% above baseline is usually needed during carotid occlusion. At the same time, blood pressure has to be kept below normal after the carotid has been unclamped.
- *Routine hemodynamic monitoring* includes an awake arterial line and three-channel EKG with lead II (arrhythmia) and lead V (ischemia). Central venous pressure monitoring, cardiac output monitoring, and transthoracic echocardiography are rarely used as fluid shifts are usually minimal, and access to the patient is limited.
- *Clamping the carotid:* Close attention is paid to the blood pressure, which is increased to 20–40% above the baseline value. The increase in blood pressure should not be accompanied with tachycardia. The ST segment changes should be monitored. Once the target blood pressure is reached and at least 3 minutes have elapsed after heparin, the ICA can be clamped.
- *Detection of cerebral hypoperfusion:* Significant changes are seen within 5 minutes of ICA occlusion. The following are suggestive of cerebral hypoperfusion:
  - Any attenuation of raw EEG by 50%
  - Somatosensory evoked potentials (SSEPs), a decrease in amplitude by 50% or an increase in latency by 10%
  - Attenuation of motor-evoked response
  - A 50% decrease in amplitude in the β band
  - A decrease in the spectral edge frequency by 50%
  - A decrease in the MCA flow velocity by >50% as observed by TCD.
  - A decrease in rSO_2 of >17%
    If these changes are seen, then hypotension and hypocapnia should be corrected. If the changes persist despite induced hypertension or when induced hypertension cannot be tolerated by the patient, the ICA is unclamped, and a shunt is placed. Some centers routinely use a shunt to ensure distal brain perfusion.

- *Concerns with shunt placement:* Placement of the shunt increases the chances of embolic injury. A mal-placed shunt can fail to perfuse the distal brain. The placement of a shunt can complicate dissection.
- *Postclamping:* After removal of the atheromatous plaque and the closure of the arteriotomy, the ICA clamp is slowly released to test the integrity of surgical closure. Due to compensatory vasodilation in the distal cerebral circulation, especially with high-grade stenosis, the release of the clamp can result in cerebral hyperperfusion syndrome (CHS). Therefore, the blood pressure is lowered to slightly below the baseline values. CHS presents unilateral headaches and eye pain that, in extremis can lead to intracranial hemorrhage.

ANESTHESIA FOR CEA

The operating Room Setup is the Same for Regional and General Anesthesia

- Positioning equipment and shoulder roll for intubation.
- Arms tucked to the side, extension needed on arterial and IV lines, and neuromuscular monitoring limited to face or feet under drapes.
- *Intubating equipment:*
  - ETT: Covering the ETT tube tip and cuff with 5% lidocaine ointment can minimize postoperative coughing and bucking.
- *Drugs required:*
  - Propofol is the induction agent of choice. The hypotension with propofol requires boluses of pressors. Narcotics, benzodiazepines, and muscle relaxants are needed as for any general anesthesia. With poor cardiac functions, consider etomidate as the alternative to propofol.
  - Pressor drugs and pumps for phenylephrine and vasopressin infusions may be needed. Vasopressin may be necessary for angiotensin-converting enzyme (ACE) inhibitors treated patients.
  - Atropine and/or glycopyrrolate might be required for bradycardia during sinus manipulation.
  - Antihypertensive drugs might be necessary after clamp release.
- Access to blood gas and ACT point-of-care analyzers.

Preoperative Assessment

- Baseline neurological examination
- Cardiovascular function:
  - Baseline blood pressure and hypertension
  - The status and severity of ischemic heart disease
  - Left ventricular function: exercise tolerance and echocardiography
  - Cardiac rhythm

Table 2: Advantages and disadvantages of regional and general anesthesia for carotid disease.

	Advantages	Disadvantages
Regional	• Simplicity • Less hemodynamic stress • Functional testing possible • Avoids response to intubation and extubation • Costs of EEG/EP • Quicker • For patients with poor cardiac reserve	• Cooperative patient • Intraoperative hypertension • Limited airway access • Difficulties in managing complications: Agitation, seizures, and nerve injuries (phrenic or recurrent laryngeal nerve) • Uncomfortable
General anesthesia	• Better surgical conditions • Airway secure • Optimum hemodynamics • Optimum CO_2	• Hemodynamic changes can be significant • Greater use of vasopressors • Intubation/extubation stress • EEG or neuromonitoring needed • Cerebral perfusion monitoring • Neurological can be exam delayed

- An assessment of comorbidities: peripheral vascular disease, diabetes, end-stage renal disease, smoking, obesity, and hyperlipidemia.
- Current medical treatment
- Anticoagulation status
- Airway and vascular access

Regional versus General Anesthesia for CEA (Table 2)

Regional anesthesia provides better postoperative pain relief and transient improvement in cognition after surgery. As compared to GA, a lower incidence of strokes on MRI and lower complication rates for pneumonia and MI have also been reported.

Regional Technique

Three possible approaches: (1) Superficial cervical plexus block, (2) Deep cervical plexus block, or (3) Cervical epidural. The latter is seldom used:
- *Superficial cervical plexus block:* Local anesthetic drugs are injected at the mid-point of the posterior border of the sternocleidomastoid muscle. The technique is safe and simple in experienced hands.
- *Deep cervical plexus block:* Block of C2 to C4 nerve roots. Landmarks: Draw a line 1.5 cm behind and parallel to the line joining the mastoid and the C6 transverse process (Chassaignac's tubercle). Feel for the C2, C3, and C4 transverse processes and inject 5 mL of the local anesthetic agent at C4, C3, and C2 processes (2, 4, and 6 cm below the mastoid)

using C6 as the guide. Alternately, a single injection can also be made at the C4 transverse process.
- *Technical problems with cervical plexus block:* (1) Pain relief is inadequate and local supplementation is usually needed. (2) Pain is encountered during carotid sheath manipulation, and the topical application of local anesthetics can lead to cranial nerve palsies. (3) Pain may persist along the mid-line due to some bilateral innervation.

Complications: The Complications of the superficial and deep cervical plexus blocks are:
- Seizure from vertebral artery injection.
- Respiratory distress from phrenic nerve paralysis
- Loss of voice from recurrent nerve paralysis
- Hypotension and respiratory distress due to high spinal block.
- Conversion to GA.

Ultrasound-guided cervical plexus block: Placement of the blocks under ultrasonic guidance can enhance safety but does not affect the need for supplemental topical anesthesia for CEA.

Conduct of regional anesthesia for CEA:
- The principles of blood pressure management and anticoagulation are no different under regional or GA. Proponents of regional technique assert the superiority of clinical exams over instrumental monitoring. The regional technique requires a cooperative patient, surgeons who are comfortable with the patient being awake, and the capability to intervene rapidly if complications occur. The clamp duration under regional anesthesia is usually brief, lasting <30 minutes; therefore, careful patient selection is essential.
- Under regional anesthesia, neurological monitoring is somewhat simplified. Chances of hypotension are decreased. Cognitive tests can be undertaken by voice commands. Motor functions can be assessed by squeezing a squeaky toy attached to the contra-lateral palm. During clamping, the patient can be observed for any change in neurological function, such as level of consciousness, slurred speech, contralateral motor weakness, and seizures.
- Sedation is titrated to ensure comfort and compliance. Low-dose remifentanil/propofol infusion may be given. Steroids are administered in some centers to decrease brain edema due to an accidental cerebral injury.
- Aggressive blood pressure management is needed after the CEA.

General Anesthesia

- *Premedication:* Sedative premedication is seldom given unless the patient is highly anxious. The patient continues with antihypertensive and antiplatelet drugs. Oral hypoglycemic and ACE inhibitors are avoided on the morning of surgery. Anticoagulation, in high-risk in-hospital cases, such as recent TIA, IV heparin is substituted and stopped 6 hours before surgery.

- *Induction:* Awake A-line is placed to maintain tight hemodynamic control. Ideally, surface EEG should be in situ before induction, as changes during induction could reveal the monitor's performance. Hypotension is meticulously avoided at induction. If propofol is used as an induction agent, phenylephrine boluses (40-80 μg) is prophylactically given with the drug. Patients with poorly controlled hypertension, ACE inhibitors, and contralateral CEA could become hypotensive at induction. Patients on ACE inhibitors might become severely hypotensive at induction and require vasopressin to support their blood pressure. For rapid volume recruitment, 5-10° of Trendelenburg position can be used.
- *Narcotics and benzodiazepines are given before arterial line placement:* In patients at risk of hypotension, etomidate can be used as an alternative to propofol. Intubation is achieved with muscle relaxants. A facial neuromuscular monitor can be used as the forehead is usually accessible during the procedure. After intubation, ventilation is adjusted to ensure normocapnia or mild hypercapnia. Hypothermia is avoided. An esophageal temperature probe is placed. The procedure is usually brief, and hypothermia can delay neurological examination at emergence.
- *Additional monitors:* Immediately after induction, neurological monitors such as TCD, EEG, and evoked response monitors should be placed, and baseline data should be obtained. Care should be taken that the devices remain operational if the table needs to be turned. Ventilation is adjusted to maintain a $PaCO_2$ of 35-40 mm Hg.
- *Blood gas and ACT* values are determined after induction.
- *Maintenance:* In most instances, volatile anesthetics are used to maintain anesthesia. However, if the EEG signals are weak, TIVA (propofol/remifentanil/phenylephrine) can improve the signal. Raw and processed EEG should be carefully monitored for changes from the baseline and by comparing the two hemispheres.
- *Anticoagulation:* After the carotid artery is exposed, before carotid clamping IV, heparin, usually 5,000 units or 70-100 U/kg, is given. The generally accepted value of ACT is twice the baseline. Meanwhile, the mean blood pressure is raised to 20-40% above baseline values. EKG is monitored for any ST changes.
- *Clamping the artery:* Once the appropriate level of hypertension and anticoagulation is achieved, the carotid is clamped. Over the next minute, EEG changes are carefully observed, and any change in the ipsilateral EEG is reported to the surgeon. If changes persist, then placement of the shunt might be necessary.

- *A shunt* is a small tube that bypasses the occluded carotid artery to perfuse the distal brain. The distal end of the shunt is inserted first and allowed to bleed back, and the lower end is inserted afterward to avoid embolism by debris, clot, or air. The placement of a shunt permits the perfusion of the distal brain without increasing the blood pressure or when collateral blood flow is inadequate despite increased pressure. It also helps during complicated carotid reconstruction and repair by extending the clamp time safely. However, shunt placement carries additional risks of thromboembolism, air embolism, and vascular injury. There can be technical failures of the shunt due to kinking or occlusion.
- *Declamping the carotid artery:* In preparation for clamps release, the blood pressure is decreased to 10–20% below the baseline values to reduce the chances of hyperperfusion syndrome. Once the carotid artery has been sutured, the clamps are released. The ECA is released first, then the CCA, and finally the ICA. When released in this sequence, the chances of ICA embolization are decreased.
- *Emergence and extubation:* CEA poses the risk of postoperative bleeding because it is surgery on a major artery with anticoagulation. Hematomas are likely in patients on antiplatelet drugs and those who are hypertensive at extubation. The incidence is about 2.5%, with half the patients requiring wound exploration.
- *Smooth emergence from anesthesia without coughing and bucking is critical:* Five percent lidocaine ointment on the tube effectively attenuates the cough response. In a case of >4 hours, it is possible to supplement 2–3 mL of intratracheal lidocaine (2%). Other strategies include low-dose IV remifentanil infusion, IV lidocaine bolus, small doses of hydromorphone after respiration has been established, or a small bolus of fentanyl (25 µg increments) guided by respiratory rate.
- Postoperative neurological assessment in the operating room:
  - A severe headache is suggestive of hyperperfusion syndrome.
  - Absent superior temporal artery pulse suggests ECA embolism.
  - Potential neurological injuries:
    - *Stoke:* Hemiparesis, or facial asymmetry.
    - *Nerve injuries:* Hoarseness of voice, facial asymmetry, tongue deviation, or Horner syndrome.

Postoperative Management

- In the intensive care unit with an hourly neurological review
- Pain control with narcotics for the first 24 hours.
- IV fluids at 1 mL/kg/h.
- Blood pressure is just below/at baseline values.
- Aspirin and dipyridamole can be started 24–48 hours after surgery.

Complications of CEA

- Neck hematoma, which can lead to airway compromise. If at risk of bleeding, consider repeating ACT and partially reverse heparin (which has a half-life of about 90 minutes).
- Postoperative TIA or stroke.
- *Cerebral hyperperfusion syndrome:*
  - Unilateral headaches or eye pain
  - Seizures
  - Intracranial hemorrhage is possible.
  - It can be fatal in 50% of cases
- *Cranial nerve injuries:*
  - *Cervical sympathetic:* Horner's syndrome
  - *VII cranial nerve:* Facial asymmetry
  - *Recurrent laryngeal nerve:* Hoarseness
  - *Hypoglossal nerve:* Deviation of the tongue.

CASE REPORTS FOR FURTHER DISCUSSION

Case 1: An 81-year-old male presented with a change in dizziness, dysarthria, nausea, and mental status. He had a significant history of hypertension, hyperlipidemia, hypothyroidism, renal insufficiency, and past multiple strokes. He is being treated with aspirin and dipyridamole. On examination, the blood pressure was 162/81 mm Hg, and the heart rate was 77 bpm. A higher function exam revealed disorientation in time and place. His motor exam was non-focal. There was no sensory deficit. Laboratory findings revealed mild leukocytosis (12,600/μL) and some renal impairment (serum creatinine of 1.5 mg/dL). CT, CTA, and MRI studies revealed infarcts in the posterior cerebral circulation with a persistent trigeminal artery supplying the basilar artery. A decreased flow was observed in the left carotid artery. Two days after admission, the patient became aphasic and somnolent. Repeat MRI showed limited diffusion in the left frontoparietal region. Carotid duplex studies showed 80–99% stenosis of the left ICA. The patient was subjected to deliberate hypertension and posted for left CEA with a bovine patch graft. *What are the additional concerns during CEA in patients with recent strokes? Do you want to continue with anticoagulation? What are your options? How will you monitor and reverse anticoagulation should bleeding be encountered in such a case?*

Case 2: A 67-year-old patient with a remote history of stroke was due for right CEA under regional anesthesia. Preoperative history and exam were otherwise unremarkable. The patient was premedicated with 10 mg of diazepam PO on the day of surgery. A nerve stimulator guided a deep cervical plexus block at three levels, C2 to C4. 5 mL of 0.75% ropivacaine was injected at each level. While the superficial cervical plexus block was being done, the patient complained of feeling unwell and having difficulty breathing. There were no symptoms of local anesthetic toxicity. The patient rapidly developed left hemiparesis and left facial nerve palsy, lost consciousness, and was apneic and severely hypotensive (SBP of 60 mm Hg). *What is the differential diagnosis of sudden collapse during cervical plexus block? How will you manage such a case? How do you treat an overdose of local anesthetic drugs?*

Case 3: A 71-year-old man was due for right CEA. Past medical history included a history of hypertension, coronary artery disease, and stroke some ten months previously. His medications included aspirin, nifedipine, and bendrofluazide. His baseline blood pressure was 180/90 mm Hg. During an uneventful surgery, he was administered 3,000 u of heparin, which was reversed with 30 mg of protamine. He was extubated and sent to the recovery room. However, he continued to be hypertensive, and a peak systolic blood pressure of 260 mm Hg was recorded. He was treated with hydralazine. One hour after surgery, a neck hematoma was observed. At 5 hours, the patient's voice became hoarse, but there was no respiratory distress. An hour later, there was no change in his condition, and he was transferred from the recovery to the step-down unit. Nine hours after surgery, the patient acutely decompensated with stridor and respiratory distress. A complete respiratory arrest followed. *What are the risk factors for hematoma formation after carotid surgery? What are the warning signs of impending respiratory failure in these cases? What are the typical findings on laryngoscopy? How will you manage such a case?*

Case 4: A 60-year-old male patient underwent left CEA due to mild stenosis and ulceration of the ICA. The carotid bifurcation was at the level of C4 vertebra. During surgery, limited tissue dissection was done, and the Accessory nerve was not visualized. No shunt was needed. The patient recovered uneventfully from anesthesia. There were no neurological deficits immediately postoperatively or six weeks after surgery. Two months after surgery he developed left shoulder pain. Examination revealed the atrophy of the superior portion of the trapezius muscle. Electromyography (EMG) studies revealed complete denervation of the muscle. The nerve functions did not return even after 5-year of follow-up. *What are the cranial nerves that can be injured during carotid surgery? When do these injuries usually present? What could be the cause of such delayed nerve palsy?*

Case 5: A 57-year-old male presented with a brief bout of pectoral jerks. In the past, he had sustained a right frontal stroke with some degree of residual weakness on the contralateral side. He was found to have 70%

stenosis of the right ICA on angiography. CT revealed infarcts on the right, and a smaller left frontal infarct. He underwent right carotid endarterectomy. Seven days after surgery, he was discharged. At discharge, he was prescribed phenytoin due to suspected seizures. A day after discharge, he was readmitted with right frontal headaches, confusion, and agitation. The CT scan revealed no new infarction. The right ICA was patent on angiography; however, there was a new irregular narrowing of the branches of the anterior and middle cerebral arteries. EEG revealed periodic lateralized epileptic discharges that were localized over the right side. His clinical condition resolved over the next seven days. *What is the relationship between arterial narrowing and blood flow in vivo? What is cerebral hyperperfusion syndrome? How is it managed?*

CASE REPORT REFERENCES

Case 1: Greenway MRF et al. Carotid endarterectomy in a patient with severe internal carotid artery stenosis with persistent trigeminal artery and ischemia of the anterior and posterior circulation. Case Rep Neurol Med. 2017;2017:7193734.

Case 2: Carling A et al. Complications from regional anaesthesia for carotid endarterectomy. Br J Anaesth. 2000;84(6):797-800.

Case 3: Munro FJ et al. Airway problems after carotid endarterectomy. Br J Anaesth. 1996;76(1):156-9.

Case 4: Tucker JA et al. Accessory nerve injury during carotid endarterectomy. J Vasc Surg. 1987;5(3):440-4.

Case 5: Brick JF et al. Cerebral vasoconstriction as a complication of carotid endarterectomy. Case report. J Neurosurg. 1990;73(1):151-3.

FURTHER READING

1. Bozzani A et al. Intraoperative Cerebral Monitoring During Carotid Surgery: A Narrative Review. Ann Vasc Surg. 2022;78:36-44.
2. Bissacco D et al. Modifications in Near Infrared Spectroscopy for Cerebral Monitoring During Carotid Endarterectomy in Asymptomatic and Symptomatic Patients. Ann Vasc Surg, 2021.
3. Malcharek MJ et al. Warning criteria for MEP monitoring during carotid endarterectomy: a retrospective study of 571 patients. J Clin Monit Comput. 2020;34(3):589-95.
4. Harky A et al. General Anesthesia Versus Local Anesthesia in Carotid Endarterectomy: A Systematic Review and Meta-Analysis. J Cardiothorac Vasc Anesth. 2020;34(1):219-34.
5. Knappich C et al. Associations of Perioperative Variables With the 30-Day Risk of Stroke or Death in Carotid Endarterectomy for Symptomatic Carotid Stenosis. Stroke. 2019;50(12):3439-48.

Vignette: Did the Hominid Brain Grow Larger Due to Greater Blood Flow?

In hominids, the dominant blood flow to the brain is through the carotid arteries. The carotid arteries traverse the skull in the carotid canal. Therefore, the diameter of the canal corresponds to the blood flow. When hominid fossil skulls over the last 3 million years are investigated, measurements show that the volume of the cranial cavity increase has increased by three-fold. Still, the diameter of the carotid canal has increased by seven-fold. The disproportionate canal enlargement suggests modern human brains are more generously perfused than our ancestors.

Vignette: The Marvelous Brains—Avian Intelligence

The phrase "bird-brained" has a strong negative connotation. It implies that someone is "annoyingly stupid." Yet, some aspects of avian cognition can be compared to those of primates. Birds can find food under harsh conditions, hunt animals sometimes much larger than themselves, hide seeds for winter needs, use tools, understand cause–effect relationships, and recognize themselves in a mirror. Besides these, birds migrate across great distances, have homing capabilities, have inspiring parenting traits, live in complex colonies, and have amazing vocalization skills. The organization of the avian neocortex, the pallium, differs from that of mammals and lacks the six cortical layers. However, a recent report suggests that the pallium has similar connectivity to the mammal forebrain. The forebrains of the higher functioning birds (crows, parrots, and macaws) have more neurons than the forebrains of some nonhuman primates. Therefore, being bird-brained is not an insult after all! Has anyone ever questioned the intelligence of chimpanzees or gorillas? So why put down the birds?

Chapter 38: Carotid Artery Stenting

INTRODUCTION

Carotid arterial stenosis is the pathological narrowing of the arteries due to the deposition of atheromatous plaques. The arterial narrowing results in a decrease in blood flow which can be reversed by carotid endarterectomy (CEA) or angioplasty and stenting (CAS). Extracranial stenting the artery is a more straightforward procedure that can usually be undertaken under sedation. An intracranial stent, on the other hand, requires general anesthesia. The CAS patient is typically elderly, with significant cardiovascular disease, diabetes, smoking history, and possibly stroke. The potential complications of CAS risk surgery are severe bradycardia from carotid sinus stimulation and embolic stroke. Distal emboli entrapment devices and transcarotid artery revascularization (TICAR) procedures have decreased the embolic risk. CAS and CEA have comparable survival and stroke rates in asymptomatic patients. However, CAS may be inferior to CEA in elderly (>70 years) symptomatic patients due to increased mortality and strokes in the first 30 days but not after that.

NEUROANESTHETIC CONCERNS

- Stent indications and contraindication
- *General concerns during radiological procedures:*
  - Vascular access
  - Imaging methods
  - Radiation safety
  - Contrast types
  - Contrast allergies
  - Renal protection
- Steps in the placement of endovascular stents
- *Anesthesia for stent placement:*
  - Anesthetic objectives
  - Preoperative assessment
  - Monitored anesthesia care (MAC) versus general anesthesia (GA)
  - Setup of the interventional radiology (IR) suite
  - Neuromonitoring
  - Hemodynamic monitoring

- Postoperative management
- Postoperative complications

Carotid Artery Stenting Indications
- Symptomatic patients with any of the following factors:
    - Severe cardiopulmonary disease.
    - Recurrent stenosis
    - Contralateral carotid occlusion
    - Ipsilateral isolated anterior cerebral circulation
    - Neck surgery or radiation treatment

Carotid Artery Stenting Contraindications
- Complete occlusion
- Tortuous Internal carotid artery
- Diffuse carotid disease

Concerns with Interventional Radiology Cases

Arterial Access
- *Femoral artery:*
    - *Advantages:*
        - Most common site of vascular access
        - *Highly ergonomic:* Right side easy instrumentation and compression
        - Large vessel and easily palpable
        - No surrounding nerve plexuses
        - Relatively superficial with easy access
    - *Disadvantages:*
        - Access is limited in obese patients.
        - It can lead to concealed retroperitoneal hemorrhages.
        - Affected by proximal vascular pathologies and surgeries.
        - Requires recumbency and delays ambulation.
        - Greater risk of infection in the groin.
- *Alternative sites for vascular access* (**Table 1**): Femoral punctures require closure devices to enable early ambulation. Upper extremity access, usually through the right radial artery, has been developed to hasten ambulation. The radial approach is widely used during coronary angiography. For cerebral angiography, the approach is more demanding. The left vertebral and carotid arteries are more accessible from the left arm than from the right. The arm needs to be placed on a separate board for the procedure. The procedure is usually ultrasound-assisted. A mixture of nitroglycerin and verapamil dilates the radial artery or its branch. The vasodilators may cause systemic effects. Radial access offers greater ease of monitoring and tamponading any hemorrhage. Injuries

CHAPTER 38 Carotid Artery Stenting

Table 1: Advantages and disadvantages of arterial access for angiographic procedures.

	Axillary artery	High brachial	Brachial	Radial
Advantages	• Large • Easily palpable	• Large • Easily palpable • Easy access	• Large • Easily palpable	• Medium size • Easily palpable • Easy access
Disadvantages	• Hematoma • Surrounding nerve plexus injuries possible	• Hematoma • Surrounding nerve injury and frequent complications	• Nerve injury and hematoma possible • Distal emboli • Hand ischemia frequent complications	Access to cerebral circulation limited
Clinical use	Abandoned	Rarely used	• Used for cardiac procedures • Easy closure • Early ambulation	• Used for cardiac procedures • Easy closure • Early ambulation

to radial and median nerves can occur, causing persistent pain. Other complications include arterial occlusion (1-10%) and rarely pseudoaneurysm formation.

Imaging Technology

Radiological imaging techniques include (a) high-resolution fluoroscopy and (b) high-speed digital subtraction angiography (DSA) with road mapping functions.

- *High-resolution fluoroscopy:* The INR procedure requires real-time tracking of catheter position and/or contrast injections. The system is designed to permit X-ray interrogation with very small radiation doses to the operator and the patient. Modern fluoroscopic devices have an image resolution of 0.3 mm and acquire images at 30 frames per second. The digital feed is manipulated to give road mapping functions, enable measurement, and digitally reconstruct images in three dimensions. Standardized contrast injections can also measure contrast transit time and assess regional blood flow. Crude CT imaging is also possible with some scanners.
- DSA enables the visualization of opacified vessels by contrast injection. DSA involves the subtraction of images obtained before and after the injection of radiocontrast. Any displacement of the cerebral vessels due to the movement of the head profoundly degrades DSA images. Hence, the patient must remain immobile during imaging **(Fig. 1)**.

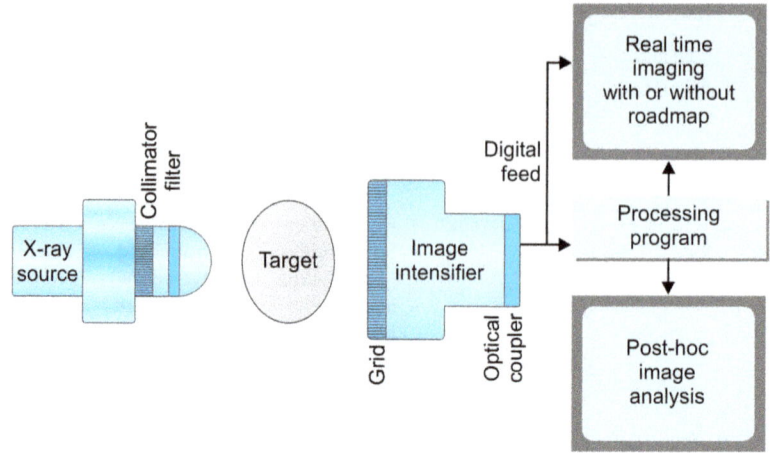

Fig. 1: Digital subtraction imaging system used for cerebral angiography.

- *The road mapping function* enables the radiologist to observe the advance of the catheter against the background map of the patient's cerebral vessels "in real-time".
- There have been many recent advances in angiography. These include the three-dimensional reconstruction of angiographic images with spin angiography. Stereoscopic examination of angiographic images that can be further manipulated on the screen in three dimensions can help to define the anatomy of the lesions precisely. Mechanized injections of radiocontrast with high-quality imaging can determine flow patterns within the vascular lesions and estimate regional blood flow.

Radiation Safety

- *Units of exposure:*
  - 1 Gray (Gy) = 100 rad
  - 1 Ray (rad) = energy of 0.01 J/kg
  - 1 Sievert (Sv) = Dose in rads absorbed × quality factor (Q)
  - Q depends on the radiation—for X-rays, Q = 1; for alpha rays, Q = 0.1
  - 1Sv: 100X Rontgen equivalent man (REM)
  - 0.01Sv: Full body CT Scan dose
  - 0.1Sv: Minimum dose associated with risk of malignancy
  - 1 Sv: Maximum safe lifetime dose. It causes radiation sickness but is not fatal. The dose has a 5% risk of malignancy during life.
- *Safe tissue exposure limits*
  - Whole body = 5 rem/year
  - Lens of the eye = 15 rem/year
  - Skin (hands and feet) = 50 rem/year
  - Thyroid or other organs = 15 rem/year

CHAPTER 38 Carotid Artery Stenting

- *Exposure mrem/min decreases with distance:* Direct beam = 4,000; at 1 feet = 40; at 2 feet = 10; at 6 feet = 0
- *Safety precautions:*
  - *Guiding principle:* As low as reasonably achievable (ALARA).
  - Imaging rooms are designed to minimize exposure to enhance safety.
  - *Minimize exposure:*
    - *Maintain distance and apply the inverse square law:* A fourth of exposure at twice the distance.
    - The desired minimum distance is 6 feet, preferably 10 feet.
    - Keep away from the IMI of the c-arm.
  - *Monitoring exposure:* Training and radiation badges
  - *Protective devices:* Lead aprons, lead gloves, lead glasses, and lead screen
    - The lead apron has a thin sheet of lead that can crack and needs periodic inspection.
    - Front only aprons do not protect the back from X-ray exposure.
  - Fluoroscopy poses a greater risk of radiation.

Radiocontrast Agents

Table 2 shows contrast agents used in neurological imaging.

Management of Allergic Reactions to Contrast Agents

- *Pretreatment is necessary with a history of contrast allergy:*
  - Change to noniodinated contrast.
  - Prednisolone 50 mg, 24-, 12-, and 2-hour pre-exposure
  - Cimetidine 300 mg PO 1-hour pre-exposure
  - Diphenhydramine 50 mg IV 5-minute pre-exposure
- *Presentation of iodinated contrast allergy:*
  - *Classic triad:* Urticaria, bronchospasm, and hypotension
  - *Other manifestations:* Facial and laryngeal edema and pulmonary edema
- *Diagnostic markers:*
  - *Serum:* Tryptase (peak 2-3 hours), histamine (peak 5-10 minutes), 11b-PGF2, and methylhistamine
  - *Urine:* 11β-PGF2, N-methylhistamine, and leukotriene E4 (LTE4)
  - Cutaneous testing
- *Differential diagnosis:* Vasovagal
- *Treatment:*
  - Epinephrine 10 µg/kg repeat as necessary 5–10 minutes
  - IV fluids
  - Diphenhydramine 50 mg IV
  - Hydrocortisone 250 IV

Table 2: Contrast agents used in neurological imaging.

	Ionic iodinated contrast agent	Nonionic iodinated contrast agents	MRI contrast agents
Contrast agent	Iodine	Iodine	Gadolinium
Examples	• Iothalamate (Conray) • Diatrizoate (Angiografin)	Iohexol (Omnipaque) is commonly used in various strengths	Magnevist, Omniscan
Main properties	• High osmolarity • High viscosity • Nonmetabolized • Renal excretion • Diffuse across capillary membranes but not BBB • Accumulate in tumors and injury sites	• Low osmolarity • Less toxic • Renal excretion • Less osmotic diuresis	• High osmolarity • Diffuse across capillary membranes but not BBB • Accumulate in tumors and injury sites
Side effects	• Pain on injection • Endothelial damage • Osmotic diuresis • Cross placenta	• High viscosity • Often diluted • Less platelet inhibition and anticoagulation • Expensive	Side effects are seen in 1% of patients
Clinical use	Limited	Usual	In MRI or with severe iodine allergy

(BBB: blood–brain barrier)

- Cimetidine/ranitidine H2 blocker 300 mg infused over 20 minutes.
- Inhaled β-adrenergic agents for bronchospasm.
- O_2/intubation as needed.
- Follow-up:
    - Recurrence may occur 8–12 hours after the initial reaction.
    - Diagnostic follow-up and immune testing.

Prevention of Iodinated Contrast Nephropathy

- Limiting the dose of contrast agents
- Hydration
- *Sodium bicarbonate:* Start infusion before surgery and continue afterwards. Dosing varies across centers; 3 mL/kg/h to a max of 9 mL/kg/h of 154 mEq/L.
- N-acetyl cysteine 600 mg (IV) before exposure to contrast agent and 600 mg PO afterward.

Surgical Approach Overview

- The right femoral artery access is usually preferred.
- A 6 French femoral sheath is first deployed.

- A coaxial guiding catheter is deployed in the CCA through the femoral sheath.
- A preliminary digital subtraction angiogram is done to verify the need for stent placement and to select the appropriate embolic prevention device (EPD) and stent.
- *Deployment of the EPD:*
  - EPD is positioned in the straight segment of the ICA.
  - The device can be a wire net, occluding balloon, or a flow diversion method.
  - EPD size is critical—a small device may lead to emboli passing by, while a larger one may injure the vessel or trigger vasospasm.
  - Care is taken to avoid plaque rupture or dissection of the vessel inadvertently.
  - Once the EPD has been deployed, balloon angioplasty is sometimes done before stent deployment.
- The stent is navigated over the EPD wire and positioned 1 cm above the stenotic region, covering the entire stenotic length.
- Usually, self-deploying stents are used.
- During stent deployment, sinus bradycardia and even cardiac arrest are possible. Atropine should be at hand to treat such a complication.
- Post-procedure, an angiogram ensures adequate dilation and rules out surgical complications such as vasospasm or dissection.
- Dilation is usually considered to be complete if, after stenting, the narrowing is 50% or less.
- Catheters and sheath are withdrawn, and the femoral arteriotomy site is closed.

Anesthetic Management

Objectives

- Provide a level of sedation that permits prompt neurological assessment.
- Ensure immobility.
- Optimally manipulate systemic blood pressure and prevent bradyarrhythmia.
- Provide emergency care for catastrophic complications.

Preoperative Assessment

Most carotid artery stenting (CAS) is done under light MAC. Complex lesions and those with intracranial stenosis might require GA.

Preoperative requirements for any MAC case include the following:
- The ability of the patient to cooperate:
  - Adequate cognition

- Pain tolerance
- Manageable anxiety
- Good communication
- Medically stable and able to remain supine during surgery:
  - No shortness of breath
  - Fluid overload
  - Chest pain
- No significant drug allergies, including contrast agents
- Surgery of limited duration
- *Assess comorbidities:*
  - *Significant cardiac disease:* CHF, unstable angina, ejection fraction (EF) <30%, and recent myocardial infarction (MI)
  - *Significant carotid disease:* Recurrent stenosis and contralateral carotid stenosis
  - Significant pulmonary disease
  - Radiation, surgery, or infection in the neck
  - Contralateral laryngeal nerve palsy
  - History of snoring and obstructive sleep apnea (OSA).

MAC versus GA for carotid stenting: The potential bias in patient selection due to sicker patients being assigned to the general anesthesia group confounds the interpretation of outcome studies comparing MAC and general anesthesia. Studies show a better outcome, fewer complications, and shorter in-hospital stays with MAC than general anesthesia. The choice of the anesthetic technique has to be individually assessed, **Table 3**.

Premedication

The critical concern during a stenting procedure is that antiplatelet treatment is continued five days before surgery. However, if this is not possible, then a loading dose of Plavix and aspirin can be given on the day of stent placement **(Table 4)**.

Setup of the INR Suite

- INR suite is often in a peripheral location.
- Rapid assistance is difficult due to the risk of radiation exposure and sterile barrier.
- Setup for any other case requiring general anesthesia.
- IV atropine at hand for possible bradycardia
- Regular EKG and noninvasive blood pressure (NIBP) monitoring
- Consider A-line under local anesthesia because:
  - Close monitoring of BP is needed.
  - Bradycardia during sinus manipulation
  - Conversion to GA is possible in an emergency.

CHAPTER 38 Carotid Artery Stenting

Table 3: Comparison of sedation versus general anesthesia for carotid stenting.

	MAC	General anesthesia
Anesthetic management	Simple but may require active intervention	Can be demanding due to comorbidities
Patient cooperation	Essential	Not needed
Hemodynamic changes	Minimal	Significant
Clinical neurological examination	Possible	Not necessary
Neuromonitoring	Not essential	Necessary
High-risk cases	• Uncooperative • Language barriers • Pain sensitive • Anxious • Aphasic • Unable to lie flat	• Cardiovascular morbidity • Significant respiratory disease • Unable to cooperate

Intraoperative anesthetic concerns	• Disinhibition
	• Seizure
	• Stroke
	• Vascular injury
		• Hemodynamic:
		  – BP management
		  – Bradycardia
		• Maintain mild hypercapnia until stenting

Table 4: Common antiplatelet drugs.

	Aspirin	Clopidogrel (Plavix TM)	Antiplatelet antibodies (Abciximab TM)
Mechanism of action	Inhibition of prostaglandin synthesis by cyclooxygenase inhibition	Prevent ADP binding to glycoprotein receptors IIb and IIIa, inhibiting platelet activation	Antibody to glycoprotein receptors IIb and IIIa
Dose	50–325 mg/day	300 mg loading dose +75 mg/day	0.15–0.25 mg/kg, followed by an infusion of 0.125 mg/kg/min
Half-life	1–2 hours	8 hours	10–30 minutes
Correction strategy	Platelet transfusion	Withheld for most neurosurgical procedures, 1 week; may be permitted for stenting. Reversed with platelet transfusions.	Platelet transfusion
Contraindication	Renal and hepatic failure; drug interactions	Allergic reactions	Allergic reactions

- Intubating equipment at hand as needed.
- A nasal trumpet is avoided due to antiplatelet therapy and the risk of bleeding.
- EEG monitoring in some centers.

Monitored Anesthesia Care

- Fentanyl/midazolam is usually sufficient to ensure cooperation.
- Propofol infusion as needed.
- Dexmedetomidine infusion if the airway is at risk.
- Low-dose remifentanil if in persistent pain.
- Infiltration of groin site with local anesthetic drugs.
- Glycopyrrolate treatment at the time of sinus manipulation.

General Anesthesia

- It is rarely needed for carotid stenting.
- EEG monitoring is desirable.
- Maintain blood pressure during induction and intubation.
- Relative hypercapnia and hypertension are necessary.
- The procedure is usually brief.
- Anticipate and treat bradycardia during sinus manipulation.
- Post-stenting blood pressure at or below the baseline value
- Careful extubation

Postoperative Care

- Frequent neurological monitoring
- Blood pressure at or slightly below the baseline value
- Postoperative duplex scan
- Plavix and aspirin continued

Complications of Stent Placement

- Embolic protection device (EPD) impaction
- Embolic stroke
- Stent thromboisis or occlusion.
- Vasospasm
- Vessel dissection
- Cerebral hyperperfusion syndrome
- Intracranial hemorrhage (ICH)
- Delayed stenosis

T-CAR: Trans-carotid Revascularization Procedure

- Indicated in high-risk carotid surgery cases.
- The procedure shown in **Figure 2** is designed to reduce the risk of embolic stroke.
- Neck and groin access is required for the procedure, which limits the anesthesiologist's access to the patient.

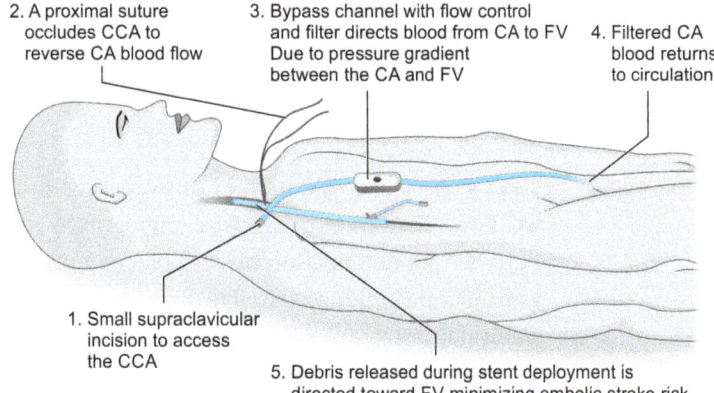

Fig. 2: The transcarotid revascularization procedure. (CCA: common carotid artery; CA: carotid artery; FV: femoral vein)

- Possible to do under sedation but given comorbidities, general anesthesia with endotracheal intubation might be preferable.
- If under GA, EEG monitoring will be necessary.

CASE REPORTS FOR FURTHER DISCUSSION

Case 1: Two days after right carotid surgery, a 67-year-old patient developed left hemiparesis and hemineglect, and CT revealed a new watershed infarct on the right side. CT angiography revealed intimal dissection and high-grade stenosis distal to the endarterectomy site. A stent placement was proposed to treat stenosis and dissection. *How does the history of recent stroke affect anesthesia technique selection? If general anesthesia is used, how can you monitor cerebral perfusion? What precautions can you take to decrease the risk of embolic stroke during the procedure?*

Case 2: A 69-year-old obese male presents with vertebral-basilar ischemia. He is due for right vertebral stenting. Access to the groin is limited, and the patient requires a head-up tilt for comfort. Surgeons want to proceed through the radial artery. *What are the problems in accessing cerebral arteries via the radial route? What are the additional concerns in a morbidly obese patient for angiography? If the patient could not lie flat, would you consider general anesthesia? How will you position the patient for radial cannulation? What is the Allen's test?*

Case 3: A 57-year-old patient with Moyamoya disease had a previous left encephalo-duro-arterio- synangiosis (EDAS) procedure about 10 years ago. The patient developed new-onset tingling and numbness on the right side. CT angiography revealed severe stenosis of the ipsilateral external carotid artery (ECA). The surgeons wanted to stent the external carotid.

What are your concerns for a patient with Moyamoya disease? What is the difference between the ECA and the ICA stenting in a normal person and one with EDAS? How will you manage blood pressure before and after stenting?

Case 4: A 74-year-old patient presented with intermittent dizziness and weakness for a month. Cerebral angiography revealed 86% stenosis of the right ICA. In anticipation of stent placement, the patient was treated with aspirin and clopidogrel for five days. The procedure was carried out under general anesthesia and systemic heparinization. The cerebral protective device was not used during balloon dilation and stent placement. The stent was successfully deployed. Protamine was not administered to reverse the effect of heparin. Low-molecular-weight heparin was administered postoperatively. Post-procedure, the patient had bouts of hypotension that resolved with fluid administration. On the first postoperative day, the patient complained of blurred vision in the right eye. Fluorescein angiograms revealed occlusion of the central artery of the retina. *What role can an anesthesiologist play in improving the outcome of embolic injury in this case? How are ischemic events managed during INR procedures? Does retrobulbar block improve retinal perfusion? What is the role of hyperbaric oxygenation?*

Case 5: A 79-year-old man was admitted with episodes of transient ischemic attack. There was a history of right hemiparesis, for which he was treated with aspirin and atorvastatin. MRI revealed a left hemispheric infarct with severe stenosis of the left carotid artery. He was pretreated for five days with aspirin and clopidogrel and was due for stenting under sedation. Immediately after the femoral puncture, heparin 5,000 u was injected, and 1,000 u/h was infused. A cerebral protective filter was placed, and the ICA was dilated with balloon angioplasty. Stent deployment followed but was not satisfactory, and an in-stent thrombus was evident. Additional heparin (2,000 u) was given intravenously, and tPA was injected into the thrombus with a microcatheter. Once recanalization was achieved, a larger balloon at a higher pressure was used to dilate the stent. Carotid revascularization was achieved without any neurological side effects. The patient was investigated, and he was found to have cyp2C19 gene that enhances the metabolism of clopidogrel. *What are the pros and cons of stent placement under regional anesthesia in symptomatic patients at risk of stroke? If this patient had a difficult airway, how would you proceed? How will you assess the suitability of using clopidogrel in a patient with enhanced drug metabolism?*

CASE REPORT REFERENCES

Case 1: Doss VT, Arthur AS, Watridge C, Elijovich L. Acute carotid stenting for treatment of stuttering transient ischemic attacks after recent carotid endarterectomy. J Neurointerv Surg. 2014;6(6):e35.

Case 2: Layton KF, Kallmes DF, Cloft HJ. The radial artery access site for interventional neuroradiology procedures. Am J Neuroradiol. 2006; 27(5):1151-4.

Case 3: Schmidt E et al. External carotid stenting for symptomatic stenosis in a patient with patent EDAS for Moyamoya disease. BMJ Case Rep. 2014; 2014:bcr-2014-011328.

Case 4: Shang F et al. Retinal artery embolization after carotid artery stenting: report of a case and review of literature. Int J Clin Exp Med. 2016;9(6):12294-300.

Case 5: Hu W et al. Acute in-stent thrombosis after carotid angioplasty and stenting: a case report and literature review. Interv Neurol. 2018;7(5):265-70.

FURTHER READING

1. Burton BN et al. Association of primary anesthesia type with postoperative adverse events after transcarotid artery revascularization. J Cardiothorac Vasc Anesth. 2020;34(1):136-42.
2. Gekka M et al. Efficacy of carotid artery stenting performed under general anesthesia with somatosensory evoked potential monitoring. J Stroke Cerebrovasc Dis. 2021;30(10):106007.
3. Hasan B et al. A systematic review supporting the society for vascular surgery guidelines on the management of carotid artery disease. J Vasc Surg. 2022;75(1S):99S-108S e42.
4. Marmor RA et al. Anesthetic choice during transcarotid artery revascularization and carotid endarterectomy affects the risk of myocardial infarction. J Vasc Surg. 2021;74(4):1281-9.
5. Teter K et al. Risk factors for and intraoperative management of intolerance to flow reversal in TCAR. Ann Vasc Surg. 2022;79:41-5.

Vignette: The History of Stroke and its Treatment

Around the 4th century BCE, Hippocrates used the term "apoplexy" to describe what is now referred to as a stroke. Apoplexy means to "strike down". Galen refined the concept and elaborated on the clinical description of stroke. Johann Jakob Wepfer used the term "stroke" in 1658 and attributed the clinical syndrome to hemorrhage or occlusion of the cerebral arteries. In 1928, Moniz performed the first cerebral angiogram. Michael E DeBakey did the first carotid endarterectomy in 1953. The first percutaneous balloon angioplasty was done in 1979 by Klaus Mathias. Mathias also did the first stenting of the carotid artery to treat an intimal flap in 1989.

Vignette: Winston Churchill's Strokes

Few other characters rise from the ashes of the Second World War, as does the British Prime Minister, Sir Winston Churchill. It was foreseeable that his high-stress lifestyle with age, alcohol, and smoking was likely to cause a stroke. In August 1949, unknown to the public, Churchill suffered his first stroke. He was rendered hemiparetic on the left side, and his speech became dysarthric. He was diagnosed with a thrombotic stroke or a small lacunar hemorrhage of the lenticulostriate branches of the right middle cerebral artery. He was incapacitated for three days but recovered within two weeks. Despite this warning, Churchill did not change his ways.

In June 1953, he was 79 years old. The post World War time was hectic, and Queen Elizabeth had just been crowned, so Churchill was under considerable stress. On the afternoon of June 23, his physician noted that his speech was slurred and advised rest. But Churchill went on to deliver a speech that evening. Immediately afterward, he sat down and had to be assisted to his bedroom. By the following day, his speech and hemiparesis had worsened, but Churchill refused to take rest. Unassisted, he walked into and chaired a two-hour cabinet meeting the next day, yet no one noticed any difference. However, his condition deteriorated over the following days. He was hemiparetic, with impaired speech and difficulty in swallowing. He had sustained a stroke in the same arterial distribution four years earlier. Shielded from the public view, he was sent to his country state to recover. By November, he had recovered and returned to public duties, but subtle neurological deficits remained. Churchill retired as Prime Minister in April 1955. In 1963 he fractured his hip and passed away two years later. Churchill's strokes reveal the state-of-the-art management of the disease in the 1950s and the tenacity of the man who never gave up.

Chapter 39: Cerebral Arteriovenous Malformation Resection

INTRODUCTION

Cerebral arteriovenous malformation (AVM) is a rare vascular abnormality of the brain occurring in 1.5% of the population. It has a peak incidence in the third decade and has no gender bias. Multiple AVMs with an autosomal dominant inheritance are found in Osler Rendu Weber disease or hereditary hemorrhagic telangiectasia. Histologically, AVMs are characterized by a tangle of vessels in which the arteries and veins communicate without the intervening capillaries. The symptoms arise due to bleeding, compression of the brain structures, and changes in regional blood flow. The most frequent presentations are hemorrhage (50%), seizures (25%), and headaches (15%). AVM hemorrhage carries an annual risk rate of 2-4% bleeds/year. AVMs can be treated by endovascular embolization or by surgical excision. This chapter discusses the clinical presentation and the treatment of these lesions.

NEUROANESTHETIC CONCERNS

- *Preoperative assessment:*
  - Incidence of cerebral AVMs
  - Cerebrovascular effects of AVMs
  - Clinical syndromes
- Endovascular versus surgical resection
- *Operative care:*
  - The hemodynamic goal during AVM resection
  - Induction
  - Maintenance
  - Postresection management
  - Emergence
- *Surgical complications:*
  - Hemorrhage
  - Normal perfusion pressure breakthrough (NPPBT)
  - Incomplete resection

PREOPERATIVE ASSESSMENT

- *Incidence of AVMs:*
  - *Incidence:* 1/100,000 per year
  - *Prevalence:* 10/100,000 population
  - *Peak incidence:* 20–29 years
  - *Mean age:* 31 years.
  - 10% under 10 years
- *Presentation in adults:*
  - As an incidental finding in 15%
  - *Hemorrhage* is the most frequent presentation, seen in 50% of the patients..
    - Generally, intraparenchymal, but it can be subarachnoid or intraventricular.
    - Unlike significant subarachnoid hemorrhages with aneurysms, minor bleeds from AVMs do not usually cause vasospasm.
    - Overall, all risk of rebleed ≈ 2–4%/year.
    - Lifetime risk % = 105 – age.
    - *Clinical risk factors:*
      - The incidence of rebleeding is ≈6% in the first year.
      - The Rebleed rate is higher in men than in women.
      - Rebleed likely with hemorrhage as the presentation
    - *Radiological risk factors for bleeding:*
      - Size <3 cm
      - Single feeding artery
      - Aneurysms within AVM
      - Deep venous drainage
      - Venous thrombosis
      - Venous varix
  - *Seizure:* 25%
  - *Headaches:* 15%
  - *Focal neurological deficits:* 5%
  - *Tinnitus:* 2%
- *Presentation in children:*
  - Congestive heart failure
  - Hydrocephalus
  - Seizures

Investigations

- *Digital subtraction angiography (DSA):* As the gold standard, DSA helps define the size and nature of the lesion, the feeding arteries, and the draining veins.
- *Computed tomographic (CT) imaging:*
  - *Non-contrast CT:* Due to the hyper-density of blood, non-contrast CT scans do not have the sensitivity to detect the source of bleeding.

- In the absence of bleeding, AVMs do not cause midline shifts, limiting the diagnostic value of non-contrast images.
  - In contrast-CT, the AVMs appear as "a bag of worms".
  - CT angiography (CTA) permits visualization of the vessel components in the malformation and enables endovascular treatment.
- *Magnetic resonance imaging (MRI):*
  - *MRI:* T2 images can define the extent of the lesion.
  - *MRA:* Dynamic MRI images enable differentiation between hemorrhage and the pathological lesion.
- *Wada testing:*
  Wada test is needed to guide operative and endovascular interventions. The test involves the intra-arterial injection of anesthetic drugs for the localization of brain functions. Amytal is the agent of choice. The arterial injections can be given into the internal carotid artery for locating the speech center in a given hemisphere. Super-selective Wada testing is done using microcatheters that can determine if the sacrifice of a particular arterial feeder will affect language or other cortical functions.

Surgical Management

- *Surgical resection:* Surgical resection is effective but carries the risk of intra-operative hemorrhage, NPPBT and neurological injury. These complications can be decreased with staged embolization.
- *Endovascular embolization:* Staged endovascular embolization decreases the severity of hemodynamic changes due to the closure of the arteriovenous (AV) fistula in preparation for surgery to reduce blood loss, or it could be the definitive treatment. Graded ablation is possible. However, partial obliteration can predispose to bleeding.
- *Radiosurgery:* Small AVMs can be treated by stereotactic radiosurgery. Radiosurgery needs multiple procedures over months and can cause edema, cyst formation, hemorrhage, and necrosis.
- *Choice of treatment:* Spetzler–Martin AVM grading scale and suggested treatments are given in **Table 1**. Scores of 1–2 require microsurgery. A score of 3 requires embolism and microsurgery. The higher scores require careful individual assessment and multi-modality treatment.

Table 1: Spetzler–Martin arteriovenous malformation grading scale and suggested treatments.

Diameter	Location	Venous drainage
<3 cm = 1	Noneloquent = 0	Superficial only = 0
3–6 cm = 2	Eloquent = 1	Deep = 1
>6 cm = 3		

(Total score: 1–2: microsurgery; 3 = multimodality, e.g., embolization and surgery; 4–5: observe, critical assessment, and multimodality review)

ANESTHESIA FOR ENDOVASCULAR EMBOLIZATION

- The primary goals for MAC are to alleviate pain and discomfort, allay anxiety, and ensure patient immobility during surgery. Patient immobility is essential, whether conscious or deep sedation is used. Movement cannot only degrade the image quality but can also result in vascular injury.
- Sedation should permit rapid arousal for neurological testing.
- The procedures are not generally painful. There is an element of pain associated with distention or traction on the vessels; contrast injection into the carotid artery is frequently described as "burning".
- Discomfort might be due to prolonged periods of lying still, bladder catheterization, and, to a lesser extent, the femoral puncture site.
- *Sedation scores:* Most sedation scores require responding to verbal commands or noxious stimuli. Due to the remote location of the head, communication with the patient may be limited, and it might be difficult to elicit the glabellar tap, **Table 2**. Thus, close monitoring of the patient for movements and respiratory function is critical.
- Anesthetic drugs are selected to meet the above goals of sedation, analgesia, and anxiolysis and to ensure comfort and relative immobility. The strategy for conscious sedation is establishing a neurolept anesthesia base by titration of 1-2 µg/kg of fentanyl and 1-2 mg of midazolam after obtaining intravenous access and establishing and providing supplemental oxygen.
- A small bolus of propofol is required for bladder catheterization in males. The propofol bolus also helps to assess the airway under deep sedation and determine if a nasopharyngeal airway will be needed. The placement of the urinary catheter can cause significant discomfort in some men that can be minimized by 2% lidocaine jelly. The placement of the nasopharyngeal airway after anticoagulation can result in bleeding. It is better to insert the airway at the start of the procedure using a topical local anesthetic. It is also to be inserted cautiously in patients on antiplatelet drugs.

Table 2: Ramsay sedation score.

Sedation score	Awake or asleep	State/response
1	Awake	Restless
2	Awake	Cooperative
3	Awake	Responds to verbal commands
4	Asleep	Brisk response to light glabellar tap or loud sound
5	Asleep	Sluggish response to glabellar tap or loud sound
6	Asleep	No response to glabellar sound or loud sound

Table 3: Pharmacokinetics of sedative hypnotics.

	Dexmedetomidine	Propofol	Midazolam
Commercial name	Precedex	Diprivan	Versed
VDss (L)	120	250–300	80–120
T1/2α (min)	6	2–4	6–15
T1/2β (min)	2 hours	30–60 minutes	100–150 minutes
Protein binding	94%	97–99%	95%
Metabolism	Liver	Liver	Liver
Cl (L/min)	0.7	1.5–2	0.5–0.8
Loading dose	0.5–1 µg/kg in 10–20 minutes	Optional for sedation	10–50 µg/kg
Maintenance dose	0.2–0.7 µg/kg/hr	25–200 µg/kg/min	N/A

(Cl: Clearance; VDss: steady-state distribution volume)

- When the patient is in the final position, a propofol infusion is started at low doses (20–40 µg/kg/min) and then increased slowly to render the patient immobile yet breathing spontaneously.
- Alpha-2 agonist, dexmedetomidine, offers an alternative to propofol. The airway is better maintained during sedation with dexmedetomidine. Dexmedetomidine (1 µg/kg over 10–20 minutes; loading dose with an infusion of 0.2–0.7 µg/kg/h) permits neurological examination. Further, patients sedated with dexmedetomidine may have lower blood pressure during recovery requiring inotropic support.
- Typically, the choice of sedative infusion is between propofol and dexmedetomidine **(Table 3)**. The latter is preferable if there is a history of snoring or obstructive sleep apnea. The choice is based on the practitioner's experience, the patient's need, and the procedure requirements.
- Narcotics **(Table 4)**, such as fentanyl or remifentanil, can be used for analgesia if the respiratory rate is >10–12 breaths/min.

Microsurgical Resection

Unlike aneurysms, surgical resection of an AVM is usually an elective procedure. Emergency surgery is usually due to large intracranial bleeds that require urgent treatment. AVM surgery is typically more prolonged than aneurysm clipping as it often requires extensive tissue dissection, **Table 5**.

Table 4: Pharmacokinetics of narcotics.

	Sufentanil	Fentanyl	Alfentanil	Remifentanil
Potency versus fentanyl	7–10×	1×	0.1–0.2×	0.8×
VDss (L)	98	375	36	35
T1/2α (min)	1	3	2	1
T1/2β (min)	2.5 hours	4 hours	1.5 hours	5–8 minutes
Cl (L/min)	0.75	1	0.3	0.3
Octanol: water partition coefficient	1,800	810	130	18
Sedation doses	5–10 µg bolus	50–100 µg bolus	250–500 µg bolus	0.25–1.25 µg/kg/30 s

(Cl: Clearance; VDss: steady-state distribution volume)

Table 5: Comparison of the salient feature of anesthesia for cerebral arteriovenous malformations (AVM) and aneurysms.

	AVM	Aneurysm
Patient age	<40 years	Bimodal young or >50 years
Patient profile	Usually healthy	If old comorbidities are common
Surgery	Elective	Usually emergency
Acute rebleed	<6%/year	1–2%/day for 0–2 weeks
Bleeding risk	Modulated by several factors	Directly related to transmural pressure
Pre induction A-line	Desired	Required
Temperature control	Normothermic	Mild hypothermia
Ventilation	Mild hyperventilation	Normocapnic ventilation or mild hypercapnia to increase collateral blood flow
Induced hypertension	To test vascular bed after resection	Transiently during temporary clipping
Postoperative angiogram	High-resolution imaging in INR suite	In the OR with C-arm
Major postoperative concern	Hemorrhagic stroke	Ischemic stroke

(INR: interventional neuroradiology)

Anesthetic Goals

- Given the fragility of the dysmorphic vessels constituting the AVM and the possibility of concurrent aneurysms in as many as 10% of these lesions, it is desirable to ensure hemodynamic stability at induction.
- Maintain normocapnia to mild hypocapnia to improve the perfusion of the potentially ischemic zone around the AVM nidus.
- Maintain normothermia to facilitate coagulation.
- Maintain mild arterial hypotension to decrease bleeding during resection.
- Maintain low airway pressure and gently elevate the head ≈5° to facilitate the venous return and decrease venous bleeding.

CHAPTER 39 Cerebral Arteriovenous Malformation Resection

- Use mannitol to decrease the pressure under the retractors that could impede venous return.
- At the end of the resection, test the vascular bed with IV phenylephrine by increasing the mean blood pressure transiently to 20% above the baseline value.

Preoperative Assessment

- Patients are usually young and healthy.
- They may have a history of headaches and focal neurological deficits.
- Seizures are a frequent presentation that requires anti-seizure medication.
- *Laboratory tests:* Due to potential blood loss, baseline hematocrit and coagulation profile must be assessed.
- Deliberate hypotension may be needed to decrease blood loss; hence any significant cardiac disease must be ruled out.

Intraoperative Management

- Pre-induction arterial line for monitoring blood pressure is highly desirable but not essential if precautions are taken to ensure hemodynamic stability during induction and intubation. Pre-induction arterial line might be necessary with large AVMs, significant intracranial hemorrhage, raised intracranial pressure (ICP), emergency surgery, or in patients with other medical indications.
- *Induction drugs selected to ensure hemodynamic stability:* Propofol is the agent of choice, given with the background sedation with midazolam and fentanyl. Lidocaine bolus (1-1.5 mg/kg) can blunt intubation response and mitigate pain due to propofol injection.
- Anesthesia should aim for a low normal heart rate and blood pressure for the given patient. Target systolic blood pressure during surgery is about 10% below the baseline.
- *Bleeding during AVM resection:*
  - It is likely to be venous and is therefore affected by local pressure, venous return, cardiac output, and pressure in the feeding arteries.
  - Airway pressure should be minimized, and the head mildly elevated to encourage venous return.
  - Mannitol administration relaxes the brain tissue and minimizes retractor pressure.
  - Hypothermia could impair coagulation and is therefore avoided. Furthermore, unlike aneurysm surgery, ischemic brain injury due to temporary arterial occlusion is unlikely; thus, hypothermia is generally avoided.
- Attention should be paid to the color of the blood in the draining veins. Once arterial feeders are ligated, the color of the blood in the draining veins changes from arterial to venous in a characteristic manner.

- After resection, meticulous attention is paid to the AVM vascular bed. Gelfoam, surgicel, and hemostatic matrix like Floseal (a mixture of bovine gelatin and human thrombin) are all deployed to ensure a dry bed.
- Once satisfactory hemostasis is obtained in the surgical field, mean arterial pressure is raised by 20% of the baseline value to test for hemostasis. After testing, the mean blood pressure is kept 10–20% below the baseline value during closure and extubation.
- Before extubation, high-definition images are obtained in the angiography suite to ensure complete resection of the lesion.

Postoperative Imaging

- Due to the risk of bleeding from dysplastic AVM vessels, it is essential to ensure complete resection of the lesion. Such verification requires better imaging in the angiography suite than the C-arm X-ray devices in the operating room. Post-resection imaging requires:
  - Preparation of the INR suite
  - Total intravenous anesthesia (TIVA) for transport and imaging
  - Monitoring during transport
  - Ensure the patient remains warm, as hypothermia can delay emergence and impair neurological assessment.
- *Other measures:*
  - Continue with TIVA, as the angiographic procedure is usually short.
  - Anti-emetic measures usually include ondansetron.
  - Routine oropharyngeal with endotracheal suctioning, if needed.
  - Assessment and reversal of muscle paralysis
- *Strategies to avoid coughing and bucking include:*
  - Lidocaine IV bolus or infusion
  - A fine mist of lidocaine can be delivered into the endotracheal tube with a 26-gauge needle.
  - Supplemental long-acting narcotics
  - Short-acting narcotic (remifentanil) infusion
  - Dexmedetomidine infusion
  - Avoid any increase in blood pressure:
    - *Target:* At 10% below the baseline
    - *Maximum spike:* Not >20% above the baseline
  - Ensure adequate antiemesis.

Postoperative Complications

Normal Perfusion Pressure Breakthrough

- Unique post AVM resection hemorrhage complication.
- Residual dysplastic vessels cannot constrict like normal arteries.
- Vasoparalysis in the AVM bed prevents constriction.
- Increased local perfusion pressure due to the removal of the AVM.
- Bleeding can occur at normal blood pressure even with complete resection.

CHAPTER 39 Cerebral Arteriovenous Malformation Resection

- Careful blood pressure control is necessary.
- Frequent postoperative neurological monitoring
- Early CT scans when bleeding is suspected.

CASE REPORTS FOR FURTHER DISCUSSION

Case 1: A 55-year-old male presented with progressively worsening headaches and seizures for the last six years, which were poorly responsive to treatment. CT scan reveals a highly calcified paraventricular right frontal AVM. CTA reveals superficial and deep afferents with drainage into the superficial sagittal sinus. Surgical resection was planned. *Would you place an arterial line before or after induction in a patient with no history of hemorrhage or an increase in ICP? Would you hyperventilate such a patient?*

Case 2: Under general anesthesia, a 39-year-old woman underwent resection of a right arteriovenous malformation (3 × 3 × 2 cm). At the end of the surgery, the mean arterial pressure was increased to 100 mm Hg with phenylephrine to test hemostasis. The patient emerged from anesthesia without any neurologic deficits. Six hours after the surgery, the patient complained of severe headache, vomited, and became lethargic. The right pupil was dilated. An immediate CT scan revealed an extensive hemorrhage at the AVM site with a midline shift. *How are AVM vessels different from normal blood vessels? What precautions do you take during AVM surgery to decrease the chances of excessive bleeding?*

Case 3: A 2-year-old girl sustained a fall. The clinical exam revealed left upper extremity weakness. During investigations, she was found to have a large (4.5 cm) right-sided AVM with multiple feeders from internal carotid arteries and anterior, middle, and posterior cerebral arteries. The lesion had an early venous return suggesting a significant shunt drained into superficial and deep veins. The surgical treatment was deemed risky. Hence, the child was observed. At the age of 4 years, she developed dense left hemiplegia. MRI was suggestive of extensive cerebral ischemia with a minor acute infarct. Cerebral steal due to AVM was suspected, and a revascularization procedure was planned. *What is a cerebral steal? How does cerebral steal affect the surrounding brain tissue? What precautions will you take during surgery to increase blood flow in a patient with ongoing cerebral ischemia? Given that volatile anesthetics vasodilate cortical vessels, will you use them in this case?*

Case 4: A 27-year-old female patient was recovering from an intracranial bleed with gross impairment of consciousness. She was due for an elective embolization of a large left cerebellar AVM under general anesthesia.

General anesthesia was maintained with nitrous oxide and isoflurane. Heparin was administered to decrease thromboembolic complications. During embolization, her blood pressure suddenly increased from 110/70 to 150/90 mm Hg, and her heart rate decreased from 120 to 50 bpm. Extravasation of contrast was evident. Methacrylate glue was injected through the microcatheter to seal the vascular leak. However, the microcatheter had become attached to the brain tissue. The patient was due for an urgent craniotomy to remove the catheter. *Given the hemodynamic changes suggestive of the raised ICP, will you change the anesthetic drug selection? Will you reverse heparin? How would you manage this case of intracranial hemorrhage if the microcatheter impaction was not an issue? How does the management of embolic and hemorrhage complications during cerebral angiography differ?*

Case 5: A 32-year-old, 22-week pregnant, otherwise healthy patient presents with severe headache, nausea, and vomiting. A CT scan revealed an acute hematoma with an estimated volume of 22 mL. Angiography revealed a left cerebral AVM fed by the middle and posterior cerebral arteries. The patient was due for the excision of the malformation. *Would you consider pretreatment with steroids before surgery? Would you hyperventilate this case if an increase in the ICP was suspected? Would you monitor the fetus during surgery?*

CASE REPORT REFERENCES

Case 1: Florian IA et al. Intracranial gorgon: Surgical case report of a large calcified brain arteriovenous malformation. Am J Case Rep. 2020;21:e922872.

Case 2: Joshi S et al. Chapter 181: Normal Perfusion Pressure Breakthrough. In: JL Atlee (Ed). Complication in Anesthesia, Philadelphia: Elsevier Saunders; 1999.

Case 3: Ellis MJ et al. Large vascular malformation in a child presenting with vascular steal phenomenon managed with pial synangiosis. J Neurosurg Pediatr. 2011;7(1):15-21.

Case 4: Redhu S et al. Successful anesthetic management for microsurgical excision of ruptured cerebellar arterio- venous malformation with trapped endovascular microcatheter. J Anaesthesiol Clin Pharmacol. 2014;30(3):403-5.

Case 5: Guerrero-Dominguez R et al. Anaesthetic management for craniotomy in a pregnant patient with rupture of a cerebral arteriovenous malformation: case report. Revista Colombiana Anestesiología. 2015;43(S1):57-60.

CHAPTER 39 Cerebral Arteriovenous Malformation Resection

FURTHER READING

1. Chui J et al. Postoperative hemodynamic management in patients undergoing resection of cerebral arteriovenous malformations: a retrospective study. J Clin Neurosci. 2020;72:151-7.
2. Dabus G et al. Analysis of potential time-saving in brain arteriovenous malformation stereotactic radiosurgery planning using a new software platform. Med Dosim. 2022;47(1):38-42.
3. Shellikeri S et al. Association of intracranial arteriovenous malformation embolization with more rapid rate of perfusion in the perinidal region on color-coded quantitative digital subtraction angiography. J Neurointerv Surg. 2020;12(9):902-5.
4. Teig MK. Anesthetic management of patients undergoing intravascular treatment of cerebral aneurysms and arteriovenous malformations. Anesthesiol Clin. 2021;39(1):151-62.
5. Wang AT et al. Anesthetic management of awake craniotomy for resection of the language and motor cortex vascular malformations. World Neurosurg. 2020;143:e136-48.

Vignette: My Stroke of Insight

"My Stroke of Insight" is a personal account of an intracranial hemorrhage narrated by a neuroscience researcher, Jill Bolte Taylor. The researcher sustained a brain hemorrhage due to a ruptured arteriovenous malformation at the age of 37 years. In the book, she provides a graphical minute-by-minute description of her symptoms from hemorrhage to hospitalization. During these 4 hours, she alternated under the left (linear, logical information processing) and the right (image-driven abstract perception of reality) sides of her brain. Her experience is also available as an online talk. It is educational to see a disease evolve from within and how it affects cognition.

Vignette: Egas Moniz and the First Cerebral Angiography

After graduating with honors in medicine in 1899 and his training in neurology and psychiatry in 1903, Egas Moniz was more interested in Portugal's national politics than medicine. However, the rise of the Salazar dictatorship in Portugal led him to abandon politics and return to medical research in 1919. Moniz started his experiments with cerebral angiography in cadavers and dogs late in his career. Due to the radiolucency of the brain tissue, plain X-rays of the skull were of limited value in diagnosing brain pathologies. In 1916, in the US, Dandy pioneered air injection in the ventricles to delineate brain tumors. Jean Sicard, in 1921, in Paris, demonstrated the compression of the medulla by using lipiodol. However, for cerebral angiography, Moniz required the contrast compound to be radiopaque, harmless, and non-fatty to avoid embolic stroke. He experimented with lithium bromide, strontium bromide, sodium bromide, and sodium iodide. Lithium injections caused considerable pain and were abandoned. His first four angiographic attempts with percutaneous injections failed. In two patients, the injections were extravascular; one hemorrhaged the fourth had poor-quality images. In his second attempt, he used surgical exposure of the carotid artery. He initially injected strontium bromide; although the images were good, the patient died of a massive stroke eight hours later. Therefore, he recommended using 5-6 cc of 25% sodium iodide for the procedure, and to avoid any accidental injection of air or letting the blood enter the needle to prevent clot formation and embolization. Cerebral angiography opened new avenues for the diagnosis and treatment of neurological diseases. Moniz was nominated for the Noble Prize thrice and eventually won it in 1949. However, it was not for angiography that is widely used today but for prefrontal leucotomy, which has long been abandoned!

Chapter 40

Clipping of Cerebral Aneurysms

INTRODUCTION

Clipping of brain aneurysms is usually undertaken under general anesthesia as an urgent or emergent procedure. Their peak incidence is 40–60 years of age. Risk factors for developing aneurysms include an underlying connective tissue disorder, hypertension, smoking, and substance abuse. These must be assessed during the preoperative review. With the wider availability of imaging technologies, patients are often asymptomatic and present with unruptured aneurysms. However, aneurysm clipping after SAH carries a significant perioperative risk that depends on the severity of the bleeding. Compared to coiling, the benefits of aneurysm clipping are lesser rebleeding and recurrence rates and better survival. However, clipping carries greater risks of early postoperative complications. The most critical consideration of clipping aneurysms is tight perioperative control of arterial blood pressure.

NEUROANESTHETIC CONCERNS

- *Preoperative assessment:*
  - The severity of the disease
  - Comorbidities
  - Baseline neurological examination
  - Cardiovascular function
  - Medical management
- *Treatment options:* Clipping versus coiling.
- *Management of clipping:*
  - Operative approach
  - *Setup of the OR:* Hemodynamic monitoring
  - *Anesthesia:*
    - Induction
    - Blood pressure management
    - Extubation
- Postoperative complications.

PRE-ANESTHETIC CONCERNS

Cerebral aneurysms: Abnormal focal dilation of an intracranial artery.

CHAPTER 40 Clipping of Cerebral Aneurysms

- *Types: Saccular, fusiform, mycotic, and dissecting*
- *Incidence:*
  - 2% of the general population harbors brain aneurysms.
  - The incidence of subarachnoid hemorrhage (SAH) is about 10 per 100,000 of the population.
  - Aneurysmal bleeding accounts for 3-5% of all strokes.
  - 50-80% of aneurysms remain unruptured.
  - Most aneurysms are between 3 mm to 2.5 cm in size.
  - 15% of patients with aneurysm rupture die before hospitalization.
  - Rupture is fatal in 50%, and 66% of those who survive have a poor outcome.
- *Patients at risk of developing brain aneurysms have a history of:*
  - Age >40 years
  - *Gender bias:* Females: males::3:2
  - Smoking
  - Hypertension
  - Alcohol and drug abuse (cocaine)
  - Familial history
  - Ruptured aneurysms are 2x more common in African American and Hispanic populations.
- *Congenital syndromes:*
  - Polycystic kidney disease
  - Marfan syndrome
  - Ehlers-Danlos syndrome
  - Fibromuscular dysplasia
- Moyamoya disease
- Infection and head trauma

CLINICAL PRESENTATION

- *Ruptured aneurysms:*
  - *Most common presentations:*
    - *Thunderclap headache:* "Thunderclap" is an acute-onset severe headache peaking within seconds or minutes.
    - *Sentinel hemorrhage:* 40% of patients have had a history of recent severe headaches during the previous month.
    - Nausea
    - Vomiting
    - Neck rigidity
    - Altered cognition.
    - Signs of increased ICP:
      - *Neurological symptoms:* Confusion, blurred vision, altered behavior, motor weakness.
      - Hypertension and bradycardia, and altered breathing.

- Less common presentations:
  - Mild headache
  - Seizures
  - Focal signs (facial droop, speech, and hemiparesis)
  - Cognitive and behavioral changes
  - Mimic myocardial infarction (MI) with EKG changes.
- Unruptured aneurysms:
  - Incidental finding
  - Headache
  - Dizziness
  - Transient ischemic attack (TIA)/ischemic stroke
  - Isolated cranial nerve palsies
  - Seizures
- Aneurysms with increased rupture risk:
  - Posterior circulation aneurysms
  - Anterior communicating artery aneurysms
  - Large aneurysms
  - History of hypertension, smoking, and cocaine abuse

RADIOLOGICAL FINDINGS

- *Unruptured aneurysm:*
  - Incidental findings during workups for other complaints
  - MRI/MRA and CT angiography useful
  - Digital subtraction angiography remains the gold standard.
- *Ruptured aneurysms:*
  - Non-contrast CT scan 90–100% sensitivity under 6 hours but decreases after that.
  - MRI T2 FLAIR (fluid-attenuated inversion recovery) is highly sensitive for blood.
  - *Lumbar puncture (LP):* High opening pressure, blood in cerebrospinal fluid (CSF) that does not clear in the 4th tube, xanthochromia (most sensitive indicator), crenated red blood cells (RBCs) in CSF seen after 6 hours of SAH
  - If CT and LP are negative, no workup is usually needed.
  - CT angiography (CTA) may be negative for aneurysms <3 mm.
  - If the digital subtraction angiography (DSA) is negative, repeat the angiogram in 10–14 days. About 20% of the patients will reveal an aneurysm with a repeat angiogram.
- *Hunt and Hess grade:*
  - *I:* Mild headache or asymptomatic
  - *II:* Moderate-to-severe headache, neck rigidity, and cranial nerve deficits only
  - *III:* Drowsiness, confusion, and mild (usually motor) deficits

- *IV:* Stupor with severe deficits
- *V:* Moribund
- *Fisher grade CT scans:*
  - *1:* No bleed evident
  - *2:* Thin layer of subarachnoid blood <1 mm
  - *3:* Thick layer of subarachnoid blood >1 mm
  - *4:* Intracerebral or intraventricular blood

PATHOPHYSIOLOGY

- *Biomechanics of aneurysm rupture:*
  - *Transmural pressure (TMP):* The pressure gradient across the wall of an aneurysm is the TMP. It is the effective pressure that leads to erosion of the aneurysmal dome.
  - The TMP is the difference between the mean arterial pressure (MAP) and the ICP. Thus, factors that increase MAP or decrease the ICP increase the TMP. A decrease in the ICP can occur during surgery with the rapid infusion of mannitol, aggressive hyperventilation, or if the ICP drain is left open at a level below the patient.
  - Thus, measures to decrease the ICP in these cases should be judiciously used and are best avoided until the bone flap has been raised.
  - Mathematical modeling shows that the relationship between the wall shear stress and the hemodynamics of the lesion is complex. The low wall shear stress increases the chance of rupture.

Treatment Options and Risks

Brain aneurysms are treated either by clipping or by coiling (**Table 1**). These treatments require general anesthesia.
- *Clipping:* Titanium clips are applied to the base of an aneurysm after craniotomy exposure.
- *Coiling:* Coiling is the technique to obliterate an aneurysm by placing coils within its lumen. Memory-conforming platinum coils deployed with electrolytic detachment are used to embolize aneurysms. Coiling is effective when the neck is narrow relative to its dome. However, if the dome-to-base ratio <2:1, a balloon or a pipeline stent-assisted deployment is needed to deposit the coils.
- *Flow-diverting stents:* Normal stents have a 10% surface area, while flow-diverting stents have a 30% surface area. When applied to the base of the aneurysm, they decrease flow into the lesion and result in thrombosis.
- *Vascular sacrifice* with aneurysm bypass is undertaken when safe coiling is not possible.
- *Trapping:* Craniotomy for trapping an aneurysm involves isolating and bypassing the vessels of a thin-walled or fusiform aneurysm that cannot

Table 1: Studies on aneurysm rupture risk treatment outcomes.

Trial name/year	Subjects enrolled	Outcome
2003: International Study of Unruptured Intracranial Aneurysms (ISUIA)	4,060 enrolled; 1,917 craniotomies, and 451 endovascular treatments.	Rupture is likely in posterior circulation; the risk increases with size: 0–7, 7–12, 12–24, and >25 mm; the risk is 0, 2.5, 15, and 40% in ACA, while it is 2.5, 15, 20, and 50%, respectively, for PCA aneurysms
2005: International Subarachnoid Aneurysm Trial (ISAT)	9,559 enrolled, but only 2,143 followed up: Selection bias possible	Coiling improves survival than clipping has fewer complications at 1 year after ruptured aneurysm. Coiling higher rebleeding but less seizures
2010: Small Unruptured Aneurysm Intracranial Verification Study (SUAVe)	446 Japanese adults with 540 aneurysms <5 mm; 1,307 aneurysm year follow-up	Annual rupture risk was 0.5% for a <5 mm aneurysm. Multiple aneurysms <5 mm, those >4 mm, age >50 years, or history of hypertension needed treatment
2011: Pipeline Embolization Device for Intracranial Treatment of Aneurysms (PITA)	28 of 31 patients with ICA aneurysms with wide neck >4 mm, dome-to-neck ratio <1.5 or failed Rx	28/30 patients were successfully treated with a pipeline device, while 2 serious strokes. Pipeline flow diversion provides effective aneurysm Rx
2012: Unruptured Cerebral Aneurysm Study (UCAS)	5,720 unruptured saccular aneurysms >3 mm followed up for 11,660 aneurysm years in Japanese adults	The rupture rate is 0.95%/year, which increases exponentially with size, with PCA vs. ACA or MCA location, and with daughter sac.
2017: Pipeline for Uncoilable or Failed Aneurysms (PUFAs)	107 treated with pipeline embolization device (PED) 109 enrolled	PED leads to progressive vascular remodeling over time. When followed over 0.5, 1, 3, and 5 years, a 95% obliteration rate can be achieved. 6% complications and no deaths.
2018: Nationwide study (Korea)	Retrospective data review with data imputations, 26,411 patients, 11,777 clippings and 14,634 endovascular Rx	No significant impact on mortality by the two RX after 7 years

(ICA: Internal carotid artery; MCA: Middle cerebral artery, ACA: anterior cerebral artery; PCA: posterior cerebral artery)

be clipped. Endovascular trapping is possible with or without a surgical bypass.
- *Clipping versus coiling of aneurysms:* Clipping carries higher earlier morbidity and mortality, but coiling has greater rates of recanalization, delayed rupture, and higher retreatment rates. Clipping might be associated with greater cognitive dysfunction in patients >50 years of age.
  - *Clipping is preferred* in younger patients, very small or very large aneurysms (<2 mm or >20 mm), those with mass effects (such as III

CHAPTER 40 Clipping of Cerebral Aneurysms

cranial nerve palsy), and failure to coil or with a residual flow in the lesion despite coiling.
- *Coiling preferred:* Age >75 years, significant comorbidities, narrow neck of the lesion, posterior circulation, surgically inaccessible lesion, patients on Plavix, and failed clipping.

- *The decision to treat an aneurysm:*
  - Ruptured aneurysms, irrespective of size
  - Unruptured aneurysm >7 mm
  - Aneurysms in the posterior circulation
  - Aneurysm with a secondary lobe
  - Increasing size over time
  - Life expectancy >5 years
- *Potential complications of coiling:*
  - Thromboembolism perforation
  - Coil migration
  - Vascular injury
  - Retroperitoneal bleed
  - Limb ischemia
- *Potential complications of clipping:*
  - Vasospasm
  - Ischemic stroke
  - Seizures
  - Hemorrhage
  - Imperfect clip placement
  - Cognitive dysfunction in elderly

Preoperative Assessments

- *Key issues:* Presentation: Ruptured/unruptured? If ruptured, assess for vasospasm, raised ICP, and myocardial dysfunction.
- *The medical review includes aneurysm risk factors such as* hypertension, cardiovascular disease, smoking, substance abuse, and comorbidities with specific syndromes.
- *Exam:* Careful airway assessment is necessary. Impaired cognition and neck rigidity could affect airway assessment. Photophobia and blurred vision may lead to the patient covering his eyes or face.
- Neurological assessment to document deficits that could worsen after surgery and any evidence of raised ICP.
- Assessment of vascular access.
- *Cardiovascular status:* Pre-existing cardiovascular disease, cardiac rhythm, pump failure, pulmonary congestion, and edema.
- Electrolyte imbalances and renal failure in high-grade hemorrhages
- *Complete blood count (CBC):* Anemia, infection, and platelets; coagulation and biochemical profile; EKG, echocardiogram, and

chest X-ray (CXR, particularly in SAH cases for infection, congestion, pneumothorax, and central lines).

Neurogenic Stunned Myocardium

- High Hunt and Hess grades associated with neurogenic stunning of the myocardium (NSM).
- NSM manifests as a global myocardial dysfunction, while Takotsubo syndrome manifests with regional wall motion abnormality.
- Neurological injury (hypothalamic ischemia) leads to a massive surge of catecholamines with consequent myocardial injury.
- Peak incidence 2–14 days after SAH.
- Clinical congestive heart failure (CHF), EKG abnormalities, and ECHO reveals decreased myocardial functions.
- The increase in troponins is disproportionately less than ECHO findings.
- Treatment is supportive for CHF.
- Cardiac functions usually recover.
- 10% lead to MI.

Hemodynamic Management

- In patients with unprotected aneurysms the systolic blood pressure should not exceed 150 mm Hg. Therefore, it is necessary to prevent any spike in systolic blood pressure in response to noxious stimuli such as *intubation, lumbar CSF drain placement, pinning, skin incision, and extubation.*
- Deliberate hypotension is seldom used routinely during aneurysm clipping due to alteration in aneurysm geometry.
- If a blood pressure decrease is needed to decompress the aneurysm, temporary clipping can decrease the regional arterial pressure. In high-risk cases, the carotid artery is dissected and can be occluded to enable proximal control of the blood flow.
- In the case of intraoperative aneurysm rupture, a rapid decrease in blood pressure may be precipitously needed. A bolus of propofol or adenosine can achieve the reduction.
- A patient with high Hunt and Hess grades is not extubated. Care is needed for patients who have not woken up when transported to and from the CT scanner.

Hemodynamic Monitoring

- Aneurysm clipping requires aggressive control of blood pressure throughout the perioperative period. Furthermore, cardiac functions often decline after significant SAH, probably due to massive catecholamine surge. There can be a substantial increase in serum troponins and a decline in ejection fraction, resulting in frank CHF.

- *EKG:* At least two-channel EKG monitoring lead II for arrhythmia and lead V for any ischemia should be undertaken.
- *Arterial cannulation:* Patients with SAH should ideally have an optimally functioning radial artery catheter for pressure monitoring and blood sampling. The lines should be optimally damped so as not to underestimate or overestimate the blood pressure. The dorsalis pedis artery can yield higher systolic pressures. Arterial pressures should be compared with noninvasive blood pressure, and appropriate correction should be applied when necessary.
  - *Accessory monitors:*
    - *Pulse contour analysis for cardiac output:* The area under the arterial pulse is related to cardiac output. It is possible to derive reasonable cardiac output assessment from arterial pulse contour analysis. This method could underestimate the cardiac output compared to the classical thermal diffusion method. However, it could help monitor the relative changes in output over time.
    - *Pulse pressure analysis for preload:* A method for determining volume preload by pulse pressure analysis is shown in **Figures 1A and B**. A delta down pressure of 5 mm Hg or a 13% decrease in delta pulse pressure suggests the need for fluid therapy.
    - *Central venous pressure (CVP):* Monitoring CVP, or less frequently the pulmonary artery (PA) pressure, is important to manage the fluid input-output balance in the settings of neurogenic pulmonary edema. The PA catheter is usually reserved for a patient with evidence of impaired myocardial functions.
    - *Role of transesophageal echocardiography (TEE):* Traditionally, TEE has played only a sporadic role in neuroanesthesiology. The limited use of TEE is partly because of the restricted access to the patient's head during surgery and the reported complications with TEE probes that can cause swelling and pressure necrosis of the tongue. The smaller TEE probes can reduce the chances of injury; thus, TEE should be considered a monitoring option when myocardial contractility is significantly impaired.

Hemodynamic Response to Intubation

- Aneurysm surgery is perhaps the most frequent neurosurgical operation requiring aggressive blood pressure control during intubation.
- *Intubation response:* The sensory arm of the intubation response is the glossopharyngeal and vagus nerves. The parasympathetic and sympathetic systems mediate the efferent response to intubation. The response to intubation is essentially parasympathetic in children (bradycardia), while it is mainly sympathetic in adults (tachycardia and hypertension). It usually manifests in 5 seconds after laryngoscopy and

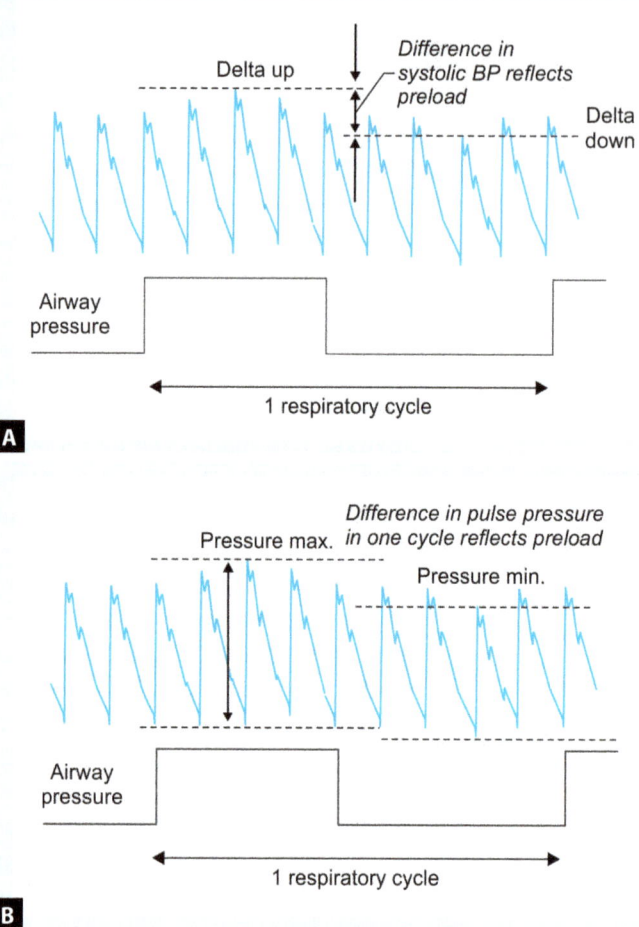

Figs. 1A and B: Two methods of determining preload from variations in arterial blood pressure during a respiratory cycle: (A) The peak difference in systolic blood pressure reflects the preload; (B) The peak difference in pulse pressure reflects the preload.

plateaus over the next 45–60 seconds. It is affected by several factors, such as the level of anesthesia, underlying cardiac status, history of hypertension, and duration of intubation.
- *Treatment strategy:*
  - Ensure depth of anesthesia. A typical combination of drugs used for induction of anesthesia in otherwise healthy aneurysm patients includes fentanyl (1–2 µg/kg), the dose of midazolam (0.03–0.05 mg/kg), lidocaine (1 mg/kg), and propofol (2–3 mg/kg). Induction of anesthesia should ensure the absence of eyelash reflex and the ability to ventilate effectively before using muscle relaxants. Volatile anesthetics may be supplemented at this stage. Once the paralysis is achieved, a test laryngoscopy can be done.

- *Test laryngoscopy* can be done during which the larynx is only visualized, but intubation is not done. The laryngoscope is withdrawn if the heart rate or blood pressure changes.
- *If a response is seen, consider the following:*
  - Supplemental propofol bolus
  - IV narcotics, fentanyl/remifentanil: fentanyl 50-100 µg bolus is used. The usual dose of remifentanil is 1 µg/kg. In patients with no concurrent narcotics, remifentanil 0.25–0.5 µg/kg is inadequate to prevent hypertensive response to laryngoscopy, while 1.25 µg/kg can cause hypotension.
  - Beta-blockers (esmolol/labetalol)
  - IV lidocaine bolus
  - Judicious use of volatile anesthetics
  - Antihypertensive drugs (labetalol, nicardipine, and hydralazine)
  - Superior laryngeal nerve block at the greater cornu of the hyoid bone is possible but rarely used.
  - The challenge in such a patient is increased in the setting of vasospasm. When one has to minimize the hypertensive response to prevent any rise in TMP yet avoid hypotension, that can decrease cerebral perfusion.

Furthermore, attention should also be paid to the ICP when monitored. In the case of ruptured aneurysms with ICP monitoring, any rise in ICP should be managed by elevating the head of the bed, correcting any hypercapnia, ensuring adequate muscle paralysis, and, if necessary, carefully draining the CSF in consultation with the neurosurgeons.

Thus, the dose of anesthetic drugs must be adjusted to the patient's condition, the response to anesthetic drugs, and the response to test laryngoscopy.

Maintenance of Anesthesia

- Immediately after intubation, the focus should shift to optimizing cerebral hemodynamics.
- The head position should be gently elevated.
- Hyperventilation should be avoided.
- Mannitol infusion should be timed to end when the bone flap is lifted.
- The ICP should be monitored in patients with external ventricular drain cases for as long as possible. A lumbar drain is placed in patients with raised ICP while removing the ventricular drain to enable surgery.
- Volatile anesthetic agents, such as sevoflurane, cause dose-dependent vasodilation. However, their effects are manageable under one-minimum alveolar concentration (MAC). At higher concentrations, the vasodilatory effects are greater and potentially increase the ICP.

Therefore, it may be helpful to restrict the use of volatile agents to <1 MAC. Volatile agents could also lead to cerebral steal in the setting of cerebral vasospasm. Thus, the safe plan would be to limit the use of volatile agents to <1 MAC and to supplement with total intravenous anesthesia (TIVA) with propofol and remifentanil as needed.
- To respond to any acute hemodynamic change, pressors and depressors are readily available with adequate flush volume. The response has to be unequivocal and quick, as the aneurysm has little protection from the surrounding parenchyma once surgically exposed. Keeping two lines, one for pressor and one for depressor drugs can help to prevent and minimize pharmacological interactions.

Transient Circulatory Arrest

Transient deliberate hypotension/circulatory arrest is sometimes needed to facilitate clipping the aneurysm. This is usually achieved by a bolus of adenosine (6–12 mg). Adenosine has a very short half-life, estimated from 1-10 seconds. It causes bradycardia by suppressing cardiac pacemaker activity. In high doses, it also causes profound systemic hypotension by peripheral vasodilation. Potential complications include bronchospasm and supraventricular arrhythmias. While it is reasonably safe to use in healthy aneurysm cases, its uses in those with impaired myocardial functions and arrhythmia must be carefully evaluated.

Intraoperative Hypothermia

- Temporary arterial occlusion is often used during aneurysm surgery. Some centers use mild hypothermia (34°C) to prevent neurological injuries during arterial occlusion. Surgeons may request EEG silence with either pentobarbital or propofol for the same reason.
- Hypothermia is often induced by a cold mattress set at 4–10°C. The water mattresses can be cooled rapidly but it takes time to rewarm them. Therefore, the temperature in the rewarming mattress has to be raised to 34°C as soon as the core temperature reaches 34.5°C. Once the aneurysm is exposed, the mattress temperature is raised to 42°C. Once it is clipped, forced air rewarming begins. Rewarming with both these devices can take time (approximately 0.1°C/10 min).

Clipping the Aneurysm

- During temporary clipping, the surgeons might request mild hypertension (at or 10-20% above baseline) to increase collateral perfusion.
- Usually, the temporary clipping lasts for under three minutes and can be repeated after a five-minute interval. These time points are recorded and reported to the surgeons.

CHAPTER 40 Clipping of Cerebral Aneurysms

- For intraoperative vasospasm after clipping, topical papaverine, hypercapnia, and judicious hypertension can be used to improve blood flow.

Extubation and Immediate Recovery Period

- Most elective aneurysm surgery patients are extubated after surgery. A plan should be in place by the time intraoperative angiography is completed. See Appendix 18.
- Rewarming is initiated once the aneurysmal dissection is completed.
- Sevoflurane can be replaced with desflurane. The latter has a much lower blood gas partition coefficient, enabling early wakeup.
- The target blood pressure depends on the presence or absence of vasospasm, other untreated aneurysms, and intraoperative angiographic findings suggestive of any arterial occlusion.
- Pressor and depressor drugs should be at hand.
- Antiemetics are administered.
- Paralysis is reversed after the head has been released from the pins.
- Smooth extubation strategies could include:
  - *Lidocaine:* IV bolus, IV infusion, and intratracheal lidocaine
  - Low-dose remifentanil infusion
  - Judicious dosing of long-acting narcotics
  - Dexmedetomidine infusion
- Response to simple verbal commands is assessed before extubation. Once extubated, a more detailed examination can be done depending on the state of cognition. A CT scan is usually undertaken if the patient is not extubated.

Postoperative Care in ICU

- Intensive care unit (ICU) admission is needed because continuous vital sign monitoring and hourly neurological examination is required.
- Head elevation at 20° and caution with lumbar drain
- Deep vein thrombosis (DVT) prophylaxis with stockings, pneumatic compression, and subcutaneous heparin can be started on day 2.
- Ranitidine or another H_2 antagonist
- Analgesics
- Antipyretics
- Pressors and depressors as needed for blood pressure control.
- Nicardipine or nimodipine is helpful in the setting of vasospasm.
- Antibiotics
- Anticonvulsants

CASE REPORTS FOR FURTHER DISCUSSION

Case 1: A 72-year-old woman with a history of multiple intracranial aneurysms and past surgical treatments developed a new-onset headache and diplopia for two days. She was scheduled for an angiogram under sedation with noninvasive monitoring. For the procedure, she was given minimal sedation and could cooperate fully. The right femoral artery was cannulated for catheter access, and the angiographic catheter was guided to the junction of the right subclavian and vertebral arteries. At that point, 12 mL of the contrast was injected approximately 37 cm proximal to the treated basilar apex aneurysm. Immediately upon injection, the contrast leak was evident from the aneurysm, and the blood (with contrast) filled the third and lateral ventricles within 2 seconds. The patient lost consciousness. An anesthesiologist was summoned. When he arrived, the patient was unresponsive, hemodynamically stable, and breathing spontaneously. *Will you intubate the patient? If so, how? After intubation, the blood pressure increases to 249/138 mm Hg. How will you manage?*

Case 2: An otherwise healthy 46-year-old man complained of a persistent headache for several years. In recent months, though, he has developed left lower limb weakness. Investigations reveal a 5 × 4 × 4 cm right middle cerebral artery (MCA) aneurysm. The patient was due for aneurysm clipping under surgery. Due to his good physical condition, it was determined that the blood pressure reduction needed for clipping was achieved by rapid ventricular pacing. *What are the methods of reducing blood pressure to facilitate the clipping of aneurysms? What are the limitations of rapid ventricular pacing? How will you set up for the procedure?*

Case 3: A 49-year-old female patient with a 30-pack-year active smoking history and heavy coffee and occasional alcohol consumption was admitted in the emergency room. The patient was poorly compliant with her blood pressure treatment. She presented with a 3-week history of severe headache, nausea, and vomiting. On examination, she was alert and oriented, with slight neck stiffness. MRI revealed a small SAH with a ruptured 6-mm aneurysm at the right M1 and M2 junction and an unruptured right M2 aneurysm. *What are the generally accepted pressure limits of treated and untreated aneurysms? What is TMP? What precautions will you take to minimize TMP across the aneurysm dome?*

Case 4: A 70-year-old woman with a history of well-controlled hypertension presented with acute headache and change in sensorium for the last several hours. CTA showed an acute SAH and a 9-mm right anterior communicating artery aneurysm. She was posted for an emergency clipping of the aneurysm. Her pre-induction blood pressure was 128/52 mm Hg with a heart rate of 52 bpm. Anesthesia was induced and maintained with propofol/remifentanil with rocuronium for intubation. EtCO$_2$ was maintained at 30–35 mm Hg. She was given mannitol at the skin incision. Blood pressure remained stable at 100–130/50–60 mm Hg with a pulse rate of 60–80 bpm. During dissection, the aneurysm ruptured, and massive bleeding resulted. At that time, the blood pressure was 110/50 mm Hg with a pulse rate of 80 bpm. The surgeons requested an immediate decrease in blood pressure with a bolus injection of adenosine. *What are the contraindications to the use of adenosine? What dose will you use? What are the possible side effects? What is the outcome of intraoperative rupture of intracranial aneurysms? What about bolus injection of propofol?*

Case 5: A 68-year-old woman, in otherwise good health, had a 10-month history of headaches and was diagnosed with a 21-mm saccular aneurysm without a discrete neck arising from a significant length of the feeding artery. Due to the complex nature of the aneurysm, clipping was to be assisted by endovascular occlusion using a balloon catheter. *What additional precautions will you take while clipping the aneurysm assisted with balloon occlusion? When would you administer heparin? Would you reverse it after the clipping was completed?*

CASE REPORT REFERENCES

Case 1: Welch TL et al. Real-time cine angiography visualization of cerebral aneurysm rupture in an awake patient: anatomic, physiological, and functional correlates. Mayo Clin Proc. 2017;92(9):1445-51.

Case 2: Ping Y et al. A case report on middle cerebral artery aneurysm treated by rapid ventricular pacing: A CARE compliant case report. Medicine (Baltimore). 2018;97(48):e13320.

Case 3: Nica DA et al. Multiple cerebral aneurysms of the middle cerebral artery. Case report. Romanian Neurosurg. 2010;17(4):449-55.

Case 4: Jang E et al. The use of adenosine for temporary cardiac arrest during intraoperative cerebral aneurysmal rebleeding: J Clin Case Rep. 2016;6(11):844.

Case 5: Fernandes ST et al. Treatment of complex intracranial aneurysm: Case report of the simultaneous use of endovascular and microsurgical techniques. Surg Neurol Int. 2016;7(Suppl 41):S1060-4.

FURTHER READING

1. Bhardwaj A et al. Com- parison of ketofol (combination of ketamine and propofol) and propofol anesthesia in aneurysmal clipping surgery: a prospective randomized control trial. Asian J Neurosurg. 2020;15(3):608-13.

2. Cebral JR et al. Understanding angiography-based aneurysm flow fields through comparison with computational fluid dynamics. AJNR Am J Neuroradiol. 2017;38(6):1180-6.
3. Kim M et al. Anaphylactic shock after indocyanine green video angiography during cerebrovascular surgery. World Neurosurg. 2020;133:74-9.
4. Thongrong C et al. Appropriate blood pressure in cerebral aneurysm clipping for prevention of delayed ischemic neurologic deficits. Anesthesiol Res Pract. 2020;2020:6539456.
5. Yoshida A et al. Prevention of trigeminocardiac reflex-induced severe bradycardia during cerebral aneurysm clipping surgery by topical anesthesia of the dura surface and atropine administration: a case report. JA Clin Rep. 2022;8(1):2.

Vignette: The First Cerebral Aneurysm Clipping

On March 23, 1937, Walter Dandy clipped the first cerebral aneurysm at Johns Hopkins. The patient was a 43-year-old man who presented with a painful right third cranial nerve palsy. What is remarkable is that Dandy diagnosed and treated the internal carotid artery aneurysm without the benefit of an angiogram.

Vignette: A Brief History of Interventional Radiology

Egas Moniz's angiography in 1923 showed the benefits of the technique. Sven Ivar Seldinger, in 1953, developed the wire-guided percutaneous catheter placement technique that opened a new era in angiography. In 1963 Charles Dotter accidentally opened a stenotic iliac artery while performing retrograde catheterization of renal arteries. In doing so, he grasped the value of using catheters to treat vascular diseases and has been called the Father of Interventional Radiology. A year later, Dotter formally demonstrated the effectiveness of balloon angioplasty. In 1965 the first embolic materials were developed for the controlled occlusion of arteries. Copper coils were first directly inserted into an aneurysm during craniotomy by Mullan in 1974. Sadek Hillal, in 1989 used short stainless steel coils to embolize cerebral aneurysms. In 1991 Guglielmi developed platinum coils that could be electrostatically detached and completely pack aneurysms. The 1990s saw the development of stents. The combination of stents to assist coil placement and the development of flow-diverting stents have greatly improved the treatment of brain aneurysms. While advances in image processing, such as 3-D reconstructions, have also helped improve clipping outcomes.

Chapter 41

Treatment of Cerebral Vasospasm

INTRODUCTION

Cerebral vasospasm is a temporary, focal, or diffuse narrowing of the intracranial arteries. The spasm is due to smooth muscle contraction triggered by exposure to subarachnoid collection of blood. Such spasms typically occur after subarachnoid bleed but can occur after trauma, surgery, infection, or inflammation. In the US, about 30,000 patients have subarachnoid hemorrhage (SAH) each year. About 20-40% patients with SAH have vasospasm. Characteristically after SAH, the spasm can present with new neurological deficits, increased doppler flow velocity, or arterial narrowing on angiography. Cerebral vasospasm can have severe cardiovascular, respiratory, and endocrine effects. A third of the patients with clinical vasospasm have a fatal outcome. These patients require careful systemic review and aggressive hemodynamic management.

NEUROANESTHETIC CONCERNS

- Preoperative assessment
- Pathology of cerebral vasospasm
- Rationale for IA vasodilator therapy
- Interventional neuroradiology (INR) setup
- Pharmacology of IA vasodilators
- Anesthetic management of the case
- Postoperative management
- Complications.

Preoperative Assessment

- *Cerebral vasospasm* is the focal or diffuse narrowing of cerebral arteries that typically occurs between 5 and 7 days after SAH but can occur from 4 to 21 days.
- Cerebral vasospasm can be *asymptomatic*. About 70% of SAH patients show angiographic narrowing between 7 to 14 days. However, vasospasm is less frequently *symptomatic*, as evidenced by delayed ischemic neurological deficits (DIND) in 20-30% of SAH cases.
- The incidence of vasospasm is proportional to the amount of blood in the subarachnoid space. See Fisher grades in **Table 1**.

Table 1: Possibility of vasospasm after SAH based on CT assessment.

Fisher Scale			Modified Fisher Scale		
Grade	SAH on CT scan	Possibility of vasospasm	Grade	SAH on CT scan	Possibility of vasospasm
N/A	N/A	N/A	0	No SAH or intra-ventricular hemorrhage	0%
1	None	21%	1	Minimum SAH only	24%
2	<1 mm	25%	2	Minimum SAH + blood in lateral ventricles	33%
3	>1 mm	37%	3	Thick SAH only	33%
4	Diffuse/None; Intraventricular or intra-parenchymal bleed	31%	4	Thick SAH + blood in lateral ventricles	40%

(CT: computed tomography; SAH: subarachnoid hemorrhage)

- Clinical vasospasm peaks 1–2 days after the peak of angiographic vasospasm on days 5–7.
- Clinical DIND is a diagnosis by exclusion of other potential causes of neurological deficits without any detectable changes on CT scans.
- These symptoms typically include:
  - Changes in cognition
  - Impaired speech
  - Pronator drift
  - Motor weakness.

Pathology of Vasospasm

Blood in the subarachnoid space triggers a perivascular inflammatory response. *Early:* Perivascular inflammation, impaired vascular reactivity, smooth muscle necrosis, and endothelial cell swelling, with the loss of tight junctions and eventual necrosis. *Late:* Proliferation of muscle cells with thickening of the arteries. Spasm is severe enough to lead to tissue infarction. Endothelin-1 plays a critical role in vasospasm evolution. The role of arterial wall thickening versus smooth muscle spasm is debated.

Differential Diagnosis of Vasospasm

Delayed ischemic neurological deficit is often a diagnosis based on exclusion. New neurological deficits after SAH can be due to:
- Rebleed
- Stroke
- Edema
- Hydrocephalus
- Seizures

- Electrolyte imbalance
- Hypoxia
- Sepsis.

Diagnosis of DIND
- Diagnosis is usually confirmed by measuring the middle cerebral artery (MCA) velocity on TCD. MCA velocity <120 cm/s is normal, 120–200 cm/s suggests mild-to-moderate vasospasm, while velocity >200 cm/s or an increase in 50 cm/s/24 hr suggests severe vasospasm.
- The extent of arterial narrowing can grade spasm as mild (<25% narrowing), moderate (25–50% narrowing), or severe (>50% narrowing) angiographically.
- CT angiography (CTA), magnetic resonance angiography (MRA), or conventional angiography further confirms the diagnosis.
- A decline of alpha waves on EEG or a decrease in the total *power of processed EEG is also seen with DIND.*

Investigations
High-risk patients: Fisher grade 3 requires daily neurological examination and alternate-day TCD for early detection. If a new neurological deficit occurs, rule out other causes.
- *Arterial blood gas (ABG):* Hypoxia, hypercapnia, hyponatremia, and anemia
- *Complete blood count (CBC):* For infection/sepsis
- *Computed tomography (CT):* For new bleed, edema, infarct, or hydrocephalus.
- *Electroencephalography (EEG):* Seizures.

Management
- *Preventive measures:* Treatment of unruptured aneurysms, early recognition and treatment after sentinel hemorrhages, clot removal or fibrinolysis, and cerebrospinal fluid (CSF) drain to mitigate the progression of the disease.
- *Routine intensive care:* Placement of A-line, central venous pressure (CVP), or pulmonary artery (PA) catheter if there are cardiac concerns, and ventricular drain to monitor and treat increased intracranial pressure (ICP). Patients are regularly treated with enteral nimodipine if there is a risk of vasospasm hypotension.

Pharmacological Interventions
- Triple-H therapy (hemodilution, hypervolemia, and hypertension) versus deliberate hypertension alone:
  - In recent years, the benefits of triple H treatment were not supported in clinical trials and deliberate hypertension alone has been used as

the alternative. If triple H therapy is used, a trial lasting for 6 hours is first undertaken:
  - *Hemodilution:* Infusion of crystalloid and albumin aimed at a target hematocrit (Hct) of 33 g/dL
  - *Hypervolemia:* Infuse crystalloid and albumin at 200–250 mL/h. Consider DDVAP if the urine output is>200 mL/h
  - *Hypertension:* Blood pressure (BP) is increased to reverse neurological deficits: If the aneurysm is unprotected, the target systolic BP (SBP) is 150 mm Hg. A protected aneurysm can withstand SBPs of 180–220 mm Hg. Phenylephrine, dopamine, levophed, and vasopressin are used alone or in combination for increasing BP.
- Intra-arterial drugs used for cerebral vasospasm treatment, including experimental treatments, are listed in **Table 2**.
- *Angioplasty:* Large proximal arteries can be dilated mechanically.
  - *Indications:*
    - Failed medical management.
    - Failed or in combination with intra-arterial verapamil treatment.
    - Recurrent vasospasm despite treatment
    - Moderate to severe vasospasm on angiography
    - Prophylactic angioplasty in high-risk patients
    - Post-clipping vasospasm
    - After treatment of a ruptured aneurysm
  - *Potential complications:*
    - Perforation
    - Dissection
    - Clip displacement
    - Arterial occlusion
- *Intra-arterial (IA) vasodilator treatment:* IA vasodilator treatment is undertaken if neurological symptoms do not resolve in 6 hours after maximum medical management. Several vasodilators, such as papaverine, verapamil, nicardipine, and nitroglycerin, have been used to treat cerebral vasospasm. Complications include hypotension, increased ICP, seizures, and focal neurological deficits, particularly with papaverine. Spastic arteries can be dilated by balloon angioplasty or with stent placement. Surgical complications of endovascular interventions also include vasospasm, dissection, and perforation.
  - *IA verapamil:* Verapamil blocks voltage-gated calcium channels. IA verapamil is widely used for the treatment of medically resistant cerebral vasospasm. IA verapamil relieves angiographic vasospasm. Small doses of up to 5 mg do not decrease the heart rate and have minimal effect on the BP. However, large doses of the drug (20–30 mg) are often used and lead to bradycardia and hypotension, sometime several hours afterward.
  - Other drugs for IA treatment are listed in **Table 2**.

Table 2: Treatment of cerebral vasospasm.

Treatment	Rationale for treatment	Advantage	Side effects/ Status
Calcium channel blockers			
Nimodipine	Vasodilator/ neuroprotectant	Oral or IV; Long half-life 9 hours	Hypotension/ in use
Nicardipine	Vasodilator/ possible neuroprotectant	Common antihypertensive	Hypotension/in use
Verapamil	Vasodilator/ neuroprotectant	Safe and effective with IA administration	High doses cause hypotension/in use
Rho kinase inhibitor			
Fasudil	IV Fasudil decreases cerebral vasospasm	It maintains BP and decreases the incidence of ischemic injury	Investigational
Phosphodiesterase inhibitors			
Milrinone	Vasodilator/anti-inflammatory action	IA injections effective	Short half-life; infusions are needed; It is useful with CHF
Papaverine	Potent vasodilator	Profound vasodilation after IA injections	Severe complication; seldom used
Cilostazol	Vasodilator and antiplatelet effects	Decreases incidence of vasospasm	Experimental
Endothelin 1 antagonist			
Clazosentan	ET-1 antagonist	Preliminary data supportive of improved outcome	Not supported in randomized control trials and abandoned
Miscellaneous drugs			
Estrogen	Vasodilation by downregulating endothelin and upregulating NOS	Vasodilation	Preclinical
Magnesium	• Vasodilator • Neuroprotectant • Antiseizure/ sedative	Clinical experience in obstetric cases	Not effective and could provide sedation
Statins	Anti-inflammatory properties	Improvement reported in early studies	Not supported in recent trials
EPO	Neuroprotective effects	Neuroprotection	Preclinical
Nitric oxide	Potent vasodilator	Vasodilation	Unproven
Heparin	Nonspecific	Neuroprotection	Investigational

(BP: blood pressure; CHF: congestive heart failure; EPO: erythropoietin; ET: endothelin 1; FDA: Food and Drug Administration; IA: intra-arterial; NOS: nitric oxide synthase)

Table 3: Hemodynamic targets during aneurysm treatment.

Aneurysm	Treated	Untreated
ABP (systolic mm Hg)	180–220	150
CVP (mean mm Hg)	6–10	8–12
PCWP (mm Hg)	6–10	12–20

Anesthetic Management

- IA vasodilator treatments can be done under sedation. However, general anesthesia will be required for uncooperative patients or those requiring angioplasty or stent placement.
- *INR suite set up:*
    - Prepare the suite for high-risk general anesthesia with invasive monitoring.
    - Necessary intubation, monitoring equipment, cardiovascular drugs, and fluids should be available.
    - Extended anesthetic circuits might be necessary to enable free movement of the table for groin and cerebral imaging.
- *Preoperative assessment:*
    - Vasospasm patients show a range of cognitive dysfunction. They might be restless, aphasic, unable to comprehend and communicate, or they may be sedated and ventilated.
    - A careful review of cardiovascular status is necessary. SAH can cause myocardial injury with low ejection fraction and conduction blocks. The patient might be in fluid overload and/or overt respiratory failure.
    - Despite poor cardiac function, they might be on high-dose pressors to maintain the target BP.
    - They may require ventilation during transport.
    - They are transferred from the ICU with multiple infusion pumps, ventricular drain, A-line, CVP, or PA catheter. The ventricular drain has to be clamped during transport to avoid uncontrolled drainage of the CSF.
- *INR suite and transport:* Before transport, prepare the INR suite and ensure that the staff is available to receive the case. Prepare sufficient volumes of drug infusions for the procedure before starting from the ICU.
- For a patient unable to cooperate with the procedure or if stents are to be deployed, general anesthesia with endotracheal intubation is required.
    - General anesthesia can help control the $PaCO_2$, improve the quality of the images by decreasing the movements, and provide better

control of the situation if there are unanticipated complications such as vascular injury or rupture.
- The concerns with general anesthesia are hypotension at induction or during treatment, an increased dose of vasopressors, the need for prolonged ventilation, and the inability to extubate at the end of the procedure.
- *Intraoperative care:* The major challenge during the procedure is to prevent hypotension due to IA vasodilator therapy due to poor myocardial function, prophylactic calcium channel blockade, and background anesthetics. High-dose vasodilator treatments, e.g., 50 mg of verapamil, may be needed in some cases. Super-selective vasodilation can decrease the chances of systemic side effects but is less frequently undertaken. Hypotension is usually treated by increasing the vasopressor infusion rate.
- *Postoperative care:* Deliberate hypertension treatment of cerebral vasospasm with or without IA vasodilator treatment usually lasts for three days. If the patient remains intubated, the neurological examination is challenging due to the need for sedation. Additional postoperative monitoring may be necessary, such as a TCD exam, or microdialysis may be needed in these cases. On the other hand, leaving the patient intubated ensures that the airway is protected, and one can intervene rapidly in any adverse neurological and cardiac event.
- *Microdialysis guided management of SAH patients:*
  - Cerebral microdialysis (CMD) monitors tissue metabolite concentrations by dialyzing interstitial fluid across a semipermeable membrane.
  - The technique monitors the concentrations of several compounds.
  - The pathological threshold values for concentrations of these compounds in detecting brain injury in the first 72 hours are as follows:
    - *CMD lactate:* >4 mmol/L
    - *CMD pyruvate:* <120 µmol/L
    - *CMD glucose:* <0.7 mmol/L
    - *CMD glutamate:* >10 µmol/L
    - *CMD glycerol:* >50 µmol/L
    - *Derived values:* CMD lactate: pyruvate ratio >40.

Complications of IA Vasodilator Treatment

- Vessel dissection/perforation
- Raised ICP
- Seizures
- Embolic stroke

- Bradycardia/hypotension
- Relapse and need for repeat treatment.

CASE REPORTS FOR FURTHER DISCUSSION

Case 1: A 59-year-old female patient with a history of hypertension and heavy smoking of 1.5 packs per day for 30 years complained of occasional dizziness and headache. Investigations revealed two aneurysms: A 5-mm left MCA bifurcation and a 3-mm left internal carotid artery (ICA) aneurysm. There was no evidence of any intracranial bleeding. The patient underwent an uneventful pterional craniotomy for the MCA bifurcation aneurysm. She was ambulant on day 2. CT scan on day 6 was negative for SAH. However, immediately after surgery, she resumed smoking. On day 6, she became aphasic. A repeat CT scan showed no change from the earlier one in the day. Cerebral angiography showed narrowing of the M1 and the MCA bifurcation, consistent with vasospasm. Serial TCD revealed an increase in flow velocity in the M1, and MRI showed evidence of ischemia on day 8. The spasm gradually reversed over the next two weeks with functional improvement. The patient returned to work at the end of the year. *What are the predictors of cerebral vasospasm after aneurysm clipping? What are the hemodynamic targets during vasospasm treatment in a patient with an untreated aneurysm? What are the concerns in anesthetizing an aneurysm patient who smokes heavily?*

Case 2: A 37-year-old man with no significant medical history other than excessive alcohol intake became acutely confused. The CT scan, 4 hours after the onset of symptoms, revealed left thalamic hemorrhage with extensive intraventricular bleeding and hydrocephalus. He was intubated and ventilated. An external ventricular drain (EVD) was placed. The EVD was removed after a week, and a lumbar drain was inserted. Ten days after the operation, his condition had minimally improved; however, repeat CT revealed a new hemorrhage. Angiography on day 13 revealed a thalamic arteriovenous malformation, but the endovascular treatment was aborted due to vasospasm. The patient was medically managed. Nimodipine, volume expansion, and low-dose norepinephrine were used to treat vasospasm. Some three weeks later, he was extubated and transferred to the ward. A follow-up four weeks after the initial event revealed no lesion on CT and angiography. A spontaneous resolution of the lesion seems to have occurred. *What measures will you take to blunt the hemodynamic response to laryngoscopy in a patient with intracranial hemorrhage (ICH)? What are the complications of an EVD? How will you prevent excessive drainage of CSF? What is the role of volume expansion in the treatment of cerebral vasospasm?*

Case 3: A 52-year-old man underwent complete coil embolization of a ruptured intracranial aneurysm at the right A1 and A2 junction. The rupture resulted in a significant ICH (Hunt and Hess and Fisher, grade 3). Post-procedure, he was prescribed aspirin and nimodipine to prevent vasospasm. However, on ultrasound assessment, the Doppler flow velocities continued to increase over the next few days but without gross neurological deficits. By day 6, angiography revealed a significant vasospasm involving both anterior cerebral arteries. Verapamil 10 mg was injected into each ICA. On return to the ICU, the patient developed dense monoplegia of the left lower extremity. The CT scan revealed coil displacement with a new right anterior cerebral artery (ACA) infarct. Repeat angiography revealed herniated coil loop blocking the A2 segment. *Given the conflicting treatment requirements, in this case, the risk of further displacement of coils and vasospasm, would you use vasodilators to augment blood flow? What anesthetic steps can you take to increase collateral blood flow? Justify the selection of cerebral vasodilating drugs, verapamil, and nimodipine, for IA and intravenous administration.*

Case 4: A young sickle cell crisis patient presented with left hemiparesis following a SAH. Angiography revealed multiple aneurysms. The bleeding was attributed to a right supra-clinoid ICA aneurysm. The aneurysm was coiled. It was found that the left ICA was occluded distally with retrograde flow through the posterior communicating arteries. The CT scan revealed early bifrontal infarcts. Over the next week, the patient improved. However, on day 8, his condition worsened with the recurrence of left hemiparesis. There was no evidence of fresh bleeding or hydrocephalus. Angiography revealed severe diffuse right-sided vasospasm involving the carotid and vertebral systems. The blood flow on the left hemisphere was also critically compromised. IA injection of verapamil (5 mg) reversed the angiographic spasm. Consent was obtained from the family for bilateral continuous IA verapamil infusion. Microcatheters were located in the right internal carotid and vertebral arteries. Verapamil, 2 mg/h in the right vertebral artery and 4 mg/h in the ICA, was infused for 22 hours. Intravenous and IA heparin was also infused. Post-treatment angiograms revealed significant angiographic improvements. *What are the risks of long-term catheter placement? Under what circumstances is it acceptable to place such catheters? How will you manage a case for long-duration catheter infusions? What monitoring will you recommend?*

Case 5: A 33-year-old woman underwent uncomplicated cesarean delivery. Her history was significant for migraines and protein S deficiency. Four days after delivery, she developed a severe headache and facial droop. 2 weeks later, she developed left upper extremity weakness. The initial CT scan was normal, but subsequent MRI revealed subacute left putaminal hemorrhage with minimal SAH. On examination, her BP was normal. She had left spastic hemiparesis with an upgoing plantar reflex. Later that day, she developed right lower limb weakness. Repeat MRI revealed new areas of ischemia, and MRA revealed multiple regions of focal vasoconstriction and dilation in all vascular territories. High-dose methylprednisolone was given with the provisional diagnosis of vasculitis. The patient was confused and agitated. On the 22nd postpartum day, she was posted for balloon angioplasty and IA verapamil treatment. *What are the advantages and disadvantages of general anesthesia versus sedation in such a case? How will you manage the blood pressure? After verapamil, the patient becomes severely bradycardic; what are the differential diagnoses?*

CASE REPORT REFERENCES

Case 1: Marco CM et al. A case report of cerebral vasospasm following elective clipping of unruptured aneurysm: pathogenetic theories and clinical features of a dangerous underestimated event. Sci Reposit. Surg Case Repts. 2020;2613-5965.

Case 2: Tseng WL et al. Vasospasm after intraventricular hemorrhage caused by arteriovenous malformation. Asian J Neurosurg. 2015;10(2): 114-6.

Case 3: Chen SH et al. Coil herniation following intra-arterial verapamil infusion for the treatment of cerebral vasospasm: case report and literature review. Interv Neuroradiol. 2015;21(2):184-7.

Case 4: Sigounasa D et al. Continuous intra-arterial infusion of verapamil for treatment of severe vasospasm after subarachnoid hemorrhage. Interdiscip Neurosurg. 2019;19:100622.

Case 5: Fugate JE et al. Fulminant post-partum cerebral vasoconstriction syndrome: Arch Neurol. 2012;69(1):111-7.

FURTHER READING

1. Athiraman U et al. Evidence for a conditioning effect of inhalational anesthetics on angiographic vasospasm after aneurysmal subarachnoid hemorrhage. J Neurosurg. 2019; p. 1-7.
2. Barpujari A et al. Pharmaceutical management for subarachnoid hemorrhage. Recent Trends Pharm Sci Res. 2021;3(2):16-30.
3. Doring, K et al. Ultrasound-induced release of nimodipine from drug-loaded block copolymer micelles: in Vivo analysis. Transl Stroke Res; 2022.
4. Ginanneschi F et al. Somatosensory evoked potentials and transcranial color Doppler monitoring in subarachnoid hemorrhage. J Stroke Cerebrovasc Dis. 2021;31(2):106214.
5. Lee JW et al. The effect of anesthetic agents on cerebral vasospasms after subarachnoid hemorrhage: a retrospective study. Medicine (Baltimore). 2018;97(31):e11666.

CHAPTER 41 Treatment of Cerebral Vasospasm

Vignette: The History of Vasospasm after Subarachnoid Hemorrhage

In 30 AD, Aulus Cornelius Celsus, a Roman scholar and physician, described SAH as the condition with "violent pains in temple and occiput" characterized by "strong shivering, nervous relaxation, dimness of sight, vomiting, and suppression of voice." In 1817, Sir John Hunter described three states of the arteries: the natural state, a relaxed state, and a narrowed state due to the contraction of the muscle. The later state reflected vasospasm. Robertson, in 1949 hypothesized the correlation between subarachnoid blood clots and cerebral infarction due to vasospasm. The first cerebral angiograms showing vasospasm after SAH were reported by Arthur Ecker in 1951. In his paper, Ecker revealed 12 cases of cerebral vasospasm in which the arteries were so severely narrowed that there was no contrast in the lumen. At the presentation, his findings were rejected by the audience. Only one person seemed to be listening. Ecker thanked the person for his attention. The man stuttered, "I don't speak English!"

Deep Hypothermic Circulatory Arrest

Chapter 42

INTRODUCTION

The deep hypothermic circulatory arrest (DHCA) technique uses hypothermia (core temperature of 28-29°C) to stop systemic circulation safely for 30 minutes. Various cardiac, aortic, vascular, and neurosurgical procedures can be undertaken during DHCA. Clipping of complex aneurysms was the primary neurosurgical application of the technique. With an arrest time of 30 minutes, the technique permitted the safe clipping of aneurysms. However, advances in endovascular treatments have rendered DHCA largely obsolete for aneurysm clipping due to its complexity and potential complications.

NEUROANESTHETIC CONCERNS

- Transient circulatory arrest methods
- Indications for DHCA
- *Preoperative:* High-risk aneurysm with impending rupture
- Control of hemodynamics during induction and intubation
- Lumbar drain placement
- Positioning and pinning
- Surgical exposure
- Anticoagulation after dissection
- Cardiopulmonary bypass and deep hypothermic circulatory arrest
- Neuroprotection and brain temperature monitoring during arrest
- Rewarming and circulatory support
- *Complications:* Bleeding, brain bulge, coagulation failures, neurological injury, and intracranial hemorrhage
- Postoperative care

TRANSIENT CIRCULATORY ARREST METHODS

- *Objectives:*
  - Facilitate dissection of the aneurysmal sac
  - Placement of clip
  - Reduce bleeding and increase visibility in the case of rupture.
- *Methods to reduce aneurysm blood flow:*
  - Temporary clipping

- Adenosine bolus
- Rapid ventricular pacing
- Endovascular balloon occlusion
- Deep hypothermic circulatory arrest
- Temporary carotid artery clamping.

INDICATIONS AND RATIONALE OF DHCA

Deep hypothermic circulatory arrest (DHCA) safely stops blood flow, enabling dissection and clipping of a complex aneurysm. DHCA is a high-risk procedure indicated when conventional approaches to aneurysm clipping/coiling have failed or are unsuitable.

- With the availability of stent-assisted coil embolization, the indications of DHCA are limited to:
  - Aneurysms of the posterior circulation, which are large (>10 mm) or giant (>25 mm) in size, with complex vascular pattern
  - DHCA is sometimes indicated when the lesion does not decompress completely on temporary clipping due to unclipped feeding arteries, calcification, luminal thrombus, or coil.
- Rationale:
  - Circulatory arrest permits dissection of the aneurysm by creating space due to the decompression of the lesion.
  - No flow conditions during dissection permit surgery, even when there is potential for injury to the aneurysmal sac during dissection.
  - Circulatory arrest should not exceed 45 minutes. Ideally, it should be under 30 minutes. Therefore, each step has to be carefully planned.

Preoperative Assessment

- Preoperative assessment is no different than any high-risk neurosurgical operation. However, due to the potential for complications, physicians likely to be involved downstream should participate in the preoperative case discussion and planning.
- Patients with valvular heart disease, patent foramen ovale (PFO), or other congenital heart conditions may require additional care during cardiopulmonary bypass.
- DHCA needs an operating room with sufficient space to accommodate the necessary equipment, such as a fluoroscope, transesophageal echocardiogram (TEE) machine, operating microscope, brain lab for image navigation, and cardiopulmonary bypass (CPB) machine.

Anesthetic Goals

- Blood pressure is kept within 10–20% baseline while off bypass and an adequate cerebral perfusion pressure of 50 mm Hg during bypass.

- Monitoring and maintaining a stable metabolic profile.
- Monitoring brain and core temperatures to ensure adequate hypothermic neuroprotection.
- Ensuring adequate paralysis during circulatory arrest
- Effective coagulation management and timely delivery of heparin, protamine, and other coagulation products as needed.
- Smooth rewarming.
- Safe transport to and care in the neuro-critical care unit.
- Extubation in the neuro-critical care unit.

Monitoring

Electrocardiogram (ECG), noninvasive blood pressure (NIBP), arterial line, bilateral hemispheric electroencephalogram (EEG)/Bispectral index (BIS)/Sedline, SaO_2, $EtCO_2/O_2$/anesthetics, TEE, central venous pressure (CVP)/pulmonary artery catheter (PAC), multisite temperature monitoring, urine output, and neuromuscular transmission monitor.

Induction

- The sequence of events for deep hypothermic circulatory arrest is shown in **Figure 1**. A large bore (18G or 16G) IV access is obtained at induction. Sedation (midazolam/fentanyl) is needed to place the pre-induction A-line. Care is taken to ensure smooth induction, typically with lidocaine, propofol, and rocuronium. A test laryngoscopy may be needed before intubation.
- After intubation, a urinary catheter, TEE probe, external defibrillator pads, and central venous or pulmonary artery catheters are placed. BIS or EEG monitors are placed to monitor the depth of anesthesia.
- Mechanical ventilation is adjusted to achieve a $PaCO_2$ of around 35 mm Hg. Volatile anesthetics are titrated to ensure narcosis; however,

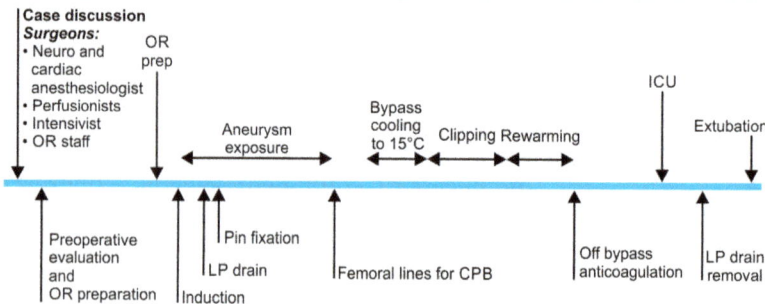

Fig. 1: Sequence of events during a deep hypothermic circulatory arrest for aneurysm clipping. (CPB: cardiopulmonary bypass; ICU: intensive care unit; LP: lumbar puncture; OR: operating room)

nitrous oxide is avoided. A lumbar drain is used to monitor and drain cerebrospinal fluid (CSF).
- Fentanyl is supplemented as needed (to a total dose of 10–50 µg/kg) in anticipation of pin fixation.
- Temperature monitoring is critical to both cooling and rewarming. Besides esophageal temperature, nasopharyngeal, tympanic, rectal, urinary and axillary temperatures are monitored to ensure even cooling and rewarming.
- Surgery is preferably done in the supine position if a thoracotomy is needed to initiate CPB.
- Prophylactic antibiotics and steroids (dexamethasone 10 mg) are administered 1 hour before the incision. Mannitol (1 g/kg over 30 minutes) is started at the craniotomy. The depth of anesthesia is gradually increased to burst suppression by the time surgical dissection is completed.

SURGICAL EXPOSURE AND INSTITUTION OF BYPASS

- The patient is draped for craniotomy, sternotomy, and groin access. Initially, the neurosurgeons proceed with the craniotomy and expose the aneurysm. Meticulous hemostasis is needed for the procedure.
- Once the aneurysm is exposed, the femoral artery and vein are exposed below the inguinal ligament. Femoral bypass is instituted using 21 French arterial and venous cannulas. The patient is heparinized. Flow is instituted. Cooling (target temperature 16–18° C) and arrest are achieved.
- After cardiac arrest, the aneurysm generally collapses due to the decrease in arterial pressure. It is carefully dissected. During the flow arrest, the aneurysm can be incised. Intramural thrombi are removed. The neck of the aneurysm is clipped with one or more clips. Flow is then reinstated to check for any bleeding from the clip site. Restoration of flow changes the geometry of the vessels. Should the clip be repositioned, the pump is momentarily stopped, and the clips repositioned.
- If there is no bleeding, rewarming is begun. The arrest time for clipping the aneurysms should ideally not exceed 30 minutes.

REWARMING AND RECOVERY

- Rewarming is started after satisfactory clip placement. Once heart functions return, the cannulas are removed. Inotropic support is provided as needed. Anticoagulation is reversed. The skull and skin flaps are closed.
- A postoperative CT scan of the head is done.
- The patient is transferred to the ICU while still intubated.
- Sedation is next withdrawn, and the patient is extubated when awake.

OUTCOME OF DEEP HYPOTHERMIC CIRCULATORY ARREST

- A good prognosis is expected in the following:
  - The younger patients, <60 years. Bypass-related complications increase in the elderly due to vascular disease.
  - A circulatory arrest time of <30 minutes
  - Good cardiac functions at the baseline
  - *Smaller aneurysms:* Giant aneurysms >3 cm often contain thrombi and are associated with poor prognosis.
- Half to two-thirds of patients have good functional outcomes after DHCA for aneurysm clipping.

TRANSIENT CIRCULATORY ARREST WITH ADENOSINE

High-dose Adenosine

Adenosine is an antiarrhythmic drug. A 3–6 mg bolus dose is used for treating supraventricular tachycardia. However, in larger doses, adenosine can cause a profound decrease in heart rate and blood pressure. Doses of 30–90 mg can cause transient severe bradycardia, sinus arrest, and profound hypotension **(Table 1)**.

Contraindications to High-dose Adenosine

- Adenosine allergy
- Bronchial asthma
- Second- and third-degree atrioventricular (AV) block
- Sick sinus syndrome

Complications of High-dose Adenosine

- Sustained cardiac pause.
- Supraventricular arrhythmias
- Bronchospasm
- Seizures
- Ventricular tachycardia
- *In awake patients:* Flushing, dizziness, numbness, dyspnea, and nausea

Table 1: Adenosine doses used for various clinical indications.

Dose	Cardiovascular effects	Applications
3–6 mg	Suppresses AV conduction	Antiarrhythmic agent
12–24 mg	Transient asystole (HR <40), severe hypotension (SBP <60 mm Hg)	Aneurysm surgery
30–90 mg	Cardiac arrest (10–15 seconds), profound hypotension SBP <40 mm Hg	Embolization of AVMs

(AV: atrioventricular; AVM: arteriovenous malformation; HR: heart rate; SBP: systolic blood pressure)

Clinical Use of Adenosine Arrest

- *For transient hypotension:* For example, intraoperative aneurysm rupture. Adenosine 6–12 mg boluses are given. This dose is unlikely to have prolonged cardiovascular effects and can be undertaken with routine monitoring with ECG and A-lines in such cases.
- For profound hypotension: For high-dose adenosine (30–90 mg), in addition to routine monitoring, central venous access should be obtained, and pacing pads applied to treat arrhythmias. If hypotension is needed for a more extended period with high-dose arrests, then a repeat bolus dose can be administered, or adenosine infusion can be used. Alternatively, another shorter-acting hypotensive agent (such as nitroprusside or esmolol) can be used. Rebound hypertension may occur during wakening that needs to be treated.

CASE REPORTS FOR FURTHER DISCUSSION

Case 1: A 42-year-old male complained of abnormal sensations on the right side of his face. No neurological deficits were evident on examination. Angiography revealed a single, large 22 mm left internal carotid artery aneurysm. Coiling was unsuccessful, and the patient failed the test occlusion of the carotid artery. Surgical clipping under deep hypothermic circulatory arrest was planned. *What are the current indications for deep hypothermic circulatory arrest? What is a "test occlusion of the carotid artery", and the significance of failing the test? How is anesthesia for such a test managed?*

Case 2: A 53-year-old, 164 cm, 53 kg female patient with a history of hypertension and smoking (1 pack/day) presented with headache, photophobia, and altered sensorium for the last three weeks. The patient had a Grade 3 SAH. On angiography, she had a 5-mm middle cerebral artery (MCA) bifurcation aneurysm, a 3-mm posterior cerebral artery (PCA) aneurysm, and a 10-mm basilar apex aneurysm. Laboratory, ECG, and echocardiography reports were within normal limits. The surgeons requested DHCA with femoro-femoral bypass for clipping the basilar apex aneurysm. *How does the presence of multiple aneurysms affect your management? What additional monitoring will you have in place in planning for the procedure?*

Case 3: A 43-year-old female, 154 cm, 43.6 kg, with no significant medical history, had a giant (26 × 29 mm) basilar artery aneurysm. Aneurysm clipping was planned under deep hypothermic circulatory arrest. After successful clipping of the aneurysm and adequate rewarming, cannulae were removed. Protamine was used to reverse anticoagulation. Excessive bleeding was encountered at this time in the surgical field. Protamine, fresh frozen plasma, and platelets were infused, but bleeding persisted. *What are the possible causes of coagulopathy? How will you monitor coagulation? Will you consider antifibrinolytic drugs in such a case?*

Case 4: A 69-year-old man presented with right retro-orbital pain, diplopia, and worsening headaches. On examination, the plantar reflex was bilaterally upgoing, and there were severe gait difficulties. On angiography, the left internal carotid artery (ICA) was occluded, and on the right side was a 1.6-diameter partly thrombosed aneurysm of the posterior communicating artery. The left vertebral artery was stenosed, and the distal right vertebral artery was poorly perfused. The patient had a significant medical history of coronary artery disease, and coronary angiography revealed depressed myocardial functions (ejection fraction of 40%) with multivessel disease involving the distal segment of the right coronary artery with 90% stenosis of the mid-circumflex artery. He was due for aneurysm clipping under hypothermic circulatory arrest and concomitant coronary artery bypass surgery. *What is the appropriate sequence of surgical events? Where can you monitor temperature, and what are the advantages and disadvantages of each site? The patient developed mild left hemiparesis that resolved over time; what was the likely cause? Besides hypothermia, what neuroprotective strategies could have been used in this case?*

Case 5: A 30-year-old postpartum female presented with a 3-week history of seizures and right-sided weakness starting 3 hours after the delivery of her fourth child. She had a remote history of similar headaches and weakness at the first child's birth. On examination, she was drowsy with right-sided hypertonic hemiparesis. The CT scan revealed intracranial hemorrhage in the left temporal lobe and a calcified left middle cerebral artery trifurcation aneurysm with an ill-defined neck. Given the absence of a defined neck, the large size, and the history of calcification, she was due for deep hypothermic circulatory arrest using the thoracic approach. During the procedure, she was cooled to 16°C, and thiopental was infused to protect the brain. After successful clipping, she was rewarmed. She was ventilated overnight and extubated the next day. There were no changes in her neurological examination from baseline. On the 13th postoperative day, she presented with acute chest pain but no shortness of breath. *What is the differential diagnosis? What predisposing factors for pulmonary embolism (PE) exist in this case? How will you rule out PE? How will you prevent it?*

CASE REPORT REFERENCES

Case 1: Castro H et al. Técnica de hipotermia profunda y paro circulatorio total para clipaje de aneurismas cerebrales gigantes. Rev Col Anest Febrero. 2010;38(1):111-23.

Case 2: Kim YR et al. Deep hypothermic total circulatory arrest (DHCA) under total intravenous anesthesia for giant basilar aneurysm clipp- ing-A case report. Anesth Pain Med. 2009;12(4):326-34.

Case 3: Taki W et al. Circulatory arrest with profound hypothermia during the surgical treatment of large internal carotid artery aneurysm—case report. Neyrol Med Chir (Tokyo). 1998;38:725-9.

Case 4: Bose B et al. Clipping of cerebral aneurysm under hypothermic cardiac arrest and simultaneous coronary artery bypass grafting: case report. J Neurol Neurosurg Psychiatry. 2002;72:394-5.

Case 5: Thomas AN et al. Anaesthesia for the treatment of a giant cerebral aneurysm under hypothermic circulatory arrest. Anaesthesia. 1990;45:383-85.

FURTHER READING

1. Habertheuer A et al. How to perfuse: concepts of cerebral protection during arch replacement. Biomed Res Int. 2015;2015:981813.
2. Lawton MT et al. The future of open vascular neurosurgery: perspectives on cavernous malformations, AVMs, and bypasses for complex aneurysms. J Neurosurg. 2019;130(5):1409-25.
3. Linardi D et al. Temperature management during circulatory arrest in cardiac surgery. Ther Hypothermia Temp Manag. 2016; 6(1):9-16.
4. Veerhoek D et al. Anticoagulation management during pulmonary end-arterectomy with cardiopulmonary bypass and deep hypothermic circulatory arrest. Perfusion. 2021;36(1):87-96.
5. Wang X et al. Giant cerebral aneurysms: comparing CTA, MRA, and digital subtraction angiography assessments. J Neuroimaging. 2020;30(3):335-41.

Vignette: When it Comes to Brains, the Size Does Not Matter

Among all animals, the sperm whale has the biggest brain, weighing about 8 kg. These whales are the largest animals both in size (20 m) and weight (30–60,000 Kg). However, when corrected for body weight, the ratio of brain weight to body weight is <1/1,000. While the brain-to-body weight ratio is easy to determine, it correlates poorly with a given animal's intelligence. For example, the brain weight to body mass ratio of humans and mice is about the same, 1/50, while that of elephants is 1/580. The ratio is challenging to understand when one compares the human brain's functionality to that of the a mouse or the complex social behavior of an elephant to that of a rodent.

Chapter 43

Management of Traumatic Brain Injury

INTRODUCTION

In 2019, traumatic brain injury (TBI) accounted for 222,000 hospitalizations and 65,000 deaths in the USA. The worst outcome was in patients over 75 years of age, who accounted for about 30% of hospitalizations and deaths. The hospitalization rate was two times, and the fatality rate was three times greater in the males than in the females. About 7% of the hospitalizations and 4% of the deaths were in children under the age of 17 years. Moderate to severe TBIs were due to falls, gunshot injuries, assaults, and motor vehicle accidents. Five years after severe TBI, 22% of adult patients with TBI either died or did not improve, while 30% worsened, but only 26% improved. The healthcare cost of TBI was 75 billion per year by 2010 estimates. Developing guidelines for managing TBI is challenging due to difficulties in synthesizing information across clinical trials. Before recommending any intervention, the study design, clinical details, and analysis must be carefully assessed. While the general guidelines for TBI management are widely accepted, many therapeutic targets and novel monitoring techniques are yet to be standardized. Thus, newer guidelines are being developed on a rolling basis based on constantly emerging data.

NEUROANESTHETIC CONCERNS

- *Pathophysiology of traumatic brain injury (TBI):*
  - Primary and secondary injuries
  - Prevention of secondary injury
  - Strategies to decrease secondary brain injuries.
- *Preoperative assessment:*
  - TBI severity assessment
  - Initial management
  - Impending brain herniation
  - Conservative management
- Surgical intervention
  - Intraoperative:
    - Operating room preparation
    - Induction and intubation

- Drug selection
    - Management goals
- Surgical interventions
- Postoperative care
- Complications
- Outcome

Pathophysiology

TBI is a structural injury and/or physiological disruption of brain tissue after the application of an external force. The injury results in either a new intracranial lesion, a deterioration of neurological functions, or a worsening of an existing one. It manifests as unconsciousness, memory impairment, altered mental state, or a new neurological deficit.

- *Focal TBI:* Contusion; epidural, subdural, and intraparenchymal hematoma
- *Diffuse TBI:* Axonal injuries, microvascular injuries, and hypoxic-ischemic injuries
- *Combined:* Most TBIs share components of focal and diffuse injuries
- *Primary injury:* Direct result of mechanical forces such as acceleration/deacceleration forces, blast injury, and penetrating injuries
- *Secondary injury:* Commonly due to ischemia, hypoxia, cerebral edema, raised intracranial pressure (ICP), hydrocephalus, and infections..

Avoiding secondary injuries:
- Assure cerebral tissue perfusion and oxygenation:
    - *Avoid hypoxia:* Supplement oxygenation.
    - Avoid hypotension.
    - *Avoid increase in ICP:*
        - Hyperventilation
        - Head elevation
        - Unobstructed cerebral venous return
        - Osmotic diuretics
        - Avoid coughing and bucking.
    - Monitor ICP
    - Ventricular drainage
    - Craniotomies
    - Craniectomies
- *Avoid increase in oxygen demand:*
    - Avoid seizures.
    - Avoid hyperthermia.
    - Ensure adequate sedation.
    - Mild hypothermia.

- *Decrease tissue injury:*
  - Avoid hyponatremia and electrolyte imbalances.
  - Correct coagulopathy
  - Treat infections
  - Treat SIADH (syndrome of inappropriate antidiuretic hormone secretion)

PRE-OPERATIVE ASSESSMENT

- Clinical features
  - Most TBIs are mild and go unreported.
  - Of those admitted, 40% are associated with alcohol intake.
  - 8% have major trauma.
  - 30% have some degree of cervical spine injury.
- Head injuries are due to:
  - Traffic accidents (50%)
  - Falls (25%)
  - Assaults (15%)
  - Sports injury (10%)
- *Some characteristic signs/symptoms of direct head injury:*
  - Bone step or a palpable discontinuity of the skull
  - *Raccoon's eyes:* Periorbital ecchymosis
  - *Battle sign:* Bruising over the mastoid.
  - Hemotympanum
  - Cerebrospinal fluid (CSF) rhinorrhea
  - CSF otorrhea.
- *Assessment of severity:* Classification of head injuries based on coma scales **(Table 1)** and other parameters **(Table 2)**.
- *Cranial nerve examination (Table 3):*
  - *Ophthalmic:* Ocular deviation, pupillary size, and response
  - *Trigeminal/facial:* Facial symmetry and corneal reflex
  - *Lower cranial:* Gag reflex (Cranial nerves IX and X), caloric response testing (VIII CN)

INITIAL MANAGEMENT

- *Airway:*
  - *Oxygen supplementation:* Target SaO_2 of 95%
  - *Intubation:*
    - *Indications:*
      - GCS of <8
      - Risk of aspiration
      - Before transferring to another center

CHAPTER 43 Management of Traumatic Brain Injury

Table 1: Glasgow Coma Scale (GCS) in adults, children, and infants.

Score	Adults	Children	Infants
Best eye opening			
4	Spontaneous	Spontaneous	Spontaneous
3	Verbal	Verbal	Verbal
2	Pain	Pain	Pain
1	None	None	None
Best verbal response			
5	Oriented converses	Appropriate speech	Appropriate interaction
4	Disoriented converses	Inappropriate speech	Inappropriate
3	Inappropriate speech	Moaning	Cries to pain
2	Incomprehensible	Irritable/inconsolable	Moans
1	None	None	None
Best motor response			
6	Normal response	Normal response	Normal response
5	Localizes pain	Localizes pain	Withdraws to touch
4	Withdraws to pain	Withdraws to pain	Withdraws to pain
3	Abnormal flexion	Abnormal flexion	Abnormal flexion
2	Abnormal extension	Abnormal extension	Abnormal extension
1	None	None	None

Table 2: Clinical features of head injury with increasing severity.

	Mild	Moderate	Severe
GCS	13–15	9–12	≤8
Loss of consciousness	<1 hour	<24 hours	>24 hours
Post-traumatic amnesia	<1 hour	<24 hours	>24 hours
Clinical presentation	• Fully alert • Attentive	• Persistent confusion • Behavioral change • Decreased attentiveness • Focal signs	• Impaired consciousness • Stupor • Coma • Discharge from nose or ear
History	• Headache • Transient loss of consciousness • Nausea • Vomiting • Transient amnesia	• Headache • Loss of consciousness for a short duration • Dizziness • Photophobia • Vomiting • Amnesia	• Worsening headache • Sustained loss of consciousness • Slurred speech • Disorientation • Seizures • Photophobia • Sustained vomiting
Clinical examination	Minimal finding	• Significant findings • Pain localization • Nystagmus • Drowsiness • Unsteady gait	• Dilated or asymmetric pupils • Impaired pain localization, decorticate, or decerebrate positioning • No response to pain

Table 3: Cranial nerve examination in conscious and unconscious patients.

	Conscious patient	Unconscious patient
CN I: Olfactory N	Smell tests	Usually not tested
CN II: Ophthalmic N	Visual field test	Blink reflex
CN III, IV and VI: Oculomotor N, Trochlear N, and Abducens N	Position and movements of the eye, pupil size and response, tracking eye movements	Position and movements of the eye, e.g., during brainstem testing. Pupil size and response
V and VII: Trigeminal N and Facial N	Symmetry of facial touch, blowing cheek and smile	Corneal reflex, facial grimacing in response to local pain, blink reflex
VIII: Vestibulocochlear N	Symmetry of hearing	Cold caloric response testing
IX and X: Glossopharyngeal N and Vagus N	Symmetry of gag reflex	Symmetry of gag reflex
XI: Accessory N	Shrugging shoulders	Usually not tested
XII: Hypoglossal N	Tongue movement/deviation	Asymmetry of tongue

- *Rapid-sequence intubation:*
    - Inline traction if emergent
    - *Induction agents:*
        - None may be needed in an unconscious patient.
        - Propofol for smooth induction
        - Etomidate to ensure hemodynamic stability.
    - Succinylcholine or rocuronium for muscle relaxation
    - Propofol, midazolam, and fentanyl are used for sedation after intubation.
    - Prolonged muscle relaxation is avoided, as it could interfere with the neurological examination.
- *Ventilation:* Targets:
    - PaO_2 around 100 mm Hg
    - $PaCO_2$ 35–45 mm Hg
    - If an impending herniation is suspected, ventilate to a $PaCO_2$ of 25–35 mm Hg for 30 minutes.
- *Two large-bore peripheral IVs:*
    - Normal saline is preferred due to isotonicity.
    - If 3% hypertonic saline is used, the dose limit is typically 250–500 mL, as guided by serum sodium.
- *Hemodynamic goals:*
    - Judicious use of fluid and pressor of choice norepinephrine
        - Systolic blood pressure (SBP) >100 mm Hg
        - Mean arterial pressure (MAP) >70 mm Hg

- If blood pressure permits, raise the head of the bed by 30°.
- Urinary catheter
- *Lab screen:* Arterial blood gas (ABG), complete blood count (CBC), metabolic, and coagulation
- *Immediate diagnostic imaging:*
  - C-spine/skull X-ray often in ER
  - *Imaging:* CT of head/C-spine

Impending Herniation

- *An urgent response is necessary if:*
  - The patient is unresponsive to pain.
  - Showing decorticate or decerebrate posturing.
  - Pupils are unequal.
  - *Cushing's triad:* Bradycardia, hypertension, and abnormal breathing
- *Immediate treatment:*
  - Place the head in a neutral position.
  - Transient hyperventilation
  - Hyperventilation to $PaCO_2$ of 25–35 mm Hg for 30 minutes.
  - Mannitol 20–25% (0.25–1 g/kg over 15 minutes)
  - *Hypertonic saline:* 3% saline up to 500 mL or 23% saline 10 mL bolus over 10 minutes
  - Ensure adequate sedation; if needed, consider muscle relaxation.
- *Post-traumatic seizures:*
  - Incidence of early seizures (<7 days) up to 20% of TBIs; late seizures (>7 days) up to 40% of TBIs. On admission, 5% of TBI patients have seizures, while 15% of severe TBI patients have seizures.
  - *Risk factors for persistent seizures after TBI:* Intracranial hematoma, depressed skull fracture, GCS of <10, penetrating injuries, early onset seizures (<24 hours), and history of alcohol abuse.
  - *Consider seizure prophylaxis:*
    - *Fosphenytoin:* 20 mg/kg
    - *Levetiracetam:* 20 mg/kg

CONSERVATIVE MANAGEMENT

- Continue with the above management.
- *Institute-appropriate neuromonitoring:*
  - Insert A-line and central venous pressure (CVP).
  - Assess severity and treatment response to institute ICP monitoring.
  - *Therapeutic targets:*
    - SBP >100 mm Hg
    - CVP 8–12 mm Hg
    - Ensure cerebral perfusion pressure (CPP) of ≥60 mm Hg
    - SaO_2 >95%

- PaCO₂ 35–45 mm Hg
- Temperature ≤38.5°C
- Hb ≥7 g%
- Platelets ≥75,000/μL
- International normalized ratio (INR) ≤1.5
- Blood sugar 140–180 mg/dL or 8–10 mmol/L
- *Sodium:* 135–145 mEq/L
- *Magnesium:* ≥1.5 mg/dL
- *Potassium:* 4 mEq/L
– *Advanced neuromonitoring:*
  - *Cerebral perfusion monitoring:*
    - Transcranial Doppler (TCD)
    - Thermal diffusion
    - Laser Doppler
    - Microdialysis
  - *Cerebral oxygen monitoring:*
    - Near-infrared spectroscopy (NIRS)
    - Tissue interstitial oxygen saturation
    - Jugular venous oxygen saturation
  - *Cerebral function monitoring:*
    - Frequent clinical examination
    - Electroencephalogram (EEG)
    - Somatosensory-evoked potential (SSEP)
  - *Deep vein thrombosis (DVT) prophylaxis:* Stocking/compressive devices

SURGICAL MANAGEMENT

Indications

- *Epidural hematoma:* GCS <9, unequal pupils, midline shift >5 mm, hematoma thickness >15 mm, and bleed volume >30 cc
- *Subdural hematoma:* GCS <9, neurologic deterioration, midline shift >5 mm, and hematoma thickness >10 mm
- *Traumatic cerebral injury:* Injury volume >20 mL, midline shift >5 mm, neurologic deterioration, cisternal compression, and refractory intracranial hypertension
- *Posterior fossa surgery:* Any posterior fossa bleed, distortion of the 4th ventricle, and hydrocephalus
- *Depressed fracture:* >1 cm, intraparenchymal bleed, dural breach, CSF leak, and pneumocephalus

Operating Room Setup

- *Induction agents:* Propofol and etomidate; narcotics: fentanyl; muscle relaxants: succinylcholine, rocuronium

CHAPTER 43 Management of Traumatic Brain Injury

- *Airway management devices:* Laryngoscopes, stylet, bougie, and glide scope
- *Routine monitoring:* ECG, noninvasive blood pressure (NIBP), SaO_2, temperature, ventilatory parameters, and neuromuscular blockade
- *Invasive monitoring:* A-line, CVP, and urinary catheter for output
- Adequate IV access tools, fluids, and blood warmers
- *Fluids:* Normal saline, hypertonic saline, and mannitol
- Infusion pumps for total intravenous anesthesia (TIVA) and pressors
- Suction and nasogastric (NG) tube [for possible upper gastrointestinal (GI) bleeding and routine stomach decompression]
- Point-of-care monitoring for biochemistry and hemoglobin; thrombo-elastography (TEG)/rotational thrombo-elastometry (ROTEM)
- Sample tubes for hemogram and coagulation testing

Management Concerns

Intubation concerns:
- Need rapid-sequence intubation (RSI)
  - Cricoid pressure is potentially dangerous if the spine is injured.
  - Inline traction is needed for C-spine injury if the collar is removed.
  - Nasal intubation is avoided if a skull-base fracture is suspected.
- Positioning may be suboptimal.
- Associated facial trauma.
- If intubated, confirm position and cuff leak.
- ICP concerns
- Hypertensive response to intubation
- Intubation can be challenging in uncooperative or intoxicated patients.

Induction

- In critically ill patients, an awake A-line enables the treatment of blood pressure changes during induction rapidly.
- *The induction agent of choice is propofol (1.5–2 mg/kg):*
  - Lidocaine pretreatment blocks pain and ICP response.
  - A supplemental dose of narcotics could help decrease the propofol dose and blunt the intubation response.
  - Prophylactic phenylephrine can prevent hypotension.
- *Muscle relaxation:* Typically, succinylcholine (1–2 mg/kg) is used, but if contraindicated, rocuronium (0.8–1.2 mg/kg).

Positioning

- Head in a neutral position, mildly elevated, and avoid excessive neck flexion.
- Check tube position and bilateral air entry.

- *Appropriately zero the arterial line:*
  - If the head is elevated, zero pressure is set at the external auditory meatus.

Maintenance of Anesthesia

- Although volatile agents are widely used, they can cause cerebral vasodilation and increase ICP.
- Besides providing a smooth induction, propofol reduces cerebral blood flow, lowers ICP, and preserves flow metabolism coupling and autoregulation.
- Adequate muscle relaxation avoids coughing and bucking and decreases airway pressure with mechanical ventilation.
- *After induction:*
  - Mannitol
  - Anticonvulsants
  - Antibiotics
- *Fluid selection:*
  - Saline (isotonic) is preferred to lactated ringer (mildly hypotonic)
  - The benefits of colloids (such as albumin) are unclear.
  - The target for Hb for transfusion is not specified.
  - *Potential hazards of anemia (Hb <7 g%):*
    - Inadequate oxygen delivery
    - Cerebral hyperemia
    - Inflammation
    - It can impair blood–brain barrier (BBB) functions.
    - Predispose to venous sinus thrombosis.
    - Potentiates systemic hypotension, resistance to pressors.
  - *Hyperosmolar therapy:*
    - *Mannitol:*
      - In a 0.25–1 g/kg to decrease ICP.
      - It can cause fluid loading.
      - It can cause a rebound increase in ICP.
      - Severe TBI may be refractory to mannitol.
    - *Hypertonic saline (3, 7.5, or 21%):*
      - Improves trauma outcome.
      - Decreases ICP
      - Requires monitoring of serum Na.
- *Coagulopathy:*
  - Seen in a third of severe TBIs.
  - Increases mortality.
  - *Risk factors for coagulopathy:*
    - Severe head injury (GCS <8)

- *Injury severity score ≥16:* The score is the sum of the squares of the three highest grades of the injury (0-5) in nine body regions (face, head, neck, spine, chest, abdomen/pelvis, upper and lower extremities, and externally). A score of 16 implies severe injury.
    - Presence of cerebral edema
    - Subarachnoid hemorrhage
    - Midline shift
  - TBI releases tissue factor that activates thrombotic and fibrinolytic cascades resulting in disseminated intravascular coagulation (DIC).
  - Tranexamic acid can improve survival.
  - The role of factor VIII concentrate is unclear.
- *Institution of postoperative monitoring:*
  - Implanting ICP bolt
  - Implanting microdialysis probes
  - Paratrend tissue oxygen tension monitor
  - Laser Doppler blood flow
  - Thermal diffusion blood flow monitor
  - Jugular venous oximetry

POSTOPERATIVE MONITORING

- Routine postoperative ventilation
- Post-procedure CT scan
- ICP monitoring
- Intracranial invasive monitoring
- EEG/SSEP
- Close hemodynamic monitoring
- Measures to decrease secondary injury.
- Mild hypothermia
- Antibiotic prophylaxis
- Antiseizure treatment
- Deep venous thrombosis (DVT) prophylaxis
- Prevention of stress ulcers.

COMPLICATIONS OF TBI

- *Neurological:*
  - *Seizures:* Early or late
  - *Impaired cognition:* Attention deficits, personality changes, and impaired memory
  - Spasticity
  - *Cranial nerve palsies:*
    - Olfactory
    - Trigeminal

- Facial
- Vestibulocochlear
- Neuropathic pain
- Hydrocephalus
- Early or late CSF fistula
- Deficits/coma/brain death
- *Endocrine*:
  - Diabetes insipidus
- *Infective*:
  - Meningitis
  - Intracranial abscess
  - Subdural empyema
  - Aspiration pneumonia
  - Urinary tract infection
- Cushing's ulcers
- DVT and pulmonary embolism (PE).

OUTCOME OF TRAUMATIC BRAIN INJURY

Long-term predictors of survival with TBI:
- *Age:* A linear increase in mortality with age
- Worse prognosis in men
- Adverse outcomes are directly related to injury scores.
- Pupillary response
  - Worse prognosis if bilateral impairment or unilateral with no pupillary reaction
- *Glasgow Coma Scale:*
  - A linear increase in mortality when GCS increases from 3 to 15.
  - *GCS of 3:* Mortality is 80–90%
  - *GCS of 8:* Mortality is 25%
- *Injury assessment on CT scan: A poor prognosis if:*
  - Presence of subarachnoid hemorrhage
  - Extensive diffuse injury
  - Massive focal injury

CASE REPORTS FOR FURTHER DISCUSSION

Case 1: A 38-year-old man was repeatedly hit on the head by fists and kicks for an uncertain time until he escaped. There was no loss of consciousness, but the patient has no recollection of the beating. Several hours later, he arrived at the hospital with a GCS of 15, complaining of blurred left-eye vision. On examination, he had a minor contusion over the right eye. The clinical examination and X-ray were negative. The patient returned to the ER two days later. He complained of increasing headaches, nausea,

CHAPTER 43 Management of Traumatic Brain Injury

vomiting, and difficulty in upper limb coordination. The CT scan revealed a nose fracture but no intracranial injury. Neuropsychometric assessment revealed impaired recent memory, impaired executive function, impaired attention, and slow response to visual stimuli. *If this patient were to undergo exploration and reduction of the nasal fracture, what would be the anesthetic concerns? Will you delay surgery? For how long? What are the risks?*

Case 2: An 18-year-old boy presented to the ER with a stab injury to the head. He complained of increasing headaches and vomiting. On examination, the patient was hemodynamically stable. He was able to move both the upper and lower extremities. There was a 20 cm-long knife that was deeply embedded in the skull. The CT scan revealed the blade embedded about 5 cm in the occipital lobe. *The patient is due for a craniotomy to remove the knife, so what are your concerns? How will you intubate this patient?*

Case 3: A 17-year-old female patient was involved in a motor vehicle accident. She had sustained multiple injuries and was intubated on-site, sedated, and mechanically ventilated. On arrival at the ER, her GCS was 5. She was hemodynamically stable, able to breathe spontaneously, with bilateral breath sounds and basal rales on the left side. She had bilateral flexion response to pain, and the pupils were equal and reactive. The CT scan revealed bilateral frontotemporal contusions, hematoma, laceration of the left occipital lobes, and extensive cerebral edema but no mid-line shift. Investigations revealed left basal lung contusion, a contained splenic rupture, fracture of the mandible and clavicle, and displacement of the distal epiphysis of the radius. None of these injuries were to be treated surgically immediately. She was transferred to the neuro-intensive care unit (ICU) for conservative management. Her hemoglobin was 8.4 g%. However, 24 hours later, the left pupil dilated, the CT scan showed worsening edema, and obliteration of the left ventricle and midline shifted to the right. She was posted for an emergent left decompressive craniotomy. *Given the seriousness of her injuries, how would you manage her anemia? Would you anticipate coagulation problems? If excessive intra-operative bleeding occurs, how will you manage coagulation following TBI?*

Case 4: A 22-year-old combat soldier was ambushed with AK-47 assault rifles. He was not wearing a helmet. After the incident, he was found lying on the ground bleeding from the head. On arrival at the forward medical post, he was fully conscious. Later, at a tertiary care hospital, his condition deteriorated. He developed anisocoria and lost consciousness. The CT scan showed intracerebral hematoma with mass effect and midline shift, ventricular obliteration. He was due for urgent surgery to remove the hematoma and a decompressive craniectomy. There was no evidence of direct injury to the brain by the bullet. *What is the mechanism* of high-velocity gunshot injury to the tissue? How should these injuries be managed, given that tangential high-velocity gunshot wounds lead to brain edema? When would it be ideal for intubating such a case?

CASE REPORT REFERENCES

Case 1: Staba UC et al. Mild traumatic brain injury: case report. J Psychol Clin Psychiatry. 2015;3(1):00116.

Case 2: Fahde Y et al. Penetrating head trauma: 03 rare cases and literature review. Pan Afr Med J. 2017;28:305.

Case 3: Martiniuc C et al. Polytrauma with severe traumatic brain injury: case report. Romanian Neurosurg. 2010;17(1):108-13.

Case 4: Robles LA. High-velocity gunshot to the head presenting as initial minor head injury: things are not what they seem. Am J Emm Med. 2012; 30(9):2089e5-7.

FURTHER READING

1. Froese I et al. Cerebrovascular Response to Propofol, Fentanyl, and Midazolam in Moderate/Severe Traumatic Brain Injury: A Scoping Systematic Review of the Human and Animal Literature. Neurotrauma Rep. 2020;1(1):100-12.
2. Iaccarino C et al. Management of intracranial hypertension following traumatic brain injury. J Neurosurg Sci. 2021;65(3):219-38.
3. Kumar A et al. Comeback of ketamine: resurfacing facts and dispelling myths. Korean J Anesthesiol. 2021;74(2):103-14.
4. Shriki J et al. Sedation for Rapid Sequence Induction and Intubation of Neurologically Injured Patients. Emerg Med Clin North Am. 2021;39(1):203-16.
5. Svedung Wettervik T et al. Autoregulatory or Fixed Cerebral Perfusion Pressure Targets in Traumatic Brain Injury: Determining Which Is Better in an Energy Metabolic Perspective. J Neurotrauma. 2021;38(14):1969-78.

Vignette: Lincoln's Gunshot Injury

A 41-caliber derringer was used to shoot Abraham Lincoln. The gun had a muzzle velocity of 400 feet(s), which was low compared to other civil war weapons. At postmortem, the lead ball weighed 6.314 g. It was 13.3 mm at the broadest and 7.2 mm front to back. Autopsy findings later revealed that the bullet shattered the skull, carried bone fragments deep into the wound, punctured the lateral sinus, and entered the occipital lobe and the lateral ventricle. It crossed the mid-line to be lodged in the right frontal white matter. There was also a large contralateral subdural hematoma, and the ventricles were found to be full of blood.

Immediately after he was shot, Lincoln was rendered unconscious. He was found to be pulseless and was not breathing. Whether he had arrested right away remains controversial. Within an hour, his left pupil had dilated. Lincoln was transferred to the Petersen House across from the Ford Theater. On reaching the house, he was cold, suggesting he was in shock. The surgeons repeatedly probed his skull wound and kept removing blood clots from his skull to prevent pressure from building in his brain. His breathing was labored, and he initially responded to clot removal. By the third hour, his face twitched, and his pupils dilated. His pulse ceased nine hours after the injury. As he closed Lincoln's eyes for the last time, Edwin Stanton said the famous words, "Now he belongs to history."

It is now generally believed that Lincoln would survived with modern treatment possibly with a good outcome.

Chapter 44

Brain Herniation

INTRODUCTION

Treatment of brain herniation requires urgent and effective interventions. However, many treatment modalities, both medical and surgical, fail to impact the outcome in rigorous prospective case-controlled studies. The benefits of monitoring and pharmacological interventions also remain somewhat unproven. However, the lack of proof does not imply the ineffectiveness of the treatment. It could reflect the factors that affect the outcomes that are challenging to control in clinical trials. The key goals in managing impending herniation are early recognition, expeditious reduction of ICP, and restoring cerebral perfusion and tissue oxygenation. Urgent surgery is needed to treat the precipitating causes, such as intracranial bleeding, malignant infarction, or hydrocephalus. The ICP should be kept below 22 mm Hg, and the cerebral perfusion pressure should be maintained at 60–70 mm Hg. It is necessary to prevent secondary injury due to hypoxia, hypotension, electrolyte imbalance, hyper-/hypoglycemia, seizures, or infection. A protocol-driven multidisciplinary team approach is required to improve the chances and quality of survival.

NEUROANESTHETIC CONCERNS

- Pathology of brain herniation:
  - Monro-Kellie Doctrine
  - Cerebral edema
  - Herniation Syndromes:
    - Sub-Falcine
    - Transtentorial
    - Central
    - Upward transtentorial
    - Tonsillar
- Care for raised ICP
- ICP monitoring
- Specific management:
  - Osmotic diuresis
  - Steroids and loop diuretics

- Pharmacological burst suppression
- Hypothermia
- Decompressive craniotomy.

PATHOLOGY OF BRAIN HERNIATION

Monro-Kellie Doctrine

The net intracranial volume is the sum of three incompressible components: (1) brain tissue (85%); (2) Blood (10%), of which the venous blood is 7%, and arterial blood is 3%; and (3) cerebrospinal fluid (CSF 5%). Expansion of any component's volume is possible if another component's volume is reduced. Otherwise, it increases intracranial pressure (ICP) with a corresponding reduction in cerebral perfusion pressure (CPP). Resulting in a cycle of increasing edema, leading to an increase in tissue volume, increasing ICP, decreasing CPP, increasing ischemia, and increasing edema. Either edema, CSF, or blood volume has to be reduced to interrupt this cycle. Alternatively, the skull has to be breached by a decompressive craniectomy to permit tissue expansion.

Cerebral Edema

Cerebral edema is an increase in the water content of the brain tissue. The brain tissue water content differs in gray (80%) and white matter (68%). Radiological evidence of edema can be detected when the water content of the gray matter increases by 2%. Still, an increase of almost 9% is required to see edema in the white matter.

Types of Cerebral Edema

- *Cytotoxic brain edema* is the swelling of cells due to the failure of ionic (Na^+/K^+) pumps. Typically, it is seen with hypoxic–ischemic brain injuries. It affects both gray and white matter. On imaging, the distinction between the two is lost. The blood-brain barrier (BBB) remains intact. The fluid increase is mainly intracellular water and Na^+. The extracellular fluid volume is not increased. It responds poorly to steroid treatment, but osmotic diuretics might be transiently effective.
- *Vasogenic brain edema* is due to the disruption of the BBB near tumors, trauma, hematoma, or abscesses. The fluid collects mainly in the interstitium. It predominantly affects the white matter, enhancing the contrast between the gray and the white matter in imaging studies. The edema fluid is rich in proteins. Steroid treatment is effective, but the response to osmotic diuretics may be poor if barrier permeability is extensively compromised.
- *Mixed edema* has the features of both cytotoxic and vasogenic edema.
- *Interstitial edema:* Periventricular edema due to leakage of CSF is seen with hydrocephalus. The fluid collects in the extracellular space.

The BBB is intact. The fluid is protein depleted. The edema responds poorly to steroids or with minimal response to osmotic diuretics.
- *Hydrostatic brain edema* is due to increased arterial pressure and impaired autoregulation. The BBB is intact such that the edema fluid is protein depleted. The water and Na$^+$ content of the interstitial tissue is increased. Edema is seen in white matter tracts. The edema responds poorly to steroids or with minimal response to osmotic diuretics.
- *Hypo-osmolal edema* is due to a decrease in serum osmolality, such as hyponatremia. It can also occur with SIADH (syndrome of inappropriate antidiuretic hormone secretion), diabetic ketoacidosis, hypotonic fluids, and rapid correction of hyponatremia. An increase in water content predominantly affects the white matter tracts. The edema responds poorly to steroids or with minimal response to osmotic diuretics.

Primary and Secondary Injuries

Primary injury represents direct injury to the neural tissue during the impact, such as avulsion, contusion, or laceration. *Secondary injury* represents the progressive loss of neural functions due to indirect mechanisms such as hypoxia, hypoperfusion, or edema. These mechanisms trigger a complex neurochemical cascade that eventually leads to cell death.
- *Ischemic brain injury:* Transient cerebral hypoperfusion is a common clinical entity. Syncope may affect 3-4% of the population and increases with age and debility. Global cerebral hypoperfusion after cardiac arrest results in significant morbidity and mortality. Acute severe hypotension can cause watershed lesions between adjacent arterial irrigation.
- *Cell vulnerability to hypoxia and ischemia:* White matter is more tolerant of ischemia. The third, fifth, and sixth layers of gray matter, the Ammon's horn, the hippocampus, globus pallidus, the Purkinje cells, and dentate nuclei in the cerebellum, and inferior olives are vulnerable to hypoxia.
- *Watershed regions of the brain:*
    - A Watershed lesion between the anterior cerebral artery (ACA) and middle cerebral arteries (MCA) causes transcortical motor aphasia. If bilateral, it causes weakness of the upper extremities.
    - A watershed lesion between the posterior cerebral artery (PCA) and MCA causes transcortical sensory aphasia. If bilateral, it causes cortical blindness.
    - Deep watershed infarcts generally lie between the lenticulostriate artery (LSA) and the MCA **(Fig. 1)**, present with hemiplegia, and typically carry a poor prognosis.

Herniation Syndromes (Table 1)
- The skull is divided into supra- and infratentorial compartments by meningeal investments. The falx cerebri divides the skull into left

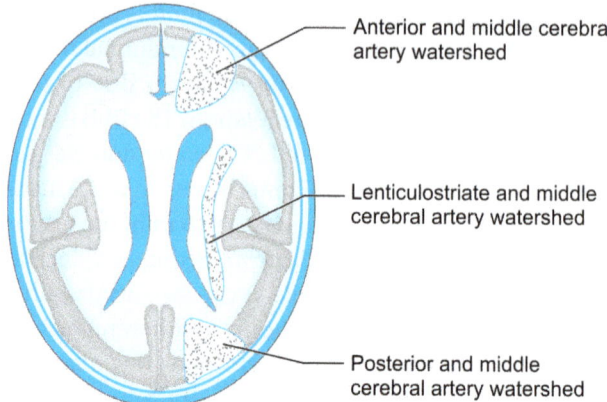

Fig. 1: Watershed zone in the cerebral circulation.

Table 1: Mechanisms and consequences of brain herniation (See Further reading 4)

Herniation	Mechanism	Effect
Subfalcine:		
• Herniation of cingulate gyrus under anterior falx cerebri • **Most common herniation**	Anterior cerebral artery compression or stroke	• Contralateral lower limb weakness and weakness of the face • Sensory sparing • *Speech:* Dysarthria/aphasia • Urinary incontinence
	Ischemia or infarction of cingulate gyrus	• Weakness of the lower limbs • Cerebral edema • Compression of foramen of Monro • Ipsilateral ventricular compression • Contralateral hydrocephalus • Increased ICP • Predispose to other types of herniations
Transtentorial herniation:		
• Temporal lobe herniation • Caudal displacement of hippocampus and uncus • Obliteration of the quadrigeminal cistern • Second most common herniation	CN III palsy	• Initial constriction then dilation of pupil • Ptosis • Lateral downward deviation of the eye • Fixed dilated pupils
	Compression and stroke of distal posterior cerebral (Calcarine) artery	• *Visual symptoms:* Impaired vision, diplopia, reading and facial recognition impaired • Contralateral homonymous hemianopia • Impaired response to visual threats • Infraction of the temporal and occipital lobes

Contd...

Contd...

Transtentorial herniation:		
	Compression of aqueduct of Silvius	• Hydrocephalus • Increased ICP • Worsening herniation
	Ipsilateral peduncular compression	Contralateral weakness
	Compression of thalamus and brain stem	• Respiratory abnormalities • Fixed unequal pupils • Impaired consciousness

Central herniation:		
• Both temporal lobes herniate through tentorial notch • All basal cisterns are obliterated • Results in the classic Cushing's Triad: hypertension, bradycardia, irregular breathing 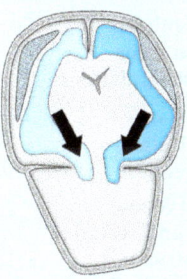	**Compression of thalamus and upper brain stem**	• Impaired consciousness • Abnormal breathing • Fixed unequal pupils
	Compression of CN III, thalamus, and hypothalamus; posterior cerebral artery occlusion, hypothalamic and basal infractions	• Impaired consciousness • *Abnormal breathing:* Deep sighs or Cheyne-Stokes breathing • Meiosis 1–3 mm • Hyperactive pain response • Absent pain localization • **Decorticate posture**
	Compression of the mid brain and upper pons	• Unconscious • Hyperventilating • Irregular pupils fixed 4–5 mm • Extensor plantar reflex • **Decerebrate posture**
	Late compression of the brain stem	• Absent corneal reflex • Absent oculovestibular reflex • Absent oculocephalic reflex • **Decerebrate posturing**
	Compression of the medulla	• Flaccidity • Fixed unreactive pupils • Slow breathing • **Brain death**

Contd...

Contd...

Cerebellar tonsillar herniation:

• Downward displacement of the cerebral peduncles through the foramen magnum • Compression of the cisterna magna 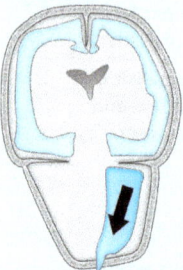	**CSF flow obstruction**	• Acute hydrocephalus • Low spinal CSF pressure
	Posterior cerebral, vertebral, and anterior spinal arteries	Brainstem and cerebellar ischemia and stroke
	Compression of the brainstem and medulla oblongata	• Deconjugate eye movements • Lower cranial nerve palsies • Respiratory arrest • Cardiac arrest

Transalar herniation:

• Middle cranial fossa content herniation over the greater wing of sphenoid bone. • Rare	**Descending:** Frontal lobe herniates	Orbital gyri herniation early
	Ascending: Temporal lobe herniates	Compresses the internal carotid artery
	Occurs with Subfalcine or transtentorial herniations	See above

Upward transtentorial herniation:

• Tissue impacted in incisura • Sudden decrease in ICP with ventricular tap • **Extremely rare** 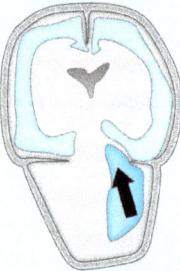	**III ventricular obstruction**	• Acute hydrocephalus • Increased ICP
	Cerebral venous outflow and posterior and superior cerebellar arterial occlusion	• Nausea, vomiting, headache • Dizziness, vertigo • Loss of coordination • Ataxia
	Cerebellar compression	• Cerebellar signs • Impaired movement and coordination
	Brain stem compression	• Unconsciousness • Respiratory abnormalities • Cardiovascular instability • Loss of brainstem reflexes

(CSF: cerebrospinal fluid; ICP: intracranial pressure; PCA: posterior cerebral artery)

and right compartments. The tentorium divides it into supra- and infratentorial compartments. The latter two communicate through the tentorial hiatus. In addition, herniation can occur through the foramen magnum and any skull defect.
- There are nerves, arteries, and veins that run on the edges of the meningeal investments that can be compressed to cause nerve deficits or injuries or obstruct flow in blood vessels to cause injury.

- CSF venous return can be impeded by herniation of brain tissue resulting in hydrocephalus or isolated ventricular dilation. Obliteration of ventricles and cisterns is often seen in the early stages of herniation.
- Finally, direct compression or ischemia of vital structures in the midbrain, pons, and medulla is seen in later stages, usually with fatal outcomes unless promptly treated.

Clinical Features of Raised ICP

- *In adults:* Early morning headache, nausea, vomiting, photophobia, altered consciousness, and focal deficits. The examination might reveal increased blood pressure, decreased heart rate, papilledema, and changes in respiration. Consciousness in adults is usually by the Glasgow Coma Scale (GCS, **Table 2**). *GCS can help predict the outcome after cardiac arrest.* A good recovery can be anticipated if, at 24 hours, the GCS motor score improves by 3 or eye movement improves by 2. Recovery of pupillary reaction within 6 hours after an arrest also predicts a good outcome.

  Cushing's triad: Bradycardia, respiratory irregularities, widened pulse pressure (increased systolic and decreased diastolic pressure).

  Respiratory patterns with brain herniation:
  - *Cheyne–Stokes:* Increased ICP or metabolic causes
  - *Hyperventilation:* Brainstem dysfunction or functional
  - *Cluster breathing:* High medullary or lower pontine lesion
  - *Apneustic breathing:* Basilar artery stroke.
  - *Ataxic breathing:* Medullary lesion or often preterminal
- *In pediatric patients:* The best eye and best motor are assessed the same way as in adults. However, the best verbal response is judged by the nature of crying: Inconsolable (2), intermittently consolable (3), and consolable (4). Alternately, interactions can be graded as restless (4), moaning (3), and inappropriate (2).
- *In infants:* Raised ICP usually presents with bulging of the fontanelle, dehiscence of the sutures, increased head circumference, and a high-pitched cry.

Table 2: Glasgow coma scale.

Score	Best motor	Best verbal	Eye opening
1	None	None	None
2	Extensor (decerebrate)	Incomprehensible	To pain
3	Flexor (decorticate)	Inappropriate	To speech
4	Pain withdrawal	Confused	Spontaneous
5	Pain localization	Oriented	
6	Obeys		

Care for Raised ICP

- Head elevation 15–30° when possible
- Prevent secondary injury. Avoid
  - Fever >38.5°
  - Hypoxia
  - Hypercapnia
  - Hyper or hypoglycemia
  - Pain
  - Ongoing seizure activity
  - Avoid hypotonic fluids.
  - Electrolyte imbalance
  - Avoid hypotension SBP <90 mm Hg.
- Hypertonic mannitol or saline infusions
- Target serum osmolality 309 mOsm/L; may require fluid restriction and diuretics.
- Adequate sedation and muscle relaxation.

SPECIFIC MEASURES

ICP Monitoring

- *Direct methods*
  - External ventricular drain
  - Lumbar CSF drain
  - Other approaches are less-used probes/micro-transducers
  - Intraparenchymal
  - Epidural
  - Subdural
  - Subarachnoid
- *Indirect methods*
  - *Clinical exam:* Vital signs, breathing, posture, coma scale, and pupils
  - *MRI and CT:* Alteration, distortion, and displacement of brain structures
  - Pupillometry
  - Tympanic membrane displacement
  - Optic nerve sheath diameter
  - *Transcranial Doppler:* Assessment of pulsatility index
  - Near-infrared spectroscopy with decreased oxygen saturation
  - Electroencephalogram.

Hyperventilation

Temporizing measures to decrease ICP and vasoconstrictor response are lost over time as CSF pH corrects. Intubation and ventilation are also indicated to protect the airway; with irregular breathing, hypoxia; and/or hypercarbia. Ventilation decreases CO_2, causes vasoconstriction, and decreases intracranial blood volume.

- *Advantages:* Improves oxygenation, decreases ICP, and permits deep barbiturate sedation. Inverse steal blood flow is directed to ischemic regions, called "Robin Hood syndrome".
- *Disadvantages:* Stress of intubations, coughing, and bucking during tube care can raise ICP; positive-pressure ventilation can increase intrathoracic pressure and hence ICP; it can shift the oxyhemoglobin dissociation curve to the left to decrease O_2 unloading and may precipitate cerebral ischemia in healthy regions of the brain; The trend in treatment is avoiding aggressive hyperventilation except temporarily in an emergency.

Steroid and Loop Diuretics
- Steroids are ineffective in most situations except for tumor-induced increases in ICP.
- Loop diuretics, such as furosemide, can increase free water clearance to help reduce edema. When the diuretic is given with mannitol, it can decrease cardiovascular loading, and with steroids, it can decrease sodium retention.

Pharmacological Burst Suppression
Pentobarbital is the drug of choice and is titrated to burst suppression.
- *Advantages:* Provide sedation needed with intubation; decreases abnormal excitation and even normal excitation-related metabolic activity; vasoconstriction decreases intracranial volume; redistributes blood flow to ischemic regions; scavenges free radicals; lysosomal stabilization; reduces cerebral edema.
- *Disadvantages:* Benefits unproven; cardiovascular depression; prevents neurological examination; delays declaration of brain death; prolongs the need for ventilation and the risk of respiratory infections..

Hypothermia
- *Rationale:* For each °C reduction in brain temperature, the $CMRO_2$ decreases by about 6%. A target core temperature of 32–34°C for 24 hours should be instituted soon after diagnosis.
- *Benefits:* Hypothermia decreases $CMRO_2$, decreases ICP, decreases CBF, decreases CSF formation rate, and is the only clinically proven neuroprotective intervention.
- *Indications:*
  - Cardiac arrest after the return of spontaneous circulation
  - Neonatal Hypoxia/ischemia
  - *Others are unproven:* Traumatic brain injury, stroke, aneurysm surgery, spinal cord injury, and hepatic encephalopathy.
- *Relative contraindications for hypothermia:* Significant intracranial bleeding, hypotension refractory to treatment, infections, coagulopathy, pregnancy.

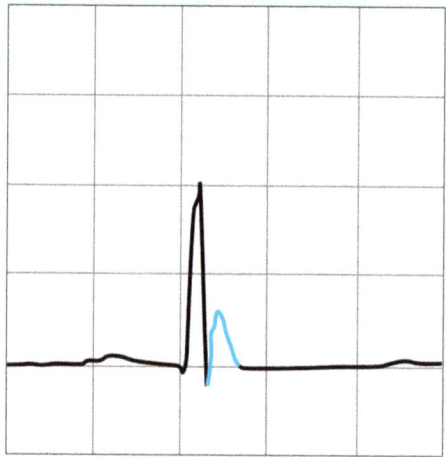

Fig. 2: Elevation of the J point or Osborn wave (blue).

- *Methods*:
  - Surface cooling devices are commonly used. Icepacks over major arteries can lower the temperature.
  - Vital signs are monitored; ventilation and cardiovascular support are provided to maintain desired $PaCO_2$ and blood pressure.
  - Bradycardia <40 may require treatment.
  - *Osborn waves* are seen with hypothermia. Their significance is unknown. Osborn wave is the upward deflection of the J point which is the junction of R and S waves in the lateral leads **(Fig. 2)**.
  - Check the skin for frostbite.
    - Rewarming is gradual over 4–8 hours. Maintain paralytics and sedation to decrease the chances of shivering until 35°C.
    - Hypothermia is terminated if severe hypotension, malignant arrhythmias, or increased bleeding are encountered.
- *Complications*:
  - Seizures are common.
  - Myoclonic status epilepticus carries a grave prognosis.
  - Pulmonary infections
  - Deep venous thrombosis and pulmonary embolism
  - If the coma after injury lasts for >6 hours, the prognosis is poor, and only 22% are likely to regain consciousness.

Decompressive Craniectomy

Indications, see chapter 45 for details:
- Traumatic brain injuries
- Malignant stroke

- Subarachnoid hemorrhage
- Intractable cerebral edema.

CASE REPORTS FOR FURTHER DISCUSSION

Case 1: A 31-year-old male with no significant medical history sustained a sudden cardiac arrest. CPR was immediately started. Medical responders found him in ventricular fibrillation (VF), and he was defibrillated. His family history was significant for a sibling with sick sinus syndrome requiring a pacemaker placement at the age of 22 years. Laboratory and toxicological screens were negative. Since no neurological recovery was observed after hemodynamic stabilization, hypothermia protocol with a targeted cooling to 32°C was initiated. As cooling began, ventricular fibrillation runs required frequent cardioversions. Isoproterenol infusion was started to suppress ectopy and enable hypothermia. *What are the contraindications of deliberate hypothermia? What could be the rationale for the use of isoproterenol? How could it have helped? If there is hemodynamic instability, could you continue with hypothermia?*

Case 2: A 62-year-old man with a history of diabetes, hypertension, and chronic renal failure sustained a cardiac arrest. Basic life support was rapidly instituted. However, due to a lack of definable rhythm, no cardioversion was done, and chest compressions continued. He regained spontaneous rhythm an hour later. His biochemical screen showed severe hyperglycemia and hyperkalemia. Blood urea nitrogen (BUN), serum creatinine, and cardiac enzymes were also raised. Coagulation tests, including the platelet count, were in the normal range. Chest X-ray (CXR) revealed bilateral pulmonary edema, and a non-contrast CT did not show a hemorrhage. Hypothermia protocol using surface cooling with ice packs and a cold fluid irrigation blanket, with a target temperature of 33°C, was initiated. A few hours later, the patient had a bout of epistaxis. The coagulation screen now revealed a platelet count of $111 \times 10^9/L$ with an international normalized ratio (INR) of 1.23 and an activated partial thromboplastin time (APTT) of 41 seconds. Vitamin K and fresh frozen plasma (FFP) were given. *What is the etiology of coagulation failure with hypothermia? What are the possible contributory factors in this case? How will you investigate this problem?*

Case 3: A 43-year-old woman with no significant medical history sustained a sudden pulseless cardiac arrest. The return of circulation took an estimated total of 39–59 minutes. Over the next hour, her hemodynamics stabilized. Her pupils were pinpoint and unresponsive to light; however, her corneal reflex was intact. The laboratory tests were within normal limits. Deliberate hypothermia protocol was initiated with cold saline infusion and surface cooling to a target temperature of 33°C. During hypothermia, she had a bout of upper gastrointestinal bleeding, which responded to endoscopic treatment with epinephrine. The patient was rewarmed at 0.3°C/h. She developed polyuria with 8 L urine output on the third post-treatment day. Her serum sodium increased from 142 to 195 mEq/L. MRI revealed severe brain edema but no hemorrhage. She responded to desmopressin; however, there was no neurological improvement. *What are the causes of diuresis in ICU patients? How will you diagnose diabetes insipidus? What is nephrogenic DI? What is the treatment of choice? When is the treatment started?*

CASE REPORT REFERENCES

Case 1: Badertscher P et al. Case report: electrical storm during induced hypothermia in a patient with early repolarization. BMC Cardiovasc Disorders. 2017;17:277.

Case 2: Cho HJ et al. Therapeutic hypothermia complicated by spontaneous brain stem hemorrhage. Am J Emergency Med. 2013;31:266.e1-3.

Case 3: Choi SS et al. Unexpected fatal hypernatremia after successful cardiopulmonary resuscitation with therapeutic hypothermia: a case report. J Korean Med Sci. 2012;27:329-31.

FURTHER READING

1. Desai A. Hyperosmolar therapy: a century of treating cerebral edema. Cl in Neurol Neurosurg. 2021; 206: p. 106704.
2. El Hazzaz R et al. [Impact of the use of systemic corticosteroid therapy on the effectiveness of immune checkpoint inhibitors]. Bull Cancer. 2021;108(6): 635-42.
3. Esquenazi Y et al. Critical Care Management of cerebral edema in brain tumors. J Intensive Care Med. 2017;32(1):15-24.
5. Maiese K. Brain Herniation: Patient education Merck Manual Professional Version 2019 https://www.msdmanuals.com/en-in/professional/neurologic-disorders/coma-and-impaired-consciousness/brain-herniation
6. Riveros Gilardi B et al. Types of Cerebral Herniation and their imaging features. Radiographics. 2019;39(6):1598-610.
7. Tadevosyan A et al. Brain herniation and intracranial hypertension. Neurol Clin. 2021;39(2):293-318.

Vignette: Edwin Smith Papyrus: Head Injuries in Ancient Egypt

The Edwin Smith papyrus was a 15.3-foot long scroll dating back to 1650–1550 BCE. It was purchased by Edwin Smith, an American Egyptologist, in 1862. The scroll contained 569 lines in 26 columns but has since been cut down. The papyrus was transcribed by mostly one person with the help of an assistant. The text ends mid-sentence suggesting that it was a copy of an earlier text. The text focuses on trauma and surgery, indicating that it was a manual for military use. It contains 48 illustrative case histories, 27 of which are neurological. These include deep scalp wounds and skull fractures. It describes the examination of head injuries by inspection and palpation. It classifies their outcomes as (1) one I can treat, (2) one I am content with, and (3) one that cannot be treated.

Chapter 45

Decompressive Craniectomy

INTRODUCTION

Decompressive craniectomy is the emergent removal of a part of the skull. It decreases the pressure on the brain tissue to improve tissue perfusion. It is usually done when there is an inexorable expansion of tissue volume due to edema refractory to medical treatment. Common indications include severe traumatic brain injury, a massive stroke, and aneurysmal subarachnoid hemorrhage.

NEUROANESTHETIC CONCERNS

- *Medical management of raised ICP.*
- *Decompressive craniectomy*
- *Indications*
- *Anesthetic concerns:*
  - The urgency of the operation
  - Potential or actual ongoing herniation
  - Major neurological morbidity
- Comorbidities
- *Intraoperative:*
  - Possibly intubated and sedated.
  - Monitoring
  - Tight brain
  - Blood loss
  - ICP management
- Postoperative computed tomography (CT) examination
- Postoperative care
- Potential complications.

Medical Management of Increased ICP

- The principles of conservative management apply throughout the perioperative care of patients undergoing decompressive craniectomy.
- Therapeutic intervention is usually necessary with ICP >20 mm Hg.
- *General measures:*
  - Rule out any other causes of raised ICP, such as pain, hypoxia, hypoventilation, impaired venous drainage, hypertension, or hypotension.

- Elevate the head to 30–45° to increase venous return.
- Guarded CSF drainage using a ventricular drain under monitoring.
- Maintain a target cerebral perfusion pressure (CPP) >50 mm Hg.
- Consider sedation, intubation, and mechanical ventilation.
- *Specific interventions:*
  - Optimize ventilation, avoid hypercapnia (target $PaCO_2$ of 30–35 mm Hg) and hypoxia (PaO_2 of 150–200 mm Hg)
  - Increase sedation and paralysis as needed to ventilate effectively.
  - Check arterial blood gas (ABG) values for adequate ventilation, hematocrit (27–33%), and glucose 140–180 mg/dL.
  - Mannitol (0.25–1 g/kg, q 6 hours) with furosemide (10 mg q 6 hours) if needed.
  - If the ICP remains high and serum osmolarity is <320 mOsm, consider using hypertonic saline (3% saline 20–25 mL/h or 10–20 mL bolus of 23.4%).
- *Management of refractory cases:* Reevaluate the case with CT or MRI. Rule out status epilepticus with EEG. Consider hyperventilation, aggressive diuretics, deep anesthesia, hypothermia, decompressive surgery, and controlled hypertension.
- *Hyperventilation:*
  - *Advantages:* Hyperventilation aims at $PaCO_2$ of 30 mm Hg and provides a temporary measure to decrease acute increase in ICP. Hyperventilation is of immediate benefit in the setting of brain herniation. Increased ventilation could also increase oxygenation and favorably redistribute blood to ischemic brain regions (inverse steal).
  - *Disadvantages:* Excessive hyperventilation ($PaCO_2$ of <30 mm Hg) could lead to cerebral ischemia, decrease cardiac output due to increase intrathoracic pressure, decrease critical organ perfusion, increase neuronal excitability, increase release of excitatory neurotransmitters, increase in seizures, increase in platelet adhesion and aggregation, and result in poor offloading of oxygen in tissues due to a left shift in the oxygen-hemoglobin dissociation curve. Thus, the general trend is to limit hyperventilation to emergent situations with potential brain herniation. Additional monitoring, such as jugular venous oximetry, can guide prolonged hyperventilation.
- *Hyperosmolar agents:* The two agents used are mannitol (20 and 25%) and hypertonic saline (3, 7.5, and 23.4%) **(Table 1)**. Mannitol decreases ICP by the following mechanisms:
  - With intact autoregulation, the decrease in viscosity causes vasoconstriction to decrease blood volume and ICP.

Table 1: Comparison between mannitol and hypertonic saline.

	Mannitol	Hypertonic saline
Dose	1–1.5 g/kg can be repeated q 6–8 hours	• 3% NaCl 150 mL • 7.5% 75 mL • 23.4% 30 mL
Target	Serum osmolality of 300–320 mOsm	• Na 145–150 mmol/L • Osmolarity 300–320 mOsm
Onset	10–20 minutes	5 minutes
Duration	3–6 hours	2–12 hours
BBB penetration	If breached	Yes
Rebound	Yes	No, but it has been reported
Peripheral vascular irritation	No	No, with 3%, but CVL needed for higher concentration
Relative contraindications	CHF Renal failure if the osmolar gap is >20 or serum osmolarity >320 mOsm	CHF, severe hyponatremia: Rapid Na infusion and central pontine myelinolysis
Side effects	*Rapid infusion:* Fluid overload, CHF, acidosis, and hyperkalemia *Others:* With doses >2.5 g/day ARF	Renal failure, hypernatremia, hyperchloremia, acidosis, hypokalemia, cardiac depression, heart failure, ARF, infusion-related hypotension; coagulopathy
Precautions	• Infuse over 20–60 minutes • Use filter • Monitor osmolarity and osmolar gap*	• Monitor serum sodium • Preferably infuse via CVL

*Osmolar gap = Measured osmolarity – estimated osmolarity.
(ARF: acute renal failure; BBB: blood–brain barrier; CHF: chronic heart failure; CVL: central venous line)

- It increases the serum osmotic pressure to shift water from the intracellular/interstitial compartment to the vascular compartment. Over time, it decreases ICP further by withdrawing fluid from the brain parenchyma.
- The decrease in ICP augments the net cerebral perfusion pressure and increases blood flow. Tissue perfusion is also improved by the reduction of blood viscosity due to hemodilution.
• *Mannitol:*
  - The typical dose of mannitol is 1 g/kg (range 0.5-1.5 g/kg) over 30 minutes every 4-6 hours.
  - The onset of the effect is 5-15 minutes after infusion. The Peak effect is in 20-60 minutes after infusion.
  - Effective in TBI when the CPP <70 mm Hg.

- Intermittent mannitol boluses are more effective than continuous infusions.
- Concerns with mannitol:
  - Mannitol infusions are generally safe.
  - The decrease in ICP lasts 3–6 hours.
  - Rapid infusion of mannitol due to volume expansion may lead to congestive heart failure in patients with impaired cardiac reserve.
  - Volume expansion can cause a transient rise in ICP.
  - The rapid influx of intracellular fluid into the intravascular compartment can cause hyperkalemia and acidosis.
  - Increases in ICP with mannitol infusions can occur when the blood–brain barrier (BBB) is impaired. Vasogenic cerebral edema and intracranial hypertension due to hyperemia can worsen with mannitol treatment.
  - Renal functions can be impaired if serum osmolality exceeds 320 mOsm due to osmotic nephrosis. The risk can be reduced if the osmotic gap (difference between calculated to measured osmolality) is <20 mOsm.
  - Mannitol, phenytoin, and steroids combined can lead to hyperosmolar non-ketoacidosis.
  - Rebound ICP increase occurs 12 hours after discontinuation of mannitol infusion. Ideally, mannitol infusions have to be tapered slowly.
  - Mannitol could delay the detection of diabetes insipidus.
- *Hypertonic saline:*
  - Three percent hypertonic saline can be given through a peripheral line, but a central venous line is necessary for 7.5% or 23.4%. Local complications include venous phlebitis, thrombosis, tissue ischemia, and necrosis.
  - Vascular expansion is beneficial in hypovolemic shock.
  - ICP decreases within 5 minutes and lasts for 12 hours.
  - Rebound increase unlikely.
  - *Disadvantages:* Complications increase with higher concentrations; these include:
    - Electrolyte imbalance: Hypernatremia, hyperchloremia, hypokalemia, metabolic acidosis
    - Volume expansion can lead to congestive heart failure.
    - Infusion-induced hypertension
    - Acute kidney injury
    - Cognitive changes and seizures
    - A rebound increase in ICP is possible but less likely than mannitol.

        - In hyponatremic patients, the rapid hypertonic saline infusion can cause central pontine myelinolysis.
        - Limit the rate of correction of hyponatremia to 12 mEq/L in 12 hours.
- *Steroids:* Steroids, like dexamethasone, reduce ICP with peri-tumor vasogenic edema and pseudotumor cerebri. For other conditions, such as TBI, steroids have little benefit and can increase mortality.
- *Hypothermia:* Moderate hypothermia (32–35°C) decreases cerebral metabolic rate, cerebral blood flow, rate of CSF formation, and intracranial pressure. Therapeutic hypothermia is most useful after ischemic stroke but can increase mortality after TBI. Some improvement in TBI survival is seen in pediatric patients, those in whom hypothermia is initiated within 24 hours or combined with craniectomy.
  Complications: Hypothermia increases the incidence of:
    - Infection, pneumonia, and sepsis
    - Electrolyte imbalance
    - Thrombocytopenia, coagulopathy, intracranial hemorrhage
    - Bradycardia and arrhythmias
    - Rebound increase in ICP if less than 48 hours.
- *Propofol-induced EEG silence* decreases ICP and improves blood flow but does not improve survival. High-dose propofol infusions (100 mg/kg, 48 hours) can result in "propofol infusion syndrome". The syndrome is characterized by lipemia, hyperkalemia, acidosis, rhabdomyolysis, hepatomegaly, kidney, and heart failure. Propofol is a popular sedative-hypnotic in the ICU, but its prolonged use or excessive doses require close monitoring for end-organ dysfunction.
- *Barbiturate coma:* Barbiturates, such as thiopental, pentothal, and phenobarbital, decrease the cerebral metabolic rate of oxygen ($CMRO_2$), reduce cerebral blood flow (CBF), decrease ICP, and cause cerebral vasoconstriction and redistribute blood to ischemic areas. Barbiturates are sedatives and anticonvulsants that prevent secondary brain injury and the rise in ICP due to coughing/bucking or seizure activities. At a cellular level, barbiturates scavenge-free radicals; they decrease the increase in intracellular calcium and stabilize the lysosomal membrane. However, the benefits of barbiturate coma in adults remain unproven. Some benefits are seen in pediatric TBI. Hypotension due to barbiturates could decrease the CPP despite fluid resuscitation and inotropic therapy. Currently, barbiturate coma is used after maximum medical management fails to decrease ICP. These measures include failing to respond to adequate sedation, optimum ventilation, optimum cerebral perfusion, and failure to respond to hypertonic agents. Barbiturate coma under these circumstances is indicated if there is (i) ICP of 20–35 mm Hg for 4 hours, ICP of 36–40 mm Hg for 1 hour, or ICP >40 for 5 minutes.

DECOMPRESSIVE CRANIECTOMY

Definition: Decompressive craniectomy is the excision of a skull segment with dural release to permit tissue expansion and avoid herniation.

- *Indications:*
  - Intractable increase in ICP despite full medical interventions, secondary to:
    - TBI
    - Stroke
    - Intracerebral bleed
    - Subarachnoid hemorrhage
    - Nontraumatic refractory intracranial hypertension
- *The rationale of decompressive craniectomy:*
  - Decrease intracranial pressure.
  - Improve cerebral perfusion.
  - Provide additional space for expansion of edematous brain tissue
  - Prevent herniation of brainstem
- *Preanesthetic review:*
  - Patient profile:
    - History and examination might be limited.
    - Extreme neurological injury
    - Urgent/emergent operation
    - Transfer from intensive care unit (ICU)/emergency room (ER)
    - Patients are usually intubated, sedated, and mechanically ventilated.
    - Patients may be on inotropic support, and measures to lower ICP improve cerebral perfusion.
    - Arterial and venous access may have been established.
    - An adequate level of sedation and paralysis is needed during transfer and positioning to avoid coughing and bucking, which could increase ICP.
    - Comorbidities:
      - Other injuries in the case of TBI
      - Children with Reye's syndrome may have an underlying infection and/or liver failure.
      - Complications expected from ICU stay: Deep venous thrombosis, chest infections, fluid and electrolyte imbalance, and tissue edema.
  - Investigations:
    - ABG to assess ventilation and metabolic status.
    - Complete blood count (CBC), biochemistry, coagulation screen
    - EKG/ECHO review to assess cardiac status.
    - Chest X-ray (CXR) to verify the endotracheal tube position, fluid overload, and lung condition.

CHAPTER 45 Decompressive Craniectomy

- *Monitoring:*
  - Routine monitoring.
  - An arterial line is desirable at induction to ensure close hemodynamic monitoring and frequent arterial gas sampling.
  - ICP monitor might be in-situ.
  - A central venous catheter is desirable for monitoring venous pressure, delivery of hypertonic saline and drugs, and blood volume replacement if needed.
  - Close monitoring of hemodynamic changes and ICP is required during positioning.
  - Monitor urine output to assess the effectiveness of mannitol diuresis.
- *Anesthetic management:*
  - Given the intractable increase in ICP, total intravenous anesthesia with propofol, narcotics, and muscle relaxants is preferable to using volatile anesthetics.
  - To decrease ICP:
    - Ensure adequate sedation, analgesia, and muscle relaxation.
    - Consider hyperventilation, and verify with arterial blood gas analysis.
    - Consider head elevation and use of hypertonic saline or mannitol.
    - Ensure adequate cerebral perfusion pressure.
  - *Blood loss:* Can be substantial due to large incision, bone resection, coagulopathy due to brain injury—
    - Check the history of bleeding, anticoagulation, and anti-platelet drugs.
    - Replace blood with packed cells, fresh frozen plasma (FFP), and platelets.
    - Consider factor VIII concentrate.
    - Consider anti-fibrinolytic treatment with point-of-care coagulation monitoring.
- *Surgical approaches:*
  - Unilateral (anterior or posterior), or bifrontal.
  - Large incision, so skin flap viability is an issue.
  - *The fate of the removed skull:* It might need to be replaced in 6–12 weeks
    - The skull is usually discarded if infected (e.g., due to scalp laceration in TBI).
    - Skull is stored saline in sterile refrigerated containers.
    - Or it is implanted in a subcutaneous pouch.

Postoperative Care

- *Admit to ICU:*
  - Continues with measures to decrease ICP if needed.
  - Continuous vital sign monitoring/EKG monitoring

- Neuro exam/EEG monitoring
        - Input/output monitoring hourly
        - DVT prophylaxis
    - *Medications:*
        - Anticonvulsants
        - Antibiotics
        - Antipyretics
        - Analgesics
        - Steroids
        - Ranitidine/H2 antagonists
    - *Laboratory tests:* CBC, biochemical screen, and ABG

Potential Complications

- Intractable bleeding
- Herniation under a bone edge with injury to brain tissue
- Injury after surgery to a relatively unprotected brain
- *Sunken flap syndrome:* A large craniectomy permits the sinking of the skin and compression of brain tissue with autonomic and neurological symptoms, including seizures.
- *Fluid collection:* Ipsilateral hemisphere, contralateral hemisphere, and interhemispheric - skin breakdown.

PROGNOSIS

- A high incidence (60–80%) of postoperative complications
- For TBI, two-thirds have a poor outcome, and one-third have a good outcome.
- Those who survive have a good neurological outcome.
- *Predictors of poor outcome:*
    - Persistent intracranial hypertension after craniectomy
    - Poor neurological status before surgery.

CASE REPORTS FOR FURTHER DISCUSSION

Case 1: A 16-year-old intoxicated male was brought to the ER with a stab wound in the chest. He was treated for pneumothorax, and the chest tube drained 100 mL of blood, but no other injury was evident. The next day, the patient became incontinent and developed left hemiparesis with neglect and an upgoing plantar reflex. Pupils were bilateral 4 mm reactive. A CT scan revealed an unexpected right 8 × 7 × 7 cm mass with ventricular dilation, midline shift (10 mm), and early uncal herniation. He was intubated and transferred to the neurosurgical intensive care unit. An ICP bolt revealed a pressure of 38 mm Hg and an affected cerebral perfusion pressure of 57 mm Hg. While the CT angiogram of the chest was negative. CT of the

CHAPTER 45 Decompressive Craniectomy

brain revealed an unexpected malignant middle cerebral artery infarction. TTE revealed no cardiac source of emboli. Consequently, the patient was posted for an emergent decompressive craniectomy. *Given the ICP of 38 mm Hg, what measures could you have used, if any, to treat the raised ICP? What is malignant middle cerebral artery infarction? What is the impact of decompressive craniectomy on the outcome of such cases? What precautions will you take, given the precarious state of cerebral perfusion?*

Case 2: A 20-year-old female road traffic accident victim was admitted to the ER with a Glasgow Coma Scale (GCS) score of 9. Her other injuries included a right pneumothorax that required chest tube placement. The CT scan revealed extensive intracranial injuries. These included fractures of the skull base, right temporal and parietal bones, left brain contusions, an inch-sized right frontotemporal epidural hematoma, and a small frontoparietal temporal subdural hematoma. A ventricular drain was placed, and the ICP was measured at 22 mm Hg. An emergent bilateral fronto-temporo-parietal craniectomy was planned. *How will the presence of skull base fractures affect your management of this case? Given the extensive nature of intracranial injuries, how will you prepare for surgery? During surgery, excessive bleeding is noticed, so what are the differential diagnoses? Given the possibility of lung injury, how will you optimize ventilation in the settings of extensive intracranial injuries?*

Case 3: A 58-year-old male presented for L 4–5 hemilaminectomy. His history was significant for hypertension, hyperlipidemia, and stroke with residual right-sided weakness. He was on Plavix and aspirin, which were discontinued before the procedure. On the second postoperative day, he developed sudden-onset hemiparesis with cognitive changes suggesting a right MCA stroke. He was intubated, and subsequent CTA confirmed the provisional diagnosis of large MCA infarction with no significant penumbra. Anticipating a nonsurgical course, he was restarted on aspirin and Lovenox for DVT prophylaxis. However, the next day, he was no longer responsive to pain. An emergency right decompressive hemicraniectomy was undertaken. *How will aspirin and lovenox affect your management? What are the anesthetic considerations at this stage? After an uneventful craniectomy on the eighth postoperative day, the patient's condition deteriorated suddenly, and after imaging, a diagnosis of a sunken flap was made. What is sunken flap syndrome, and how is it treated?*

Case 4: A 38-year-old man presented with a 1-hour history of sudden-onset left hemiplegia. His story was significant for smoking and febrile childhood convulsions. CTA revealed a right MCA infarct with right ICA dissection but no intracranial bleed. Thrombolysis with alteplase (0.9 mg/kg) was started two hours after admission. During the infusion, the condition of the patient deteriorated. A repeat CT scan revealed the extension of the MCA infarction but with no evidence of new bleeding. An immediate decompressive craniectomy was planned. *Given the ongoing thrombolysis, what additional precautions will you take? What additional steps can you take in the postoperative period to improve the outcome?*

CASE REPORT REFERENCES

Case 1: Lammy S et al. Decompressive craniectomy for malignant middle cerebral artery infarction in a 16-year-old boy: a case report. J Med Case Rep. 2016;10:368.

Case 2: Pérez-Alfayate R et al. Primary bilateral fronto-temporo-parietal decompressive craniectomy—an alternative treatment for severe traumatic brain injury: case report and technical note. Clin Case Rep. 2019;7(5):10319.

Case 3: Michael AP et al. Paradoxical herniation following decompressive craniectomy in the subacute setting. Case Rep Neurol Med. 2016; 20909384.

Case 4: Souper N et al. Anesthetic management of a patient with ongoing thrombolytic therapy during decompressive craniectomy: a case report. Anesth and Analg Pract. 2018;11:3048.

FURTHER READING

1. Kirkman MA et al. Challenges in the anesthetic and intensive care management of acute ischemic stroke. J Neurosurg Anesthesiol. 2016;28(3):214-32.
2. Lee JM et al. Factors affecting optimal time of cranioplasty: brain sunken ratio. Korean J Neurotrauma. 2017;13(2):113-8.
3. Liotta EM. Management of cerebral edema, brain compression, and intracranial pressure. Continuum (Minneap Minn). 2021;27(5):1172-200.
4. Robba CF et al. Tier-three therapies for refractory intracranial hypertension in adult head trauma. Minerva Anestesiol. 2021;87(12):1359-66.
5. Venkateswaran et al. Regional cerebral oxygen saturation changes after decompressive craniectomy for malignant cerebral venous thrombosis: a prospective cohort study. J Neurosurg Anesthesiol. 2019;31(2):241-6.

Vignette: The Brain–Heart Rivalry

Since antiquity, the significance of the brain has taken second place to heart. The Egyptians considered the brain to be the marrow of the skull. Almost all the organs were preserved during mummification, but the brain was discarded. The removal was done through the nose, not unlike the modern-day trans-sphenoidal hypophysectomies. On the other hand, the heart was carefully preserved to be weighed in the afterlife. The weight of the heart determined the fate of the individual. Such was the import of the heart. The Greeks carried on the bias in favor of the heart. For them, the heart was the seat of the soul. Even today, we use the phrase "to learn by heart," which reveals the bias, knowing that cognition resides in the brain.

Chapter 46: Cerebrospinal Fluid Leak

INTRODUCTION

A cerebrospinal fluid (CSF) leak is due to a dural tear in the cranium or the spine. The loss of CSF due to the leak results in intracranial hypotension. The hypotension is associated with a CSF pressure of less than 60 mm H_2O or 4.5 mm Hg in the lateral position. CSF leaks are seen in 5/100,000 population. The most frequent cause of CSF leak is trauma which is sometimes iatrogenic. Such leaks predispose to infections. They typically present with postural headaches and neurological symptoms due to pressure on cranial nerves. CSF leaks may resolve spontaneously with medical management or require the placement of a CSF drain or operative dural repair.

NEUROANESTHETIC CONCERNS

- CSF dynamics
- CSF fistula
- Cerebral hypotension
- *Preoperative assessment:*
  - Postural headache
  - Hypertension
  - Cranial nerve involvement
  - Infection
- Conservative management
- Blood patch
- Surgical repair
  - Role of hypotension
  - Perioperative CSF drainage
  - Intraoperative localization of the leak.
- Postoperative care

CSF Dynamics

- *CSF as a biomechanical cushion:* The brain is suspended in CSF, which protects it from mechanical injury. Suspension in the CSF also prevents compression of dependent regions that could impair neural functions.

- *CSF circulation:* Production: Most (80%) CSF is secreted by the choroid plexus in the lateral and third ventricles. Other sites of CSF formation include the choroid plexuses in the fourth ventricle. CSF is formed by ultrafiltration and active secretion. The critical step in the production of CSF is the active secretion of sodium, which leads to a concurrent chloride efflux. The Na^+ content of plasma and CSF are nearly identical. However, compared to plasma, CSF is rich in Cl- but poor in K^+, Ca^{++}, proteins, albumin, glucose, and red and white cells **(Table 1)**.
- *Circulation:* The volume of CSF in adults is about 135 mL and the rate of synthesis is 0.3–0.35 mL/min. CSF is turned over three times a day. The CSF is separated into three compartments: (1) ventricles (35 mL), (2) cranial subarachnoid space (25 mL), and (3) spinal subarachnoid space (75 mL). After production in the lateral ventricles, the CSF passes through the foramen of Monro into the third ventricle. From the third ventricle, it drains into the fourth through the aqueduct of Sylvius. From the fourth ventricle, the CSF drains into the subarachnoid space through the midline foramen of Magendie and the lateral foramen of Luschka.
- Posture, arterial pulsations, and respiratory movements affect CSF circulation within the skull. The movement of CSF in the spinal space is much slower. The specific gravity of CSF at 37°C is 1.007, its viscosity is 1.006 centipoise, and its density is 1.003 g/mL. These factors affect the distribution of hyperbaric, isobaric, and hypobaric drugs.
- *Reabsorption:* In the subarachnoid space, the CSF is reabsorbed through the arachnoid villi. It is suspected that significant amounts of CSF are also reabsorbed through the spinal nerve sheaths into the lymphatic.

Table 1: Composition of CSF and plasma.

	CSF	Plasma		CSF	Plasma
Na^+	138	138	Lactate	1.6	1
K^+	2.8	4.5	Pyruvate	0.08	0.11
Ca^{++}	2.1	4.8	Proteins	26	18
Cl^-	119	102	Albumin	0.2	3.6
H_2O	99%	93%	Osmolarity	295	295
PaO_2	43	104	RBCs	0	
$PaCO_2$	47	41	Lymphocytes	0–5	
pH	7.33	7.41	Neutrophils	0	

(CSF: cerebrospinal fluid)

Pathophysiology

Excessive draining of CSF, either after trauma, surgery, or dural tap, can lead to intracranial hypotension. Usually manifesting with orthostatic headache, it can be associated with photophobia and cranial nerve deficits in severe cases. The problem is generally self-limiting, requiring bed rest, hydration, analgesics, caffeine, and, in extreme cases, an epidural blood patch.

- *CSF leak/fistula:*
  - *Etiology:*
    - *Traumatic:* Head injury, 70%; postoperative (e.g., trans-sphenoidal hypophysectomy, skull base, and spine surgery, 30%)
    - *Traumatic CSF fistula:*
      - 2–3% of all TBIs and 15% of penetrating TBIs result in CSF fistulae.
      - Increases infection risk 10-fold
      - Infection risk increases with the persistence of the fistula
  - *Nontraumatic:*
    - *Normal pressure:* Congenital defects, bone erosion, or focal atrophy
    - *High pressure:* Hydrocephalus, tumors, and skull base infections.

Characteristics of CSF Leak

- *Clinical features:*
  - Discharge of clear, salty, and nonirritating fluid
  - Anosmia in 5%
  - *Double-ring sign on the linen:* A ring of blood surrounded by clear fluid
  - *Reservoir sign:* Abrupt release of pooled CSF with sitting up.

Differential diagnosis: Pseudo-CSF rhinorrhea can be due to excessive mucus secretion after skull base surgery.

Confirmation of CSF

- Glucose >30 mg/dL is suggestive of CSF
- β-2 transferrin confirms CSF leak.

Investigation

- *Plain X-ray and CT:* Pneumocephalus is seen in 20%
- *Water-soluble contrast (Iohexol):* CT may show contrast leak or accumulation.
- MRI may indicate an underlying cause. T2-weighted images with spin-echo can track the CSF flow. MRI spin-echo sequence protocols can track CSF formation and circulation.
- Radionucleotide studies.

Management of CSF Leak

- Prophylactic antibiotics
- *Nonsurgical Rx:* Bed rest, stool softeners, acetazolamide, and cautious fluid restriction
- *Surgical:*
  - CSF tap
  - Continuous lumbar drainage
  - Surgical closure of the defect
    - *Closure indicated for:*
      - Leaks >2 weeks
      - Meningitis
      - Delayed onset leaks.

Intracranial Hypotension Syndrome

The clinical syndrome is usually due to excessive CSF drainage characterized by postural headache, low CSF pressure, and diffuse parenchymal enhancement on MRI.

- *Symptoms:*
  - Postural headache is worse in the upright position and relieved in the supine position.
    - Hearing impairment
    - Tinnitus
    - Visual disturbances
    - Muscle twitching/spasms
- *Investigations:*
  - MRI:
    - Diffuse leptomeningeal and parenchymal enhancement
    - Brain descent
    - Pituitary enlargement
    - Small ventricles
    - Subdural hematomas
    - Spinal MRI may show a CSF leak close to localized pain if any.
- *Confirmation:*
  - Radioisotopic localization of the leak
  - Co-registering data with MRI.

Conservative Treatment

- Bed rest
- Decrease straining
- Decrease CSF formation with acetazolamide
- Fluids
- Analgesics

- Caffeine
- Lumbar drain
- Epidural blood patch.

Anesthetic Management

- *Preoperative considerations:*
  - Headache and other neurological symptoms
  - Bacterial meningitis
  - Pneumoencephalus
  - Preoperative localization of the site of the leak
- *Intraoperative considerations:*
  - Smooth induction and intubation
  - The role of intraoperative systemic hypotension in decreasing leak is debatable
  - Intraoperative localization of leak may require IV fluorescein
  - Valsalva maneuver used to test for a leak
  - A lumbar drain is placed to reduce CSF pressure
  - Avoidance of coughing and bucking at extubation.
- *Postoperative care:*
  - Supine bed rest: avoid head elevation
  - Lumbar drain management
  - Infection prevention.

CASE REPORTS FOR FURTHER DISCUSSION

Case 1: A 27-year-old woman presented with a gradually increasing headache. The headache was in the frontotemporal region, made worse on standing, and associated with nausea and vomiting. There was no history of any trauma or surgery. She was seen by a physician and was found to have severe hypertension with systolic blood pressure (SBP) >200 mm Hg. She was hospitalized and treated for hypertension treatment. The CT scan of the head and renal ultrasounds were negative. She was discharged on atenolol and amitriptyline. Despite treatment, the headaches persisted. MRI imaging two weeks after discharge revealed leptomeningeal enhancement but no other abnormalities. Radioisotopic cisternography identified a low cervical CSF leak. A lumbar blood patch with 12 mL of blood helped to resolve the symptom for nearly two days. Subsequently, a C6–C7 blood patch was performed. Her headache decreased, and she resumed normal activities. *What is the role of intrathecal saline treatment for cerebral hypotension? What are the complications of an epidural blood patch?*

Case 2: A chronic low back pain patient underwent L2–L5 laminectomies and foraminotomies. However, during surgery, the dural sac was ruptured.

The tear was surgically repaired. The patient had a postoperative CSF leak on the second postoperative day. Lying flat and treatment with diuretics (acetazolamide and furosemide) had no effect. A lumbar drain was placed and 350 mL of CSF was drained over the next three days before the drain was removed. A CT scan was done. *What is the role of diuretics in the treatment of CSF leaks? How are the actions of furosemide and acetazolamide different? Why was the CT scan of the head done? What is the rationale of lumbar drain placement when there is already a CSF leak?*

Case 3: One day after revision spine surgery for lumbar disc prolapse at L4–5 and L5–S1 levels, the 34-year-old patient developed acute-onset lower limb numbness, weakness, and urinary incontinence. Urgent MRI revealed an extensive fluid collection from T12–L2, which was some 8 mm thick. There was evidence of cord compression. An unguent decompressive laminectomy was to be done. *What are your preoperative concerns in such a case?* During surgery, a sizeable subdural collection of CSF was seen. The sac was decompressed. To test the integrity of the dural repair, the surgeons request Valsalva at 40 cm of water. *What are your concerns? What are the hemodynamic effects of the Valsalva maneuver?* After surgery. they leave a lumbar drain; *what precautions will you take at extubation?*

Case 4: A 47-year-old with a history of intracapsular excision of vestibular schwannoma and past radiation therapy underwent revision surgery due to the recurrence of the tumor. MRI revealed a tumor recurrence with cerebellar compression and surrounding brain edema. A preoperative ventriculoperitoneal (VP) shunt was placed to drain the CSF. The retrosigmoid approach was used to excise the tumor completely. The postoperative MRI revealed complete excision with patchy CSF collection. The patient was seen three months later when he complained of progressive headaches and worsening dizziness. Repeat MRI showed a massive CSF leak extending on the posterolateral aspect of the skull to the first cervical vertebra. The patient is due for the repair of the posterior fossa dural defect. *Do you anticipate any difficulty in intubation consequent to a large volume of CSF collected at the occiput and upper cervical spine? Would you request preoperative drainage of CSF to assist with the positioning in such a case?*

Case 5: At the age of 30 years, a patient underwent trans-sphenoid hypophysectomy. A CSF leak was noticed during surgery, and a fat graft was applied to seal the defect. The patient recovered uneventfully after that. Twenty-eight years later, she underwent a robotic-assisted hysterectomy and oophorectomy. The surgery required a steep head-down tilt for several hours. After surgery, she developed a nasal discharge of clear fluid that was considered to be due to allergic rhinitis. The discharge continued, and three weeks later, the patient was admitted to the hospital with headache, photophobia, and neck rigidity. The nasal discharge was positive for β2-transferrin. MRI and CT studies revealed a 2–3-mm defect in the sella with dural enhancement. An endoscopic repair of the CSF leaf was planned. *Besides the β-transferrin test, how will you differentiate between CSF leak and allergic rhinitis? How does anesthesia for endoscopic repair differ from traditional surgery using a nasal speculum?*

CASE REPORT REFERENCES

Case 1: Nipatcharoen P et al. High thoracic/cervical epidural blood patch for spontaneous cerebrospinal fluid leak: a new challenge for anesthesiologists. Anesth Analg. 2011;113(6):1476-9.

Case 2: Hussein M et al. Continuous lumbar drainage for the prevention and management of perioperative cerebrospinal fluid leakage. Asian J Neurosurg. 2019;14(2):473-8.

Case 3: Nentwig MJ et al. Spinal subdural hygroma as a post-operative complication in revision spine fusion: a case report. J Surg Case Rep. 2019;11:1-3.

Case 4: Iannella G et al. Massive cerebrospinal fluid leak of the temporal bone. Case Rep Otolaryngol. 2016:7521798.

Case 5: Dowdy JT et al. Late onset of CSF rhinorrhea in a postoperative transsphenoidal surgery patient following robotic-assisted abdominal hysterectomy. J Invest Med High Impact Case Rep. 2014:1-6.

FURTHER READING

1. D'Antona L et al. Clinical presentation, investigation findings, and treatment outcomes of spontaneous intracranial hypotension syndrome: a systematic review and meta-analysis. JAMA Neurol. 2021;78(3):329-37.
2. Feng J et al. Systematic review and meta-analysis of the effect of continuous cerebrospinal fluid drainage on keyhole surgery during the perioperative period. Ann Palliat Med. 2021;10(10):11129-40.
3. Jiam NT et al. Presentation and management of post-operative cerebrospinal fluid leaks after sphenoclival expanded endonasal surgery: a single institution experience. J Clin Neurosci. 2021;91:13-9.
4. Kim DH et al. Usefulness of imaging studies for diagnosing and localizing cerebrospinal fluid rhinorrhea: a systematic review and meta-analysis. Int Forum Allergy Rhinol, 2021;12(6):828-37.
5. Missale F et al. Cerebrospinal fluid leak repair: usefulness of intrathecal fluorescein for correct topographic identification of the skull base defects. World Neurosurg. 2022;160:e267-77.

Vignette: The History of Choroid Plexus

The earliest description of the choroid plexus in the lateral ventricles was provided by Herophilos (335–280 BCE). The term choroid was used to describe the structure by Galen in the first-century AD. Vesalius, in 1543, described the choroid plexus in the lateral ventricles and hypothesized that the choroid was the source of fluid in the ventricles. In 1664, Thomas Willis described the choroid plexus of the fourth ventricle. Ridley, in 1675, described the choroid plexus of the third ventricle and completed the description of the whole system. Besides secreting two-thirds of the CSF, the choroid plays a vital role in neurodevelopment. The choroid plexus is relatively large in fetal life. In the mouse embryo, almost 30% of the ventricular wall area is covered by the choroid, while it covers twice as much area in the human embryo. The most recent interest in the choroid arises from the neuroectodermal progenitor cells that could help understand developmental diseases and dementia.

Chapter 47: Cervical Decompression

INTRODUCTION

Decompression is the surgical enlargement of the spinal canal to relieve pressure on the nerves or the cord. The narrowing of the canal, or spinal stenosis, can affect any spine region. Spinal stenosis can be due to degeneration, herniated disc, osteophytes, arthritis, thickened ligaments, tumors, or injuries. The symptoms include pain, numbness, tingling, disturbances of gait, and bladder or bowel dysfunction. The decompressive procedure needed in a given case depends on the nature of the pathology. Common decompressive procedures include foraminotomy, laminectomy, laminoplasty, or discectomy. They could be simple single-level procedures or demanding multi-level interventions which affects their anesthetic management.

NEUROANESTHETIC CONCERNS

- *Preoperative assessment:*
  - Neurological deficits
  - Airway assessment
  - *Intubation:* Awake/asleep
  - *Monitoring:* A-line awake/asleep
  - Evoked potential (EP) monitoring.
- *Preparation:* Setup for the following:
  - Intubation
  - Processed electroencephalogram (EEG)
  - Total intravenous anesthesia (TIVA)
  - Blood loss in cervical and single-level decompression is minimal. However, if bleeding is expected, then consider the following:
    - Cell saver
    - Antifibrinolytic drugs
  - Point-of-care monitors.
- Positioning after induction.
- Hemodynamic monitoring and cord perfusion.
- *Electrophysiological monitoring:*
  - Somatosensory evoked potential (SSEP) and motor evoked potential (MEP)

- Processed EEG
- Management of attenuation of evoked potentials
- *Emergence:*
  - Smooth extubation
  - Postoperative pain management

Preoperative Assessment

- Assessment of comorbidities
- Fasting history, history of reflux, potential risk of aspiration
- Careful airway assessment, even if awake fiberoptic intubation is planned.
  - Mallampati grade, jaw protraction, state of dentition
  - A nasal fiberoptic might be needed if mouth opening is limited.
  - Separately assess for the degree of flexion of the neck and the atlanto-occipital extension. These can be tested by placing the hand behind the neck when flexed and assessing atlantoaxial (AA) extension.
  - Assess the range of neck movements at the onset of symptoms, such as pain or numbness in the arms.
  - The ability to say the high-pitched vowel "E" indicates a free movement of the vocal cords.
- If the patient has a collar:
  - If the collar cannot be removed, oral intubation is exceedingly challenging.
  - In most cases, the collar can be removed, and the head can be supported by inline traction to permit oral intubation.
- The patient's ability to cooperate with awake fiberoptic intubation.
- Review and documentation of baseline neurological deficits **(Table 1)**.

Table 1: Symptoms of cervical disc herniation.

Level	Signs and symptoms
C1-2	Neck and occipital pain, unilateral numbness/abnormal sensation of tongue. Fatigue, dizziness and nausea
C2-3	Pain radiating down the arm with weakness and numbness. Decrease range of motion
C3-4	Backache middle of the scapula, pain radiating down arm into fingers with numbness and tingling, muscle spasms
C4-5	Pain, tingling, numbness and weakness of deltoids/shoulder and radial side of the hand
C5-6	Pain, tingling, numbness, and weakness of later side of the arm and hand
C6-7	Pain, numbness and weakness extending from arm to the middle finger
C7-T1	Pain, numbness and weakness extending from arm to the little finger

Monitoring
- Routine anesthesia monitors are placed at the start of induction.
- An awake placement of an A-line has the following advantages:
  - Awake blood pressure is higher than after induction, and the line placement is easier awake.
  - It enables prompt treatment of hypotension at induction.
  - It avoids delays in positioning the patient after induction.
- Baseline-evoked somatosensory and motor potentials are recorded soon after induction, often before positioning; thus, infusions for TIVA should be at hand along with processed EEG monitoring. A single dose of rocuronium can be used initially yet permitting baseline testing.

Awake Fiberoptic Intubation
- Background sedation to alleviate anxiety is necessary. Fentanyl, midazolam, low-dose remifentanil, and dexmedetomidine are often used. Low-dose glycopyrrolate helps decrease secretions. Scopolamine (which provides amnesia), if available, is preferable.
- *Local anesthesia* involves the suppression of glossopharyngeal and vagal afferent nerves. Both can be achieved by nebulized lidocaine (4%).
- *Glossopharyngeal nerve block:* Topical lidocaine or prilocaine applied in the mouth, the base of the tongue, and the posterior pharynx.
- *Superior laryngeal nerve block:* Pledgets with 2% lidocaine behind the tonsils where the nerve is submucosal or by injection of 2 mL of 1% lidocaine anterior and superior to the greater cornu of the hyoid bone just beyond the mylohyoid diaphragm.
- Supraglottic anesthesia is assessed by the severity of the gag response to the oral airway; William's airway gives better directional control but is narrower than the Ovassapian airway. Remove the endotracheal tube (ETT) connector while using William's airway. If no gag is evident, proceed with a transtracheal block.
- *Inferior laryngeal nerve and vagal block by:*
  - Transtracheal injection of 3–4 mL of 4% lidocaine or
  - By injection through the biopsy port advanced of the bronchoscope.
  - An epidural catheter with a forward injection port can be passed through the biopsy port to direct the jet of local anesthetic.

Postintubation Check
Secure the ETT. Check for power in the lower and upper limbs and inject an induction agent. Anticipate an exacerbated hypotensive response due to background sedation and topical local anesthetics and correct it immediately.

Video Laryngoscopic Intubation

Basic Technique

- Hyper-angulated video laryngoscopic (VLS) blades, such as Glidescope, can permit intubation with minimal cervical spine movement.
- The optimum position is mid-sniffing; the external auditory meatus should be below the manubrium sterni.
- Insert the VLS in the midline over the tongue, under direct view. The classical approach with the lateral entry of the laryngoscope, such as the Macintosh blade, could injure the tonsils or the lateral pharynx. Once the tip is at the base of the tongue, alternately view the advance of the VLS blade directly and on-screen until the tip of the epiglottis is seen. Then, under continuous on-screen visualization, advance the VLS blade into the vallecula.
- The stylet of the endotracheal tube should match the curve of the VLS blade. The application of gel could help with the withdrawal of the stylet. The styleted tube is introduced after visualization of the laryngeal inlet. It is introduced into the mouth from the side under vision until it reaches the pharynx. It is then rotated along the mid-line to align with the curve of the VLS. Once the tip of the endotracheal tube is at the laryngeal inlet, the stylet is withdrawn, which advances the endotracheal tube beyond the vocal cord. Blindly advancing the rigid styleted tube could lead to injury. The endotracheal tube is maneuvered to its final position under direct visualization.

Problems with VLS

- *Inadequate access to the airway:*
  - *Cervical collar limits access and mouth opening:* Discuss with the surgeon if the collar can be removed; if needed, consider intubation with inline traction.
  - Extreme cervical deformities such as ankylosing spondylitis
  - Limited mouth opening may be due to abnormalities in the temporomandibular joint (TMJ)
  - *A small mouth opening:* Consider VLS devices with smaller blades.
  - If oral access is limited, consider nasotracheal instead of orotracheal placement of the ETT.
- *The inability to visualize the larynx can be due to the following:*
  - Inappropriate blade selection relative to the airway
  - Check position to rule out extreme flexion or extension of the neck.
  - The blade needs to be inserted further.
  - The blade may be posterior to and beyond the laryngeal inlet.
- *The inability of the tube to reach the vocal cords can be due to the following:*
  - Crowded oropharyngeal space.

- Incompatibility of the curve of the stylet and the VLS blade may make intubation challenging. Correct the curve of the stylet.
- The tube might be posterior to the larynx.
  - Lift the base of the tongue.
  - Apply cricoid pressure.
- Consider bougie-assisted intubation using VLS.
• *Inability to advance the endotracheal tube, consider:*
  - Verify the size of the tube relative to that of the larynx.
  - Extreme angulation of stylet
  - Angulation of spine
  - *Angulation of the trachea:* Keep the stylet in position and rotate the endotracheal tube while advancing; apply cricoid pressure or move the larynx.

Complications of VLS

- Dental injuries—upper incisors
- Soft tissue injuries by laryngoscope to—lips, buccal mucosa, tongue, hypopharynx, and epiglottis
- Perforation of the palatopharynx by a stylet
- Injuries to the epiglottis, larynx, and trachea

Postintubation Management

- *EP monitoring and TIVA:* The anesthesia regimen used for TIVA should be discussed with electrophysiologists, and significant changes to the background infusions must be communicated to them. Volatile anesthetics and nitrous oxide are avoided. **Table 2** shows the usual doses of drugs used for TIVA.

Table 2: Infusion targets for total intravenous anesthesia.

Drug	Dose range	End point
Propofol	80–150 µg/kg/min	BIS 40–60
Remifentanil	0.3–2 µg/kg/min	HR <80, no noxious response evident
Rocuronium	0.15–0.3 mg/kg/h	TOF 2 twitch/no gross motor response with EP monitoring
Sufentanil	0.1–0.5 µg/kg/h	HR <80, no noxious response evident; curtail infusion at least 30 min from the end
Dexmedetomidine	0.2–0.7 µg/kg/h	
Phenylephrine	0–80 µg/min	To maintain target blood pressure

(BIS: bispectral index; HR: heart rate; TOF: tetralogy of Fallot)

- *Pharmacokinetic consideration in TIVA:*
  - *Context-sensitive half-life:* The elimination half-life is proportional to the duration of the infusion. Thus, the infusion rate has to be adjusted for the duration of the infusion.
  - *Target site infusion rates:* The infusion rate is determined by computing the drug infusion rates using patient parameters and target drug concentrations to achieve desired serum concentrations.
  - *Effect-site target infusion:* Instead of the serum concentration, the infusion is adjusted to the predicted concentration at the effect site using pharmacokinetic modeling and patient parameters.
- If remifentanil is used, long-acting narcotics should be titrated to prevent postoperative pain toward the end of the case. Low-dose remifentanil (0.02–0.03 µg/kg/min) might be helpful to smoothen wake-up at extubation.

Smooth Extubation Strategies

- A smooth extubation is necessary due to the potential risk of bleeding. Patients at risk of vigorous bucking at extubation includes smokers, younger and more robust individuals, or when anesthesia levels are rapidly decreased. Sufentanil infusions usually have smoother extubation.
- *At the start of wound closure*, 30–45 minutes before anticipated extubation. Consider the following:
  - Monitor and reduce minimal alveolar concentration (MAC) of any volatile agents.
  - Reduce remifentanil to 0.02–0.03 µg/kg/min.
  - Reduced propofol/dexmedetomidine infusion rates appropriately.
  - Titrate judicious amounts of narcotics 5–10 minutes before extubation.
- *Just before extubation, consider the following:*
  - Examine the eyes for puffiness (fluid overload), redness (corneal injury), and pupillary size (visual impairment).
  - Assess airway leak pressure, particularly after prolonged prone spine surgery.
  - Consider IV lidocaine bolus.
  - *Intratracheal lidocaine (2%: 2–3 mL):* Use a #26 G needle to ensure small droplet size that is less likely to cause coughing.
  - Consider placing a nasal trumpet after topical lidocaine application.
  - Before reversing paralysis, suction the oropharynx.
  - Suctioning is best done before putting the rigid collar.
- Check for and reverse neuromuscular blockade.
- Reduce anesthetics drug infusions to wake-up doses.

CHAPTER 47 Cervical Decompression

- Assess the return of adequate spontaneous ventilation.
- If awake and tolerating the tube, test for movement of the limbs before extubation.

CASE REPORTS FOR FURTHER DISCUSSION

Case 1: A 29-year-old previously healthy male presented with acute-onset right upper and lower limb weakness of 8 days. The weakness rapidly progressed to incontinence and difficulty breathing, requiring intubation and mechanical ventilation. The MRI revealed a C2–C3 intradural extramedullary lesion on the ventral surface of the upper cervical cord with compression of the spinal cord between C2 and C4. The neurological symptoms rapidly worsened to quadriparesis with greater involvement of the upper than the lower and proximal versus the distal muscle groups. A C2, C3, and C4 laminectomies were planned with SSEP and MEP monitoring. *Given the pre-existing weakness, what is the choice of anesthetic drugs? The baseline median SSEPs have increased latency and morphology, and MEPs are poorly recordable. After positioning, there is a complete loss of SSEP and motor potentials. What precautions can you take during the turning of the patient to minimize the risk of spinal injury? Discuss the advantages or disadvantages of the head supports (prone view, sponge block, and pinning) used in prone positioning. The SSEP and MEP returned with repositioning of the head. What precautions will you take during surgery to minimize the risk of secondary cord injury?*

Case 2: A 55-year-old male with chronic back pain radiating to the legs and difficulty standing and walking was due for a two-level lumbar laminectomy. During surgery, bilateral ulnar and posterior tibial nerve SSEPs were monitored along with spontaneous electromyography of L1 and L2 root muscular innervations. Anesthesia was maintained with 1-MAC sevoflurane, narcotics, and muscle relaxants. During decompression, SSEPs were lost. The surgeons proceeded with surgery to complete decompressing the spinal cord. The SSEPs returned on completing L3 nerve root decompression, which took about half an hour. *Discuss the use of muscle relaxants during EP monitoring. What are the pros and cons of using supplementary-processed EEG during evoked potential monitoring? How will you deal with the loss of SSEPs?*

Case 3: A 6-year-old boy with progressive kyphosis and multiple skeletal abnormalities diagnosed with Maroteaux–Lamy syndrome or mucopolysaccharidosis VI (arylsulfatase deficiency) presented for corrective surgery with SSEP monitoring. There was no reported change in SSEP during the procedure; however, the patient could not move his lower limbs on awakening. He underwent surgery for the removal of the Harrington rod. After surgery, motor power was restored to the lower limb proximally. *This six-year-old cannot cooperate but is due for an EP examination a week after surgery. How would you manage the case?* It was decided that he should undergo transcranial magnetic stimulation (TMS). *What are the pros and cons of using TMS compared to conventional EPs?*

Case 4: A 49-year-old female presented with neck pain for several months, with severe pain radiating down the second and third fingers. Her neurological examination was essentially normal. However, she had a large C6-7 central disc herniation on the MRI. Anterior cervical C6-7 discectomy was undertaken with cage insertion and plate fixation. On wake-up, upper extremity sensory and motor examination was relatively normal. However, there was severe motor weakness (0/5) of the lower limbs with hyperactive reflexes and ankle clonus. Cervical spine MRI revealed C6-7 high signal intensity STIR signal suggestive of cord edema secondary to cord reperfusion injury. A diagnosis of white cord syndrome was made. She was treated with methylprednisolone 30 mg/kg/15 minutes with 5.4 mg/kg/23 h and was scheduled for an emergency C3-7 spinal cord decompression. *What is the role of steroids in spinal cord reperfusion injury? What are the pros and cons of electrophysiological monitoring in this case?*

CASE REPORT REFERENCES

Case 1: Alkhatib M et al. Sudden onset temporary loss of SSEP and MEP as a result to positional neck changes in an intradural extramedullary cervical spine schwannoma: a case report. Interdiscip Neurosurg. 2020;21:100717.

Case 2: McNamee GA et al. Loss of lower extremity somatosensory evoked potentials during lumbar laminectomy and instrumented fusion: a case report. J Neurol Stroke. 2016;4(1):00121.

Case 3: Rosenberg JR. Somatosensory and magnetic evoked potentials in a postoperative paraparetic patient: case report. Arch Phys Med Rehabil. 1991;72:154-6.

Case 4: Jun DS et al. A case report: white cord syndrome following anterior cervical discectomy and fusion: importance of prompt diagnosis and treatment. BMC Musculoskelet Disord. 2020;21(1):157.

FURTHER READING

1. Gadomski BC et al. Intubation Biomechanics: Clinical Implications of Computational Modeling of Intervertebral Motion and Spinal Cord Strain during Tracheal Intubation in an Intact Cervical Spine. Anesthesiology. 2021; 135(6):1055-65.
2. Park JW et al. Comparison of a New Video Intubation Stylet and McGrath(R) MAC Video Laryngoscope for Intubation in an Airway Manikin with Normal

Airway and Cervical Spine Immobilization Scenarios by Novice Personnel: A Randomized Crossover Study. Biomed Res Int. 2021;2021:4288367.
3. Singleton BN et al. Effectiveness of intubation devices in patients with cervical spine immobilization: a systematic review and network meta-analysis. Br J Anaesth. 2021;126(5): 1055-66.
4. Swain A et al. Intubating Laryngeal Mask Airway-assisted Flexible Bronchoscopic Intubation Is Associated With Reduced Cervical Spine Motion When Compared with C-MAC Video Laryngoscopy-guided Intubation: A Prospective Randomized Cross Over Trial. J Neurosurg Anesthesiol. 2020; 32(3):242-8.
5. Zhang AS et al. Cervical Myelopathy: Diagnosis, Contemporary Treatment, and Outcomes. Am J Med. 2022;135(4):435-43.

Vignette: The First Use of Intravenous Narcotics

Soon after William Harvey in 1628 demonstrated the role of the heart in blood circulation, blood was considered to the body's principal life force. Several bizarre experiments were initiated to treat disease conditions. One school of thought was to inject known poisons in minute amounts into blood to treat diseases. In this context, Sir Robert Boyle (famous for his gas law) and Sir Christopher Wren (the renowned architect who designed St. Paul's Cathedral in London) injected dogs with a tincture of opium in 1656. They used a quill and an animal bladder to inject the opium to induce sleep. In doing so, they were the first to use intravenous narcotics.

Chapter 48

Acute Spinal Injury

INTRODUCTION

An estimated 18,000 spinal cord injuries occur in the US annually, and about 300,000 people live with such injuries. There is a 4-fold male preponderance. Seventy percent of these are due to accidents or falls, and 60% involve the cervical spine. A spinal injury has catastrophic consequences on the life of an individual. The outcome and costs depend on the patient's age and the injury's level and severity. About 30% of patients require hospitalization each year. Pneumonia and septicemia are ultimately the leading cause of death. Initial stabilization with collar, blocks, and board, and adequate resuscitation, are crucial. Life-saving interventions take priority while maintaining traction. The airway is secured to ensure ventilation and prevent aspiration. Neurogenic and spinal shock is treated to ensure cord perfusion. The initial assessment may be misleading, and follow-up exams may better document the extent of the injury. Imaging studies and stabilization surgery are undertaken when deemed safe. This chapter briefly describes the clinical presentation while focusing on managing these injuries.

NEUROANESTHETIC CONCERNS

- Spinal trauma
- Initial resuscitation
- Indication for surgery
- Airway management
- Intraoperative monitoring
- *Prevention of secondary injury:*
    - Cord perfusion
    - Hypothermia
- *Complications:*
    - Spinal shock
    - Autonomic hyperreflexia
    - Others

Spinal Trauma

Spinal injuries frequently affect young, healthy mobile individuals. Two-thirds of the patients with spinal injuries have multiple injuries. Spinal injuries occur in 10% of patients with severe head injuries.

Etiology

Almost 50% of spinal injuries are due to motor vehicle accidents (MVA), while others are due to falls (20%), sporting accidents (15%), and physical violence (15%). Spinal injuries are rarely associated with pre-existing pathologies, such as degenerative diseases or metastasis.
- Of all spinal injuries, 50% involve the cervical spine, 30% involve the thoracic, and 10% involve the lumbar spine.
- The high incidence of cervical spine injuries is attributed to its frail structure and excessive mobility. C-6 is the most common level of spinal injury.
- The upper spine (C1-4) is more frequently involved in children, while the lower cervical spine (C5-8) is more likely to be involved in adults.
- The lower thoracic spine (T11-12) is a frequent injury site as the rib cage support is relatively lacking compared to other thoracic levels.

Pathophysiology

Biomechanically, the spinal column can be divided into three support columns, known as the: (1) anterior, (2) middle, and (3) posterior pillars. The column concept was first described by Holdsworth in 1963 and latter modified by Denis in 1983.
- *The anterior pillar* is the anterior longitudinal ligament and the vertebral body.
- *The middle pillar* is the posterior longitudinal ligament.
- *The posterior pillar* is the spinous processes, ligamentum flavum, and interspinous and supraspinous ligaments.
  Loss of more than one pillar makes the spinal column unstable. Mechanically, spine injuries can be classified as flexion, extension, rotational or craniocaudal compression.

Whiplash injury: Most common nonfatal motor vehicle accidents (MVA); traumatic injury to the soft tissue in the cervical spine in the absence of apparent structural damage; symptoms are often delayed and may be nonspecific, such as headache or back pain.

Primary injury: It represents direct injury to the cord at the time of impact; examples include avulsion, contusion, and laceration.

Secondary injury: Represents the progressive loss of cord functions due to indirect injuries such as hypoxia, hypoperfusion, or edema. These

Table 1:: Functional impact of the level of spinal cord injury.

Level of injury	Syndrome	Impact
C4	Tetraplegia with respiratory insufficiency	Severe injury with ventilator dependency
C6	Tetraplegia	Severe injury without ventilator dependency
T6	Paraplegia	Paraplegia with significant autonomic disturbances
L1	Paraplegia	Paraplegia with significant less autonomic disturbances

mechanisms trigger a complex neurochemical cascade that eventually leads to cell death. The key to managing spinal cord injury patients is maintaining cord perfusion and preventing secondary injury.

Clinical Evaluation

- In a conscious individual, spinal trauma often presents with local pain, evidence of injury, tenderness, or muscle spasms. A step deformity of the spinous processes might be palpable. Clinical examination is often able to detect neurological deficits.
- Acute spinal trauma may result in complete or partial loss of cord functions the consequences of which depend on the level of injury (**Table 1**).
- *Complete transection of the cord:* Results in spinal shock with total loss of sensations, flaccid areflexia, loss of anal sphincter tone, and sometimes priapism. These signs should be sought in any unconscious patient with a suspected head injury. Unconscious patients may also demonstrate abnormal breathing patterns. The injuries above T6 lead to loss of sympathetic control with vagal dominance. This loss of autonomic control is known as neurogenic shock. Spinal shock can be at any level; the higher the level, the more severe the manifestations. It is the transient loss of sensory, motor, and autonomic control. This results in initial areflexia, which tends to recover over time.
- *Partial transection of the cord:* Some residual function (sensory or motor) is evident two to three levels below the injury site. However, it excludes sacral sparing (perianal sensation, voluntary sphincter tone, or toe flexion). It usually results in one of the following four syndromes:
    1. *Central cord syndrome* is associated with greater loss of motor power in the upper than in the lower limbs, variable sensory loss, and frequent retention of urine.
    2. *Cord hemisection* results in ipsilateral paralysis with contralateral loss of pain or temperature sensations.
    3. *Anterior cord syndrome* results in motor paralysis, impaired pain, and touch but intact proprioception and vibratory sensations.

4. *Cauda equina syndrome* due to lumbar injury results in loss of bladder and bowel control, lower motor neuron type of lower limb paralysis, and patchy sensory loss.

Resuscitation

- Whenever possible, the movement of cervical trauma patients must be undertaken by trained personnel. The cervical spine is usually immobilized using *a hard collar*. The patient is log-rolled onto *a board*. The head is secured by straps between *two blocks*. This stabilization remains in place until spine injury is ruled out. If removed for critical intervention, in-line traction has to be maintained.
- In the case of airway obstruction, a nasal or oral airway can be cautiously placed at minimal risk of displacing spinal fragments. Nasal airway is avoided if an skull base injury is suspected. The choice of airway management technique depends on urgency, coexisting injuries (e.g., facial trauma), equipment availability, and operator skills **(Table 2)**.
- *Awake fiber-optic* intubation represents the safest way for intubating a patient with a suspected spine injury. Cricoid pressure is avoided as it can displace unstable fracture fragments.
- *Respiratory insufficiency* in a patient with a spinal injury may be due to an associated head injury, intoxication, high cervical injury with loss of phrenic nerve function (C3-C5), airway obstruction due to secretions or trauma, aspiration, or direct chest trauma. Mechanical ventilation should be instituted for a target PaO_2 of 80 mm Hg and $PaCO_2$ of 30–35 mm Hg.
- Shock after spinal injuries can be due to trauma to spine or elsewhere in the body. Hemorrhage elsewhere and cardiac injury must be ruled out before shock is attributed to spinal injuries. Spinal injury can result in neurogenic or spinal shock. Neurogenic shock is typically seen with

Table 2: Intubation techniques for C-spine injuries.

Technique	Advantage	Disadvantage
Awake		
Fiber-optic	Safety: reduced aspiration and hypoxia risk	Time/equipment
Blind nasotracheal	Minimal movement	Cooperative patient
Tracheostomy	Helpful with a facial injury	Anterior cervical approach to spine difficult
Under anesthesia		
DL with online traction	Minimal movements	Familiar method
Intubating LMA	Minimal movement	Skill/training
Glidescope	Minimal movements	Skill/training
Retrograde intubation	No visualization is needed.	Trauma

(DL: direct laryngoscopy; LMA: laryngeal mask airway)

Table 3: Spinal versus neurogenic shock.*

Feature	Spinal shock	Neurogenic shock
Mechanism	Spinal injury with loss of sensation, motor power, and reflexes	Loss of sympathetic tone with resulting vasodilation and distributive shock
Severity	It depends on the level and extent of the injury	Injuries above T6 that block the sympathetic response
Paralysis	Flaccid paralysis	Variable
Reflexes	Absent	Variable
Onset	Immediate	Immediate
Duration	Early recovery, days	Sustained—weeks
Hemodynamic effects	Hypotension/bradycardia	Hypotension/bradycardia
Temperature regulation	It depends on the level and extent of the injury	Impaired—hypothermia
Treatment	Fluid, pressors and inotropic measures	Fluid, pressors and inotropic measures

*Other causes of shock may coexist with spinal and neurogenic shock

injuries above T-6 that can affect the sympathetic out flow (T1-5). It can result in unopposed vagal action. Thus, neurogenic shock results in vasodilation, with hypotension and brady cardia. It requires treatment with fluids, pressors and anticholinergic drugs. Spinal shock is due to the loss of sensory, motor, and autonomic functions. This results in flaccid paralysis and transient suppression of reflexes. The state of spinal shock can resolve in 48 hours and could result is hyperactive reflexes. In spinal shock, generally the injury is partial, and recovery is more likely that after neurogenic shock. Treatment also requires judicious fluids, pressor and inotropic drugs. There is greater risk of ileus, poikilothermia, and thromboembolism (*see* **Table 3**).

Radiology

- *X-ray:* Spinal injuries are usually screened by five-view series of radiographs: Anteroposterior, lateral, two supine obliques, and odontoid views (for the cervical spine). Radiological abnormalities may not be evident in 15% of spinal injuries. Spinal radiographs should be checked for the following:
  - *Alignment* of the vertebral bodies and spinous processes
  - *Bone characteristics* such as density, contour, anterior and posterior vertebral height, and spinous and transverse processes
  - Width and distortion of *intervertebral and interspinous spaces*
  - Evidence of damage to *soft tissues* in the retropharyngeal space, mediastinum, and retroperitoneum
- *Computed tomography* is needed when there is a suspicion of injury despite a negative radiology screen.

- *MRI:* The use of MRI in acute spinal trauma has been limited. The limited value of the MRI is mainly due to the time required for scanning and the logistics of transporting the patient into a strong magnetic field. However, MRI can demonstrate the extent of subtle neural and vascular injury not revealed by computed tomography.

Stability of the Spine

Once an injury to the spine has been detected, it is essential to ascertain whether the lesion is stable. However, structural stability does not imply the absence of neurological injuries, e.g., due to hematoma.
- A *cervical lesion* is considered unstable if: more than one pillar is disrupted, the subluxation is >3 mm, the space is narrowed or widened, or when the interspinous distance is increased.
- A *thoracolumbar lesion* is considered unstable if: there is a loss of more than one pillar or kyphosis of >40°.

SURGICAL MANAGEMENT

Acute surgical management is aimed at the decompression and/or stabilization of vertebral fractures.

Preoperative assessment:
- Surgery is considered urgent or emergent if cord compression is suspected.
- *Associated injuries:* Neurological, orthopedic, thoracoabdominal.
- *Agitation:* It can be due to hypoxia, pain, other neurological injuries, intoxication, or drug use.
- Full stomach
- C-spine stability, cervical collar, or head in traction
- Selection of intubation equipment and techniques:
  - Bougie assisted with direct laryngoscopy with minimal jaw lift.
  - Glide scope selection of appropriate size is essential. It can also be used to guide bougie/fiberoptic scope.
  - Bullard's laryngoscope
  - *Airtraq:* It is bulky with a small screen in the line of intubation.
  - Intubation LMA such as Fasttrack
  - Pantex AWS has a 12 cm long cable with an end camera.
  - *Fiberoptic devices:* Multichannel fiberoptic devices with a proximal camera or disposable distal digital camera models.
  - The blind nasal technique is rapid and requires no equipment but skill. Hazardous with face or skull base trauma.
  - Retrograde intubation
  - Tracheostomy. It is rapid, safe and reliable, but traumatic.

OR Preparation: The operating room should be prepared for: Placement of a pre-induction A-line, awake intubation, central venous pressure (CVP) placement for monitoring and resuscitation, adequate peripheral venous access, infusion pumps for total intravenous anesthesia (TIVA) and pressor support, fluids, blood, fresh frozen plasma (FFP), and Bispectral Index (BIS) and evoked potential monitoring. Evoked potential monitoring, if needed and time permits.

Induction and Intubation

- The method to secure the airway will be determined by the needs of the individual case and the urgency of the situation.
- Fractures and injuries to the face, an uncooperative patient, children, or a full stomach can make intubations challenging. With cervical spine injuries, cricoid pressure and tracheostomy pose additional risks due to possible displacement of the bones.
- The advantage of awake intubation is that the patient's neurological condition can be documented after intubation before inducing general anesthesia. However, the method requires time, expertise, and patient cooperation.
- Alternately, asleep fiber-optic or Glidescope intubation offers an alternative method when awake intubation is not possible. Other intubation devices listed above can also be used. Induction with propofol can lead to hypotension; therefore, phenylephrine is often used with the drug during induction. Anesthesia is best maintained with propofol/narcotic-based TIVA when electrophysiological monitoring is necessary. However, relieving cord compression may supersede electrophysiological monitoring to avoid setup delays in an urgent situation.

Prevention of Secondary Injuries

- The primary strategy to prevent secondary injury is to avoid hypotension and hypoxia. High-dose methylprednisolone (30 mg/kg bolus followed by 5.4 mg/kg/h) may improve the outcome if given within 8 hours of injury.
- The benefits of other measures, such as hypothermia, hyperbaric oxygen, 21-aminosteroid, superoxide dismutase, and pentoxifylline, remain unproven in clinical studies.
- The best practical means of preventing secondary injury are avoiding hypotension, maintaining adequate oxygenation, and preventing hyperglycemia and electrolyte imbalance. Cord functions must be monitored closely, clinically, or electro-physiologically to detect any change promptly.

Postoperative care: For major spine trauma, a case can be made for careful postoperative monitoring that guides hemodynamic targets, ensures tissue oxygenation, maintains a safe milieu, permits mild hypothermia, and detects any new injury.

Complications

- *Respiratory insufficiency* may require prolonged ventilator support for lesions above C6. A tracheostomy is needed if intubation lasts >2 weeks.
- *Spinal and neurogenic shock: Hypotension and bradycardia* usually occur with lesions >T6 due to loss of sympathetic innervation to the heart.
- *Autonomic hyperreflexia:* Patients with lesions higher than T6 demonstrate a massive sympathetic response to noxious stimuli, such as a distended bladder. The sympathetic discharge results in hypertension, bradycardia, and cutaneous changes. Due to vagal dominance, patients may develop bradycardia, heart block, and rarely asystole. Avoidance of noxious stimuli, judicious use of vasodilators, and anticholinergic drugs are required to treat autonomic hyperreflexia.
- Urinary incontinence requires bladder catheterization and often results in *urinary tract infections*.
- Recumbency can lead to *bed sores*, loss of bone mass, *renal calculi*, increased risk of *deep venous thrombosis*, and *pulmonary embolism*.
- *Hyponatremia* is seen in the first week of the injury.
- Chronic infections may lead to *anemia*.
- Drug *dependency* can result due to phantom pains.

Outcome

- Approximately 90% of all patients with spinal cord injuries survive.
- 50% of these can be successfully rehabilitated.

CASE REPORTS FOR FURTHER DISCUSSION

Case 1: A 72-year-old man presented with acute upper gastrointestinal (GI) bleeding from a peptic ulcer. He underwent an uneventful subtotal gastrectomy. The intubation and extubation were unremarkable during surgery, and the blood loss was 250 mL. The surgery lasted about 2 hours. He was sent to the surgical intensive care unit (SICU) for recovery. Around 10 hours after surgery, the patient was found to have flaccid paralysis of both legs with bilateral upper limb weakness. There were no sensations below the T4 level. On review of his medical history, he said he had intermittent pain in the neck and shoulder. CT scan revealed multiple herniated discs from C3 to C6 with spinal stenosis confirmed on MR imaging. The patient was due for anterior spinal discectomy with fusion. *What are your concerns* in this case when there is a history of recent GI surgery? How will you protect the spine from further damage during intubation?

Case 2: The patient, a 73-year-old tourist, was on a sailing trip with several physicians. He fell from his bunk bed. During the fall, he sustained a minor head trauma but remained conscious. After the fall, the patient was completely quadriplegic with no sensation below C4, although he could speak and breathe. The other physicians on the cruise stabilized his C-spine using an unhinged cabin door. Gradually, his sensation and motor function returned from distal to proximal in the lower limb. Over the next several hours, his arm showed a similar recovery. On admission to the hospital on the same day, the patient had 4/5 hemiparesis on the left side with the loss of fine movements on the right. There was no bladder or bowel dysfunction. He was ambulant two days later, and five days later, he could take an intercontinental flight.

Further investigations revealed the instability of the C-spine with 4/5 weakness of the left biceps. The patient was scheduled for anterior spinal fixation. *Due to the instability of the C-spine, the surgeons requested awake fiber-optic intubation. How will you proceed? There was no problem in passing the scope; however, difficulty was encountered in advancing the endotracheal tube over the fiber-optic device. What would you do?*

Case 3: A 35-year-old female patient who is 21 weeks pregnant presented to the ER with a 1-day history of severe interscapular pain and weakness in the lower limbs. Over the last 24 hours, despite bed rest, the patient's weakness continued to worsen. On arrival at the hospital, she had 2/5 motor power in the upper limbs, with flaccid paralysis of the lower limbs and C7 T1 sensory level. The MRI showed a C3 to C6 hematoma with severe spinal cord compression. The fetal heart rate was 140 bpm. Her other investigations were within normal limits, and the airway was class 1.

She was due for posterior decompression under general anesthesia. *What are the additional concerns in a pregnant patient while intubating? What is the effect of a prone position on fetal blood flow? Will you monitor the fetus at 21 weeks?*

Case 4: A 50-year-old man sustained a complete C6 C7 spinal cord transection three years ago in a road traffic accident. Ten days earlier, he developed a severe headache and a hypertensive response during a flexible cystoscopy as an outpatient procedure without anesthesia. A diagnosis of autonomic hyperreflexia is made, and he is now due for the same examination under anesthesia. *What are the other diagnostic features of autonomic hyperreflexia? If the case was under general anesthesia, what precautions would you take? What are the pros and cons of epidural and spinal anesthesia?*

Case 5: An 85-year-old woman with depression and dementia was brought to the ER with a self-inflicted knife wound to the neck. A kitchen knife was deeply embedded in the neck along the mid-line. She was somnolent, hypotensive, and bradycardic. CT imaging revealed that the knife had completely penetrated the spinal cord with a fracture of T1 and suspected injuries to the thyroid and esophagus. At the time, injuries to the trachea, carotid arteries, and jugular vein were unclear. She was due for surgery under general anesthesia to remove the knife and assess and repair the injuries. *How will you proceed with such a case? Will you wait for additional investigations? How will you intubate with the knife embedded in the neck?*

CASE REPORT REFERENCES

Case 1: Zhang Q et al. Paraplegia after gastrectomy in a patient with cervical disc herniation: a case report and review of literature. Case Rep Anesthesiol. 2014;2014:718690.

Case 2: Wenger M et al. Traumatic cervical instability associated with cord oedema and temporary quadriparesis. Spinal Cord. 2003;41:521-6.

Case 3: Samali M et al. Anesthetic management of spontaneous cervical epidural hematoma during pregnancy: A case report. J Med Case Rep. 2017;11:171.

Case 4: Foaleng A et al. Combined use of epidural analgesia and intravenous lignocaine for enhanced recovery in a tetraplegic patient with autonomic hyperreflexia: a case report. Int J Case Rep Short Rev. 2019;5(5):020-3.

Case 5: Kim K-H et al. Stabbing neck injury with complete spinal cord transection and neurogenic shock: A case report. Clin Surg. 2018;3:2113.

FURTHER READING

1. Cuthbertson J et al. Spinal immobilization in disasters: a systematic review. Prehosp Disaster Med. 2020;35(4):406-11.
2. Shea C et al. Trauma indicators in spinal cord injury rehabilitation outcomes: a retrospective cohort analysis of the national trauma data bank and national spinal cord injury database. Arch Phys Med Rehabil. 2022;103(4):642-48.e2.
3. Vedantam A et al. A prospective multi-center study comparing the complication profile of modest systemic hypothermia versus normothermia for acute cervical spinal cord injury. Spinal Cord. 2022;60(6):510-5.
4. Wang TY et al. Management of acute traumatic spinal cord injury: a review of the literature. Front Surg. 2021. 8: 698736.
5. Yang CH et al. Elevated intraspinal pressure in traumatic spinal cord injury is a promising therapeutic target. Neural Regen Res. 2022;17(8):1703-10.

Vignette: Bypassing the Injured Spinal Cord: Towards Thought-Controlled Devices

Faced with complete spinal injuries, the chances of neurological recovery are exceedingly poor. While neurorestorative research continues, there is a good likelihood that brain-computer interfaces (BCI) might help restore at least some functions in these individuals. At the heart of the BCI system is the acquisition of the cortical signals either by surface EEG recordings or through implantable electrodes, processing the EEG signals by filtering out the noise and translating them, and then converting the translated signals to a meaningful output. Once the device is functioning, the person has to be trained to use it. The process can be aided by artificial intelligence, decreasing training time. Devices such as thought-controlled speech, wheelchairs, prosthetic limbs, or entire exoskeletons can profoundly affect the quality of life of paralyzed and injured patients.

Chapter 49

Intraoperative Evoked Potential Changes

INTRODUCTION

Advances in neurosurgery have increased the reliance on intraoperative electrophysiological (EP) monitoring. EP monitoring is not mandatory and is primarily determined by the surgeon's needs. The well-accepted indications for EP monitoring are posterior decompression of the cervicothoracic spine, complex spine surgery, scoliosis correction, intradural spine surgery, and revision surgery. While the commonly used EP techniques are somatosensory-evoked responses, motor-evoked responses, brainstem auditory-evoked responses, nerve monitoring, and electromyography. These techniques prevent injury and help guide surgeons and anesthesiologists. While operational aspects of the monitoring techniques are beyond the scope of the usual anesthetic practice, it is essential to interpret the results of such monitoring correctly. Technical, anesthetic and neurosurgical factors can lead to the attenuation of electrophysiological responses during surgery. Knowing how to detect and correct attenuated responses is essential for intraoperative care.

NEUROANESTHETIC CONCERNS

- Evoked potentials
- Type of monitoring
- Choice of anesthesia
- Anesthetic management
- Depth of anesthesia monitoring
- Attenuation of signal
  - Assessment
  - Corrective steps

Evoked Potentials

Evoked potentials are the changes in the electroencephalogram (EEG) in response to electrical, visual, or auditory stimulation. The amplitude of these responses is much lower than the background EEG. Therefore, to determine these changes, a burst of stimuli, typically in the hundreds, is needed to separate the evoked response from background EEG activity. Changes in EPs are usually characterized by the changes in amplitude (microvolts) or latency (milliseconds) of specific waves seen in healthy individuals. Somatosensory evoked potential (SSEPs), transcranial motor evoked potentials (MEPs), brainstem auditory evoked response (BAER), and rarely, visual evoked responses (VERs) are used for intraoperative monitoring.

- To monitor EPs, the nerves are stimulated 100–250 times. The response to each stimulus is aggregated. By doing so, background electrical noise, which is random, is canceled out, while signals generated in response to stimulation are aggregated and augmented.
- The EEG changes in response to stimulation can be upward (negative, designated as N) or downward (positive, designated as P). However care is needed during interpretation as the display orientation can be flipped. The waves are further assigned a number that designates the time elapsed milliseconds after stimulation. For example, a P300 signal is a downward wave 300 ms after the stimuli.
- Motor evoked potential monitoring requires a constant level of partial paralysis. Excessive electromyographic (EMG) artifacts from the scalp may indicate the light level of anesthesia or inadequate paralysis that interfere with SSEP monitoring. Intense paralysis masks the local EMG response needed to confirm stimulation. Thus, EP monitoring requires a level of partial paralysis (typically 1–2/4 twitches) that has to be determined in consultation with the electrophysiologists.
- *Factors that affect EPs include the depth of anesthesia, particularly volatile anesthetics, and decreased core temperature.*
- A significant SSEP change requiring intervention includes a 10% increase in latency or a >50% decrease in peak amplitude.

Indications of EP Monitoring

- *Intraoperative EPM is frequently used during the following:*
  - Spinal instrumentation for the correction of skeletal abnormalities
  - Spinal tumor surgery
  - Carotid endarterectomy (CEA)
  - Brainstem tumor surgery, such as for vestibular schwannomas
  - Excision of peripheral nerve tumors
  - Assessment of cortical functions
  - Assessment of depth of anesthesia
- *Beyond the operating rooms, EPs can be used to determine the following:*
  - The site and location of intracranial/spinal pathologies
  - Diagnosis and monitoring of neurological diseases.

Problems with Evoked Response Monitoring

- *Practical problems:*
  - *Resource intensive:* Requires a trained technician, equipment cost, and time.
- *Resource intensive requires total intravenous anesthesia (TIVA):*
  - Drugs, pumps, and preferably processed EEG monitoring.
- Evoked potential set up can extend the duration of surgery.
- Measurements can be affected by factors unrelated to injury:
  - Background electrical noise
  - Loss of contact between electrical components
  - Changes in type and depth of anesthesia
  - Core temperature
- Possibility of injury to patient and staff due to needles
- *Conceptual problems:* There are two main problems with EP monitoring in neurosurgery—
  - The loss of signals at baselines, such as by tumor or nerve compression, makes monitoring additional changes difficult.
  - The change in the nerve function after injury may be delayed.

FREQUENTLY MONITORED EVOKED RESPONSES

Somatosensory Evoked Responses

For SSEP monitoring in the upper extremities (median and the ulnar) and the lower extremity (tibial/peroneal), nerves are stimulated **(Table 1)**.

The fasciculus cuneatus transmits the upper limb impulses. The fasciculus gracillis transmits lower limb impulses. The anterior spinal artery perfuses the dorsolateral fasciculus, which contains both tracts. Therefore, lower limb SSEP monitoring permits monitoring of any direct injury to the cord as well as cord perfusion.

Motor Evoked Potentials

- Transcranial electrical stimulation of the cortex transmits the impulses through the lateral cord (D wave) to generate a distal motor response

Table 1: Somatosensory evoked potential (SSEP) monitoring sites in the upper and lower limb.

Upper limb		Lower limb	
Stimulation sites	Recording sites	Stimulation sites	Recording sites
Median nerve (wrist)	Erb's point ↓	Saphenous nerve (thigh)	L4/5 ↓
Radial nerve (elbow)	C5, C2 ↓	Deep peroneal nerve (popliteal fossa)	T10 ↓ C2/C5 ↓
Ulnar nerve (wrist)	Cortex	Posterior tibial nerves (Medial malleolus)	Cortex

in the muscle (compound motor potentials). Therefore, MEPs provide a method for monitoring surgical injury and anterior spinal artery perfusion. Electrical stimulation for MEPs can be painful, and the resulting motor response can interfere with surgery; thus, the depth of anesthesia has to be carefully monitored, and the level of paralysis maintained between 1 and 2 twitches. MEPs are to be used with care in patients with a history of seizures, skull defects, metal implants in the head or neck, or implanted pacemakers. Contractions of the masseter muscles can result in tongue bites; thus, a bite block is required during MEP monitoring.
- Descending motor response (DMR) is a less frequently used mode of motor stimulation that is useful when conventional MEPs are unavailable. To elicit DMR, the spinal cord or a peripheral nerve below a lesion is stimulated, and the recording is obtained from the caudal region. DMR can be mediated by a sensory nerve and does not represent an isolated motor response.
- While consistent D waves can be recorded from the spinal cord's lateral aspects, although, it requires surgical exposure. Compound motor potentials can be recorded from the muscles; however, these are polymorphic and somewhat difficult to interpret. Amplitudes of the peak are used to assess motor activity, and sometimes the absence or presence of the wave is all that is noted. *Compared to the SSEPs, the MEPs are more sensitive to the effects of anesthetic drugs.*

CAUSES OF DETERIORATION OF EP RESPONSES

- *Technical:*
  - Electrode disconnections
  - Contact deterioration.
  - Lead displacement
  - Movement artifacts
  - Electrical noise
- *Anesthesia-related:*
  - Increase in anesthetic concentration or dose.
  - Hypothermia
  - Inadequate or excessive paralysis
  - Systemic hypoxia, acidosis, hypocapnia, and hypercapnia
- *Surgical causes:*
  - Direct:
    - Positioning
    - Nerve compression due to retraction
    - Surgical injury to the nerve
    - Local loss of conductivity due to injury
    - Local hypothermia (irrigation)

- *Indirect causes:*
  - *Ischemia:* Sensitivity to ischemia—VERs > MEPs > SSEPs > BAERs
  - Systemic hypotension

MANAGEMENT

Evoked potential deteriorates over minutes after injury.
- *If a sudden change occurs:*
  - Review preceding surgical intervention.
  - Rule out any equipment failure.
  - Check the position of limbs.
  - Review if there is any change in anesthetic drug dosing or administration of muscle relaxants.
  - Acute hypoxia or hypercapnia.
  - Rule out hypoxia, hypercarbia, or metabolic conditions.
- *If the change is slow:*
  - Evaluate for hypothermia.
  - Assess the cumulation of anesthetic drugs.
  - *Consider metabolic changes:*
    - Acidosis
    - Hypoxia
    - Hypercarbia
    - Blood sugar, acid-base, and electrolytes
- *If a surgical injury is suspected:*
  - Release the retractors.
  - Check X-ray for instrumentation and/or change in position.
  - Reverse instrumentation.
  - Consider waking up and abbreviating the surgery if deficits persist.

CASE REPORTS FOR FURTHER DISCUSSION

Case 1: A 30-year-old male patient with severe kyphosis and L1-L2 vertebral subluxation was scheduled for corrective surgery with tibial and median nerve monitoring. The patient was positioned on an open-frame hinged table for the surgery. After prone positioning, a baseline recording was obtained. After that, the frame was adjusted to enable exposure. As the frame was extended, the lower extremity MEP and SSEP signals were lost. The frame was returned to the neutral position, and MEP and SSEP returned to the baseline. *Will you proceed with surgery? The surgeons plan for decompression and instrumentation. The signal might be lost again as the frame is extended to enable instrumentation. What precautions will you take before extending the frame?*

Case 2: A 14-year-old female patient was undergoing kyphoscoliosis correction with anterior and posterior spinal fusion under general anesthesia. Anterior fusion was undertaken in the lateral position and was achieved uneventfully. The estimated blood loss was 600 mL. Central venous pressure (CVP) remained at 9 mm Hg. A total of 2.2 L of IV fluid was given. SSEP and MEP signals remained unchanged from the baseline. However, when positioned prone for posterior fixation, there were several bouts of severe hypotension with BP decreasing from 100/60 to 40/20 mm Hg. These hypotensive episodes coincided with the testing of motor potentials. The patient was treated with boluses of dopamine and phenylephrine. Hypotension was attributed to electrically induced sympathectomy. The cervical electrodes were repositioned, the motor response could be monitored without hypotension, and surgery continued uneventfully. *Where is the cervical sympathetic chain? Besides hypotension, what are the other effects of cervical sympathectomy? What criteria will you follow to treat systemic hypotension? What could be the rationale for using dopamine? What are the dose-related autonomic effects of dopamine?*

Case 3: A 15-year-old female presented with right thoracic idiopathic spinal scoliosis. There were no medical or neurological concerns. During posterior decompression (T4–T11) and the rod placement, the left-sided SSEPs were lost, but motor-evoked potentials remained intact. Causes of signal loss were evaluated and addressed, but the deficits persisted. As per protocol, the rod was removed. The patient recovered from anesthesia and had no clinical neurological deficits. Postoperative MRI revealed no spinal cord injury or edema. However, the SSEP deficits persisted for several days afterward. A repeat CT scan revealed a burst left pedicle, with a bone fragment impacting the dorsal spinal cord at the T10 level. The patient was scheduled for repeat spinal instrumentation a week after the surgery. *What precautions will you take for EP monitoring in a patient with known spinal deficits? What anesthetic drugs can you use to enhance EP monitoring?*

CASE REPORT REFERENCES

Case 1: Graham RB et al. Loss of intraoperative neurological monitoring signals during flexed prone positioning on a hinged open frame during surgery for kyphoscoliosis correction: case report. J Neurosurg Spine. 2018;29:339-43.

Case 2: Hays SR et al. Transient hypotension as a complication of monitoring transcervical motor evoked potentials. Anesthesiology. 1999;90:314-7.

Case 3: Tomé-Bermejo F et al. Identification of risk factors for the occurrence of cement leakage during percutaneous vertebroplasty for painful osteoporotic or malignant vertebral fracture. Spine (Phila Pa 1976). 2014;39:E60-3.

FURTHER READING

1. Bala E et al. Motor and somatosensory evoked potentials are well maintained in patients given dexmedetomidine during spine surgery. Anesthesiology, 2008;109(3):417-25.
2. Biricik E et al. A comparison of intravenous sugammadex and neostigmine + atropine reversal on time to consciousness during wakeup tests in spinal surgery. Niger J Clin Pract. 2019;22(5):609-15.
3. Kondo T et al. Intraoperative responses of motor evoked potentials to the novel intravenous anesthetic remimazolam during spine surgery: a report of two cases. JA Clin Rep. 2020;6(1):97.
4. Sloan TB et al. Intraoperative neurophysiological monitoring during spine surgery with total intravenous anesthesia or balanced anesthesia with 3% desflurane. J Clin Monit Comput. 2015;29(1):77-85.
5. Toossi A et al. Effect of anesthesia on motor responses evoked by spinal neural prostheses during intraoperative procedures. J Neural Eng. 2019; 16(3):036003.

Vignette: The First EEGs Were Too Good to be True!

Richard Canton was a man of outstanding achievements. He was a physician, scientist, teacher, and, later in life, the Lord Mayor of Liverpool in England. In 1875, Canton first reported recording electric currents from the exposed brains of rabbits and monkeys by using a sensitive galvanometer. He also observed a paradoxical increase in the current amplitude with sleep. The signals were increased at the onset of death but disappeared afterward. Canton's findings that the signals increased during sleep generated skepticism and were less ignored until Hans Berger cited them in 1929, over half a century later.

Chapter 50

Posterior Fossa Surgery

INTRODUCTION

The posterior fossa is the region of the skull between the tentorium cerebelli and the foramen magnum. Besides containing vital structures such as the pons, medulla, and cerebellum, it also contains the IV ventricle and neural tracts. Due to its small size and predisposition to ventricular obstruction, small increases in tissue volume or blood can rapidly increase intracranial pressure resulting in tissue and brain herniation. The posterior fossa is a frequent site for primary and secondary brain tumors. These operations require sitting, prone or lateral positions. Brainstem and lower cranial nerve monitoring are necessary during surgery. Hemodynamic changes and venous air embolism can occur. Postoperative complications include macroglossia, pneumocephalus, and nerve injuries.

NEUROANESTHETIC CONCERNS

- Posterior fossa anatomy
- Anatomical concerns
- Pathological lesions and indications of posterior fossa surgery
- Preoperative assessment
- Monitoring
- Choice of anesthetic technique
- *Positioning:* Surgery in the sitting position
- Intraoperative management
- Immediate postoperative concerns
- Delayed complications.

Posterior Fossa Anatomy

- *Boundaries:*
  - *Superior:* Tentorium cerebelli
  - *Inferior:* Foramen magnum
  - *Anterior:* Dorsum sellae and occipital bone (basilar part)
  - *Posterior:* Occipital bone
  - *Lateral:* Occipital bone
- *Contents:*
  - Cerebellum

- Brainstem
- Lower cranial nerves
- Venous sinuses
- Fourth ventricle.

Clinical Significance

- Emissary veins that connect the sinuses to the extracranial veins traverse the occipital bone. Surgical disruption of these non-retractile communications can lead to air embolism.
- In adults, the volume of the posterior fossa is 150 cm^3, about 50% of which is the cerebellar volume (80 mL). The posterior fossa volume is about a tenth of the intracranial volume. Consequently, a slight increase in the tissue volume, blood, or CSF, causes a rapid increase in pressure within the fossa with cerebellar or brainstem herniation.
- Compression of the fourth ventricle by tumors can also lead to hydrocephalus and a rise in intracranial pressure (ICP).
- *Signs of cerebellar herniation* are primarily due to brainstem and upper spinal cord compression, these include the following:
  - Headache, vomiting, head tilt, neck stiffness, and flaccid paralysis
  - Hemodynamic instability
  - Deviation of the eyes and vertical nystagmus
  - Cerebellar fits present as opisthotonos with muscle spasms.
  - Vocal cord paralysis, paroxysmal coughing, and irregular respiration
  - Cardio-respiratory arrest.

Pathological Lesions

- *Cerebellar lesions:*
  - In the adult age group:
    - *Metastasis:* Solitary intraparenchymal lesions are always metastatic
    - Hemangioblastoma
    - Glioma
    - Abscess
    - Hemangioma
    - Hemorrhage
    - Cerebellar stroke
  - In the pediatric age group:
    - 60–70% of all pediatric brain tumors are in the posterior fossa
    - The three most common tumors are (30% each):
      1. Medulloblastoma
      2. Astrocytoma
      3. Glioma.

- Cerebellopontine angle (CPA) lesions:
  - *Vestibular schwannomas:* 80–90%
  - *Meningiomas:* 5–10%
  - *Others:* Epidermoid cysts, metastasis, and neuromas.

Indications for Posterior Fossa Surgery

- *Tumors:*
  - *Mid-line:* Cerebellar vermis, fourth ventricle, pineal, and brainstem
  - *Lateral:* Cerebral lesions and cranial nerve tumors (acoustic neuromas)
- Aneurysms
- Microvascular decompression of cranial nerves
- Electrode implantation for cerebellar nerves
- *Brainstem decompression:*
  - Arnold-Chiari malformations
  - Syringomyelia.

Preoperative Assessment

- *General condition:*
  - Nausea/vomiting can impair sensorium due to electrolyte imbalance. Dehydration can lead to hypovolemia and hypotension.
  - *Extremes of age:* Avoid sitting position.
- *Neurological assessment:*
  - *Cerebellar symptoms:* Two syndromes:
    - *Lateral lesions:* Classic cerebellar signs
      - Hypotonia
      - Intention tremors
      - Dysdiadochokinesia, dysmetria, dysarthria
      - *Ocular signs:* Nystagmus, gaze paralysis, and skew deviation of the eyes
      - Late hydrocephalus
    - Mid-line lesions and fourth ventricle tumors:
      - Early hydrocephalus
      - Truncal ataxia
      - Wide base gait
      - Nystagmus
      - Papilledema
  - Cranial nerve paralysis (**Table 1**) with impaired bulbar functions
  - A ventriculoartrial (VA) shunt can lead to air embolism. It is a contraindication for sitting position surgery.

Table 1: Rapid assessment of V–XII cranial nerves.

Cranial nerve	Origin	Name	Pathological signs
V	Pons	Trigeminal	Loss for corneal reflex
VI	Pons	Abducens	Loss of lateral movement of the eye
VII	Pons	Facial	Loss of smile
VIII	Pons	Vestibular	Loss of hearing
IX	Medulla	Glossopharyngeal	Loss of gag reflex
X	Medulla	Vagus	Loss of swallowing
XI	Medulla	Spinal accessory	Inability to shrug shoulders
XII	Medulla	Hypoglossal	Tongue deviation

- A ventriculoperitoneal (VP) shunt can lead to over-drainage of CSF in the sitting position. Resulting in pneumocephalus and delayed wake-up after surgery.

Cardiovascular assessment:
- Cardiovascular instability can be due to the following:
  - Hypovolemia secondary to:
    - Dehydration due to impaired consciousness
    - Use of diuretics to decrease ICP.
  - Impaired vasomotor responses (e.g., in the elderly)
  - Orthostatic hypotension
- Arrhythmias/bradycardia due to brainstem involvement
- Presence of a "right-to-left" shunt:
  - It can lead to systemic air embolism resulting in myocardial infarction or stroke.
  - Considered to be an absolute contraindication to sitting position surgery.

Monitoring Posterior Fossa Surgery

- *Routine monitoring:* EKG, pulse oximeter, inspired and end-tidal gas composition, noninvasive blood pressure, neuromuscular transmission monitor, and invasive arterial blood pressure monitoring.
- *Specific:*
  - Precordial Doppler or transesophageal echocardiography (TEE) for early warning for venous air embolism (VAE): To test for the sensitivity of placement of precordial Doppler, inject 10 mL bolus of agitated albumin or saline, which should result in a change in the heart sounds.
  - End-tidal carbon dioxide ($EtCO_2$) monitoring:
    - Keep minute ventilation constant if at risk for VAE.

- If switching to 100% O_2 during suspected VAE, keep fresh gas flow the same.
- Avoid changing the minute ventilation to increase $EtCO_2$ as it prevents accurate interpretation of $EtCO_2$ changes.
- An abrupt $EtCO_2$ (3 mm Hg) decrease suggests air embolism. A more gradual decline is seen in other conditions, such as hypothermia or subtle changes in ventilation.
- Any decrease in $EtCO_2$ with tachycardia/arrhythmias or fall in SAO_2 is highly suggestive of VAE.
- End-tidal N_2 concentration (EtN_2):
  - An increase in EtN_2 concentration can detect VAE.
  - Occurs before hemodynamic changes or a decrease in $EtCO_2$.
  - The reduction in cardiac output blunts EtN_2 rise during VAE.
  - Therefore, predicting recovery from VAE is difficult with EtN_2 monitoring.
- Central venous pressure (CVP) monitoring:
  - The placement of a multi-hole CVP catheter could be helpful but not essential.
  - Long-arm CVPs for air aspiration require EKG guidance to locate at the superior vena cava/right atrial (SVC/RA) junction **(Fig. 1)**.
- *Cranial nerve monitoring:*
  - Facial, auditory nerve, hypoglossal, and vagus nerves are monitored.

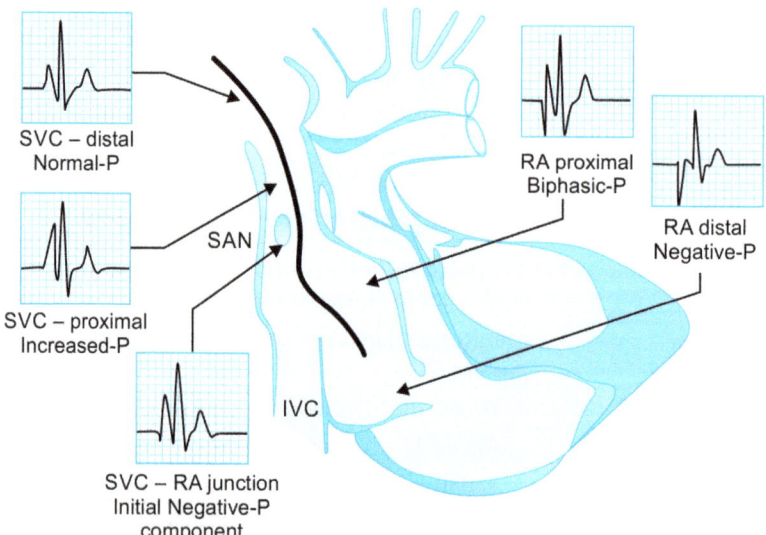

Fig. 1: EKG changes during central venous catheter placement for VAE: P-wave morphology changes from upright to inverted. (RA: right atrium; SVC: superior vena cava; IVC: inferior vena cava; SAN: sinoatrial node)

- The EMG activity of innervated muscles is monitored during surgery.
- Muscle relaxants are avoided to monitor motor nerves.
- Nerve integrity monitoring (NIM) endotracheal tube: The NIM tube has two sets of electrodes to monitor the EMG activity of the vocal cords. Placement is done using video laryngoscopy.
- A bite block is needed to avoid tongue injury during motor-evoked potential monitoring.

Anesthetic Techniques

- Posterior fossa surgery can is done in different positions (*see* **Table 1**). During positioning, care is needed to prevent injury to the cervical spine, spinal cord, cervical nerves, and the brachial plexus.
- Total intravenous anesthesia (TIVA) or volatile anesthetics can be used, as determined by monitoring needs:
  - Brainstem auditory evoked responses for monitoring VIII cranial nerve integrity are resistant to volatile agents.
  - Muscle relaxants are avoided to enable EMG monitoring.
  - TIVA with remifentanil and propofol is most commonly used as it enables electrophysiological monitoring.

Sitting Surgery

- Sitting surgery is usually for supra-cerebellar tumors.
- Due to the risk of air embolism, nitrous oxide is avoided.
- The main risk of TIVA is systemic hypotension in a sitting position.
- Therefore, volatile anesthetics are sometimes used if electrophysiological monitoring is not required.
- The level of anesthesia can be adjusted as needed.
- The advantages and disadvantages of the other positions for posterior fossa surgery are listed in **Table 2**.

SITTING POSITION

- *Contraindications for the sitting position:*
  - Patent foramen ovale
  - Right-to-left shunts
  - Severe congestive heart failure
  - Low-pressure or malfunctioning VP shunt
  - Degenerative spine diseases
  - General debility
  - Elderly.
- *Advantages:*
  - The midline position provides better surgical orientation than a lateral approach.

Table 2: Positioning for posterior fossa surgery.

Position	Indication	Advantage	Disadvantage
Supine with head tilt	• CP angle tumor • Unilateral lesions	• Hemodynamic stability • Lower risk of VAE	Blood and CSF pooling
Lateral	Unilateral lesions	Good blood and CSF drainage	Surgical exposure to midline limited
Prone	Midline lesions	• Hemodynamic stability • Excellent surgical orientation • Lower risk of VAE	• Blood and CSF pooling • Facial congestion • If head elevated, venous pooling possible
Park bench (Fig. 2)	• CP angle tumors • Unilateral lesions	• Good exposure • Blood and CSF drainage	Surgical exposure to midline limited
Sitting	Mid-line lesion	• Excellent surgical orientation. • Good blood and CSF drainage. • Good access to the patient and monitoring	• Hemodynamic and position-related complications • Contraindicated for some patients • High risk of venous air embolism

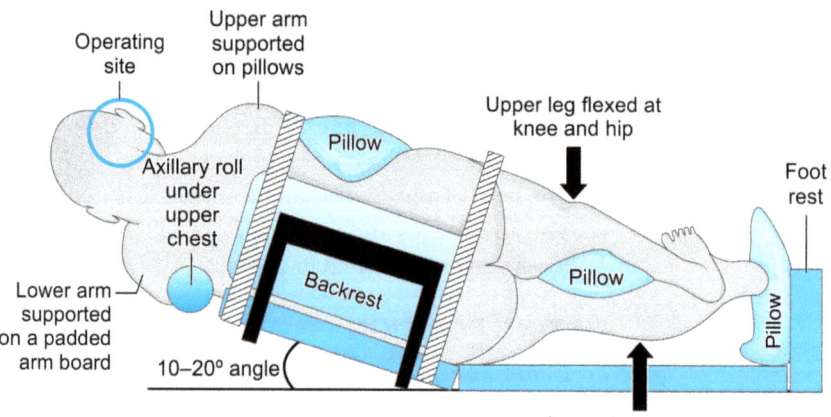

Fig. 2: Park bench position for posterior fossa surgery can avoid several problems seen with the sitting position.

- Clear surgical field, blood and CSF can drain away from the operative site.
- Lower blood pressure, better venous drainage, and less blood loss
- Decreases ICP
- Better ventilation.

- *Disadvantages:*
  - *Cardiovascular:*
    - Possible air embolism
    - Postural hypotension can be seen in as much as 30% of the cases.
    - *Cardiac arrhythmias:* Ventricular ectopy in 50% and sinus bradycardia in 25% of the cases, respectively
    - Decreased cerebral perfusion pressure (CPP)
    - Impaired autoregulation
    - Decreased cerebral blood flow (CBF) and potential for hypotensive stroke
    - Greater risk of postoperative bleeding due to concealed vascular injury due to lower regional arterial and venous pressure.
    - Venous stasis in legs and deep vein thrombosis (DVT).
  - *Airway and respiratory:*
    - Endobronchial intubation
    - Macroglossia may be due to impaired venous return and could be exacerbated by probe pressure if a TEE is used.
  - *Positioning hazards:*
    - Pins often secure the head to the mid-section of the table. Lowering the back can result in moving the head away from the pins. It can result in scalp lacerations or a release of the head from the pins.
    - If the head needs to be lowered in an emergency, the entire table should be tilted using the Trendelenburg controls.
    - The patient may slide down when the back is elevated. Care is needed to prevent such a slide that can result in high spinal injury due to excessive traction on the neck.
    - Exposure of the body in a sitting position can lead to hypothermia.
    - Pin fixation can cause intracranial injuries such as epidural hematoma.
  - *Cerebrovascular effects:*
    - Decreased CPP
      - Impaired pressure autoregulation
      - Impaired CO_2 reactivity
    - *Increased regional venous pressure:* Neck flexion with less than a 2-finger distance between the chin and chest can increase resistance to jugular venous flow and result in facial or brain edema.
  - *Increased CSF drainage:*
    - Ventricular collapse is possible and may predispose to pneumocephalus.
    - The collapse of the ventricle may displace the shunt tip.
    - VA shunt is a contraindication due to possible air embolism.

- VP shunt pressure threshold should is checked and settings adjusted.
- Increased risk of tonsillar herniation.
  - *Nerves injuries:*
    - Brachial plexuses injury is possible if the arm is not supported correctly or by a misplaced axillary roll.
    - Ulnar nerve injury is possible at the elbow.
    - Peroneal nerve injury is possible at the knee.
    - Sciatic nerve injury is possible at the hip.
    - Mid-cervical quadriplegia is possible due to excessive neck flexion.
  - *Respiratory effects:*
    - Neck flexion can lead to endobronchial tube migration.
    - Compression of the abdomen-restricted lung volumes.
  - *Other considerations:*
    - Operator fatigue, unsupported arms, and prolonged standing.

Intraoperative Concerns

- *Hemodynamic changes:*
  - Hypotension
  - Venous air embolism
  - Arrhythmias
- Surgery-triggered arrhythmias
- Ensure stable anesthesia to permit monitoring.
- Brain swelling
- Blood loss.

Immediate Postoperative Concerns

- *Hemodynamic instability:*
  - Treatment of hypertension and arrhythmias
- *Potential complications:*
  - Macroglossia
  - Lower cranial nerve palsies
  - Upper gastrointestinal (GI) hemorrhage with fourth ventricular tumors
  - SIADH (syndrome of inappropriate antidiuretic hormone secretion)
  - Febrile reaction due to blood in the subarachnoid space
- *Delayed awakening:*
  - Bleeding
  - Elevated ICP
  - Pneumocephalus
  - Brainstem injury.

Delayed Concerns
- Lower cranial nerve palsies
- Inability to close the eyes and the loss of blink requires tarsorrhaphy
- CSF leaks
- Pseudomeningocele
- Meningitis
- Behavioral changes.

CASE REPORTS FOR FURTHER DISCUSSION

Case 1: An 18-year-old otherwise healthy patient was scheduled for suboccipital craniotomy in the sitting position to remove an ependymoma. Preoperative labs and coagulation screens were within normal limits. During surgery, there was a sudden decrease in $EtCO_2$ from 36 to 20 mm Hg, but with no significant hemodynamic change. The incision site was packed with a wet sponge, and 100% oxygen was given. A tear in the occipital sinus was clipped, and surgery proceeded uneventfully. Toward the end of the case, the surgeons requested the Valsalva maneuver to assess for CSF leak and venous hemostasis. Immediately after the release of positive pressure during Valsalva, the $EtCO_2$ decreased from 30 to 9 mm Hg. There was severe hypotension with ST-T segment depressions on the EKG. A 39 mm Hg gradient was found between the end tidal and arterial PCO_2. Central venous catheter aspiration yielded 50–60 mL of air. *What is the value of precordial Doppler monitoring? What is the frequency of the ultrasound probe used to detect air embolism? What are the benefits and limitations of central venous catheters during sitting position surgery? How does the Valsalva maneuver increase the CSF pressure?*

Case 2: A 55-year-old female patient underwent a right acoustic neuroma excision in the park-bench position. During surgery, the head was fixed in pins. Bite blocks were placed between the teeth. A retro sigmoid approach was used to access the tumor. The total surgery time was 6.5 hours. At the end of the surgery, the patient was extubated. Immediately on extubation, airway obstruction was noted. She was given steroids but continued to desaturate. She was reintubated and transferred to an intensive care unit (ICU). The swelling continued to increase over the next several hours. Antihistamine, steroids, and antifibrinolytic treatment had no effect. A CT scan of the head and neck revealed tissue edema but with no hematoma or an abscess. Her condition remained unchanged for two weeks. After tracheostomy, the edema decreased rapidly within 24 hours. *What is the etiology of macroglossia after posterior fossa surgery? What was the likely cause in this case? How will you reintubate a patient with postoperative macroglossia in respiratory distress? What could be the rationale for antifibrinolytic treatment?*

Case 3: A 7-year-old patient developed headache, vomiting, and other signs consistent with a cerebellar tumor. MRI revealed a 5 × 4 × 3 cm mid-line lesion in the cerebral vermis compressing the fourth ventricle. A ventricular drain was placed. She subsequently underwent a suboccipital craniotomy for tumor excision. Postoperatively, the patient was hemodynamically stable, breathing adequately, and localizing pain. However, she was unresponsive to verbal commands. She exhibited movements suggestive of seizures. The postoperative CT scan was not diagnostic. The patient was extubated approximately 3 hours later. Although she followed verbal commands, she did not speak. Over the next several hours, there was some improvement in her speech, but the speech remained slow for many months after surgery, requiring speech therapy. *What are the possible causes of speech impairment after GETA for posterior fossa surgery? What are the causes of delayed awakening after anesthesia? How will you manage such a case? What are the signs of cerebellar dysfunction?*

Case 4: A 46-year-old with progressive deafness and gait impairment underwent an uneventful suboccipital craniotomy in the left park-bench position. Precautions were taken to ensure adequate space between the chin and the chest to avoid compromising the venous return. Vitals remained stable throughout surgery and had a net negative (900 mL) fluid balance. After extubation, face and neck swelling were noted. After 2 hours, the edema was sufficient to cause respiratory distress, requiring emergent intubation. Head and neck CT scans revealed tissue edema but no other abnormality. Doppler interrogation revealed patent veins with no obstruction to venous drainage. The swelling declined by the third day, but extubation was possible only on the 17th postoperative day. *What are the problems associated with the park-bench position? What is the minimum safe distance between the chin and the chest when the neck is flexed? What is the likely cause of the face and neck swelling in this case? How do you test for air leaks with suspected upper airway swelling?*

Case 5: An 18-year-old boy was admitted with a headache, vomiting, and unsteady gait for three days. On further questioning, there was a much longer history of intermittent headaches and episodes of dizziness. MRI revealed a mass in the vermis. A sub-occipital craniotomy in a prone position was performed. The operation lasted 8.5 hours. There was no vascular injury or significant hypotensive episodes during surgery. A tissue biopsy confirmed medulloblastoma. Postoperatively, complete motor and sensory losses were evident below the C5–C6 level. MRI revealed a long segment of the spinal cord from C2 to T1 that was hyperintense suggestive of ischemia/injury. Steroid treatment was immediately instituted, but there was no significant recovery. *Would electrophysiological monitoring have helped in this case? What are the possible causes of quadriparesis* *with suboccipital craniotomies? How would you explain such an injury in a prone position? What is the likely long-term outcome of such an injury in an eighteen-year-old patient?*

CASE REPORT REFERENCES

Case 1: Moningi S et al. Coagulopathy following venous air embolism—a disastrous consequence: a case report. Korean J Anesthesiol. 2013;65(4): 349-52.

Case 2: Vermeersch G, et al. Life-threatening macroglossia after posterior fossa surgery: a surgical positioning problem? B-ENT. 2014;10:309-13.

Case 3: Chao JY et al. Postoperative pediatric cerebellar mutism after posterior fossa surgery: a case report. AA Case Rep. 2017;8(8):213-5.

Case 4: Hsu SK et al. Delayed airway obstruction in posterior fossa craniotomy with park-bench position: a case report and review of the literatures. Surg Sci. 2012;3:526-9.

Case 5: Rau CS et al. Quadriplegia in a patient who underwent posterior fossa surgery in the prone position. J Neurosurg. 2002;96:101-3.

FURTHER READING

1. Bapteste L et al. Pulse pressure variations and plethysmographic variability index measured at ear are able to predict fluid responsiveness in the sitting position for neurosurgery. J Neurosurg Anesthesiol. 2020;32(3):263-7.
2. Himes BT et al. Contemporary analysis of the intraoperative and perioperative complications of neurosurgical procedures performed in the sitting position. J Neurosurg. 2017;127(1):182-8.
3. Klein O et al. Surgical approach to the posterior fossa in children, including anesthetic considerations and complications: the prone and the sitting position. Technical note. Neurochirurgie. 2021;67(1):46-51.
4. Kurihara M et al. Estimation of the head elevation angle that causes clinically important venous air embolism in a semi-sitting position for neurosurgery: a retrospective observational study. Fukushima J Med Sci. 2020;66(2):67-72.
5. Luostarinen T et al. Prone versus sitting position in neurosurgery-differences in patients' hemodynamic management. World Neurosurg. 2017;97:261-6.

Vignette: The History of Venous Air Embolism

The hazards of air entrainment through open veins were well-known to surgeons even before the demonstration of ether anesthesia in 1846. Seven years earlier, John Rose-Cormack wrote an authoritative dissertation on "Air in the Organ of Circulation," describing more than 40 cases of venous air embolism. Venous air embolism was well-known to surgeons even before then. It was known that the division of veins caused air entrainment, resulting in an airlock in the right atrium. It produced a hissing, gurgling sound and was rapidly fatal. There were over 50 reports of such catastrophic events between 1811 and 1885. One of the risk factors was the speed of surgery. Before anesthesia, the surgery had to be recklessly fast, and there was little time to dissect the veins carefully. This problem was made worse because surgery in the late 19th century was often done sitting with the patient strapped to chairs.

Chapter 51

Transsphenoid Hypophysectomy

INTRODUCTION

The location of the pituitary in the sella turcica permits it to be accessed extracranially through the nasal sphenoid and maxillary approaches. For decades microscopic, nasal, or sublabial transsphenoid approaches were used to excise pituitary tumors. The alternative endoscopic approach permits safer and wider access to the pituitary gland, which is particularly useful when the tumors extend outside the sella. The usual indications for Transsphenoid surgery are resection of pituitary adenoma, meningioma, cysts, or craniopharyngiomas. Endocrine disturbances may have profound systemic effects that need careful preoperative review. The airway is of particular concern both at intubation and extubation. Pituitary surgery can be challenging due to the many critical structures adjacent to the gland, with the risk of bleeding and neurological injuries. Transsphenoid surgery is highly effective for microadenomas.

NEUROANESTHETIC CONCERNS

- Pituitary tumors
- *Clinical presentation:*
  - Neurological
  - Endocrine
  - Pituitary apoplexy
- Investigation
- Treatment
- *Anesthetic management:*
  - *Preoperative assessment:* Endocrine syndromes, airway, endotracheal tube (ETT) selection
  - *Intraoperative:* Total intravenous anesthesia (TIVA)/volatile, pin fixation, hypertensive responses, hemorrhage, and cerebrospinal fluid (CSF) leak
  - *Extubation:* Strategies for smooth extubation
- Complications.

PITUITARY TUMORS

- Classified as microadenomas (<1 cm) or macroadenomas (>1 cm)
- Represent 10% of primary brain tumors
- Typically present in the third or fourth decade with no gender predilection
- 50% <5 mm at diagnosis, and ≈50% are secretory.

CLINICAL PRESENTATION

- *Neurological symptoms:*
  - Headache
  - Visual field defect and often bitemporal hemianopsia from optic chiasm compression
  - *Pituitary insufficiency:* See endocrine syndromes.
  - Compression of cranial nerves III, IV, V1, V2, and VI produces diplopia, ptosis, and facial pain.
  - Occlusion of the cavernous sinus leading to proptosis and chemosis
  - Carotid artery compression, especially with apoplexy
  - Hydrocephalus.
- *Endocrine syndromes* **(Fig. 1):**
  - Multiple endocrine neoplasia type 1
    - Autosomal dominant
    - Tumor cluster in the pituitary, pancreas, and parathyroid gland

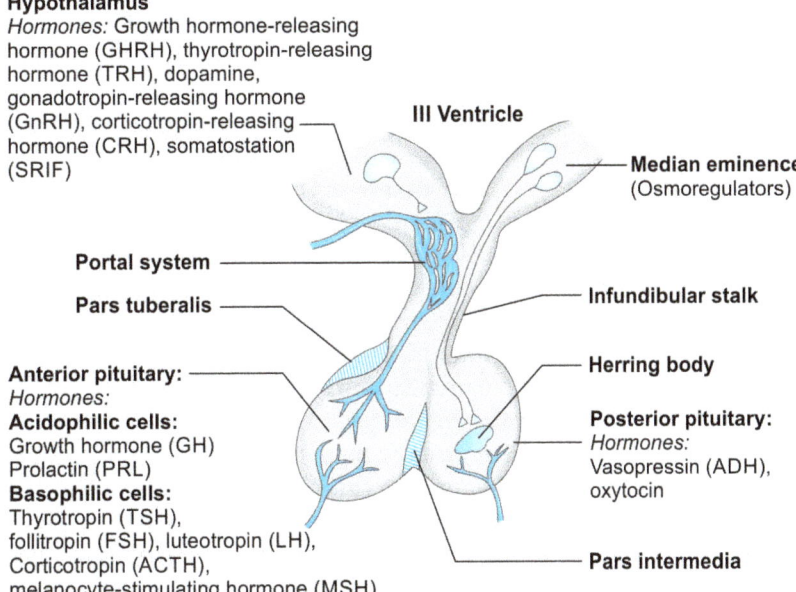

Fig. 1: Pituitary hormones and endocrine anatomy.

- *Forbes–Albright syndrome:*
  - Prolactin-secreting tumor
  - Galactorrhea, amenorrhea, sexual dysfunction, infertility, and osteoporosis
- *Acromegaly/gigantism*
  - Growth hormone-secreting tumor
  - Its clinical features include rapid growth with increased height and weight, enlargement of acral parts, joint pains, deep voice, gaps between teeth, macroglossia, thickened skin, hirsutism, hyperhidrosis, hyperglycemia, peripheral neuropathy, and cardiomyopathy. Although both gigantism and acromegaly are due to excessive growth hormone release and are characterized by abnormal growth, the difference being:
    - *Gigantism* occurs in children and young adults before the epiphyses of long bones have fused. It is earlier in onset and results in considerable increase in height.
    - *Acromegaly* occurs adults after the epiphyses have fused and thus growth is more in the acral (limbs) parts and flat bones.
- *Thyrotoxicosis:*
  - Thyrotropin-secreting tumor
  - Goiter and hyperthyroidism
- *Cushing's disease:*
  - Adrenocorticotropic hormone (ACTH) secreting tumor
  - Truncal obesity, buffalo hump, abdominal striae, easy bruising, hirsutism, hypertension, hyperglycemia, and osteoporosis
- *Panhypopituitarism:* Hypothyroid, hypoadrenalism, and hypogonadism
- *Diabetes insipidus:*
  - Decreased antidiuretic hormone (ADH)
  - Polydipsia, polyuria, decreased urine osmolality (<200 mOsm/kg), increased serum osmolality (>320 mOsm/kg), and hypernatremia (>150 mEq/L)
- *Addisonian crisis:*
  - Acute and severe hypoadrenalism primarily due to ACTH deficiency
  - Impaired sensorium, coma, cardiovascular collapse, hyponatremia, and hyperkalemia
- *Pituitary apoplexy:*
  - Hemorrhagic infarction results in rapid enlargement.
  - Often seen in pregnant patients.
  - Presents with retro-orbital pain, acute visual field defects (sometimes blindness), symptoms from mass effect of adjacent brain structures, and Addisonian crisis.
  - Treatment includes resuscitation, steroid replacement, and surgical decompression.

INVESTIGATIONS

- Complete endocrine panel and provocative tests [for growth hormone (GH), insulin-like growth factor 1 (IGF-1), ACTH, prolactin, luteinizing hormone (LH), follicle-stimulating hormone (FSH), and thyroid stimulating hormone (TSH)] undertaken before surgery.
- Inferior petrosal sinus sampling
- CT scan for bony erosion around the pituitary fossa. However, it is difficult to visualize the region due to surrounding bone.
- Visual field testing.
- Pituitary protocol MRI is a sequence of four T1, T2, T1 contrast dynamic and T1 contrast delayed images. These images are optimized for sellar and peri-sellar soft tissue imaging.

TREATMENT

- *Medical therapy* **(Table 1)**
- *Radiotherapy:* Often for residual or recurrent disease after surgery
- *Surgical approaches:*
    - Transsphenoidal, endoscopic vs. microscopic:
        - Transnasal
        - Sublabial
    - Transcranial:
        - Pterional
        - Subfrontal
        - Subtemporal
        - Combined

Anesthetic Management

Preanesthesia Evaluation

- *Medical system review:* Cardiomyopathy/CHF with GH excess; tachyarrhythmia with thyrotoxicosis; peripheral neuropathies

Table 1: Medical management of pituitary tumors.

Syndrome	Treatment	Comment
Acromegaly	Bromocriptine	Dopamine receptor agonist
	Octreotide	Somatostatin analog decreases GH
	Pegvisomant	GH receptor antagonist
Cushing's disease	Ketoconazole	Block peripheral steroid conversion
	Cyproheptadine	Serotonin antagonist
	Mitotane	Adrenal suppressant
Prolactinomas	Bromocriptine	Dopamine antagonist
	Cabergoline	Dopamine receptor agonist

(GH: growth hormone)

- *Airway assessment:*
  - An acromegalic patient with gigantism can have a large tongue and redundant soft tissues, buck teeth, large epiglottis, and infiltration of the vocal cords.
  - Joint movements may be limited; check for neck flexion, AA extension, and jaw protraction.
  - Test vocal cord adduction by asking to say "E".
  - Standard endotracheal tubes, right angle endotracheal (RAE) tubes, or armored tubes are individual preferences.
- The hormone profile should be assessed, and hormonal replacement should continue. Usually, 4-10 mg of dexamethasone is required at induction. Additional steroid (hydrocortisone) doses are rarely needed.
- Involve treating endocrinologists with significant endocrinopathies to ensure continuity of care.
- Explain line placements, steroid replacement, and postoperative difficulty in breathing due to nasal trumpets and dry mouth.
- Regarding OSA management strategy, inquire about continuous positive airway pressure (CPAP).
- Sore throat is possible in the case of difficult intubation and mouth breathing after surgery due to the packing of the nose.

Operating Room Preparation

- Endoscopic surgery may require repositioning the patient away from the anesthesia machine. Extensions to the breathing system might be needed depending on operator preferences.
- *Backup intubation technique:* Bougie, Glide scope, fiberoptic, or intubating laryngeal mask airway (LMA)
- *Proper positioning:* Shoulder roll and large laryngoscope blades
- Difficult vascular access in acromegaly patients may require ultrasound.
- The risk of bleeding greater with extrasellar extension and cavernous sinus invasion determines the size of IV access. However, torrential bleeding from accidental carotid injury can occur in any case.

Monitoring

Routine anesthesia monitors are used, and two IV lines are desired. At least one should be a large-bore IV due to bleeding risk during surgery.

Intraoperative Care

- *Induction and intubation:*
  - *A concern in these cases is agitation upon waking up. Patients at risk of agitating wakeup and difficult extubation include the following:*

younger patients, smokers, with a history of OSA, and those who are obese or have had a difficult airway, consider:
- 5% lidocaine ointment rubbed onto the tube tip and cuff helps decrease coughing and bucking at extubation.
- Consider TIVA with sufentanil propofol dexmedetomidine in those at risk of agitated wakeups.
- IV lidocaine drip
- For induction, narcotics, lidocaine, and propofol are typically used.
- Rocuronium is the usual muscle relaxant of choice.
- *Tube selection and preparation:*
    - Ordinary ETT is widely used. It is safe and cost-effective, but it can rarely kink.
    - RAE tubes have a fixed distance between the cuff and the oral curve. The selection of an appropriate RAE tube could be difficult due to conflicting needs. The enlarged mandible suggests that a larger and longer tube is needed. Conversely, the narrow vocal cords suggest the need for a smaller size.
    - Armored tubes are expensive, and if they are crimped by biting, they do not regain their diameter.
    - Once the position of the ETT has been checked, it is carefully taped at the left angle of the mouth to the lower jaw. Due to limited access to the ETT during surgery, there should be no possibility of the dislodgement of the tube after it has been tapped. The connectors are rotated to provide surgeons with clear access to the nose. Surgeons should be alerted to the position of the tube and that leaning on it could obstruct the tube.
- Preoperative stress dose of steroids
- Antibiotic prophylaxis for mixed cultures is routinely administered.
- The surgeons usually pack the pharynx with gauze to prevent aspiration and ingestion of pooled blood. At extubation, collection of blood could result in a clot causing airway obstruction while ingestion of blood could lead to vomiting.

- *During surgery:*
    - Hypertensive responses occur with pin fixation, vasoconstrictor packing, speculum placement, incision, or bone nibbling. The response can be blocked by narcotics, propofol bolus, deepening volatile anesthesia, or anti-hypertensives.
    - *Intraoperative complications:* Besides hypertension, include diabetes insipidus, hemorrhage, or CSF leak.
    - Check arterial blood gases (ABG) for electrolytes and glucose.
    - To rule out CSF leaks at the end of the procedure, the surgeons may require Valsalva to test dural integrity. They may place a lumbar drain after the procedure.

- Surgery requires minimal time for closure; for careful titration of muscle relaxant doses, small doses of paralytics might be advisable toward the end of the procedure.
- For extubation:
  - Antiemetic prophylaxis essential; careful suction of blood in nasopharynx before reversal
  - For smooth extubation, consider:
    - Low-dose remifentanil infusion
    - Low-dose dexmedetomidine
    - Small doses of fentanyl
    - Lidocaine bolus IV and/or infusion
    - Intratracheal lidocaine.

Postoperative Agitation

Consider:
- Pain and distress from nasal instrumentation
- Breathing distress due to nasal trumpets
- Hypoxia
- Residual sedative drug effects
- Disorientation
- Well-planned extubation sequence should be thought through. That includes judicious administration of sedative-hypnotics, narcotics, antiemetics, topical local anesthetics, adequate reversal of muscle relaxation, and timely suctioning.

Postoperative Care

- Humidified O_2 with a face mask as nasal O_2 use is difficult with trumpets.
- Postoperative pain, nausea, and vomiting
- *Postoperative hormone replacement:* Hydrocortisone 50–100 mg 6–12 hourly
- *Postoperative diabetes insipidus (DI):* Check serum and urine osmolality and serum sodium if urine output is >300 mL/h for 4 hours or >500 mL/h for 2 hours. Replace free water deficit [0.6 wt(kg) (1-(140/Na^+))] slowly over 24 hours. Rapid sodium correction (>1 mEq/h) can lead to central pontine myelinolysis.
- **Table 2** shows preparations of vasopressin. Dosing is based on urine-specific gravity; repeat doses are needed if specific gravity <1.008.

COMPLICATIONS

- *Infection*
- *CSF rhinorrhea:*
  - Perioperative CSF rhinorrhea occurs in under 5% of cases.

CHAPTER 51 Transsphenoid Hypophysectomy

Table 2: Treatment of diabetes insipidus.

Drug	Dose	Comment
DDVAP (desmopressin)	1–2 μg/12–24 h	IV, IM, or SC
DDVAP (nasal spray)	2.5–20 μg	Intranasal spray
DDVAP (oral tablet)	0.1–0.2 mg	PO
Aqueous vasopressin (IV)	0.2–1 U/kg/h	IV infusions; half-life: 10–20 minutes
Posterior pituitary powder in oil	0.1–0.2 mg	IM or SC
Aqueous vasopressin (IM or S/C)	5–10 U/4-hr	IM or S/C

(DDAVP:1-desamino-8-d-arginine vasopressin; IM: intramuscular; IV: intravenous; SC: subcutaneous)

- *Intraoperative CSF rhinorrhea requires:*
    - Packing of the sphenoid sinus with fat or fascia
    - Placement of a lumbar drain
    - Smooth extubation without coughing or bucking.
- *Perioperative rhinorrhea is usually diagnosed by:*
    - Salty, clear fluid without any excoriation
    - Blood ring on the pillow with a clear center
    - Positional drainage
    - Positive for β-transferrin (not present in tears) and glucose.
- Confirmed by water-soluble contrast cisternography.
- Conservative management includes bed rest, avoid straining and coughing, lumbar drain placement for 3–5 days, and antibiotics.
- Leaks >5 days may require lumbar–peritoneal (LP) shunt.
- Further surgical treatment includes intranasal glue or intracranial dural repair. Persistent CSF rhinorrhea is likely to be seen with extrasellar tumor; therefore, careful hormonal/metabolic profile review and general condition reassessment are essential. Infection risk is significant.
- Empty sella syndrome typically causes chronic headaches, endocrine disturbances, and visual impairment.
- Hydrocephalus
- Carotid and cavernous sinus tears are rare, but dangerous bleeding can occur. Such injuries are usually seen with extrasellar tumors. Resuscitation and blood transfusion may be required. Packing to stem bleeding is sufficient to control it. Urgent angiography may be needed. Endovascular embolization to control bleeding is feasible.
- Such injuries can lead to forming pseudoaneurysms that may require endovascular treatment.
- *Of note:* Should the TSS approach fail or proves inadequate, the transfrontal craniotomy might be needed. The location of the pituitary

poses an additional challenge during the procedure. Access to the tumor requires excessive retraction. Excessive retraction can result in inadequate tissue perfusion beneath the retractor. Additional doses of mannitol can reduce tissue bulk and minimize retraction. Hypotension should be avoided. Retractor blade pressure should be monitored. Postoperatively, excessive retraction may present delayed recovery or a new neurological deficit.

CASE REPORTS FOR FURTHER DISCUSSION

Case 1: A 78-year-old male patient with a history of chronic obstructive pulmonary disease (COPD) and hypertension was bought to the ER after being found to be unresponsive while slumped on the couch. He had a history of smoking. There was no history of headache, nausea, or vomiting. On examination, he was lethargic but oriented. Vital signs were stable. There was complete ptosis of the right eye and complete III and partial IV cranial palsies. Most laboratory reports were within normal limits. The blood sugar was 155 mg/dL, and the serum sodium was 130 mEq/L. CT scan was negative for mass effects or hemorrhage. MRI revealed a large pituitary tumor with extension into the cavernous sinus with possible hemorrhage. Twenty-four hours later, the patient developed marked neurological deterioration and became progressively confused. The BP decreased to 98/56 mm Hg, the pulse rate increased to 113 bpm, and the blood sugar was reported at 98 mg/dL. An endocrine workup suggested pituitary insufficiency. The patient was given hydrocortisone replacement due to transsphenoid hypophysectomy. *How does this case differ from the typical case of pituitary apoplexy? How will you replace steroids after pituitary surgery? What are the different types of steroids? Compare the effects of hydrocortisone, dexamethasone, and fludrocortisone.*

Case 2: A 29-year-old female patient presented for transsphenoid pituitary adenoma resection. She was an active smoker, consuming 1.5 packs/day. She had a pituitary resection at the age of 22 years. At the age of 26 years, she had thyroid surgery, during which she had episodes of ventricular ectopy. The patient had experienced excessive growth since the age of 3 years, and at the age of 12 years, she was 6 feet tall; at 22 years, she was 7 feet tall. At the time of surgery, she was 7 feet 7 inches in height and weighed 186 kg. Her preoperative investigations regarding cardiovascular and respiratory systems were within normal limits. Her tidal volume was 1.3 L, minute ventilation was 12.5 L, and FEV1/FVC was 54%. Her serum growth hormone concentrations (30 ng/mL) were three times the normal value. There was an inadequate cortisol response to hypoglycemia. *How will you manage impaired cortisol response? What technical difficulties*

CHAPTER 51 Transsphenoid Hypophysectomy

would you expect during intubation? Would you use nitrous oxide during pituitary surgery?

Case 3: A 51-year-old woman underwent a transsphenoid resection of a pituitary macroadenoma. During surgery, there was a CSF leak. A fat graft and surgicel were packed in the sella and the sphenoid sinus to stop the leak. An external ventricular drain was placed. Over three days, 160–180 mL of CSF was drained. The catheter was then removed. However, on the 6th postoperative day, the patient became drowsy. An urgent CT scan was done. It revealed that the ventricles and the basal cisterns were full of air. She was prescribed strict bed rest and antibiotics. Serial X-rays of the skull over the next two weeks showed reabsorption of air. The patient was discharged five days later. *What precautions can you take to decrease the chances of a CSF leak after surgery? What are the complications of lumbar CSF drain?*

Case 4: A 48-year-old, 80-kg patient diagnosed with a pituitary tumor underwent transsphenoid surgery. History was significant for acromegaly and hypertension. The airway was class 4 with a large tongue, short neck, and a 6-cm thyromental distance. The induction, intubation, and surgery were essentially uneventful. Immediately after extubation, the patient developed severe difficulty in breathing. The oxygen saturation decreased to 30%, with bradycardia and ventricular ectopy onset. Positive pressure ventilation and placement of the oral airway were ineffective. Epinephrine and succinylcholine were used to reintubate the patient. After reintubation, bilateral pulmonary edema was observed. The patient was treated with diuretics, morphine, and mechanical ventilation. The edema resolved over the next 96 hours, and the patient was extubated. *What are the possible reasons for respiratory distress in such a case? What is the risk of positive pressure ventilation with a face mask in such a case?*

Case 5: An 11-year-old patient with a suprasellar tumor was to undergo transsphenoid hypophysectomy. The operation was planned for a sublabial approach. Bilateral infraorbital nerve blocks were planned for perioperative pain relief. *What are the events during transsphenoid surgery associated with significant pain? Discuss the rationale for infraorbital nerve block for such a surgery.*

CASE REPORT REFERENCES

Case 1: Salehi N et al. Pituitary Apoplexy Presenting as Ophthalmoplegia and Altered Level of Consciousness without Headache. Case Rep Endocrinol. 2018;2018:7124364.

Case 2: Chan VW et al. Anaesthesia for transsphenoidal surgery in a patient with extreme gigantism. Br J Anaesth. 1988;60:464-8.

Case 3: Cho HL et al. Tension pneumocephalus after transsphenoidal surgery: Report of two cases. J Korean Neurosurg Soc. 2004;35:536-8.

Case 4: Albergaria VF et al. Negative Pressure Pulmonary Edema after Trans-sphenoid Hypophysectomy: Case Report. Rev Brasilleria Anesthesiol. 2008;58(4):392-6.

Case 5: McAdam D et al. The use of infraorbital nerve block for postoperative pain control after transsphenoidal hypophysectomy. Reg Anesth Pain Med. 2005;30(6):572-3.

FURTHER READING

1. Hardesty DA et al. Complications after 1002 endoscopic endonasal approach procedures at a single center: lessons learned, 2010-2018. 2021;136(2):393-404.
2. Jeon C et al. Outcome of endoscopic transcortical intraventricular biopsy of isolated thickened pituitary stalk lesions in children. J Neurosurg Pediatr. 2021. pp. 1-6.
3. Tanji M et al. Intraoperative Cerebrospinal Fluid Leak Graded by Esposito Grade Is a Predictor for Diabetes Insipidus After Endoscopic Endonasal Pituitary Adenoma Resection. World Neurosurg. 2022;158:e896-e902.
4. Wu TJ et al. Opiate Use After Endoscopic Endonasal Transsphenoidal Surgery. Am J Rhinol Allergy. 2022;36(3):339-47.
5. Zhang T et al. Superiority of endoscopic transsphenoidal pituitary surgery to microscopic transseptal pituitary surgery for treatment of Cushing's disease. Rev Assoc Med Bras (1992). 2021;67(11):1687-91.

Vignette: The History of Diabetes Insipidus

Diabetes mellitus, with its characteristic polyuria, was known to physicians in ancient Egypt, Greece, and Asia. However, in 1670, Thomas Willis noted that not all diabetic patients had sweet urine. The term "diabetes insipidus" (DI, where "insipidus" is a Latin phrase for "tasteless") was introduced in 1794 by John Peter Frank.

Peter Frank described nonsaccharine urine of some diabetic patients. In 1913, Fariniand van den Valden used posterior pituitary extracts to treat the disease. Over the next three decades, it was determined that some cases of DI were resistant to the pituitary extract. In 1947, Williams and Henry described nephrogenic DI in contrast to central DI due to pituitary insufficiency. Du Vigneaud synthesized vasopressin and won the 1955 Nobel Prize for Medicine.

Chapter 52

Endoscopic Third Ventriculostomy and Shunt Procedures

INTRODUCTION

This chapter describes the anesthetic management of surgery for treating hydrocephalus. It includes endoscopic third ventriculostomy, shunt placement and choroid plexus ablation. However, there are other applications of endoscopic neurosurgery. With the improvements in optics, similar minimally invasive endoscopic approaches are being developed for skull base, pituitary, cerebellopontine, spine, and peripheral nerve surgeries. The endoscopic procedure will play a significant part in future neurosurgery.

NEUROANESTHETIC CONCERNS

- Hydrocephalus
- Classification of hydrocephalus
- Clinical presentation
- Management:
  - Endoscopic third ventriculostomy
  - Ventriculoperitoneal (VP) and ventriculoatrial (VA) shunts
  - Choroid plexus ablation
- Anesthetic management
- Post-operative care and complications.

HYDROCEPHALUS

- The incidence is 4 in 1,000 live births.
- Presentation is in early infancy, childhood, and adulthood in the fifth to sixth decades.
- *Etiology:*
  - *Congenital:* Idiopathic, stenosis of the cerebral aqueduct, Arnold Chiari malformation, myelomeningocele, arachnoid cyst, vascular malformations
  - *Acquired:* Infection, hemorrhage, tumor, trauma, nutritional deficits.

Classification of Hydrocephalus

Communicating and noncommunicating hydrocephalus and the likely underlying pathology:

- *Communicating:* Ventricles communicate with each other. There is increased ventricular dilation due to increased CSF formation, or impaired reabsorption. The latter is due to a congenital lack of arachnoid granulations, bleeding, infection, or sometimes with no apparent cause, such as in normal pressure hydrocephalus.
- *Noncommunicating or obstructive:* CSF flow is obstructed due to specific pathologies at:
  - *Lateral ventricle:* By tumors, inflammation
  - *Foramen of Monro:* By tumors, inflammation, hemorrhage
  - *Third ventricle:*
    - *Anterior:* Due to craniopharyngioma, tumor, aneurysm
    - *Posterior:* By pineal tumor, cysts, AV malformation
  - *Aqueduct of Silvius:* Due to stenosis, tumor, inflammation, Arnold-Chiari malformation, hemorrhage
  - *Fourth ventricle:* By tumor, hemorrhage, Arnold-Chiari malformation, Dandy-Walker malformation.

Clinical Presentation

- In neonates, the sutures might not close, the fontanelle remains open and bulging, and the head circumference increases.
- *Infants:* Bulging fontanelle with the "setting sun sign" due to downward gaze.
- In extremis, patients are lethargic, nutritionally deficient, and dehydrated.
- Present with headaches, vomiting, irritability, drowsiness, and impaired cognition.
- *Cushing's triad:* Hypertension, bradycardia, and irregular respiration.
- Herniation of the brain can lead to coma, respiratory arrest, and death.

Management

- *Medical management* is possible with acetazolamide, diuretics, and anticonvulsant drugs.
- *Indication for shunt surgery:* Raised ICP, neurological symptoms, and failure to thrive.
- *Surgical treatments:*
  - Endoscopic third ventriculostomy,
  - VP or VA shunt
  - Rarely choroid ablation.

ENDOSCOPIC THIRD VENTRICULOSTOMY

- *The procedure:*
  - An endoscope is advanced through the lateral ventricle into the third ventricle.

- The floor of the third ventricle is inspected, and a determination is made whether the floor is translucent enough to permit the visualization of the basilar artery and the mammillary bodies.
- If the bodies are visible, the site of ventriculostomy is identified.
- The incision is made by diathermy, and the opening on the third ventricle floor is enlarged.
- This permits free drainage of CSF through the opening into the cistern.
• Indications:
  - Obstructive hydrocephalus due to acquired aqueductal stenosis; hydrocephalus due to a tectal, pineal, thalamic, and intraventricular tumor.
  - *Contraindication to III ventriculostomies:* Communicating hydrocephalus. Poor results are expected with poor CSF drainage due to subarachnoid hemorrhage (SAH), infections, tumors, or radiation.
  - *Complications:* The critical structures which lie along the track of the endoscope are shown in **Figure 1**. Potential complications include Hemorrhage, III, and VI cranial palsies, hypothalamic injury, basilar artery injury, and aneurysm formation.

VENTRICULAR SHUNT CSF DRAINAGE PROCEDURES

- A shunt is a device to divert CSF from the ventricle into the atrium (VA shunt), peritoneum (VP shunt), and sometimes to other locations such as the pleural cavity, gall bladder, or femoral vein.
- The device consists of a silastic catheter placed in the ventricle, a flow control valve, and a draining tube. Modern shunt devices are designed to drain at a pre-set pressure that can be regulated.
- Almost 40% of shunt devices fail within two years, and nearly all malfunction in 10 years. Thus, placement and revision of the shunt are common neurosurgical procedures.

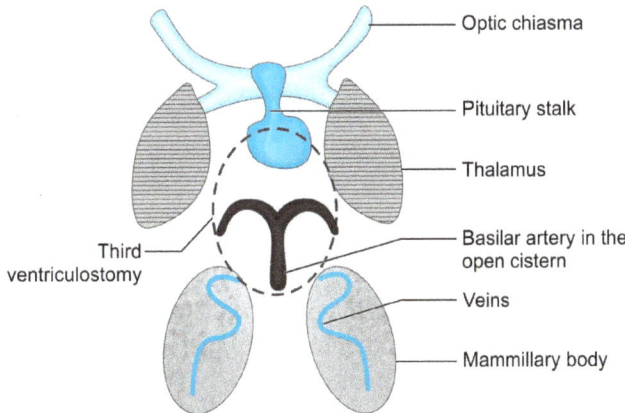

Fig. 1: The floor of the third ventricle.

Table 1: Comparison between VA and VP shunts.

	VA shunt	VP shunt
Catheter tip location	Right atrium	Paracolic gutter, away from the omentum
Frequency of use	Less frequent	More common
Overdrainage	Possible (30%)	Possible (20%)
Infection	Possible (2%)	Possible (2%)
Blockage	Less likely	More likely
Reoperation	Less likely	More likely

(VA: ventriculoatrial; VP: ventriculoperitoneal)

- **Table 1** compares the features of VA and VP shunt procedure.
- Shunt malfunction can be due to: migration, disconnection, hemorrhage blockage over drainage, and infection.

CHOROID PLEXUS ABLATION

- Coagulation of the choroid plexuses may be undertaken to decrease CSF formation.
- When used during III ventriculostomies, it improves the outcome of the procedure.
- The procedure is generally limited to pediatric patients.
- It has a success rate of about 50%.

Anesthesia Management

Preoperative Assessment

- Assess the severity of the raised ICP.
- Assess neurological deficits.
- *Comorbidities:* Neurological (such as intracranial infection, tumors, hemorrhage), developmental, C-spine abnormalities.
- A history of previous surgery.
- *Vital signs:* Pulse rate, blood pressure, and breathing may be altered by raised ICP.
- *Hydration status:* The decreased oral intake results in dehydration and hypovolemia.

Preoperative Investigations

- *Complete blood count (CBC):*
    - Hemo-concentration due to dehydration
    - Prerenal failure is possible due to dehydration.
- EKG
- *Chest X-ray:* To locate the shunt tip.

Operating Room Setup
- Routine neuroanesthetic noninvasive monitoring.
- A urinary catheter is seldom required.

Induction:
- *Intravenous induction:* Decreases ICP but may cause hypotension.
- Rapid-sequence induction is needed if inadequately fasting.
- The induction agent is usually propofol with lidocaine pretreatment.
- Succinylcholine, rarely used, can transiently increase ICP.
- Rocuronium is usually used due to its rapid onset and reversibility with Sugammadex.
- Narcotics supplements help to blunt response to laryngoscopy.
- Once intubated, the tube is secured on the side opposite the surgery.

Maintenance:
- Volatile agents (typically sevoflurane) and narcotics are used.
- Patients can have intense but transient pain during tunneling. Tunneling is usually done after CSF has been drained. It could be treated with the following:
  - Increased depth of volatile agents
  - Bolus of propofol
  - Bolus of fentanyl or remifentanil
  - Few breaths of nitrous oxide.

Reversal of Anesthesia
- *Strategies to prevent postoperative nausea and vomiting (PONV):*
  - Routine use of ondansetron
  - Bolus of dexamethasone
  - Propofol supplement toward the end of the case.
- *Strategies for smooth wakeup include:*
  - Using 5% lidocaine ointment on the endotracheal tube (ETT) cuff and tip decreases the chance of coughing and bucking during extubation.
  - Use of a small dose of fentanyl
  - Low-dose remifentanil
  - IV bolus of lidocaine
  - Intratracheal lidocaine
  - Use of lidocaine infusion.

Complications
- *Early:*
  - Bleeding
  - Sub-arachnoid hemorrhage (SAH)
  - Infection
  - CSF leak.

- *Late complications due to VA or VP shunts:*
  - Blockage of the lower end
  - Valve malfunction
  - Shunt migration
  - Infections
  - Excessive CSF collection

CASE REPORTS FOR FURTHER DISCUSSION

Case 1: After an unremarkable term birth, the patient developed a progressive head enlargement. At six months, he was diagnosed with, and surgically treated for, a sizeable intraventricular choroid plexus papilloma causing hydrocephalus. However, despite the excision of the tumor, the hydrocephalus persisted. A month later, a VP shunt was placed. The patient developed focal seizures that were adequately controlled with anticonvulsant drugs. Over the next few years, the frequency of seizures progressively increased. By age 7, there was continuous seizure activity in specific brain regions. MRI revealed a decrease in the ventricular size and no hydrocephalus. At the age of 11 years, the child, who still had continuous seizure activity, began to develop nausea and headaches. He was found to have obstructive hydrocephalus with suspected blockage of the proximal end of the shunt. The child is now due for a third ventriculostomy with ventricular shunt placement. *How does the placement of a shunt affect intracranial compliance? For a given increase in intracranial volume, will the increase in ICP be greater or lesser if there was a previous shunt?*

Case 2: A 4-week-old male infant presented with a 2-day history of worsening irritability, poor feeding, and noisy respiration. The child had been diagnosed with a lumbar myelomeningocele antenatally. After a cesarean section delivery at 36 weeks, the defect was corrected 24 hours after birth. He was discharged from the hospital at two weeks of age. No ventricular draining device was put in, and weekly head circumference measurements were advised. However, about two weeks later, the child's condition had neurologically deteriorated with respiratory distress. On examination, the anterior fontanelle was tense, the head circumference had increased, and there was a setting sun sign suggestive of raised ICP. The pulse oxygen saturation was maintained on 100% oxygen. He was treated with dexamethasone and nebulized budesonide, and epinephrine. He was due for video laryngoscopy and VP shunt placement the next day. *What are the differential diagnoses of respiratory distress at this age? How do you manage stridor?* During the night, his condition deteriorated, and an emergency ventricular drain was put in. 15 mL of CSF was drained. The stridor disappeared. *What are the possible causes of stridor with raised ICP? How will you treat stridor conservatively?*

Case 3: A 26-year-old female patient presented with fever and myalgia episodes, usually after showers. Similar episodes also occurred with physical exertion. No conclusive diagnosis could be made. In the past, she was diagnosed with Arnold Chiari malformation (type II) with hydrocephalus. In early childhood, she had undergone multiple shunt surgeries. The last VA shunt placement was done at the age of 12 years, around 14 years earlier. On investigation, the blood and urine cultures were negative. Due to the association with showering, water samples were tested and found negative. Over the next four years, extensive testing (including lumbar puncture) was done to detect infection, but no source could be localized. During this time, the patient developed interstitial nephritis. At the age of 30 years, an echocardiogram revealed vegetation on the tricuspid valve, raising the possibility of a delayed shunt infection. The shunt valve CSF sample was positive for *Propionibacterium acnes*.

Meanwhile, the patient's condition worsened, and she required dialysis. It was decided to remove the shunt and create an internal CSF diversion by an endoscopic third ventriculocisternostomy. *Given the history of Arnold Chiari's malformation, what are your anesthetic concerns? What additional difficulties will you anticipate with long-term VA shunt placement? What is a major intraoperative complication of the third ventriculostomy?*

Case 4: A 34-year-old female presented with headache and dizziness of 2-month duration and was diagnosed with hydrocephalus. On lumbar puncture, the CSF was clear, and the opening pressure was 255 mm water. Preoperatively, there was no evidence of any clinical or laboratory bleeding/clotting abnormalities. She was not receiving any antiplatelet drugs or anticoagulants. Her preoperative coagulation screen and platelets were normal. The shunt placement was uneventful. There was no bleeding intraoperatively when a programmable valve system was placed to drain the CSF. Follow-up CT scans on day one and day 3 showed a decrease in the ventricular size but no bleeding. On the fifth postoperative day, while micturating, the patient developed a severe headache and dizziness and soon lost consciousness. CT scan showed intracerebral hematoma with intraventricular bleed. She is due for an urgent evacuation of the hematoma. *Given the catastrophic nature of the hemorrhage and a severely raised ICP, how will you intubate this patient? Would you wait to put an arterial line? Would you do any additional testing and if so when? How will you manage anesthesia while the decompression is being done?*

CASE REPORT REFERENCES

Case 1: Gafner M et al. Refractory epilepsy associated with ventriculoperitoneal shunt over-drainage: case report. Child Nerv Syst. 2019; 35:2411-6.

Case 2: Solan K et al. Raised intracranial pressure in a neonate presenting as stridor. Paediatr Anaesth. 2006;16(8):877-9.

Case 3: Burström G et al. Subacute bacterial endocarditis and subsequent shunt nephritis from ventriculo- atrial shunting 14 years after shunt implantation. BMJ Case Rep. 2014; 2014:bcr-2014204655.

Case 4: Zhou F et al. Delayed intracerebral hemorrhage secondary to ventriculoperitoneal shunt: two case reports and a literature review. Int J Med Sci. 2012;9(1):65-7.

FURTHER READING

1. Auricchio AM et al. Management of slit ventricle syndrome: a single-center case series of 32 surgically treated patients. World Neurosurg. 2022;158:e352-61.
2. Della Pepa GM et al. Letter: Transesophageal echocardiography-guided ventriculoatrial shunt insertion. Oper Neurosurg (Hagerstown). 2020;20(1):E73.
3. Mansoor N et al. Revision and complication rates in adult shunt surgery: a single-institution study. Acta Neurochir (Wien). 2021;163(2):447-54.
4. Popal AM et al. Outcomes of ventriculoperitoneal shunt in patients with idiopathic normal-pressure hydrocephalus 2 years after surgery. Front Surg. 2021;8:641561.
5. Watahiki R et al. Magnetic resonance imaging findings of idiopathic normal pressure hydrocephalus and cognitive function before and after ventriculoatrial shunt. Asian J Neurosurg. 2020;15(3):587-93.

Vignette: The Role of Cerebrospinal Fluid in Evolution and Development of the Brain

In the last three decades, the critical role of CSF in the evolution and embryonic development of the brain is rapidly emerging. The "neuro-evo-devo" research focuses on the correlation between factors that affect the evolution of the brain and those involved in embryonic development. "Neuro-evo-devo" is an acronym for neurological- evolution-development. The research can help us understand development anomalies in children and functional and degenerative brain diseases in later life. In brief, the heart of neuro-evo-devo is to understand patterns of brain development across animal species, from invertebrates to humans. Despite the enormous diversity in the nervous systems of animals, the underlying patterns and the genes that control them seem to be highly conserved. There are very few patterns for nervous system development: Either the neural tube does not form (starfish), or the neural tube does not completely close (acorn worm), or it closes late (lancelet), or it closes very early (all vertebrates). The critical step in developing the vertebrate central nervous system is the early closure of the neural tube. The early closure of the neural tube is followed by the early development of the choroid plexus and the secretion and collection of embryonic CSF (eCSF). The formation and composition of eCSF are tightly controlled. The eCSF helps to enlarge ventricles, remove toxic products, and deliver growth factors. Enlarging the ventricles leads to the proliferation, increased survival, and differentiation of the neural progenitor cells. Abnormalities in eCSF production and composition have a profound effect on brain development.

Chapter 53

Anesthesia for Electroconvulsive Therapy

INTRODUCTION

Electroconvulsive therapy (ECT) poses many conflicting goals for anesthesia due to its brief duration. ECT requires narcosis without impairing seizure activity. It requires adequate muscle relaxation but with rapid recovery from paralysis. It requires amnesia without impairing memory. Anesthesia and ECT have a deep evolutionary relationship. ECT was the testing ground for anesthetic techniques that advanced anesthesia in the 1950s. Conversely, modern ECT would not have been possible without short-acting anesthetic drugs.

NEUROANESTHETIC CONCERNS

- Modified ECT and types of procedures.
- Indications and contraindications for ECT
- Physiologic effects of ECT
- ECT suite concerns
- *Preoperative evaluation:*
  - Cardiovascular assessment
  - Concurrent medical treatment
  - Monitoring
- Anesthetic drug selection
- Procedure
- Postoperative care.

Modified Electroconvulsive Therapy

Almost all ECT procedures in the developed world are "modified ECTs", implying that they use anesthesia and muscle relaxation to avoid awareness and injury during the provoked seizures. In very few parts of the world, unmodified treatment is still used, primarily due to the lack of anesthesia care.

Types of ECT Procedures

- *Unilateral ECT* limited to the nondominant hemisphere:
  - Less cognitive side effects

- Less hemodynamic side effects
- Less effective.
- *Bilateral ECT:*
  - *Bitemporal ECT* has more side effects compared to unilateral ECT.
  - *Bifrontal ECT:* Minimizes temporal lobe exposure to the electrical fields and decreases cognitive side effects.
- *Ultra-brief ECT:* Exceedingly short durations of electrical pulses are applied bilaterally or unilaterally. It is less productive with fewer side effects and rarely used clinically.
- *Transcranial magnetic stimulation (TMS):*
  - TMS is emerging as an alternative to ECT.
  - It is less convulsive than conventional ECT.
  - Minimal sedation or anesthesia is required.
  - Treatment can be prolonged, e.g., five sessions/week, for 4–6 weeks.

ECT Indications

- *Definitive:*
  - *Depression:*
    - Medically resistant
    - Drug side effects limit medical treatment.
    - Life-threatening depression (suicidal ideation, starvation, or dehydration)
    - Rapid improvement is required, e.g., during pregnancy.
    - Previously favorable treatment response
  - Acute catatonia
  - Mania and bipolar disorders
  - Schizophrenia with an affective difference.
- *Possible:* Neurolept drug-induced syndromes (neurolept malignant syndrome, tardive dyskinesia, and Parkinson's disease), catatonia, obsessive-compulsive disorder, and organic mood disorders.

ECT Contraindications

- *Absolute:* None. The risk of the procedure has to be weighed against the potential hazard of not doing the procedure, such as suicide or complete incapacitation due to psychiatric illness.
  - 2% of outpatients treated for depression commit suicide.
  - 4% of inpatients treated for depression commit suicide.
  - 6% of inpatients with suicidal ideation or attempts commit suicide.
- *Relative:*
  - American Society of Anesthesiologists (ASA) IV and V patients
  - Recent myocardial infarction (MI) <3 months
  - Unstable angina or congestive heart failure (CHF)

CHAPTER 53 Anesthesia for Electroconvulsive Therapy

- Recent cerebrovascular accident (CVA) <3 months
- The intracranial space-occupying lesion, brain aneurysm, or raised intracranial pressure (ICP)
- Pheochromocytoma
- Deep venous thrombosis
- Fractures or significant cervical spine injury
- Children under 16 years of age.

Physiological Effects

- *Central nervous system effects:*
  - Seizures:
    - *Seizure duration:* On EEG, a localized seizure is observed for 5–10 seconds that transitions to a generalized tonic-clonic seizure for the next 15 seconds.
    - Effective treatment requires seizure activity for 20–25 seconds.
    - *Prolonged seizures:* >180 seconds, require anticonvulsant therapy.
  - The increased cerebral metabolic rate of oxygen ($CMRO_2$), cerebral blood flow (CBF), and ICP
  - Increased blood–brain barrier permeability
  - Headache
  - Memory loss
  - Confusion and disorientation
  - Delirium
- *Cardiovascular effects:*
  - *Triphasic response:*
    - Transient parasympathetic response, 10–15 seconds: Bradycardia, asystole during electrical stimulation
    - Sustained sympathetic response due to catecholamine release with tonic-clonic seizures, peaks within 3 minutes
    - Rebound bradycardia possible
  - Hypertension, tachycardia, and increased myocardial oxygen consumption with sympathetic surge can precipitate arrhythmias, myocardial infarction, left ventricular failure (pulmonary edema), and rarely structural damage to the heart.
  - Tachycardia and ventricular ectopy may be sustained for several hours.
- *Other effects:*
  - *Musculoskeletal:*
    - Dislocation and injuries with suboptimum paralysis
    - Generalized myalgia
    - Trismus
  - Increased intraocular pressure

- Increased intragastric pressure
- Dental damage
- Tongue laceration.

ECT Suite

- Remote location
- Should be fully equipped to provide safe general anesthesia
- High-risk ECT patients might be treated in better-equipped post-anesthesia care units. However, relocation of patients to and from a psychiatric facility is a significant disadvantage.

Preoperative Assessment

- The patient may not be able to provide a reliable medical history.
- *Systemic review with emphasis on:*
  - *Cardiac review essential:*
    - Hypertension
    - Coronary artery disease (CAD)
    - CHF
    - Valvular heart disease
    - Palpitations and arrhythmias
- *Respiratory:* Chronic obstructive pulmonary disease (COPD) and bronchial asthma
- Gastroesophageal reflux
- Glaucoma
- Dental assessment
- Drug allergies
- Psychoactive drug interactions **(Table 1)**.

Table 1: Pharmacological interaction of psychotropic drugs.

Psychoactive drug	Interaction with	Consequence
Tricyclic drugs	Anesthetics	Postural hypotension, ↑ QRS and ↑ QTc duration
Tricyclic drugs	Indirect sympathomimetics	Hypertensive crisis
Monoamine oxidase inhibitors	Indirect and direct sympathomimetics	• Hypertensive crisis • Stopped two weeks before anesthesia
Selective serotonin inhibitors	Meperidine and Tramadol	Serotonin syndrome (hyperreflexia, hyperthermia, and agitation). SSRI may cause SIADH
Lithium		Nephrogenic diabetes insipidus

(SIADH: syndrome of inappropriate antidiuretic hormone secretion; SSRI: selective serotonin reuptake inhibitor)

Anesthesia for ECT

It differs from other procedures because:
- ECT suites are usually located within the psychiatric ward, so access to the procedure room is restricted. Help with supplies, manpower or equipment is slow to arrive compared to other peripheral locations.
- Unlike other surgeries, the patient is treated multiple times.
- The procedure is of exceedingly short duration and requires rapid recovery from anesthesia.
- Although the procedure is brief, there are dramatic physiological changes during stimulation.
- During ECT, minimal and precise doses of anesthetics drugs are used.
- Once the anesthetic drug doses have been determined, the same doses are used every time so as not to alter the effects of electrical stimulation.
- Since doses of anesthetic drugs are small, flushing them with a saline bolus is essential to ensure a predictable onset of effect.
- Clear communications with psychiatric and nursing teams are necessary at all times during the planning and execution of the procedure in a well-choreographed manner.
- *Steps for ECT* **(Fig. 1)**:
    - The steps are the same as for any general anesthesia.
    - ECT units may not have a central gas supply. The machine check should include checking for pressure in the gas cylinders. Availability of a resuscitation bag.
    - Vital sign monitors as per the ASA standards.
    - Routine monitoring includes ECG, pulse oximeter, end-tidal gas composition, noninvasive blood pressure, nerve stimulator, and tourniquet to isolate limb from paralytic drugs.

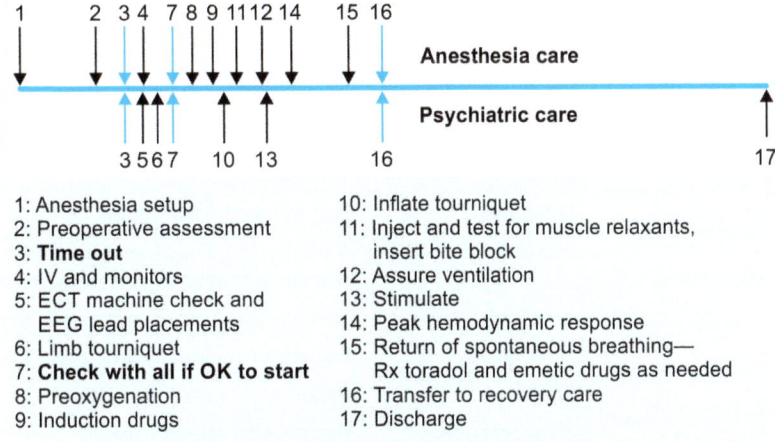

1: Anesthesia setup
2: Preoperative assessment
3: **Time out**
4: IV and monitors
5: ECT machine check and EEG lead placements
6: Limb tourniquet
7: **Check with all if OK to start**
8: Preoxygenation
9: Induction drugs
10: Inflate tourniquet
11: Inject and test for muscle relaxants, insert bite block
12: Assure ventilation
13: Stimulate
14: Peak hemodynamic response
15: Return of spontaneous breathing— Rx toradol and emetic drugs as needed
16: Transfer to recovery care
17: Discharge

Fig. 1: Typical sequence of events during an ECT.

- Invasive monitoring may be necessary in rare cases.
- Bite block, laryngoscope, endotracheal tube, and suction device
• *Frequently used drugs* **(Tables 2 and 3):**
  - Atropine 0.4 mg minimizes parasympathetic effects, avoids bradycardia, and decreases secretions. However, due to tachycardia, its use has been limited to patients with a low resting heart rate of 50 bpm.
  - *Glycopyrrolate:* 0.2 mg can be used as an alternative to atropine. It causes less tachycardia and has no significant side effects. Routine glycopyrrolate treatment has been used to minimize aerosolization and the risk of COVID-19 transmission.

Table 2: Second-line drugs used for electroconvulsive therapy.

Drugs	Main features	Comment
Induction agents		
Propofol	Short-acting, antiemetic, pain on injection	Decreases seizure duration
Etomidate	Short acting, pain on injection, proconvulsant	Myoclonic limb movements may confuse clinical seizure monitoring, increases hypertensive response, and decreases seizure threshold
Ketamine	Short-acting, LOC unclear	Delayed emergence and mild antidepressant effects
Thiopental		Delayed emergence
Muscle relaxants		
Rocuronium	Slower onset and longer effect versus succinylcholine	Supplemental anesthesia may be necessary to decrease respiratory distress due to residual paralysis
Sugammadex	Can rapidly reverse rocuronium paralysis	Early reversal block with rocuronium possible
Glycopyrrolate	COVID-19 prophylaxis	Decreases secretions, attenuates and parasympathetic surge

(LOC: loss of consciousness)

Table 3: Adjuvant drugs during ECT treatment.

Drugs	Comment
Lidocaine	Post-ECT ventricular ectopy increases seizure threshold
Esmolol	A short-acting drug, esmolol pretreatment is helpful in patients with severe hypertensive response
Labetalol	Useful with sustained sympathetic responses after seizure
Nicardipine	Boluses are useful if hypertension is with bradycardia
Ephedrine	Hypotension with bradycardia
Phenylephrine	Hypotension with tachycardia

(ECT: electroconvulsive therapy)

- *Methohexital (Brevital):* 1 mg/kg, a short-acting proconvulsant oxybarbiturate, is painful on injection, lowers the seizure threshold, and is widely used as the drug of choice.
- *Propofol:* Propofol is the alternative frontline drug, useful in patients with post-ECT agitation with methohexital or if seizures are prolonged.
- *Succinylcholine:* 0.5 mg/kg.
- *Ketorolac:* 0.25-0.5 mg/kg as indicated for myalgia.
- *Ondansetron:* 0.05 mg/kg as indicated for nausea and vomiting.
  - *Flumazenil:* 0.4 mg to reverse the effects of benzodiazepines in patients with severe catatonia. Typically, it is given 5-8 minutes before the start of the procedure.

Selection of Stimulation Threshold, the First ECT

- Establishes the anesthetic selection and dose requirements.
- Determines the strength of stimulation using—two to four increasing doses.
- The threshold for seizure is about 3-4 × less than the actual treatment.
- Provides an assessment of patient response to the procedure.
- The procedure is of a longer duration due to dose titration.
- Greater myalgia, trismus, and headache are compared to subsequent ones.

Complications

- Headache and myalgia
- Nausea and vomiting
- Dental and tongue injuries
- Post-ECT respiratory distress
- Awareness
- Pulmonary edema
- Severe bradycardia
- Sustained arrhythmias.
- Myocardial infarction
- Cardiac arrest.

Outcome

- The success of ECT for depression is 60-80%
- Benefits are seen in 20% of patients with <4 treatments, 35% with <6 treatments, and 65% with <10 treatments.
- Relapse, most likely within six months, can affect 35% of initially responding patients.

CASE REPORTS FOR FURTHER DISCUSSION

Case 1: An 89-year-old woman has had around 400 ECTs for over 60 years. Her depression began in the 1950s. With medical management and periodic ECT treatments, she functioned adequately. Between treatments, she would relapse into severe depression and a catatonic state. She had responded well to ECT treatments. There were two past adverse reactions to ECT. In one episode, she remained unconscious for 2 hours, and a decade later, there was persistent severe confusion lasting for three days. As her age progressed, her physical condition deteriorated. She suffered from hypothyroidism, anemia, hiatal hernia, bowel disturbances, Paget's disease with two episodes of hypercalcemia, chronic kidney disease, hypertension, hypercholesterolemia, and an episode of transient ischemic attack. CT scan showed a generalized loss in brain volume and attenuation of deep white matter suggestive of small vessel disease. She has had severe weight loss since the last treatments. *Given the general condition of the patient, would you proceed with ECT? What additional investigations would you request to assess the patient?*

Case 2: Upon returning from a summer camp, an 8-year-old child with an excellent academic record developed symptoms of depression. Her condition worsened despite intense medical and psychological care. Within weeks, her psychomotor retardation extended to the point of refusing to eat and becoming bedridden. She developed board-like rigidity. Neurologists assessed her, and extensive investigative workup was essentially negative. Due to her condition, possible morbidity, and the failure of medical management, she was assigned to a course of ECT treatment. *What concerns will you have in treating a pediatric patient with ECT? When would you expect the benefits of ECT after treatment? What are the potential side effects of ECT?*

Case 3: A 10-year-old child developed a progressive state of worsening fearfulness, suspiciousness, irritability, and psychiatric illness over the last month. Over the next fortnight, he refused to eat and developed psychomotor slowing. He was hospitalized with acute psychotic disorder with catatonic features. His medical workup was negative for any significant illness. He was treated with lorazepam with minimal improvement. Due to a lack of response to medical treatment, he was due for ECT treatment. *How does lorazepam affect ECT treatment? If a patient is on lorazepam, will you reverse its effect with flumazenil? What is the dose and anticipated peak effects of flumazenil? When will you restart the lorazepam treatment?*

CASE REPORT REFERENCES

Case 1: Carney S et al. Electroconvulsive therapy: a life course approach for recurrent depressive disorder. BMJ Case Rep. 2015;2015:bcr2015209763.

Case 2: Cizadlo BC et al. Case study: ECT treatment of a young girl with catatonia. J Am Acad Child Adolesc Psychiatr. 1995;34(3):332-5.

Case 3: Mohapatra S et al. Electroconvulsive therapy in a child suffering from acute and transient psychotic disorder with catatonic features. Indian J Psychol Med. 2015;37(4):465-6.

FURTHER READING

1. Gundogdu O et al. The effects of hyperventilation on seizure length and cerebral oxygenation during electroconvulsive therapy. North Clin Istanb. 2020;7(3):246-54.
2. Hickman LB et al. Postictal generalized electroencephalographic suppression following electroconvulsive therapy: temporal characteristics and impact of anesthetic regimen. Clin Neurophysiol. 2021;132(4):977-83.
3. Limoncelli J et al. General Anesthesia Recommendations for Electroconvulsive Therapy During the Coronavirus Disease 2019 Pandemic. J ECT. 2020;36(3):152-5.
4. Soehle M et al. Challenges and pitfalls in anesthesia for electroconvulsive therapy. Best Pract Res Clin Anaesthesiol. 2021;35(2):181-9.
5. Surve RM et al. Electroconvulsive therapy services during COVID-19 pandemic. Asian J Psychiatr. 2021;59:102653.

Vignette: Evolution of Electroconvulsive Therapy

The first use of electricity for medical purposes appears in ancient Egypt. The Egyptians used electrical shock by catfish to treat arthritic pains. A catfish appears on both sides of the Narmer Palette from the First Dynasty in Upper Egypt, dating to the 31st century BCE. The ancient Romans used electric eels to treat headaches and gout. In the 16th century, a Swiss alchemist, Paracelsus, used oral camphor to induce convulsion to cure lunacy. In 1744, the journal "Electricity in Medicine" described the use of electricity to cure neurologic and mental cases of paralysis. A later issue, in 1755, reported the use of electric shocks to cure hysterical blindness. In 1752, Benjamin Franklin used an electrostatic machine to cure hysterical fits. Insulin hypoglycemia and convulsive drugs were used to treat psychiatric disorders in the 1930s. Around that time, Ugo Carletti observed a butcher using electric shocks to euthanize pigs. Carletti immediately saw the potential application of electric shock to treat mental illness. He tested electrically-induced seizures in dogs, but this had high mortality. Lucio Beni recognized that the electrodes should not be applied craniocaudally, which affected the heart but bitemporally across the scalp, that locally affected the brain. The first ECT trials began in 1938.

Chapter 54: Pregnant Patient for Neurosurgery

INTRODUCTION

Neurosurgical emergencies in a pregnant patient include intracranial hemorrhage either spontaneously or due to bleeding from a vascular lesion, hydrocephalus, tumors, trauma, or disc herniations. While managing pregnant neurosurgical patients, there are several considerations. These include the nature of neuropathology, physiological changes due to pregnancy, their effect on neuropathology, the urgency to treat, duration of pregnancy, viability of the fetus, teratogenicity of the drugs, hazards of neuro investigative techniques, and the safety of anesthetic interventions for both mother and the fetus. Thus, patients' care must be individualized. The goal is to achieve the best fetal survival at minimal maternal risk.

NEUROANESTHETIC CONCERNS

- Nature of neurological emergencies in pregnant patients
- Vital physiological changes in pregnancy
- *Fetal concerns:*
  - Teratogenicity
  - Monitoring
  - Viability
  - Premature labor
- Anesthetic concerns.

Neurosurgery in Pregnant Patients

- *Intracranial hemorrhage:* 1:60,000 pregnancies
  - *Risk factors:*
    - Coagulopathy and pre-eclampsia/eclampsia
    - Aneurysms (75%)
    - Arteriovenous malformations (AVMs) (20%)
    - Cavernous malformation
    - Moyamoya disease
    - Hypertensive crisis
- *Tumors:*
  - Glioma
  - Meningioma

- Trauma
- Spontaneous subarachnoid hemorrhage (SAH)
- Hydrocephalus
- Spinal cord and nerve root compression.

Physiological Changes in Pregnancy (Table 1)

- *Respiratory volumes:* Major change is in functional residual capacity (FRC), expiratory capacity, and residual volumes that, are decreased by 20%.
- *Respiratory mechanics:* Progesterone-induced increase in minute ventilation: RR increased by 15%, tidal volume increased by 70%, minute ventilation increased by 50%, airway resistance decreased by 40%, and the $PaCO_2$ decreased, but pH is unchanged due to the HCO_3 decrease.
- *Predisposition to hypoxia:* Due to decreased FRC and a 40–60% increase in oxygen consumption.
- *Hematological:* Blood volume increased 40%; increase in serum volume is greater than the increase in red cell volume resulting in anemia of pregnancy; increase in coagulation factors.
- *Cardiovascular:* Heart rate (HR) increased by 15%, CO increased by 50%, and systemic vascular resistance (SVR) decreased by 20%. Aortocaval compression can reduce preload and mean arterial pressure (MAP) and requires left uterine displacement after 20 weeks.

Table 1: Summary of the physiological effects of pregnancy.

Physiological parameter	First trimester <12 weeks	Second trimester 13–24 weeks	Third trimester >24 weeks
Body metabolism	Normal	Increased	Increased
Blood volume	Normal	Increased	Increased
Hematocrit	Normal	Decreased	Decreased
CO	Normal	Peak increase	Increased
PVR	Normal	Decreased	Decreased
BV	Normal	Increased	Increased
BP	Normal	Increased	Decreased
Postural hypotension	None	None	Possible
Lung volumes	Normal	Normal	Decreased
FRC	Normal	Normal	Decreased
Minute ventilation	Normal	Normal	Increased
Airway resistance	Normal	Normal	Decreased
Aspiration risk	Normal	Increased	Increased
Coagulation and DVT risk	Normal	Increased	Increased

(BV: bacterial vaginosis; DVT: deep venous thrombosis; FRC: functional residual capacity; PVR: pulmonary vascular resistance)

- *Neurological:* Decreased minimum alveolar concentration (MAC) and increased sensitivity to regional anesthetics.
- *Gastrointestinal:* Progesterone slows intestinal motility and increases aspiration risk.
- *Hepatic:* Drug clearance unaffected by the volume of distribution may be increased.
- *Renal:* Increased renal blood flow (RBF; +75%) and glomerular filtration rate (GFR; +60%).
- *Metabolic:* Pregnancy-induced diabetes; decrease in blood urea nitrogen (BUN) and creatinine.
- *Drug:* Assessment of the use of prescribed and substance abuse drugs.

Maintaining Uterine Blood Flow

- *Avoid systemic hypotension:*
  - Avoid aortocaval compression.
  - Fluid preloads with a subarachnoid block (SAB)/epidural.
  - Use of phenylephrine to maintain BP.
  - Previously ephedrine (α and β stimulants) were used.
  - Avoid excessive hyperventilation.
- *Fetal monitoring:*
  - Fetal monitoring is needed at >24 weeks. <24 weeks fetal monitoring is necessary before and after a neurosurgical procedure.
  - If viable, steroid treatment should commence enhancing lung maturation.

Concerns with Teratogenicity

- Teratogenic effects are relevant in the first and early second trimesters.
- Avoid ketamine, sevoflurane, and nitrous oxide.
- Commonly used anesthetics (Propofol, muscle relaxants, narcotics) are safe.
- Anticonvulsants can cause developmental defects.
- Minimize radiation exposure < 25th weeks, with no exposure <15 weeks.
- The maximum permissible cumulative radiation exposure is five rads.
- Some common examples of teratogenic drugs include Angiotensin-converting- enzyme (ACE) inhibitors, androgenic and estrogenic hormones, antibiotics (tetracycline, doxycycline, streptomycin), antidepressants (lithium), anti-metabolites and thalidomide.

Tocolytics: Used for Preventing Premature Labor

Common tocolytics and their side-effects:
- β-adrenergic agents (can cause hypokalemia)
- Calcium channel (can cause hypotension)

- Nitroglycerine (can cause hypotension)
- Volatile anesthetics: Hypotension and cardiovascular side-effects.

Eclampsia and Pre-eclampsia

- It is the leading cause of maternal mortality, with 40% of fatalities due to brain hemorrhage.
- Pre-eclampsia is characterized by hypertension and proteinuria.
- *The eclampsia triad includes hypertension, proteinuria, and seizures:*
  - It is classified based on diastolic blood pressure as mild (95-104 mm Hg), moderate (105-125 mm Hg), or severe (>126 mm Hg).
  - Other symptoms:
    - *Renal:* Oliguria and impaired renal functions.
    - *Central nervous system (CNS):* Visual, cognitive dysfunction, and seizures (eclampsia).
    - *Liver:* Right upper quadrant pain, jaundice, and impaired liver functions.
    - *Hematological:* Increased hematocrit (contracted blood volume).

HELLP Syndrome

- Hemolysis
- Elevated liver enzymes and
- Low platelets
- HELLP carries a mortality rate of up to 30%, with deaths due to intracerebral hemorrhage (ICH) and stroke.

Pharmacological Concerns

- All induction agents (intravenous and volatile) and opioid and sedative-hypnotics cross the placenta, impairing fetal activity scores.
- Muscle relaxants and reversing agents are ionized and do not cross the placenta.
- Atropine (tertiary ammonium compound) crosses the placenta, but glycopyrrolate (a quaternary ammonium compound) does not.
- Antihypertensive (beta-blockers, hydralazine, nitroprusside, and nitroglycerine) crosses the placenta.
- Mannitol can cross the placenta and cause a hyperosmolar syndrome in a fetus with poor renal function.

Magnesium sulfate is a Ca^{++} antagonist with sedative, anticonvulsant, and antihypertensive properties routinely used in pre-eclampsia.

- No evidence of neuroprotective effects of Mg^{++} in clinical trials
- *Side effects:* Symptoms with increasing serum Mg^{++} concentrations.
  - <2 mEq/L: Normal
  - 4-8 mEq/L: Therapeutic range: Sedative, antihypertensive, and anticonvulsant effects

- 5–10 mEq/L: Conduction defects, increased PR, and wide QRS
- 10–15 mEq/L: Skeletal muscle weakness, loss of tendon reflexes
- 15–25 mEq/L: Respiratory muscle weakness
- \>25 mEq/L: Cardiac arrest.

Investigations

Specific issues: Radiation exposure consequences
- *Embryogenesis (0–2 weeks):* Stillbirth
- *Organogenesis (2–8 weeks):* Congenital abnormalities
- *Fetal development (>8 weeks):* Growth retardation, neuronal depletion, childhood cancer, and microcephaly.
- *Contrast agents:*
  - Iodinated contrast agents are safe for the fetus but can affect thyroid functions.
  - Gadolinium safety is not established and should be avoided if possible.

Surgery during Pregnancy

- Emergency surgery is undertaken whenever there is a potential threat to the mother's life or a serious neurological outcome.
- Elective surgery, such as AVMs or tumors, should be delayed until delivery or best undertaken in the second trimester when organogenesis is complete.
- In the third trimester, delivery and neurosurgical treatment can be undertaken simultaneously.

Anesthetic Management

General Anesthesia

- *Maternal concerns:*
  - Increased intracranial pressure (ICP) requires careful intubation during general anesthesia. The use of video laryngoscopy could enhance safety.
  - Key physiological changes
    - *Cardiovascular:* Increased HR, cardiac output, the possibility of postural hypotension with aortocaval compression
    - *Respiratory:* Decreased FRC, increased minute ventilation, decreased functional reserve volume, increased oxygen consumption
    - *Hematological:* Anemia of pregnancy
    - *Gastrointestinal (GI):* Gastric stasis, the risk for aspiration.
- *Fetal concerns:*
  - *Fetal monitoring:* Although the fetal heart can be monitored ultrasonically at six weeks, this is well before fetal viability.

Intraoperative fetal monitoring is helpful in the second half of pregnancy. The decision depends on an individual case. Depending on the stage of pregnancy, the heart sounds are monitored before and after the procedure to ensure viability.
- *Aortocaval compression:* Left lateral decubitus is preferred to avoid vena caval compression.
- Spine surgery can be done in the lateral decubitus position, but a mid-line approach and microscopy will be challenging.
- Hyperventilation can decrease placental blood flow; therefore, maintaining normocapnia is advisable.
- *Drug transfers across the placenta:* Anesthetic drugs and narcotics cross the placenta and can cause fetal depression if delivery is anticipated after neurosurgery. Muscle relaxants and reversing agents do not cross the placenta.
- *Teratogenicity:* The most commonly used anesthetic drugs are safe. Nitrous oxide is avoided. Total intravenous anesthesia (TIVA) with propofol/remifentanil is safe.
- *Lung maturation:* Most neurosurgical patients receive dexamethasone that accelerates fetal lung maturation. It is given 48 hours before the anticipated surgery.
- *Fetal monitoring:* For the third-trimester surgery, fetal monitoring should be available, and an obstetric team should stand by for urgent delivery.

Regional Anesthesia
- A neuraxial block carries a risk of herniation with raised ICP.
- It is possible to use regional anesthesia in pregnant patients for spine surgery no differently than for nonpregnant cases.
- The patient's condition, the surgery duration, the need for intervention, and possible blood loss must be considered.
- The technique involves fluid loading and insertion of an epidural catheter with two levels above the level of surgical intervention.
- *The benefits of regional anesthesia are as follows:*
  - Avoids airway instrumentation.
  - Reduces the cost and duration of surgery.
  - Provide postoperative pain relief.
- Regional anesthesia can be used for straightforward surgeries such as lumbar disc herniation and endoscopic spine interventions.

Monitored Anesthetic Care (MAC)
- MAC can enable simple spine surgery with local infiltration.
- Awake craniotomies and endovascular treatment, e.g., for ruptured aneurysms and AVMs, are possible with patient cooperation.

- The fetus is shielded during endovascular procedures, and a minimum amount of imaging is used. These procedures can be done under sedation. Similarly, malignant tumors can be treated with radiation with minimal sedation while shielding the fetus.

Postoperative Care
- *General postoperative care:*
  - Vital signs
  - Pain relief
  - Oxygenation
  - Fluid input/output
  - Antiemesis
- *Neurosurgical monitoring:*
  - Basic neuromonitoring at 15-minute intervals
  - *Levels of consciousness, orientation, agitation, speech, sensory and motor functions; cranial nerves:* Facial symmetry and reflex activity
- *Obstetric monitoring:*
  - Uterine tone
  - Incisional and vaginal bleeding
  - Urine output
- *Neonatal monitoring:*
  - Fetal heart sound
  - Obstetric review.

CASE REPORTS FOR FURTHER DISCUSSION

Case 1: A 27-year woman presented at 36 weeks gestation with a history of acute-onset severe headache and unilateral loss of vision in the left eye. At 19 weeks gestation, she had presented with headache, nausea, and vomiting and had been diagnosed with a prolactin-secreting pituitary tumor. She was treated with bromocriptine. MRI revealed a 2.1 × 1.3 cm-sized hemorrhagic mass with compression of the chiasma. Vision in the left eye was 20/200. Considering the imminent threat to her vision, she is due for transsphenoidal tumor resection. *How would pituitary apoplexy affect the course of pregnancy? After tumor resection, the patient has a dramatic increase in urine output. How can diabetes insipidus (DI) affect the fetus? How would you treat DI? When would you deliver the child?*

Case 2: A 23-year-old patient presented with sudden-onset severe headache with nausea and vomiting at 27 weeks of gestation. She was known to have a cerebral AVM that had been partially embolized. On examination, the patient had left hemiparesis. MRI revealed an intracranial hematoma, 2.6 cm in diameter. A digital subtraction angiography revealed an AVM supplied by branches of the anterior middle and posterior cerebral arteries. She was scheduled for an urgent cesarean section with post-cesarean resection of the hematoma and the AVM. *Could this patient have been conservatively managed to fetal maturation? What steps can you take to ensure lung maturation in a pre-term birth?*

Case 3: A 31-year-old with 39 weeks gestation presented with headache, nausea, vomiting, photophobia, and neck pain. The history was significant for a similar mild episode at 20 weeks gestation but with no neurological findings. On examination, there was neck rigidity but no focal signs. Lumbar puncture revealed blood in cerebrospinal fluid (CSF). The surgical team recommended urgent lower segment cesarean section and transfers to a neurosurgical unit for subsequent neurological care. *Do you agree with the decision to do surgery before a detailed neurological workup? For a cesarean section, what precautions would you take first?*

Case 4: A 38-year-old primigravida with 24 weeks gestation is diagnosed with L4–5-disc herniation and L5 root compression. The pain was intense and resistant to acetaminophen and nerve root injection of corticosteroids. She was posted for L4/5 discectomy under general anesthesia. *Can you do the surgery in a lateral position? What problems would you anticipate during lateral position discectomy?*

Case 5: A 30-year-old primigravida at 18 weeks gestation developed new-onset seizures. The seizures were poorly controlled with anticonvulsants. She weighed 61 kg and was 162 cm tall. Her MRI revealed a 6 mm grade III glioma in the left frontal supplementary motor area. The surgeons planned and MRI-guided complete resection to enable better control of the seizures at 27 weeks. *How will you proceed with the case? Compare the benefits of craniotomy under general anesthesia vs. an awake craniotomy. Surgeons want intraoperative neurological testing and are requesting an awake craniotomy. Will you agree? What are the risks? How do you plan to do the MRI? Are there any teratogenic risks of propofol? Would LMA and volatile agent use be advantageous or hazardous?*

CASE REPORT REFERENCES

Case 1: Tandon A et al. Endoscopic endonasal transsphenoidal resection for pituitary apoplexy during the third trimester of pregnancy. Surg Res Pract. 2014;2014:397131.

Case 2: Rispoli R et al. Rupture of an intracranial arteriovenous malformation (AVM) in pregnancy: Case report. J Stem Cell Res Ther. 2015;5:256.

Case 3: El Gawly RM. Ruptured intracranial aneurysm in pregnancy: a case report and review of the literature. Eur J Obstet Gynecol Reprod Biol. 1992;46(2-3):150-3.

Case 4: Hayakawa K et al. Surgical management of the pregnant patient with lumbar disc herniation in the latter stage of the second trimester. Spine. 2017;42(3): E186-9.

Case 5: Kamata K et al. A case of left frontal high-grade glioma diagnosed during pregnancy. JA Clinical reports (2017) 3:18. DOI 10.1186/s40981-017-0090-9

FURTHER READING

1. Bernstein K et al. Neuro-anesthesiology in pregnancy. Handb Clin Neurol. 2020;171:193-204.
2. Enomoto N et al. Pregnancy-associated hemorrhagic stroke: A nationwide survey in Japan. J Obstet Gynaecol Res. 2021;47(6):2066-75.
3. Esmaeilzadeh M, et al. Intracranial emergencies during pregnancy requiring urgent neurosurgical treatment. Clin Neurol Neurosurg. 2020;195:105905.
4. Miller EC et al. Stroke in pregnancy: A focused update. Anesth Analg. 2020;130(4):1085-96.
5. Po' G et al. Intraoperative fetal heart monitoring for non-obstetric surgery: A systematic review. Eur J Obstet Gynecol Reprod Biol. 2019;238:12-9.

Vignette: How was the Thalidomide Disaster Averted in the United States?

In the 1950s and 60s, thalidomide was prescribed in Europe for sedation and nausea.

However, it found wide use for treating morning sickness in early pregnancy. By early 1961 there were alarming reports of children being born with deformed limbs. Some ten thousand children were born worldwide with deformities, half of whom died in the first year. The defects affected the limbs, eyes, heart, and the urinary system. Though the drug was never approved for the US, it was undergoing clinical trials at the time. Some thousand physicians had access to some 2.5 million tablets released for testing in the US. An estimated 20,000 people were exposed to the drug. In an era predating cell phones, it was impossible to contact doctors to prevent the distribution of samples. President Kennedy made a public plea not to take the drug. Even after his appeal, the drug company, Richardson Merrell Pharmaceuticals, insisted on seeking FDA approval. Frances Oldham Kelsey, a pharmacologist, single-handedly denied FDA approval for the drug. As a result, some 17 children were affected by the drug in the United States, far less than the cases reported from Europe and Australia. Thalidomide is being reintroduced for the treatment of leprosy, HIV, and certain malignancies. Newer analogs of the drug are in development.

Pediatric Neurosurgery Patient

Chapter 55

INTRODUCTION

This chapter describes managing a case of craniosynostosis, a complex pediatric-neurosurgical intervention. The general anatomical and physiological differences between children and adults are listed in **Appendix 12**. The specific differences between children and adults include the relatively large size of the brain, higher blood flow, greater metabolic rate, narrow and less effective pressure autoregulation, the vulnerability to ischemic injury, a lower ICP, and the potential to increase intracranial volume in infants compared to adults due to open sutures. Management of craniosynostosis highlights the challenges of pediatric-neuroanesthesia. *Craniosynostosis* is the premature closure of the skull sutures in infancy resulting in gross deformity of the skull that impedes brain development.

NEUROANESTHETIC CONCERNS

- *Overview of concerns with craniosynostosis:*
  - Objectives and timing of surgery
  - Congenital syndromes
  - Co-morbidities
- *Management of craniosynostosis case:*
  - *Preparation for surgery:* blood harvest and respiratory care.
  - Operating room preparation
  - Airway, intubation, and ventilatory concerns.
  - Hemodynamic monitoring and vascular access
  - *Intraoperative care:* blood loss, venous air embolism (VAE), and hypothermia.
  - *Postoperative:* Fluid and electrolyte balance, nausea and vomiting, ventilation, and pain relief.

Overview

- Cranial abnormalities require a team approach for optimum perioperative management due to the wide range of clinical concerns.
- A concern in these cases is the optimum timing of surgery. Early surgery can slow the progress of developmental defects. It permits better molding

of skull bones and better brain development. However, the infant might not be able to withstand the blood loss, and there is a greater chance of subsequent reoperation. If the surgery is delayed, the bones are tough to mold and heal. The delay could affect brain development or impair hearing or vision. However, there is less likelihood of a revision surgery. Thus elective surgery is undertaken around six months to a year of age as per institutional experience.
- Synostosis (1:3,000 births) is a group of congenital disorders characterized by the premature closure of fibrous sutures between the cranial bones. The suture fusion leads to a failure of growth perpendicular to the suture with excessive growth parallel to the suture. The deformity is usually isolated (in 80%) and is not associated with recognized syndromes. Syndromic cases (20%) have a worse prognosis.

Preoperative Concerns

- *Skull deformity may make positioning and intubation difficult:*
  - Lack of symmetry with difficulty in mask ventilation and positioning for intubation.
  - A mid-cranial abnormality can result in OSA and nasal obstruction
  - Proptosis, risk of pre and intraoperative eye injury
  - Maxillary hypoplasia
  - Mandibular hypoplasia
  - Cervical deformities, immobility, and fixation.
- *Neurological:* Raised ICP, delayed milestones, seizures, hearing and vision impairment
- *Cardiovascular:* Congenital heart disease (CHD), cor pulmonale, right heart failure, excessive blood loss, and pulmonary and systemic air embolism.
- *Respiratory concerns:* Airway, intubation, obstructive sleep apnea (OSA), airway irritability, tracheobronchial abnormalities.
- It may require multistage correction.
- *Syndromic craniosynostosis:* These include:
  - *Muenke syndrome (1:30,000):* Mutation of FGFR-3 gene leads to coronal suture synostosis (30% of all cases). The facial deformity can be mild with macrocephaly, deafness, respiratory obstruction, OSA, and acral abnormalities.
  - *Apert's syndrome (1:65,000):* Mutation of fibroblast growth receptor gene (FGFR-2): Bicoronal brachycephaly, cleft palate, mid-face hypoplasia, and shallow eye socket. Respiratory concerns include OSA and difficult intubation. Neurological concerns are increased ICP, deafness, delayed milestones, and cervical spine abnormalities. Abnormal wrist, digits, and genitourinary system.

- *Pfeiffer's syndrome (1:100,000):* Due to mutation of FGFR-2 gene. Similar to Crouzon but with broad and radially deviated thumbs. Early closure of sutures may result in a clover-leaf skull. Associated with tracheobronchial abnormalities
- *Carpenter's syndrome (1:1,000,000):* Mutation of RAB-23 or MEGF8 gene with autosomal recessive inheritance. Characteristic clover leaf skull due to multiple synostosis, deafness, and mental retardation. CHD. Kyphoscoliosis.
- *Crouzon's syndrome (1:50,000):* Due to FGFR-2 gene mutation. Hypoplastic maxilla and nasal obstruction may require tracheostomy. Unlike Pfeiffer Syndrome, these patients have normal hands and feet.
- *Seethre-chotzen syndrome (1:50,000):* Mutation of TWIST-1 gene: Premature coronal suture fusion, skull and facial abnormality with wide set drooping eyes. Spinal abnormalities, syndactyly, duplication of the great toe.
- *Craniofrontal-nasal syndrome (1:120,000):* Mutation of EFNB-1 gene, X-recessive affecting females, coronal synostosis, with ocular hypertelorism, broad nose, cleft lip, and palate.

Preparation for Surgery

- *Emergency surgery may be needed for:*
  - Raised ICP
  - Potential injury to eyes
  - Threatened airway
- *Optimization needed for elective surgery includes:*
  - Treatment of respiratory infections and hyperreactivity
  - Tracheostomy if needed
  - Blood harvest for autotransfusion and erythropoietin treatment.

Preparation of the Operating Room

- *Anticipated problems with airway and intubation:*
  - Difficulties in positioning the head.
  - Asymmetric head and mandible
  - Nasal atresia and obstruction
  - Palatal abnormalities
  - Size and location of the tongue
  - Cervical abnormalities
  - Tracheobronchial abnormalities.
- *Airway equipment:* Oral airways, laryngoscopes, endotracheal tubes (cuffed/uncuffed, armored, or RAE: operator choice), face masks, and suction

- *Anesthesia machine check, breathing circuits, and monitoring equipment:*
  - Routine anesthesia monitors
  - A-line
  - CVL, femoral preferred
  - Precordial Doppler
  - Blood gas analyzer
  - ROTEM and coagulation testing tubes
- *IV fluids, blood, and products:* De-airing the lines as needed.
- *Drugs:* Anesthetic and resuscitative
- Under-body forced warm air blanket.
- *Lines:* IV with blood transfusion set and warmer.

Induction

- **Pre-medication** is seldom used.
- *Induction technique:*
  - Volatile versus intravenous induction—Selection affected by:
    - Existing venous access
    - The general condition of the patient
    - Anticipated intubation concerns
    - Increased ICP
    - Concurrent heart disease
    - Usual management includes volatile induction.
- Once sedated, necessary noninvasive monitors are placed, and IV access is obtained.
- Muscle relaxants are used for intubation once positive pressure ventilation is possible. Neuromuscular paralysis is monitored.
- The endotracheal tube is usually secured with tape, but sutures might be needed to avoid intraoperative displacement.
- *Post-intubation:*
  - Additional IV access
  - Arterial and central venous lines are placed as needed.
  - Esophageal temperature probe
  - Precordial Doppler
  - *Urinary catheter to guide fluid management:*
    - Target urinary flow >0.5 mL/kg/h
  - Surgical positioning
  - Warming devices
- *Difficult ventilation:* This can be due to the following:
  - Kinked tube
  - Secretions (monophonic wheezing)
  - Bronchospasm (polyphonic wheezing)

Monitoring
- Ventilation and hemodynamics
- Muscle paralysis
- *Temperature:* Target core temperature of 36–37°C
- *Urine output:* >0.5 mL/kg/h
- *Precordial Doppler:* As many as 80% cases have air embolism by Doppler.
- *Arterial blood gas (ABG) monitoring for:*
  - pH: Increasing acidosis.
  - The base deficit for metabolic acidosis
  - *A-a gradient:* Ventilation optimization and fluid overload
  - $PaCO_2$: Adequate ventilation and hyperventilation for ICP
  - *Expired CO_2–$PaCO_2$ gradient:* Air embolism
  - *Serum K^+ and Ca^{++}:* Particularly during blood replacement
  - *Base deficit and lactic acidosis:* Assess peripheral perfusion.
- Coagulation assessment with massive resuscitation.

Intraoperative Care
- *Positioning:*
  - Neutral position
    - To ensure adequate venous return
    - Avoid air embolism
  - Pressure points padded to avoid nerve injury during a prolonged procedure
  - *Neck:* Impediment to venous return can cause macroglossia
  - Protection of the eyes at risk of injury.
- *Vascular access:*
  - Essential to have two large-bore peripheral IVs.
  - CVL for significant blood loss is expected. Femoral preferred due to remote location.
  - *A line with:*
    - Anticipated significant blood loss/blood sampling.
    - Associated cardiac abnormalities.
    - Inability to tolerate blood loss.
- *Fluid management:*
  - Selection depends on age, physical condition, metabolic needs, and blood loss.
  - Dextrose saline is often used as maintenance fluid; hypoglycemia is a concern in the sick. Normal saline is an ideal replacement fluid for neurosurgical patients as it is isotonic. Ringer's lactate is mildly hypotonic but decreases the chances of hypocalcemia.
  - 5% albumin replacement fluid during high-volume resuscitation

- Blood replacement protocols vary. Centers may delay transfusing to conserve blood others have a higher threshold for blood replacement.
- *In neonates and in infants <10 kg:* An equal volume of fresh blood replaces the blood loss.
- *In patients >10 kg:* Any loss >20% blood volume is replaced with blood.
- *The excessive fluid requirement in children is due to the following:*
  - Higher metabolic rate
  - Greater body surface area to weight ratio
  - Limited renal tubular concentrating capacity.
  - Higher respiratory rates.

- *Blood loss and prevention strategies:*
  - Judicious use of epinephrine infiltration of incision sites
  - Cell saver
  - Monitoring and correction of any coagulation dysfunction
  - Antifibrinolytic drugs
  - *As per institutional practices:*
    - Preoperative blood harvesting and autologous transfusion.
    - Preoperative erythropoietin treatment.

- *Excessive blood loss due to:*
  - Sudden massive blood loss is possible from large venous sinuses.
  - The scalp and skull are vascular, with significant oozing.
  - Incision and tissue exposure are extensive.
  - Consumptive coagulopathy
  - Dilutional coagulopathy with fluid resuscitation.

- *Venous air embolism:*
  - Air entrainment through venous injuries
  - Accidental injection during drug/fluid injection
  - Rule out any right-to-left shunt. 50% of children at 5 years have patent foramen ovale.

- *Excessive hemodynamic lability*
  - Inadequate resuscitation
  - Low hematocrit
  - Heart failure
  - Inadequate pain relief
  - Hypocalcemia

- *Bradycardia* is a significant concern as cardiac output is rate dependent.
  - *Bradycardia can be due to the following:*
    - Oculocardiac reflex
    - Hypothermia
    - Hypovolemia

- *Hypothermia*
  - *Possible causes:*

- The relatively large size of the head
- The relatively large area of surgical exposure
- Volume resuscitation with cold blood products
- Inadequate rewarming by conventional means
  - *Prevention:*
    - Underbody warming blanket.
    - Over-body air warmer
    - Overhead heating
    - Increased ambient temperature.
    - Blood and fluid warmers
    - Low fresh gas flow and use of a circle system
    - Humidified fresh gases.
  - *Adverse effects of hypothermia:*
    - Impairs coagulation
    - Bradycardia
    - Hypotension
    - Poor pressor response
    - Delayed awakening.

Emergence from Anesthesia

- *Extubation depends on:*
  - Preoperative assessment of the airway
  - Extent and duration of surgery
  - Hemodynamic stability, pressor requirements
  - *Respiratory effort:*
    - Surgery, e.g., rib resection
    - Residual sedation and analgesic drugs
- *Pain management: Specifically, for:*
  - Cranioplasty
  - Rib resection.

Postoperative Care

- *Nausea and vomiting (70%):* Ondansetron/dexamethasone responsive.
- *Postoperative ventilation:*
  - *Difficult airway:* History of airway obstruction and OSA
  - Prolonged surgery
  - Significant resuscitation
  - Tissue edema
- *Persistent hemodynamic instability:*
  - Monitor fluid balance
  - Persistent blood loss through drains suggests potential coagulopathy
  - Hypocalcemia and acidosis

- *Postoperative analgesia:*
  - Multimodal analgesia
  - *Judicious narcotic analgesia:* Morphine, hydromorphone
  - Unlike adults, codeine is avoided in pediatric patients. Codeine is a pro-drug that is converted to morphine. The conversion rate depends on the hepatic enzyme Cyp2D6, which can show considerable genetic variability.
  - IV acetaminophen
  - Dexmedetomidine
  - Steroids
  - Ketamine.

CASE REPORTS FOR FURTHER DISCUSSION

Case 1: A 7-year-old 25 kg child presented with shortness of breath, abdominal distention, and vomiting. Four years earlier, the child underwent resection of brainstem glioma with a ventriculoperitoneal (VP) shunt placement. A revision shunt surgery was done with a programmable shunt (pressure threshold of 80 cm H_2O) in the intervening period. He was being treated with prednisolone and thyroxine. On examination, vital signs were stable with BP 90/60 mm Hg and a pulse rate of 110 bpm. There was gross abdominal distention with fluid thrill. The routine investigations, including liver function tests, were within normal limits. The child was diagnosed with a case of cerebrospinal fluid (CSF) ascites and was due for the placement of a ventriculoatrial shunt. *How will the tense nature of ascites and gross enlargement of the belly affect your clinical management of the case? What hemodynamic changes can you expect due to gross ascites? When would you drain the CSF ascites, pre- or postoperatively?*

Case 2: A 13-year-old, 45-kg girl presented with new-onset seizures. Investigations revealed a tumor in the left temporoparietal junction close to receptive speech areas. After a careful medical assessment, an awake craniotomy was planned. Other than an allergic reaction to penicillin, her systemic review and laboratory results were negative. There was no history of snoring or sleep apnea. Her physical exam was non-contributory. The airway was class I. *How will you proceed with awake craniotomy in such a case? How will you manage airway obstruction? What are your options if the need arises to convert to general anesthesia? How can you intubate a patient whose head is fixed in pins?*

Case 3: A 7-year-old girl has a history of headaches and precocious puberty. Her past medical history is significant for asthma. Investigations reveal a pineal tumor. Her clinical exam and laboratory investigations are within normal limits. She is currently on corticosteroids. The excision of the tumor is planned in the sitting position. *What are the concerns you* have in such a case? Would you need monitoring of cranial nerves? Which cranial nerves would you monitor, and how will it affect your anesthetic plan? Intraoperatively, the patient develops severe diuresis; what is the differential diagnosis?

Case 4: A 6-day-old, 3.5-kg neonate presented with new-onset seizures, vomiting, and poor feeding. The child had a normal birth and was discharged from the neonatal unit 2 days earlier. The child was intubated in the ER due to an altered sensorium. MRI revealed a large (5 × 5 cm) right temporoparietal tumor. On transfer to the neonatal ICU, the child was unresponsive, with asymmetric pupils and absent gag reflex. The blood pressure was 115/77 mm Hg, and the pulse rate was 89 bpm. An emergency bedside ventricular CSF drain was placed. The child was due for urgent tumor resection. *How will you proceed? In the course of tumor resection, excessive bleeding is encountered. How will you manage suspected coagulopathy? ABG reveals acidosis and hyperkalemia, so how will you correct the rise in serum potassium? How will you manage this case after surgery?*

Case 5: A 4-year-old child fell into the gutter, and a 12 mm thick iron spiral penetrated the skull in the frontoparietal region. There was no loss of consciousness, seizures, or any neurological deficit. He was transferred to the hospital with the iron bar in-situ. On arrival at the hospital, the vital signs were stable. The pulse was 100 bpm, the blood pressure was 100/60 mm Hg, and the respiratory rate was 18–20/minute. The Glasgow coma scale was 15/15. Neurological examination revealed no neurological deficit. X-ray skull showed that the bar had penetrated to about 3.5 cm. The laboratory screen was within normal limits. He was due for craniotomy for the removal of the bar. *What additional imaging studies will you do besides the skull X-ray? If it is not immediately available, will you wait for a CT scan before surgery? What are the anticipated risks during surgery? What are the potential postoperative complications in such a case?*

CASE REPORT REFERENCES

Case 1: Mishra RK et al. Anesthetic considerations for ventriculoatrial shunt insertion in a child with cerebrospinal fluid ascites. J Pediatr Neurosci. 2018;13(2):249-51.

Case 2: Elsey NM et al. Anesthetic care during awake craniotomy in pediatric patients. Pediatr Anesth Crit Care J. 2013;1(2):61-71.

Case 3: Thomas S, et al. Anesthetic Management of a Child Undergoing Craniotomy in the Sitting Position. Proceeding of the Society for Pediatric Anesthesia Meeting 2011. [online] Available from: http:// www5.

pedsanesthesia.org/meetings/2011annual/syllabus/submissions/lunchpblds/neuro/Neuro_ Zestos-Thomas- Rockoff.pdf.

Case 4: Sun N, et al. Cardiac arrest during emergency craniotomy for a 6-day-old neonate with elevated ICP and impending herniation from an intracranial mass. Proceeding of the Society for Pediatric Anesthesia Meeting 2014. [online] Available from: https://www2.pedsanesthesia.org/meetings/2014annual/guide/protected/syllabus/

Case 5: Karim T et al. An unusual case of penetrating head injury. J of Emerg Trauma Shock. 2010;3(2):197-98.

FURTHER READING

1. Basaran I et al. Anesthetic management of scoliosis operation in a pediatric patient with Frank-Ter Haar syndrome: a case report. Braz J Anesthesiol. 2021;71(2):181-3.
2. Delion M et al. Specificities of awake craniotomy and brain mapping in children for resection of supratentorial tumors in the language area. World Neurosurg. 2015;84(6):1645-52.
3. Meier PM et al. Craniofacial Surgery-Pediatric Considerations (Chapter 18) in A Practical Approach to Neuroanesthesia. First edition. Editors: Morgan P, Soriano SG, Sloan, TB, and Gravlee GP. Lippincott, Williams & Wilkins Wolter Kluwer Company 2013: 243-253.
4. Grau S et al. The choice of the hypnotic drug (volatile or propofol) for maintenance of anesthesia does not influence surgical conditions during cranioplasty. J Anaesthesiol Clin Pharmacol. 2018;34(2):172-6.
5. Morparia KG et al. Respiratory variation in peak aortic velocity accurately predicts fluid responsiveness in children undergoing neurosurgery under general anesthesia. J Clin Monit Comput. 2018;32(2):221-6.

Vignette: For the First Case Series for Pediatric Brain Surgery, ether was the Agent of Choice

A recent retrospective review of pediatric neurosurgical cases done by Dr. Harvey Cushing at Johns Hopkins University between 1901 and 1912 was undertaken. The review revealed that he had operated on around 40 patients. The anesthetic agent used was reported for 39 of these patients. For two operations, the records show anesthesia to be reported as "none". These were two follow-up surgeries in a patient who had a serious infection after the first surgery for tumor removal. The patient eventually succumbed to the infection. In four patients, Cushing used chloroform. In the rest, he used ether. In one of these ether cases, he used ethylene chloride. Ether was used before and after chloroform cases, and it seems to be the agent of choice at the time. In the era before endotracheal intubation, muscle relaxants, intravenous anesthetics, antibiotics, methods to control bleeding, and no brain imaging, it is remarkable that 70% of cases survived the surgery.

Chapter 56: Biopsy for Creutzfeldt-Jakob Disease

INTRODUCTION

Creutzfeldt-Jakob Disease (CJD) belongs to a group of fatal, degenerative neurological diseases in animals and humans. These diseases are caused by unique self-replicating, transmissible proteins called prions. CJD and Kuru are two such diseases that affect humans. An anesthesiologist usually encounters CJD in a patient who needs a biopsy to diagnose unexplained rapid-onset dementia. CJD is transmissible by tissue transplants and ingestion of nervous tissue. CJD does not spread through direct contact or droplet inhalation. The challenge in treating CJD patients is that prions are highly resistant to conventional sterilization methods. Given the relentless and uniformly fatal course of the disease, preventing contamination of the operating room and instruments is essential. For a case of CJD, minimum equipment should be used that should preferably be disposable. The discarded equipment and contaminated wastes should be clearly labeled. The institutional guidelines for handling such cases must be rigorously followed.

NEUROANESTHETIC CONCERNS

- Pathogenesis of CJD
  - Prion disease
  - Clinical features
  - Infection risk
- Infection control strategies
- Anesthetic management
  - Total intravenous anesthesia (TIVA) versus general endotracheal anesthesia (GETA)
- Surgical management

Pathogenesis of CJD

- CJD is a rare but transmissible form of spongiform encephalopathy caused by prions. Prions tend to infect the cortex and basal ganglia. CJD

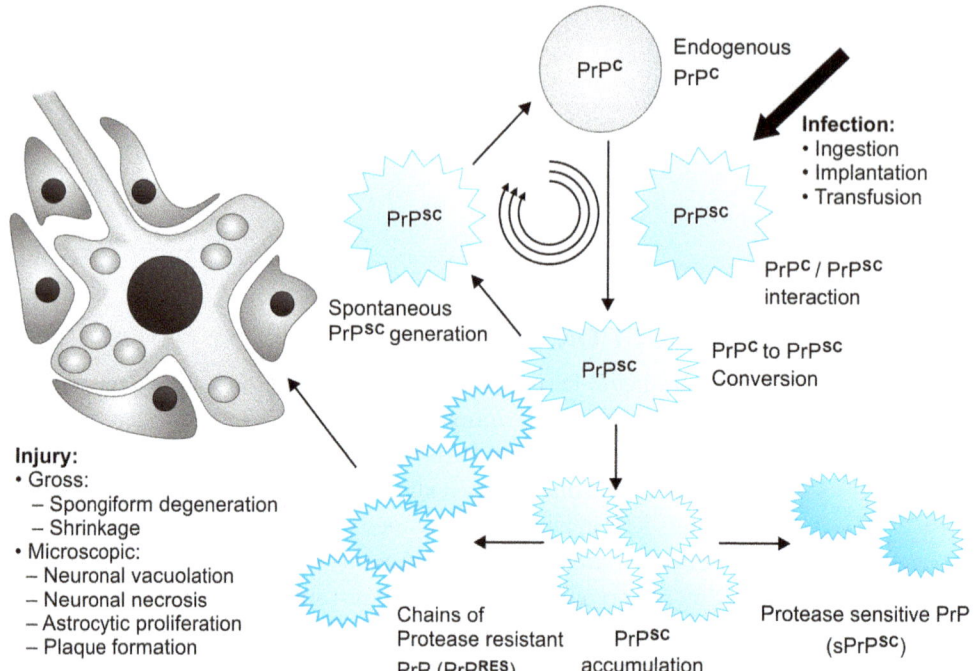

Fig. 1: The pathogenesis of Creutzfeldt-Jakob disease: Pathogenic prion protein (PrP^{sc}) transforms endogenous cellular prion proteins (PrP^c) to aggregate a protease-resistant prion's (PrP^{RES}) chain, resulting in cell injury and spongiform-damage and shrinkage of brain tissue.

is characterized by cytoplasmic vacuoles in neurons and astrocytes, with neuronal loss and proliferation of astrocytes:
- The pathological prion proteins (PrP^{SC}) can transform normal cellular proteins (PrP^c) into abnormal proteins (PrP^{SC}) to lead to the aggregation and deposition of more abnormal proteins. In doing so, they also amplify the pathological process by progressively transforming the normal proteins and depositing abnormal protein aggregates **(Fig. 1)**, leading to intractable neurological injury.
- PrP^C has a misfolded protein structure that can replicate.
- Prions that are devoid of nucleic acids are considered to be nonliving.
- They lead to the formation of an amyloid sheet.
- They elicit no immune response.
- They have a stable protein structure resistant to protease, formalin, heat, chemical degradation, and irradiation.
- No specific diagnostic tests are available.
- *Animal prion diseases:* Include mad cow disease, scrapie (in sheep and goats), feline spongiform encephalopathy, and the chronic wasting disease of deer and other animals.
- *Human prion diseases:* Include CJD and its variants, Kuru, Gerstmann-Straussler-Scheinker syndrome, and fatal familial insomnia.

CHAPTER 56 Biopsy for Creutzfeldt–Jakob Disease

Table 1: Clinical and investigative finding in Creutzfeldt–Jacob's disease.

Clinical features	Investigations
Myoclonus	MRI: Asymmetric hyperintensities or FLAIR in >2 cortical gyri or basal ganglia
Akinetic mutism	Western blotting—for protease-resistant PrP or scrapie-associated fibrils
Extra-pyramidal symptoms	Tissue histology and immunohistochemistry
Visual or cerebellar symptoms	• EEG: Periodic sharp wave complexes • CSF: Positive for 14-3-3 protein with disease less than two years duration

(FLAIR: fluid associated inversion recovery imaging)

Clinical Features

- A disease of the elderly
- A variant form may occur in younger individuals.
- Asymptomatic for 20 or more years
- Presents with cognitive defects that progress to dementia.
- Involvement of the cerebellum, pyramidal, and extra-pyramidal tracts progressively incapacitates the patient **(Table 1)**.
- Bed-bound vegetative state in weeks to months
- Relentless disease with fatal outcome
- *Variant CJD:*
  - The median age of 28 years vs. 68 years for classical CJD
  - Presents with psychiatric and sensory symptoms.
  - Ataxia, dementia, and myoclonus occur later compared to classical CJD.
  - EEG nonspecific
  - *Neuropathology:* Kuru-like amyloid plaques whose morphology is distinct from other prion diseases. The prion proteins are demonstrated by immunohistochemistry in the cerebrum and cerebellum.
  - Survival for six months or more

Infection Risk

- It is not transmitted by physical contact or droplet/airborne transmission.
- The patient does not require contact isolation.
- Contact, transplantation, or ingestion of neural tissue carries the highest risk of infectivity, especially the brain, spinal cord, and eyes. Other sources include dura and corneas.
- Cerebrospinal fluid (CSF) poses less infectivity than other neural tissue.
- Peripheral nerves are not considered infective.
- Lungs, kidneys, lymph nodes, and spleen have very low infectivity.

- Unlike CJD, vCJD is likely to be transmitted by blood transfusion. The transmission is most likely to be through the white blood cells. Removing white blood cells decreases the chances of CJD transmission. Patients with CJD should not donate blood.
- *Iatrogenic CJD:*
  - 5% of CJD cases are iatrogenic.
  - *Sources:*
    - Inadequately sterilized instruments
    - Dural and corneal grafts; injection of pituitary extracts
    - Infected blood transfusions (vCJD).

Infection Control Strategies

- Establish and implement institutional policies.
- Inform the care team, hospital personnel, and all those at risk of exposure.
- Minimize surgical procedures. CJD diagnosis is possible without a biopsy.
- Limit personnel traffic to the operating room.
- Double glove and wear face masks.
- Use dedicated or disposable surgical instruments.
- Double bag and label any CJD wastes, and discard all sharps in single-use containers that are labeled and discarded.
- Extended sterilization is required, which includes:
  - Heat sterilization at 132°C for 2 hours.
  - Treatment with 2N-sodium hydroxide, sodium hypochlorite, or undiluted bleach.
  - Tissue samples are immersed in 96% formalin for 1 hour before processing.

Anesthetic Management

- *Preparation of the OR:*
  - Plastic sheet to protect fixed hardware.
  - Basic minimal equipment
  - Use disposable equipment.
- Consider TIVA with Ambu bag ventilation to lessen equipment exposure compared to general anesthesia with volatile agents.
- Transmission through anesthesia equipment is unlikely. The anesthesia machine can be used and protected by a HEPA filter. Anesthesia equipment requires routine care and reprocessing.
- If special anesthesia equipment (e.g., bronchoscope) is needed, it should be disposable; otherwise, like other endoscopes, it should be identified, isolated, and suitably sterilized.
- Prions are found in saliva. Therefore, the suction system should be safely disposed of after use.

CHAPTER 56 Biopsy for Creutzfeldt–Jakob Disease

Surgical Management
- Safe surgery with the fewest steps and equipment requirements should be planned to minimize the risk of contamination of the neurosurgical facilities.
- All personnel should wear personal protective equipment, including gowns, face masks, visors, and double gloves.
- The manual drill minimizes fragment aerosols generated by high-speed electric or pneumatic drills.
- Tissue samples should be clearly labeled and laboratories informed.
- *Postoperative care:*
  - Cognitively impaired patients have slow emergence from anesthesia.
  - Isolation and contamination prevention protocols are to be followed.

CASE REPORTS FOR FURTHER DISCUSSION

Case 1: A 64-year-old single divorced woman with several psychosocial stressors presented with a two-month history of right upper extremity tremors, right-sided numbness, ataxia, headaches, and joint pains. Her history was significant for hypothyroidism, hypertension, and Lyme disease. The psychosocial stressors included the recent demise of her mother, solitary living, premature retirement from her job, and relocation to a new residence. She had no history of neurological injury, stroke, psychiatric problems, alcohol, or substance abuse. By the end of the first week, when an extensive neurological and laboratory diagnosis was negative, she was diagnosed with a functional neurological disorder. Accordingly, physical and occupational therapy was instituted. By the third week of admission, the patient continued to deteriorate with confusion, ataxia, and refusal to eat. She also developed an upper extremity myoclonus with generalized rigidity. She was prescribed benzodiazepines and antibiotics due to suspected catatonia and her history of Lyme disease. Her condition worsened by the fourth week of admission, and neurological tests were repeated. The EEG revealed triphasic waves, while the MRI revealed new cortical FLAIR hyperintensities. A biopsy with a provisional diagnosis of CJD was undertaken. *What are the most common neurological symptoms of CJD? What are the definitive tests that can diagnose CJD? What is the role of a biopsy in the diagnosis of CJD? Do you justify the use of an N95 mask for CJD? How is the operating room decontaminated after a CJD case?*

Case 2: A 17-year-old mother of a healthy 6-month-old child presented to the emergency department with a loss of consciousness. Over the past several weeks, she had repeated blackouts preceded by abnormal smell and vertigo. For several months, she had significant changes in mood suggestive of postpartum depression. She was treated with antidepressants. However, the patient became progressively agitated, shaky, and absent-minded.

On examination, the patient was agitated, easily distracted, and fidgety. She could not give the current date or year. Her motor coordination was clumsy. She continued to deteriorate with increasing emotional lability requiring increasing sedation. By one month after admission, she was completely dependent on nursing care. There were episodes of loss of consciousness with a vacant gaze. She was treated with sodium valproate. By the third month of admission, she was aphasic and had developed bilateral pyramidal signs with myoclonic jerks. MRI imaging four months apart revealed hyperintensities in the thalamic nuclei. The diagnosis of CJD was confirmed on autopsy. *Can the side effects of antidepressant drugs affect the diagnosis of CJD? Besides the younger age, what other clinical characteristics of the variant form of CJD differ from classical disease? How is the transmission of the variant CJD differ from classical CJD? Do you need to protect the anesthesia machine from contamination against CJD? Faced with difficult intubation, what device will you use? Is succinylcholine safe in CJD patients?*

Case 3: A 76-year-old man presented to ER with a two-week history of sudden onset confusion, memory loss, and visual and gait disturbances. The neurological symptoms were attributed to delirium due to UTI. The patient was treated with antibiotics by his general practitioner. When he failed to respond to treatment, he was directed to the ER for suspected stroke treatment. Before this illness, he was in good health with no neurological or psychological problems. On admission, he failed to respond to questions in the English language but responded to questions in a Thai dialect. He was previously fluent in both languages. His speech was slurred. He displayed dysgraphia and an ataxic gait but no myoclonic jerks. He was only able to follow simple commands. A cranial nerve exam revealed a left visual defect. The initial CT scan was negative for intracranial pathology. The patient's condition rapidly deteriorated with severe agitation, akinetic mutism, rigidity, and myoclonic jerks. Agitation made nursing difficult. He passed away 17 days after admission. An autopsy revealed histological evidence of CJD in the cerebral hemisphere, specifically in the temporal and occipital lobes and cerebellar tissue, with spongiform changes. *What are the MRI features of CJD? What are the diagnostic CSF markers of CJD? Are there special precautions that are needed to process CJD tissue samples?*

Case 4: A 4-year-old boy was admitted to the hospital with an acute hepatitis B infection. His history was significant for a past needlestick injury sustained at home. His neighbor, who was Hepatitis B and HIV-positive, was the suspected source. At the time of injury, the parents did not consider the needlestick significant. *How do you manage needlestick injuries in your hospital? In this case, will you screen the family? If the family was Hepatitis B negative, and the neighbor is suspected to be the*

CHAPTER 56 Biopsy for Creutzfeldt–Jakob Disease

source, would you consider HIV infection as well? What is the treatment for Hepatitis B?

CASE REPORT REFERENCES

Case 1: Yegya-Raman N, et al. A Case of Sporadic Creutzfeldt-Jakob Disease Presenting as Conversion Disorder: Case Reports in Psychiatry (2017). 2017:2735329. DOI: 10.1155/2017/2735329.

Case 2: Allroggen H, et al. New variant Creutzfeldt-Jakob disease: three case reports from Leicestershire: Psychiatry. 2000;68:375-8.

Case 3: Kwon GT et al. Diagnostic challenge of rapidly progressing sporadic Creutzfeldt-Jakob disease. BMJ Case Rep. 2019;12:e230535. Doi: 10.1136/bcr-2019-230535.

Case 4: Garcia-Algar O et al. Hepatitis B virus infection from a needle stick. The Ped Infectious Disease Journal. 1997; 16 (11) 1099

FURTHER READING

1. Bagyinszky E, et al. Novel prion mutation (p.Tyr225Cys) in a Korean patient with atypical Creutzfeldt-Jakob disease. Clin Interv Aging. 2019;14:1387-97.
2. Foucault-Fruchard L et al. An automated alert system based on the p-Tau/Tau ratio to quickly inform health professionals upon a suspected case of sporadic Creutzfeldt-Jakob disease. J Neurol Sci. 2020;415:116971.
3. Park HY et al. Prognostic value of diffusion-weighted imaging in patients with newly diagnosed sporadic Creutzfeldt-Jakob disease. Eur Radiol, 2021.
4. Ritchie DL et al. Variant CJD: Reflections a Quarter of a Century on. Pathogens. 2021;10(11):1413.
5. Tayyebi G et al. COVID-19-associated encephalitis or Creutzfeldt-Jakob disease: a case report. Neurodegener Dis Manag. 2021.

Vignette: The Mad Cow Disease

Mad cow disease, or bovine spongiform encephalitis (BSE), is a neurodegenerative disease of cattle characterized by weight loss, decreased milk production, unusual posture, gait disturbances, impaired coordination, and altered behavior such as showing signs of nervousness and aggression. The symptoms worsen over weeks or months, leading to coma and death. Consumption of an infected animal's brain, spinal cord, dorsal root ganglia, trigeminal ganglia, tonsils, and distal ileum can transmit the infection. The infection is due to abnormally folded proteins called prions. These proteins are not destroyed even if the beef is cooked. Prions can withstand temperatures of up to 600°C. The disease belongs to a cluster of transmissible spongiform encephalopathies (TSE), which includes scrapie in sheep and goats, chronic wasting disease of deer and elk, and the TSE of cats and minks. The human TSE examples include diseases such as Kuru, Creutzfeldt–Jakob disease, Gerstmann–Straussler–Scheinker syndrome, and fatal familial insomnia. The 1993 BSE epidemic in the UK led to the destruction of over a million heads of cattle and the shutdown of beef exports for many years. The source of infection for the epidemic has been debated. It could have jumped from another species, or it could have slowly infected the herd. The 1990 BSE epidemic possibly arose from a single source in the southwest of England and had started in 1970.

Chapter 57: Postoperative Vision Loss

INTRODUCTION

Postoperative visual loss (POVL) can occur after nonophthalmic surgery. Surgeries most likely associated with POVL are open heart surgery needing cardiopulmonary bypass, spine surgery, head and neck surgery, orthopedic surgery, and robotic pelvic surgery in an extreme Trendelenburg position. The risk factors of POVL with spine surgery are prolonged operations in the prone position, the use of Wilson's frame, obesity, male gender, excessive blood loss, hypotension, and anemia. The incidence of POLV after spine surgery is about 0.02%. Unlike cardiac surgery, the injury is not due to emboli. The primary pathology is an ischemic optic neuropathy with edema of the posterior segment of the optic nerve. The visual loss can be partial but is intractable. It is refractory to treatment. The main preventive measures include avoiding prolonged Trendelenburg position, staging surgery to decrease its duration, avoiding hypotension, and adequate colloid resuscitation.

NEUROANESTHETIC CONCERNS

- Causes of postoperative vision loss (POVL)
- Incidence of postoperative blindness
- Patient characteristics
- Risk factors during spine surgery
- Clinical manifestations
- Prevention and management

Causes of POVL

- Ischemic optic neuropathy
  - Posterior ischemic optic neuropathy (PION)
  - Anterior ischemic optic neuropathy (AION)
  - Central retinal artery occlusion
  - Branch artery emboli
- Acute glaucoma
- Lens dislocation
- Cortical blindness

- *Trauma:*
  - Corneal abrasion
  - Conjunctival injury
  - Direct optic nerve injuries.

Incidence

- *Overall (rare):* 1:2,000 general anesthetics
- *Cardiopulmonary bypass (CPB):* 0.1%, usually anterior optic neuropathy
- *Spine surgery:* <0.02%, typically posterior optic neuropathy.

Risk Factors (The Disc-at-Risk)

Patient Risk Factors

- Males
- Middle-aged
- Diabetic retinopathy
- Hypertension
- Anemia
- Other risk factors:
  - Smoker (active or within ten years)
  - Peripheral vascular disease
  - Coronary artery disease
  - Obesity
  - Sickle cell disease
  - Polycythemia

Surgical Risk Factors

- *Position:* Prone or Trendelenburg
- *Duration:* >6 hours
- Use of Wilson frame
- Hypotension
- *Blood loss with hematocrit* values of <20%
- *Massive fluid resuscitation:* >4 L

Pathological Factors

- Anatomical risk factors (**Fig. 1**):
  - Reduced blood flow in the central artery of the retina:
    - The anterior branch affects the optic nerve head.
    - The posterior branch affects the posterior segment of the optic nerve.
  - Reduced collateral blood flow through pial and posterior ciliary arteries.
  - *Reduced retinal blood flow due to:*
    - Arterial hypotension

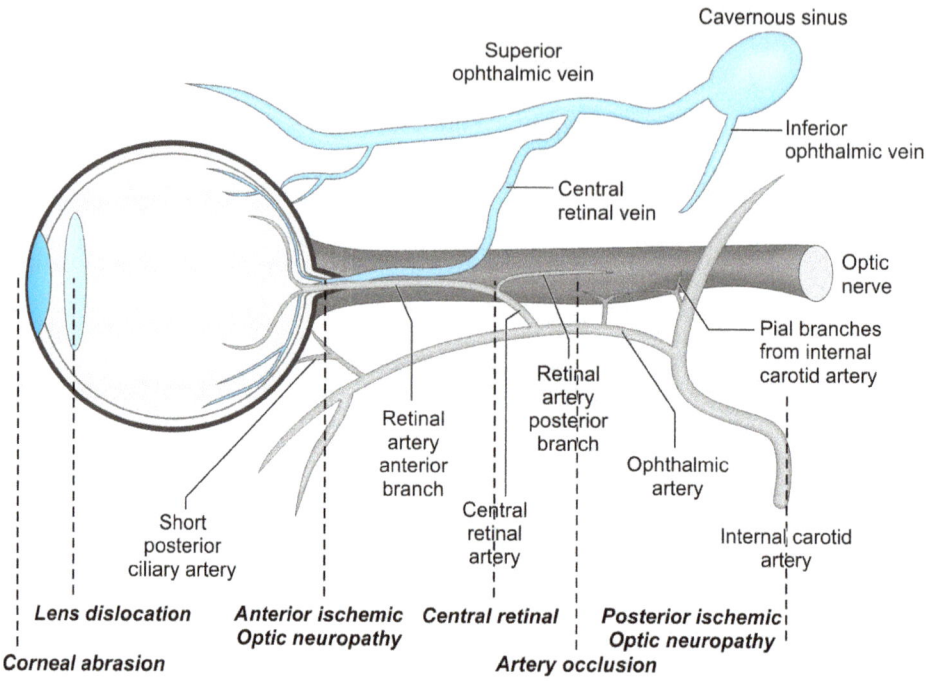

Fig. 1: Blood supply of the optic nerve and site of perioperative ophthalmic injuries.

- Increased intraocular pressure, >21 mm Hg
- External pressure on the globe
- Glaucoma
- Microvascular disease
- A significant infusion of vasoconstrictor drugs
- Blood O_2 transport:
  - Low hematocrit
  - Hypoxemia
- Edema of the nerve leads to further compression in the sphenoid canal.

Clinical Manifestations

- Pathology and some clinical features of perioperative loss of vision are shown in **Table 1** and discussed during postoperative care when these problems are usually encountered.

PREVENTION AND MANAGEMENT OF POVL

Preoperative Assessment

- Postoperative blindness in 90% is due to ischemic optic neuropathy, and 10% is due to retinal artery emboli.
- Preoperative identification of at-risk cases is listed above.
- Preoperative ophthalmic assessment in high-risk cases.

CHAPTER 57 Postoperative Vision Loss

Table 1: Perioperative causes of impaired vision.

Diagnosis	Pathological factors	Clinical features
1. Ischemic optic neuropathy		
A. Anterior ischemic optic neuropathy (AION): Occurs after cardiopulmonary bypass	*Arteritis* (giant cell arteritis) and *Nonarteritis* ischemia, emboli, diabetes, coronary artery disease, smoking, sickle cell disease affecting the anterior segment	Female > males, age >55 years, if with giant cell arteritis may be associated with pain • Acute painless loss of vision
B. Posterior ischemic optic neuropathy (PION): Occurs in prone spine cases	*Perioperative*: Prolonged surgery, hypotension, pressor use, ocular pressure, Trendelenburg position, and prone position	• Impaired light reflex, central scotoma; often bilateral
Central retinal artery occlusion (CRAO)		Acute unilateral loss of vision and decreased visual acuity
Branch retinal artery occlusion (BRAO)		Acute unilateral loss of vision and decreased visual acuity
2. Ac. glaucoma	Increase IOP due to decreased aqueous drainage	Redness, pain, blurred vision, and headache
3. Lens dislocation	Ligament breakdown	Blurred vision and irregular pupil
4. Trauma	Corneal abrasion	Pain and inflammation, light sensitivity, and blurred vision

- If extensive surgery with blood loss is expected, consider a staged procedure.
- Patients should be informed of the potential risk of POVL.

Intraoperative Care

- Avoid pressure on the globe. Repeatedly check and document the absence of pressure on the eye.
- Maintain head in the horizontal position with neck in the neutral position to ensure unimpeded venous drainage.
- Avoid hypotension, hypoxia, and significant anemia.
- Antiplatelet agents, steroids, and intraocular pressure-lowering drugs have no effect. The latter includes acetazolamide (a carbonic anhydrase inhibitor).
- Deliberate hypotension can lead to POVL, but a direct correlation is hard to establish as hypotension has been used for many years without such complications. The increased incidence of POVL in recent years could be due to more restrictive blood transfusions and a lower perioperative hematocrit.
- There is no defined threshold for the treatment of anemia, but hematocrit should be maintained at >25% in healthy patients with adequate oxygenation.

- Colloids should supplement replaced fluid with significant blood loss to prevent a decrease in oncotic pressure and a subsequent increase in tissue edema.

Postoperative Diagnosis and Care

- POVL, due to ischemia, usually presents as a painless impairment of vision.
- POVL presents within 24–48 hours of surgery.
- Onset may be delayed in ventilated/sedated patients.
- Initially, the presentation may be unilateral vision impairment, but 90% have bilateral involvement.
- *Differential diagnosis and clinical findings:*
  - *Posterior ischemic optic neuropathy:*
    - The most common cause of POVL after spine surgery
    - Impairment of visual acuity
    - Normal fundus and optic disc
    - Normal intraocular pressure
    - Progresses to complete blindness.
  - *Anterior ischemic optic neuropathy:*
    - Non-arteritic AION 80% after cardiopulmonary bypass. Painless sudden loss of vision, visual field defects, impaired color vision, swollen optic disc with splinter hemorrhages.
    - *Arteritic AION:* Pain, headaches, loss of appetite besides loss of vision
  - *Central retinal artery occlusion:*
    - Account for 10% of POVL cases
    - *Fundoscopy reveals:*
      - *"Cattle trucking" sign:* Interrupted visualization of blood vessels due to stagnant blood flow.
      - *"Cherry red spot":* Visualization of the redness of the choroid, although the ischemic retina affects the region of the fovea.
  - *Cortical blindness:*
    - A rare cause of POVL
    - Usually due to middle and posterior cerebral artery stroke
    - Bilateral painless loss of vision, homonymous - hemianopia, or quadrantanopia
    - Preservation of the pupillary reflexes and extraocular movements
    - "Blindsight" perception of movement in an otherwise dark field
  - *Glaucoma:*
    - It can be due to steroid use.
    - Usually, glaucoma is of the open-angle type.
    - It presents with redness, pain, nausea, halos around light, and blurred vision.

CHAPTER 57 Postoperative Vision Loss

- *Corneal abrasion:*
  - Blurred vision, pain, redness, irritation, photosensitivity
  - Diagnosed by fluorescein staining.
- *Lens dislocation:*
  - Painless loss of vision, rarely blurred vision
  - History of eyes surgery, severe myopia, direct trauma
  - 0.05-6% lens implants can dislocate over time.
- On suspicion of impaired vision, immediately ask for ophthalmic consultation.
- Protect the eye from further injury
- Ensure optimum oxygenation and adequate perfusion.
- Head elevation decreases intraocular pressure but could result in hypotension.

Outcome

Recognition of risk factors and preventive measures are essential to avoid POLV. Treatment with steroids, antiplatelet drugs, or intraocular pressure-reducing drugs (acetazolamide) is not effective. Some improvement is possible, but POVL is usually permanent.

CASE REPORTS FOR FURTHER DISCUSSION

Case 1: A 38-year-old male with a body mass index (BMI) of 32.4 kg/m^2 sustained traffic injuries. Radiographic investigations revealed a fracture of a second lumbar vertebra. The neurological exam revealed weakness in the lower limbs with bladder and bowel incontinence. There was no contributory past medical illness. He underwent posterior decompression approximately 72 hours after injury. The systolic blood pressure was between 90 and 110 mm Hg during surgery. His oxygen saturation was around 98%. The surgery lasted 105 minutes, and blood loss was 420 mL. The postoperative hemoglobin was 10.6 gm/dL. In the recovery room, around 12 hours after surgery, the patient complained of bilateral vision loss. Examination revealed bilateral blindness with the preservation of pupillary and corneal reflexes and normal ocular movements. There were no new neurological deficits. CT and MRI follow-up revealed bilateral infarcts in the occipital lobes. The echocardiography was negative for any potential source of emboli. *What are the differential diagnoses of perioperative loss of vision? How does cortical blindness differ from other ischemic optic neuropathies?*

Case 2: A 32-year-old female presented with weakness in her lower limbs for the last three months. Investigations revealed a giant cell tumor involving all three columns in the upper thoracic region (T2 and T3). She underwent posterior spinal instrumentation with surgical tumor resection and implantation of an expandable cage. During the 7-hour surgery, her head was placed on a horseshoe headrest, and no untoward events were reported. The systolic blood pressure remained over 90 mm Hg. The blood loss was estimated at 1,400 mL. She was resuscitated with 3,000 mL of fluids. Postoperatively, she was transfused with two units of blood. On awakening, the patient complained of severe pain in the left eye with loss of vision. On examination, there was puffiness of the eyelids with conjunctival congestion of the left eye. Visual acuity was finger counting at 2 feet. The pupil was moderately dilated, and the cornea and lens were clear. The fundus exam revealed pallor and macular edema. Retinal arteries were normal. Right-side fundus examination was normal. She was given 1 g of methylprednisolone for three days. Subsequently, visual acuity improved gradually to 6/9 by the third day. *What position-related factors could contribute to postoperative blindness during spinal surgery? What are the advantages and disadvantages of prone view and pin fixation of the head for spine surgery?*

Case 3: A 15-year-old female, 153 cm tall, weighing 50 kg, with idiopathic scoliosis, underwent anterior spinal instrumentation in the left lateral position. General anesthesia with endotracheal intubation was provided for the procedure. Her eyes were taped. Six hours later, the anesthesia was withdrawn for the wake-up test. During the wake-up test, her pupils were assessed several times. On waking up, the motor power of the upper limbs was assessed as normal. Subsequently, the general anesthesia was resumed. After the surgery, she could move all limbs on command and was extubated. She complained of severe pain in the right eye (nondependent) and could not open the eye due to severe pain. The ophthalmologist diagnosed a corneal abrasion. *What precautions could you have taken to prevent such injuries in this case? What is the outcome?*

Case 4: A 68-year-old female patient with L5 radicular pain underwent an uneventful L2 to L4 spinal fusion under general anesthesia with endotracheal intubation. The intraoperative course was unremarkable except for a transient episode of hypotension. The surgery lasted 5 hours. On postoperative day 2, the patient complained of severe eye pain and vomiting. The next day, she became hyponatremic, with altered consciousness and respiratory failure, for which she was intubated. Her intraocular pressure was measured at 45 mm Hg on the right side and 64–75 mm Hg on the left side with diffuse corneal edema, shallow anterior chamber, and fixed mid-dilated pupils. Aqueous suppressant drugs and steroid drops were instilled topically to lower the IOP. She was extubated again on day 8. Gonioscopy determined a narrow drainage angle recess for which the patient underwent bilateral laser iridectomies. *If the risk of glaucoma had been known beforehand, what precautions would have avoided such a complication?*

CHAPTER 57 Postoperative Vision Loss

CASE REPORT REFERENCES

Case 1: Goni V et al. Cortical blindness following spinal surgery: very rare cause of perioperative vision loss. Asian Spine J. 2012;6(4):287-90.

Case 2: Kumar A et al. Unilateral visual loss after spine surgery: Lesson to be learnt from unexpected devastating complication. Interdiscip Neurosurg. 2019;17:66-8.

Case 3: Yanagidate F et al. Corneal abrasion after the wake-up test in spinal surgery. J Anesth. 2003;17(3):211-2.

Case 4: Singer MS et al. Bilateral acute angle-closure glaucoma as a complication of facedown spine surgery. Spine J. 2010;10(9):e7-9.

FURTHER READING

1. Capon M et al. Visual evoked potentials monitoring in a case of transient post operative visual loss. Indian J Anaesth. 2016;60(8):590-3.
2. Chandra KN et al. Postoperative visual loss after cervical laminectomy in prone position. Rev Bras Anestesiol. 2017;67(4):435-8.
3. Greenway F et al. Consent for post-operative visual loss in prone spinal surgery: aligning clinical practice with legal standards. Br J Neurosurg. 2018;32(6):604-9.

Vignette: Reversing Blindness

There are four approaches to reversing blindness: (1) bionic eyes, (2) gene therapy, (3) stem cells, and (4) optogenetics. Bionic eyes are cameras whose information is transferred to the retina via implanted electrodes. The image perceived is fairly crude but can permit shape recognition and light perception sufficient for simple tasks. The first bionic eye was implanted in 2002, and over 300 implants were done. The technology was expensive, and the research was suspended in early 2022. Gene therapy can reverse the effects of specific mutations. It is somewhat easier for the eyes because the eyes are immunologically isolated. Gene therapy has been successful in treating blindness due to Leber's congenital amaurosis. Cell regeneration and optogenetics involve the delivery of stem cells and opsins; these technologies are in the early stages of development.

Vignette: The Tail of the Peacock

Light-sensitive organs first evolved some 600 million years ago. Their development consists of two highly conserved proteins. Crystallin is a unique heat-stable protein that covers the organ and helps to focus the light. Opsins are light-sensitive proteins. The eyes began as light sensors but have evolved into complex organs. There were two geometries: (i) the compound eye and (ii) its inverted version, the simple eye. The capabilities of the two vary with respect to their field of view, the intensity of light, and the range of color perception. The number of eye structures varies from twelve in earthworms to five in insects, eight in spiders, two in vertebrates, and many invertebrates. Given the number of creatures with multiple eyes, it is not surprising that mythological creatures are endowed with extra eyes. Whether it is Shiv's third eye or the hundred eyes of Argus Panoptes. After Hermes killed Panoptes, Hera transferred his eyes to the peacock's tail.

Chapter 58
Robot-assisted Surgery and Laser Interstitial Thermal Therapy

INTRODUCTION

Robotic-assisted neurosurgery and Laser Interstitial Thermal Therapy (LITT) are two recent advances in treating epilepsy. Robotic guidance advances electrodes and fiberoptic cables in target sites with high precision while avoiding critical anatomical structures. These procedures usually require general anesthesia. LITT is a focal cytodestructive heat treatment using a laser delivered to the target site through a stereotactically placed fiberoptic cable. Magnetic resonance (MR) imaging monitors tissue heating and thermal ablation. The procedure helps treat tumors, vascular malformations, and epileptic foci. This minimally invasive two-part procedure is undertaken under general anesthesia. In the first part, the stereotactic frame is placed to position the fiber optic cable in the operating room. In the second part, the laser creates a region of thermal ablation in the MRI suite. Pre- and post-procedure MR images document the effect of the ablation.

NEUROANESTHETIC CONCERNS

- Preoperative assessment of a patient with epilepsy
- *Anesthesia for robotic-assisted stereotactic lead implantation:*
  - The technique of electrode implantation
  - Induction of anesthesia
  - OR setup
  - Induction
  - Maintenance
  - Emergence
  - Postoperative complication.
  - Monitoring and removal of the depth electrodes.
- *MRI-guided LITT for epilepsy:*
  - *The technique of LITT:*
    - Indications
    - Principles
  - *Concerns with anesthesia for MRI:*
    - Principles of MRI

- Magnetic hazards
- MRI compatibles devices
  - Anesthesia machines
  - Monitoring equipment
  - Infusion pumps
- Postoperative care in the ICU.

Preoperative Assessment of a Patient with Epilepsy

The objectives are as follows:
- Establish a rapport with the patient and the caregivers.
- Identify any congenital syndromes.
- Ability to understand commands and cooperate during the procedure.
- Assess the severity and nature of epilepsy.
- Neurological status, any behavioral manifestations, and aura characteristics.
- Prodromal manifestations and triggering events.
- Current seizure medications and their serum levels.
  - *Side effects of antiepileptic drugs:* Sedative side effects are expected, but other serious effects are also seen: e.g., phenytoin may cause cardiac toxicity, while valproate may cause bone marrow depression.
  - *Pharmacokinetic effects of antiepileptic drugs: Hepatic enzyme induction affects the pharmacokinetics of many drugs.* The most commonly seen effect is the tolerance to competitive muscle relaxants.

Anesthesia for Robot-assisted EEG Lead Implantation

- *The technique of robot-assisted electrode implantation:*
  - *ROSA:* Robot stereotactic assistant.
  - ROSA is a precision-controlled robotic arm with six degrees of movement, i.e., able to target the desired coordinates in 3D space from multiple angles.
  - Capable of self-co-registering MRI data.
  - Navigates to an operator-determined target site while avoiding critical structures.
  - *Precision navigation is helpful* for epilepsy treatment, tumor biopsy, or LITT.
  - *In the case of epilepsy, ROSA enables:*
    - Placement of depth electrodes for superficial and depth electroencephalogram (EEG) monitoring
    - Multiple electrodes can be placed in a short time.
    - Minimizes chances of injury

- *Indications for stereotactic EEG monitoring for epilepsy treatment:*
  - Deep seizure focus.
  - Inconclusive superficial grid monitoring.
  - Bi-hemispheric exploration.
  - Assessing the neural network in an epileptic patient.
- *OR setup:*
  - Routine OR setup for general anesthesia.
  - An arterial line is indicated for any co-morbidity.
  - Noninvasive monitoring is sufficient for healthy patients.
- *Induction:*
  - If monitoring EEG, avoid benzodiazepines.
  - Induction with fentanyl, lidocaine, propofol, and rocuronium is generally satisfactory.
  - *Intubation:* Lidocaine ointment of 5% could decrease the extubation response.
- *Maintenance:*
  - Discuss the anesthetic plan with the electrophysiologists.
  - Volatile agents alone, or a combination of total intravenous anesthesia (TIVA) with a volatile anesthetic agent, can be used for EEG monitoring.
  - Muscle relaxants are permitted.
  - After induction, the patient is positioned with the head supported on a frame that permits free movement of the robotic arm.
  - Usually, several depth electrodes are implanted, which determines the duration of the procedure.
  - *Enhancing seizure activity if needed:*
    - Decrease volatile agents to 0.2–0.3 minimum alveolar concentration (MAC), and supplement with propofol as needed.
    - Consider shifting to TIVA.
    - Consider ketamine 10 mg/kg/h.
    - *Other possibilities:* In consultation with electrophysiologists, consider analeptic anesthetics: enflurane, methohexital, or etomidate infusions.
- *Emergence:*
  - After placement, the leads are carefully wrapped, giving time for planning an extubation strategy.
  - Antiemetics are administered within 30 min of the expected wake-up.
  - The neuromuscular block is reversed after the head has been removed from the pins to avoid injury.
  - Suction before reversal of neuromuscular blockade.
  - *Ensure adequate immobility to avoid any coughing or bucking before extubation; possible strategies:*
    - Low-dose remifentanil (0.03 µg/kg/min)
    - Low-dose dexmedetomidine (0.2-0.7 µg/kg/h)
    - A small bolus of narcotics (fentanyl 25 µg increments)

- Lidocaine bolus (1 mg/kg)
- Intratracheal lidocaine 2% is instilled slowly into the endotracheal tube (ETT) lumen with a 26G needle in small volumes (0.5 mL) to avoid coughing.
- Hypertension can lead to bleeding and therefore needs to be treated aggressively.
- *Postoperative care:* Possible complications include:
  - Bleeding
  - Cerebrospinal fluid (CSF) leak
  - Infections.

Monitoring and Removal of Electrodes

Stereotactic electrodes are usually left in place for about two weeks for in-hospital monitoring and mapping of seizure activity. Removal of multiple electrodes is done in the operating room. It is ideally done with adequate sedation or a laryngeal mask airway (LMA).

MRI-GUIDED LASER INTERSTITIAL THERMAL THERAPY

The Technique of Laser Interstitial Thermal Therapy

The effects of regional hyperthermia on the brain and tumor tissue are as follows:
- Hyperthermia at 38–42°C improves blood flow.
- Hyperthermia at >42°C decreases the blood flow.
- Heat at 43°C can destroy brain/tumor tissue in 10 minutes.
- Heat at 60°C can destroy brain/tumor tissue in seconds.
- *Other effects:*
  - Hyperthermia opens the blood–brain barrier (BBB) and could improve drug delivery.
  - Hyperthermia enhances immunological response.
  - Hyperthermia enhances the cytotoxicity of chemotherapeutic drugs.

Laser interstitial thermal therapy: LTTT of epileptogenic neural tissue is usually done by placing a fiber optic probe in the target site to deliver the laser beam. MRI permits thermal tissue imaging, maps heat generated at the target site by the beam, and controls heat delivery. Regions of the brain close to CSF and blood vessels act as heat sinks to redistribute heat away from the nontarget site. Deep brain tissue that lacks these heat sinks can be damaged inadvertently during thermal ablation.

Indications of Laser Interstitial Thermal Therapy

- *Epilepsy:* Thermal ablation of the anterior temporal lobe or selective amygdalohippocampectomy prevents seizure in 75% of cases of drug-resistant epilepsy. However, the ablation of deep-seated epileptic foci can damage adjacent vital structures with increased morbidity.

- *Brain tumors—primary and metastatic:* Tumors that are deep-seated, spherical, and well-circumscribed respond better to LTTE, while diffused, large vascular tumors are challenging to treat and can lead to severe complications.
- *Radiation necrosis:* Ablation of damaged tissue after radiation treatment of brain cancers

Anesthetic Concerns for MRI Procedures

The physics underlying the MRI are as follows:
- Almost 60% of the human body is made of water.
- Hydrogen nuclei of water molecules spin to generate a small magnetic field. Due to the randomness of the spin, there is no net magnetic field.
- When subjected to an intense magnetic field, usually 1.5–3 Tesla, the hydrogen nuclei orient themselves along the magnetic field. Once aligned along the field, radio-frequency waves can perturb them. The resulting transverse magnetization can be quantified and used for imaging purposes.
- MRI imaging involves the measurement of subtle changes in the radiofrequency signals due to the differences in the orientation of the hydrogen nuclei while responding to the magnetic field changes.
- *MRI has three components:* (1) magnets, (2) a shield, and (3) a computer to process data. The magnets are the primary magnet and the gradient magnet while coils enhance the radiofrequency signals.
  - *The primary magnet is usually a helium-cooled superconducting magnet with a constant active magnetic field of 1.5–3 T in strength.* When the body is introduced into the MRI magnet, most hydrogen nuclei orient longitudinally (low-energy nuclei) with a small number oriented in the opposite direction (high-energy nuclei), generating a net longitudinal magnetic field. This longitudinal field cannot be quantified. If a radiofrequency wave of a specific frequency (Larmor frequency) and amplitude (power) is applied, then 50% hydrogen nuclei-orientations can be reversed and are in phase. This generates the maximum transverse magnetization field that can be quantified.
  - *The gradient magnets are sets of magnets placed within the giant magnets that* create two perpendicular magnetic fields. These magnets are responsible for the noise of the MRI scanner. By predictably altering the magnetic field, the gradient magnets permit spatial encoding of the MR images. They can generate slices of tissue images in longitudinal, coronal, and sagittal planes.
- *Radiofrequency coils* are small caging devices that improve signal transmission and signal-to-noise ratio.

MRI Suite Hazards

The hazards posed by the MRI are as follows:
- *Strong static magnetic field:*
  - The primary magnets of the MRIs are 50,000 to 100,000 times more powerful than the Earth's magnetic field of 30 microteslas. The primary magnet can lift a car and are potentially dangerous.
  - *Projectile injury:* Hazards of ferromagnetic equipment being pulled into the magnet with 30× force due to gravity.
  - *Device dislodgement:* Implanted devices may be dislodged and cause fatal injuries.
  - Damage or malfunction of devices, such as pacemakers, may be inactivated by the magnet.
- *Gradient magnetic field:* Gradient magnetic fields can generate sufficient electric current to stimulate nerves and muscles or cause ventricular fibrillation in extreme cases.
- *Noise:*
  - Gradient magnets emit noise during cycling
  - The sound is at or above the 85-dB threshold for acoustic injury and louder than that of a lawn mower
  - *It results in:*
    - Discomfort
    - Anxiety
    - Hearing loss
  - Hearing protection around the scanner is essential.
- *Other physiological effects:*
  - A strong magnetic field centered on a column of flowing blood, such as in the transverse aorta, can generate current. This current can mimic ST elevation seen with hyperkalemia.
  - Nausea
  - Vertigo
  - Scotomas
  - Claustrophobia
  - MRI is avoided in the first trimester of pregnancy due to the unknown effects of a strong magnetic field on fetal development and possible problems with noise, stress, and exposure to anesthetic drugs.
- *Radiofrequency-induced heating:*
  - Applying a powerful radiofrequency can lead to the transverse magnetization of the tissue of interest.
  - The power of the radiofrequency used is closely monitored.
  - When radiofrequency waves come in contact with a conductive object, such as a metallic EKG lead, they can generate heat to cause skin burns.

- *Helium release and hypoxia:*
  - Scanners have up to 1,000 L of liquid helium to cool the coils.
  - In the case of an accident or emergency shutdown of the magnet, helium evaporates and has to be vented. The process is called "quenching."
  - An emergency quench is needed to turn off the magnet to remove projectiles impacted by the magnet.
  - There is a dedicated vent to handle such release outside the building.
  - If the vent is blocked. If the vent is blocked, helium may back flow into the suite causing dangerous hypoxia.
  - Rapid evacuation is therefore needed.
  - MRI suites are equipped with oxygen sensors to alert for helium release and the resulting decrease in oxygen concentrations.

MRI-Compatible Devices

The MRI suite uses the same monitoring standards as in the operating room. The equipment certification is of two types: (i) *MR conditional* poses no risk to the patient or personnel, but functionality is not tested or guaranteed, and (ii) *MRI compatible*, which implies that the equipment is safe and functions adequately in the MR environment.

- *Anesthesia machines:*
  - MR-compatible anesthesia machines use aluminum instead of conventional ferromagnetic construction. All components of the anesthesia machine, ventilator, vaporizers, and gas cylinders must be non-ferromagnetic.
  - The MRI-compatible machine provides the same essential function as any conventional anesthesia machine.
  - In the absence of MRI-compatible machines, conventional machines have been used by locating them outside the suite with anesthesia delivered by long semi-open Mapleson systems. With such devices, scavenging waste gases, often used at high flows, is a concern.
- *Monitoring equipment:*
  - Monitoring equipment, including EKG lead and cables, poses the risk of burns and malfunction.
  - MRI-compatible monitoring devices use carbon fiber or fiber-optic cables.
  - The general principle of design is to use the shortest length and well-isolated braided wiring that does not come in contact with the patient.
  - The data from the sensors is wirelessly transmitted to the monitors outside the MRI suite.

- *Specific monitoring concerns:*
  - EKG trace using MRI-compatible leads may show changes suggestive of hyperkalemia.
  - Conventional oximeter probes can lead to skin burns; therefore, MRI-compatible ones should be used.
  - Capnography data may be delayed due to long sampling lines.
  - Noninvasive blood pressure monitoring is possible with nonferrous components.
- *External infusion pumps:* Drug infusions in MRI suites are carried out by pumps outside the suite using long lines.

Anesthesia for Laser Interstitial Thermal Therapy

The anesthesia for LITT can be considered in three stages: (1) Induction and implantation of the thermal ablation probe in the ORs, (2) transport to and thermal ablation in the MRI suite, and (3) removal of the probe and the extubation of the patients in the MRI suite:
- *Setup in OR:* The setup in the OR is for any general anesthesia. After induction, the patient requires the placement of a head frame and transport to the CT scanner for imaging. Thus, anesthesia equipment and drugs for transport should be prepared, a portable monitor should be at hand, and the infusion pump for propofol should be set up.
- *Induction of anesthesia:* Anesthesia is usually induced in a transport stretcher. It is optional to place an arterial line due to ease of monitoring during transport, although it may not be helpful in the MRI suite:
  - Induction of drugs includes midazolam, fentanyl, lidocaine, propofol, and muscle relaxants, usually rocuronium.
  - Endotracheal intubation and mechanical ventilation are instituted. The ETT has to be well-secured for transport and multiple changes in position during the procedure.
  - Hemodynamic parameters have to be closely monitored after induction during head elevation. The patient is put in a nearly sitting position for placing the stereotactic frame.
  - Once the frame is in place, the patient is transported to the CT scanner under propofol anesthesia.
- Stereotactic placement of the laser probe is done on return to the operating room.
- *Transport to MRI facility:*
  - On arrival, the patient is transferred to an MRI- compatible gurney.
  - MRI-compatible monitors are placed on the patient.
  - The patients and personnel are scanned for MRI-incompatible devices before entering the suite.
  - Mechanical ventilation is undertaken using the anesthesia machine.

- Propofol infusion is usually continued although sevoflurane might be used to supplement or replace propofol.
- The thermal ablation lasts about an hour. The neuromuscular block may be augmented at this stage due to the difficulty in monitoring within the magnet.
- Hemodynamics is monitored from the control room.
- Capnography trace is observed for any spontaneous respiratory effort and the need for additional sedation or muscle relaxants.
- *Removal of the probe:*
  - After ablation, the patient is transported back to the recovery room of the MRI facility.
  - Conventional monitors are placed
  - The fiber optic probe is removed at the end of surgery.
  - Antiemetics are administered.
  - Muscle paralysis is reversed with Sugammadex in preference to neostigmine/glycopyrrolate to minimize hemodynamic side effects.
  - The patient is extubated on meeting the usual criteria.
- The patient is transported to the neuro-ICU for 24-hour observation.

Complications of Laser Ablation

- *Technical:* Catheter displacement
- Intracranial hemorrhage
- Refractory brain edema as early as an hour after treatment
- Thermal injury to adjacent vital structures
- *Neurological deficits:*
  - *Visual field defects:*
    - Homonymous hemianopsia
    - Quadrantanopia
  - Cranial nerve III and IV palsy.

CASE REPORTS FOR FURTHER DISCUSSION

Case 1: An 18-year-old male was diagnosed with periventricular heterotopia with intractable epilepsy. He underwent an uneventful LITT procedure. He had no neurological complaints on emergence from anesthesia. He was discharged the next day. Nine days later, he developed a headache with hemiparesis. CT angiography revealed a pseudoaneurysm close to bleeding. The patient's neurological condition worsened, and he was due for a craniotomy to remove the hematoma. *What factors contribute to bleeding after LITT?*

Case 2: A 62-year-old male patient presented with new-onset acute aphasia. MRI revealed a left temporal mass with a maximum enhancing diameter of 2.1 cm. The biopsy revealed glioblastoma multiforme (GBM).

He underwent an uneventful LITT ablation. He was discharged the next day. Neurological examination was no different than at baseline pretreatment. Over the next two weeks, despite corticosteroid treatment, the patient developed persistent headaches and additional difficulty performing calculations. MRI revealed hemorrhage, necrosis, and edema at the site of LITT treatment. *What are the immediate complications of LITT treatment? Would you expect steroids to be effective after such treatment? How would you treat brain edema after LITT?*

Case 3: A 55-year-old male was due for an MRI examination. He was accompanied by his son, a highly placed security officer. Both persons were instructed to remove any ferromagnetic item on them. They complied with the request. As they approached the scanner, the son felt that the jacket was being pulled into the scanner. He took off the garment. It flew into the magnet with a loaded firearm. *What are the additional hazards posed by a loaded handgun lodged into the magnet? How are such ferromagnetic objects that have been lodged in the magnet, removed?*

Case 4: A 68-year-old man had a cochlear implant and needed an MRI to follow up on a schwannoma on the contralateral side. A year before, he had undergone an uneventful MRI in a 1.5 T MRI. This time a higher resolution scan was requested in a 3 T magnet. *Will you be concerned with a repeat MRI in a more powerful magnet? What implants will you be concerned with during an MRI procedure? Will you be worried about a hip or a knee prosthesis?*

Case 5: A 40-year-old woman with suspected fibromyalgia was due for an MRI examination. Before entering the MRI suite, she was questioned about any ferromagnetic objects she might have on a person. A wand scan also cleared her. No ferromagnetic object could be detected. During the scan, artifacts were observed outside her thighs bilaterally, yet, the scan was completed. After the scan, linear redness and swelling were observed on the thigh. She was treated for second-degree burns. The burn lines corresponded to the lines on her jogging pants. Scanning and high-resolution digital imaging initially revealed no metal fibers. However, customer service noted that thin metal fibers were used in the dress. *Copper fibers are included in many exercise dresses. Would they pose a similar problem? What is the reliability of the hand wand in preventing accidents in MRI?*

CASE REPORT REFERENCES

Case 1: Barber SM et al. Delayed intraparenchymal and intraventricular hemorrhage requiring surgical evacuation after MRI-guided laser interstitial thermal therapy for lesional epilepsy. Stereotact Funct Neurosurg. 2017;95:73-8.

Case 2: Elder JB et al. Histologic findings associated with laser interstitial thermotherapy for glioblastoma multiforme. Diagn Pathol. 2019;14:19.

Case 3: Mufti S et al. A "near-miss lethal accident case" in MR suit of a tertiary care hospital. Case Rep Radiol. 2011;793570.

Case 4: Bawazeer N et al. Magnetic resonance imaging after cochlear implants. J Otol. 2019;14:22-5.

Case 5: Tokue H et al. Unexpected magnetic resonance imaging burn injuries from jogging pants. Radiol Case Rep. 2019;14 (11):1348-51.

FURTHER READING

1. Boop S et al. Robot-assisted stereoelectroencephalography in young children: technical challenges and considerations. Childs Nerv Syst. 2022;38(2):263-7.
2. Casali C et al. Robot-assisted laser-interstitial thermal therapy with iSYS1 and Visualase: how I do it. Acta Neurochir (Wien). 2021;163(12):3465-71.
3. Pan J et al. Thermal safety of endoscopic usage in robot-assisted middle ear surgery: an experimental study. Front Surg. 2021;8:659688.
4. Pangal DJ et al. Robotic and robot-assisted skull base neurosurgery: a systematic review of current applications and future directions. Neurosurg Focus. 2022;52(1): E15.
5. Troccaz J et al. Frontiers of medical robotics: from concept to systems to clinical translation. Annu Rev Biomed Eng. 2019;21:193-218.

Vignette: The Challenges of Robotic Neurosurgery

Robotic surgery has made significant advances across many other surgical specialties. In most instances, the operating paths are sufficiently wide for robotic arms to operate safely. Furthermore, the paths permit adequate imaging to monitor and guide the arm and image the target site. However, in neurosurgery, such access is minimal. In addition to the narrowness of the paths, the consequences of deviating from them can be severe. Relative to the other surgical fields, the advances in robotic neurosurgery have been relatively slow. Robotic surgery's major application has been placing EEG leads during epilepsy. The robots can reliably map the safe path for placing multiple leads while avoiding critical structures. Robotic-guided endoscopic surgery is another area of possible robot application. During endoscopy, the path for the robotic advance is fairly direct, and it is wide enough to image the ablative process. Compared to brain surgery, the situation with spine surgery is very different. During spine surgery, X-ray imaging is routinely done. Robots can therefore map out and follow trajectories for the placement of screws while being guided by intraoperative imaging. Overall, the development of robotic intracranial neurosurgery still requires better robotic tools. Tools can maneuver in smaller spaces; arms capable of sensing changes in tissue characteristics, the force of contact with tissues, and their precise orientation; and tiny cameras that can help visualize structures at short focal distances. Robots will have to be significantly more sophisticated if they want to invade the brain.

Chapter 59: Patient with Ventricular Assist Device

INTRODUCTION

About 600,000 patients are diagnosed with heart failure in the US annually, with a total of about 6 million cases. An estimated 30,000 patients await heart transplants, yet only a tenth of them undergo surgery in a year. The FDA first approved mechanical devices to assist with heart failure in 1994. Since then, left ventricular assist devices (LVAD) have provided a "bridge to transplant" or even as "destination treatment." Due to the inherent risk of thromboembolism and hemorrhage, LVAD patients often present for stroke treatment. However, these patients also present for tumor and spine surgeries. Due to the improvements and increased use, LVAD cases are likely to be an essential part of the future neuroanesthetic practice.

NEUROANESTHETIC CONCERNS

- Nature of neurosurgical interventions
- Preoperative review will reveal a complex medical history.
- Indications of LVAD
- Types of devices
- LVAD hemodynamics
- *Anesthesia:*
  - Options
  - Monitoring
  - Drug selection
- LVAD complications

NATURE OF NEUROSURGICAL INTERVENTIONS

- Thromboembolic and hemorrhagic neurological complications affect 10-30% of the patients.
- LVAD devices are improving the outcome of severe heart failure.
- They will play an increasing role in the management of heart failure.
- As survival improves, more LVAD patients may present with the following:
  - Embolic stroke
  - Intracranial hemorrhage

- Placement of VP shunts
- Brain tumors

PREOPERATIVE ASSESSMENT

- *Preoperative assessment usually provides a complex medical history:*
  - Indication of LVAD
  - Functional status of the patient
  - *Left ventricular functions are assessed by:*
    - LV functions on ECHO
    - Increased LVAD flow pulsatility
  - *Right Ventricular functions are assessed by:*
    - RV functions on ECHO
    - Central venous pressure
    - Functional status
  - Cardiac rhythm
  - *Hemodynamic status:*
    - *Target pressure:* MAP of 70–90 mm Hg
    - *Current status:*
      - Hypertension
      - Hypotension
      - Fluid overload
  - Anticoagulation: Target, drugs, and doses
  - The extent of end-organ dysfunction:
    - Neurological, Liver, Kidneys

INDICATION FOR LVAD

- *Bridge to recovery:* Acute heart failure
  - Myocardial infarction
  - Viral myocarditis
  - Postcardiotomy
- *Bridge to transplant:* Chronic heart failure: Awaiting transplant
  - Ischemic cardiomyopathy
  - Idiopathic cardiomyopathy
  - Other cardiomyopathies
  - Drug cardiotoxicity
- Destination therapy

TYPES OF DEVICES

- Biventricular vs. LV support devices
- *LVAD:*
  - *Earlier pumps* were externally located. They had a diaphragm generated pulsatile flow and are no longer used.

CHAPTER 59 Patient with Ventricular Assist Device

- *Axial flow device:* HeartMate 2:
  - Intrathoracic
  - Uses a turbine screw to push blood forwards.
  - Mechanical bearing cause friction.
  - Higher RPMs
  - Has a higher incidence of stroke.
- *Centrifugal pumps:* HeartMate 3:
  - Intrathoracic with the external drive line
  - Impeller uses magnetic levitation to minimize friction.
  - It has wide gaps to reduce flow resistance.
  - Can change flows momentarily to generate a pulse flow profile every 2 seconds.
  - Rapidly connects with battery and control units.

LVAD HEMODYNAMICS

- LVAD devices:
  - Bypass the left ventricular outflow.
  - Blood from the left ventricle is infused into the aorta downstream of the coronary artery ostia.
  - The device will not function if the aortic valve is incompetent. Placement of LVAD causes aortic incompetence in 10–30% of the patients over time.
  - There should be adequate blood flow into the left ventricles; otherwise, the negative pressure generated by LVAD can suck in the walls of the left ventricles. Increasing RPMs will further increase the ventricular collapse, dramatically decreasing Pulsatility Index and decreasing device output.
  - The aortic valve is sometimes closed to eliminate aortic incompetence and to enable the device to function.
  - Improvement in left ventricular outflow can increase the right ventricular load, increase right ventricular volume, shift in the ventricular septum, change in septal geometry, and lead to right heart ischemia and failure.
  - LVAD does not support RV functions. Measures to ensure adequate RV preload, decrease RV afterload and support RV function may be essential. In the extremes, a right ventricular assist device might be needed.
- *Pump controls:* Important to see trends rather than absolute values.
  - *Pump flow:*
    - Calculated from pump speed and in some devices corrects for hematocrit.
    - Pump outflow at a given speed depends on the following:
      - Pressure gradient between inflow and outflow
      - Left ventricular preload

- Residual cardiac function
  - *After load:* Hypertension/thrombus/Aortic incompetence
- Typically, 4–5 l/min (range 3–10 l/min)
- Flows <2.5 l/min require urgent attention and may trigger the alarm in some devices.
- *Pump speed:*
  - Revolutions per minute and hematocrit determine pump output.
  - With continuous flow devices, e.g., HeartMate 3 is set at 4000 RPM (range 3–9,000 RPM)
- *Pump power:*
  - Power required to maintain a given RPM.
  - *Typical power:* 4–9 Watts (range 0–25 W)
  - Indicates work done to maintain pump flow.
  - A linear relationship between pump speed and pump power.
  - Power consumption more significant than 10–12 W is a concern.
  - An increase in power implies an increase in afterload, usually due to hypertension. In patients with recently implanted LVAD, it can be due to mechanical flow obstruction.
  - Gradual increase in power over hours or days can be due to a thrombus, which requires investigation.
- *Pulsatility Index:*
  - Provides a measure of LV function.

$$\text{Pulsatility Index} = \frac{\text{Flow (max)} - \text{Flow (min)}}{\text{Flow (Average)}} \times 10$$

  - Systolic contraction generates a flow pulse.
  - Flow pulses are averaged over time, i.e., every 15 s.

- *PI values:*
  - PI typical values are between 3–6 but range from 1–10.
  - Unexplained PI <3 is significant **(Table 1)**
  - Patients with RVF may have stable low PI values.
  - RV failure diagnosed by low PI
  - Reduction in values suggests hypovolemia.
  - High values suggest a better LV function.
  - *PI events:*
    - Is a sudden change of PI by 50% of the baseline value.
    - Suggestive of left ventricular collapse
    - Require reduction of pump speed

- *Anesthesia concerns with LVAD patients:*
  - Overview of anesthesia techniques:
    - LVAD patients undergo a variety of procedures, sometimes in peripheral locations.

- MAC sedation is usually safe for stable patients with no recent change in their functional status.
- General anesthesia is required for patients with right ventricular failure and poor Pulsatility Index. Anesthesia is best provided in facilities where TEE is readily available and aggressive right heart support can be provided.
- The benefits for MAC vs. GA are listed in **Table 2**.
- Regional Anesthesia with ultrasonic guidance can be used when possible.
- Neuraxial anesthesia is best avoided but can be done with scrupulous attention to anticoagulation.

Table 1: Flow and pulsatility index changes with LVAD.

Decreased flow	Increased flow

• Low PI:
  – Hypovolemia:
    - Under resuscitation
    - Hemorrhage
    - Positioning
  – Right ventricular failure:
    - Decreased contractility
    - Arrhythmias
  – Increased pulmonary vascular resistance
  – Tension pneumothorax
  – Tamponade
	• Low PI:
	  – Decreased SVR:
	    - Sepsis
	    - Vasodilation: drugs
	    - Liver failure
	    - Anaphylaxis
	  – Aortic insufficiency

• High PI:
  – Hypertension
  – Partial outflow obstruction
	• High PI:
	  – Improved myocardial contractility
	  – Hypervolemia

Table 2: General vs. MAC for thromboembolectomy in LVAD patients.

Feature	General anesthesia	MAC/CS
Patient cooperation	Not needed	Essential
Procedure duration	Any duration	Only for a brief duration
Hemodynamic status	Management better	Only for stable patients
Quality of images	Better: Minimal movement	Impaired due to movements
Speed of intervention	Needs time to organize	More rapid
Hemodynamic changes	Can be significant	Generally minimal
Monitoring	IABP essential	IABP can be monitored from the femoral line
TEE	Possible	Difficult/not possible

(MAC: monitored anesthesia care; CS: conscious sedation; IABP: intraarterial blood pressure; TEE: transesophageal echocardiography)

- *Monitoring:*
  - *EKG:* Arrhythmias can affect right ventricular functions.
  - *Temp:* Hypothermia increases SVR and afterload
  - *EtCO$_2$:* Hypercarbia can increase pulmonary vascular resistance.
  - *SaO$_2$:* Hypoxia can increase pulmonary vascular resistance.
  - NIBP is challenging to assess and requires more sensitive ultrasonic sensors for pulse detection.
  - *Invasive arterial blood pressure:* Ultrasound may show the anatomical location of the artery, but due to lack of pulsations, diameter changes are minimal.
  - CVP helps to monitor right ventricular preload and assess right ventricular contractility.
  - *PAC:* Useful in monitoring Right heart functions
  - *TEE:* Essential in managing critically ill patients, can assess device malfunction, thrombi, left and right heart preload, and contractility.
- *Anesthesia:*
  - *MAC sedation*
  - Minimally disturbs hemodynamics, might be possible for specific neurosurgical procedures:
    - Burr hole for subdural bleed
    - Angiography for suspected stroke
    - Mechanical thrombectomy
    - Ventricular drain placement
  - *General anesthesia:*
    - Major intracranial surgery
    - VP/VA shunt that requires tunneling
  - *Set up:* for significant surgery
    - Arterial line necessary, CVP or PAC in patients with RVF
    - *For major surgery:* TEE should be available
    - Defibrillator pads should be placed to correct arrhythmias
    - Technical support should be available
    - CT team should be available or on standby
  - *Drug selection:*
    - The induction agent should not affect left and right ventricular preload and right ventricular contractility.
    - Etomidate/narcotic combinations suitable for induction
    - Ketamine and benzodiazepines in judicious doses can also maintain hemodynamic stability during induction.
    - Volatile agents such as isoflurane can decrease systemic vascular resistance and augment pump flow. However, they can impair myocardial contractility.
    - Adequate muscle relaxation to decrease mean airway pressure.
    - Avoid hypercarbia, hypoxia, and acidosis that can increase pulmonary vascular resistance.

- *LVAD complications:*
  - *LVAD specific:*
    - Device malfunction
    - Thrombosis
    - *Suction event:* Excessive RMPs relative to Left ventricular inflow leads to suctioning of the wall of the left ventricle.
  - *LVAD associated:*
    - *Right ventricular failure:*
      - Optimize preload guided by:
        - TEE
        - CVP
        - Fluid challenge
      - Avoid:
        - Hypovolemia
        - Hypoxia
        - Hypocarbia
        - Acidosis
      - Low-pressure ventilation
      - Treatment of arrhythmias
      - Treatment of pulmonary hypertension
        - Inhaled Nitric oxide
        - Prostacyclin
        - Inhaled milrinone
        - *Pressors:* Dobutamine, epinephrine, milrinone
    - Arrhythmias
    - Aortic incompetence

Bleeding

- *Three confronting aims for anticoagulation:*
  - Maintain proper functioning of LVAD to decrease the risk of thrombus malfunction and embolic events.
  - Decrease risk of embolic stroke and intracranial hemorrhage
  - Decrease risk of GI bleeding
- *Causes of bleeding:*
  - Surgical causes in the first two weeks
  - Development of mucosal arteriovenous malformations: GI hemorrhage common
  - Hepatic insufficiency
  - Acquired von Willebrand's disease.
- *Management of anticoagulation:*
  - The manufacturer specifies the usual anticoagulation protocol

- *In the absence of bleeding, anticoagulation consists of the following:*
  - Aspirin 81 mg PO daily
  - Oral anticoagulants (warfarin) to keep an INR of 2-3.
- In the setting of imminent surgery, these drugs are withdrawn appropriately, heparin therapy is instituted, fresh frozen plasma is used and if time permits Vitamin K is given to reverse the effects of warfarin.

Hypotension

- Noninvasive blood pressure monitoring may require sensitive instruments.
- Ephedrine, a non-specific indirect sympathomimetic, might help support the right heart while increasing blood pressure.
- Hypotension can usually be treated with phenylephrine, although an excessive increase in afterload impairs LVAD function.
- Requires judicious fluid therapy.
- It may require an increase in pump flow.
- Invasive monitoring (A-line/CVP) is desirable in patients with RV failure and for any major surgery.
- TEE should be available to assess LV, RV, and LVAD functions.

Thromboembolic Complications

- *Present with:*
  - Strokes
  - TIAs
  - Systemic emboli
  - Pump thrombosis
- Strokes and intracranial hemorrhages are the leading cause of death.
- *Risk factors:*
  - *Patient factors:* Atrial fibrillation, smoking, treatment compliance
  - Type of LVAD
  - An INR of 2.6 is suitable for minimizing bleeding and thrombotic complications.

Infections

- The second leading cause of death.
- Usually due to skin pathogens such as "Staphylococci" and fungi.
- Overall, infections occur in 30–50% of patients.
- Pneumonia 25%
- *Sepsis:* 20%
- *Driveline infections:* 20%

Liver Dysfunction
- Frequently seen early and late with LVAD placement
- Increases infection risk
- Predicts poor survival

Renal Dysfunction
- ERDS generally excludes LVAD placement
- Indicates poor short term and long term survival after LVAD placement.

LVAD Emergencies
- Device loss
  - Surgical failure
    - Dislocation
    - Vascular occlusion
  - Mechanical failure
  - *Electrical failure:* Loss of hum
- *Cardiac arrest:*
  - Prompt detection and treatment of arrhythmias
  - Vigilance is needed to avoid precipitating causes.
  - Early cardioversion
  - Cardiac compression is best avoided to decrease the likelihood of disruption of tissue device connections.
  - Resuscitation using ECMO may have to be on standby in high-risk cases.

CASE REPORTS FOR FURTHER DISCUSSION

Case 1: A 63-year-old man with ischemic cardiomyopathy who underwent LVAD placement three years previously sustained a head injury. CT scan revealed a subdural hematoma with midline shift. He was anticoagulated with warfarin. He had chronic kidney disease and an implanted defibrillator. Echocardiography revealed an ejection fraction of 20% and reduced right ventricular functions. INR was reported to be 3.4. He was scheduled for an urgent craniotomy for evacuation of the hematoma. *How will you correct coagulation for surgery? What target blood pressure will you aim for in such a case? Why is ephedrine useful in treating hypotension? If the patient proves resistant to phenylephrine, how will you treat hypotension?*

Case 2: A 62-year-old 82 kg 155 cm female present with a three-week history of headache, nausea, dizziness, and gaze disturbances. CT imaging revealed a cerebellar tumor with compression of the fourth ventricle and hydrocephalus. Her history was significant with breast cancer treatment with daunorubicin resulting in cardiomyopathy that required a HeartMate

3 placement some three years ago. She had been stable ever since. Her medications included aspirin, warfarin, losartan, and furosemide. Her pump parameters were a flow of 3.5 lpm; a speed of 5250 RPMs; a power of 3.5 watts, and a PI of 8. Her INR was 2.8. She is due to posterior fossa craniotomy in the prone position. *What monitoring will you do in this case? Where would you place the central line if you discovered her right jugular vein was thrombosed? Given that this is a planned procedure, how will you manage her anticoagulation? What is the target INR? When will you restart her anticoagulation treatment?*

Case 3: A 35-year-old male with a history of non-ischemic cardiomyopathy required a HeartMate 2 device placement. He presented to the emergency room with anorexia, abdominal pain, and bloody stool. His INR was 9.2. He was admitted to the CT ICU. The following morning, he was found to have left facial paralysis. A CT angiogram revealed distal occlusion of the middle cerebral artery. His LVAD parameters were the flow of 4.6 lpm, speed of 9200 rpm, PI of 5.4, and power of 5.7 watts. His noninvasive blood pressure was 110/72 with a mean of 90 mm Hg. Surgeons requested general anesthesia and that the blood pressure should not decrease below a mean of 80 mm Hg. *Given the urgency of the intervention, would you insist on an arterial line? What are the pros and cons of general anesthesia vs. monitored anesthesia care/conscious sedation for thromboembolectomy in LVAD patients?*

Case 4: A 14-year-old boy with dilated cardiomyopathy due for a heart transplant was implanted with an external pediatric LVAD. Despite recommended anticoagulation, three days after implantation, the child developed sudden speech disturbances; within the next four hours, he progressed to aphasia and right hemiparesis. CT scan and angiography revealed proximal occlusion of the left middle cerebral artery. CT angiography also revealed good collateral blood flow that was still perfusing 50% of the MCA distribution. The LVAD was suspected to be the source of the emboli. Before the child was transferred to the interventional radiology suite, the LVAD was replaced. Mechanical thrombectomy was undertaken under general anesthesia approximately 8.5 hours after the onset of symptoms. *What is the optimum therapeutic window for clot extraction after an embolic stroke? Does the anticoagulation required for LVAD affect the intervention time? What is hemorrhagic transformation?*

CASE REPORT REFERENCES

Case 1: Mohajerani A et al. Challenging case: Management of intracranial hemorrhage in a patient with a left ventricle assist device (LVAD): SNACC newsletter – Spring 2021.

Case 2: Patel N et al. A complicated course of brain tumor resection in a patient with left ventricular assist device. J Neuroanesthesiol Crit Care. 2021;0:1-4.

Case 3: From RP et al. Stroke and left ventricular assist device (LVAD). Open J Anesthesiol. 2013;3:51-6.

Case 4: Hak JF et al. Late pediatric thrombectomy for embolic stroke as bridge reinforcement from LVAD to heart transplantation. JACC Case Report. 2021;(4):686-9.

FURTHER READING

1. Carroll AH et al. Diagnostic evaluation and cervical spine surgery in the setting of a cardiac left ventricular assist device: challenges and a case illustration. Cureus. 2021;13(11):e19571.
2. Carroll AH et al. Management of intracranial hemorrhage in patients with a left ventricular assist device: a systematic review and meta-analysis. J Stroke Cerebrovasc Dis. 2021;30(2):105501.
3. Chen BJ et al. Bleeding risk in patients with cardiac disease from ischaemic stroke reperfusion therapy: an update. BMJ Neurol Open. 2021;3(2): e000156.
4. Ibeh C et al. Medical and surgical management of left ventricular assist device-associated intracranial hemorrhage. J Stroke Cerebrovasc Dis. 2021;30(10):106053.
5. Lai GY et al. Management and outcome of intracranial hemorrhage in patients with left ventricular assist devices. J Neurosurg. 2019;132(4):1133-39.

Vignette: The First Porcine Xeno-Heart Transplant

Only one-tenth of the patients who need heart transplants undergo surgery. Although mechanical devices have greatly improved, the lure of a biological heart remains appealing. The first xeno-heart transplant was undertaken by James Hardy in Jackson, Mississippi. On January 24, 1964, a chimpanzee's heart was transplanted into a human. It was not a great success; the recipient survived only a few hours. In 1977 Christian Bernard, the pioneering heart surgeon also experimented with a baboon-to-human heart transplant. However, despite the close primate connections, neither the chimpanzees nor the baboons are a suitable source for xeno-hearts. The pigs, on the other hand, are far more ideal than primates. They breed and grow fast, are easy to raise, can be genetically engineered, and are suitably distant from humans so as not to transfer diseases. In early 2022 the first genetically engineered porcine heart was transplanted into a human. The donor's heart lacked three immunoreactive surface antigens. The patient survived for two months. Several other genetically engineered pigs are likely to be more suitable for xenotransplantation.

Chapter 60

Post-craniotomy Pain Management

INTRODUCTION

Headache after craniotomy occurs in about two-thirds of the patients. Due to the potential respiratory depression with narcotics, it is usually inadequately treated. However, as with any other pain syndrome, such pain can be due to several factors. It is essential to evaluate, identify and treat the underlying etiology. Individual multimodality pain treatment plan is needed for optimum care instead of inflexible and inadequate conventional treatments.

NEUROANESTHETIC CONCERNS

- Incidence of pain after craniotomy
- Impact of inadequate pain management
- Pain mechanisms
- Pretreatment/preemptive analgesia
- Analgesic drugs
- Multimodality pain management.

INCIDENCE

- Clinical features of headaches with intracranial pathologies:
  - *Tumor:* Early morning headache and vomiting, worst with straining, and refractory to treatment
  - *Aneurysm rupture:* Severe acute headache described as "the worst pain ever".
  - A history of headaches such as days or weeks previously with sentinel bleeds
  - *Hypertensive bleed:* Throbbing headache
  - *Arteriovenous malformations (AVMs):* Chronic headaches may be confused with atypical migraine.
  - *Meningitis:* Headache with pain with neck flexion/movements
  - *Cerebrospinal fluid (CSF) leak:* Postural-occipital-frontal headache worse in sitting and relieved in a supine position.
  - *Frequent nonsurgical causes:*
    - Tension headaches
    - Migraine

CHAPTER 60 Post-craniotomy Pain Management

- 50% of patients with postoperative headaches have no history of pain.
- *Onset and duration of postoperative headaches:*
  - 55% of patients have moderate-to-severe pain on the first day.
  - 32% of patients have persistent pain after 48 hours.
  - Pain might persist for weeks after craniotomy.
- Pain scale for adults **(Table 1)**.
- Post-craniotomy pain management is often overlooked.
- Harner scale for assessment of chronic headaches (of 3-month duration):
  - *Grade 1:* Mild annoyance
  - *Grade 2:* Pain persists daily
  - *Grade 3:* Pain treated daily
  - *Grade 4:* Incapacitating pain.
- *Risk factors for postoperative pain include:*
  - Sub-temporal surgical approach
  - Suboccipital surgical approach
  - Infratentorial > supratentorial operations
  - Younger patients
  - Females.
- *Mechanisms of craniotomy pain:* Mostly somatic from peri-cranial tissues. Due to:
  - Tissue trauma
  - Inflammatory mediator release
  - Sensitization of pain receptors
  - Increased Aδ fiber sensitivity
  - Peri-cranial muscle spasm

Table 1: Pain scores, examples, and clinical impact.

Score	Descriptor	Example	Impact of pain
0	No pain	No pain	None
1	Minimal	Mosquito bite	Hardly noticeable
2	Mild	Skin pinch	Aware of pain when asked for
3	Uncomfortable	IM injection	Pain can be ignored most of the time
4	Moderate	Bee sting	Can function despite pain
5	Distracting	Sprained ankle	Pain excludes some activities
6	Distressing	Headache	Pain excludes many activities
7	Unmanageable	Migraine headache	Pain excludes most activities
8	Intense	Labor pain	Hard to concentrate, listen, or talk
9	Severe	Cancer pain	Cannot function and considered suicide
10	Unable to move	Crush injuries	Pain needs immediate attention

(IM: intramuscular)

- Postoperative pain is a combination of injury site pain and tension headache.
- *Pain pathways:*
  - *Trigeminal (CN-V):* Innervates the face and the dura matter:
    - *Main divisions:* ophthalmic, maxillary, and mandibular
    - Pterional craniotomy can damage the temporalis muscle and affect all three CN-V divisions. It can cause headaches with masticatory pains and orofacial dysfunction.
  - *Cervical nerves C-1 to C-3:*
    - The posterior division supplies the occipital regions.
    - Superficial divisions supply the ear and the side of the face.
  - *Cervical sympathetic nerves:* Innervation of the blood vessel can lead to vascular headaches and spasm.
  - *Other cranial nerves (minor contributions):* VII, IX, X, and XI.
- *Consequences of inadequate treatment of post-craniotomy pain:*
  - Discomfort
  - Agitation
  - Increased stress response
  - Hypertension
  - Increased intracranial pressure (ICP)
  - Increased BBB permeability
  - Increased risk of postoperative bleeding
- *Concerns with narcotic use:*
  - Narcotic receptors and their effects are listed in **Table 2**.
- *Sedation:* Interferes with:
  - *Pupillary size assessment:*
    - Normal 2–4 mm in the light
    - Normal 4–8 mm in the dark

Table 2: Narcotic receptors.

Receptor	Location	Physiological effects
μ1 (morphine)	Cortex: Lamina III and IV, thalamus, periaqueductal gray, substantia gelatinosa of the spinal cord	Supraspinal analgesia and physical dependence
μ2	Cortex: Lamina III and IV, thalamus, periaqueductal gray, substantia gelatinosa of the spinal cord	Respiratory depression, meiosis, euphoria, reduced gastrointestinal motility, and physical dependence
Δ	Brain: Pontine nucleus, amygdala, and olfactory nucleus	Analgesia
K	Brain: Hypothalamus, periaqueductal gray, and substantia gelatinosa of the spinal cord	Spinal analgesia, sedation, diuresis, dysphoria, and miosis

CHAPTER 60 Post-craniotomy Pain Management

- Miosis <2 mm
- Mydriasis >7 mm
- *Neurological exam:* Cognitive testing
  - *Respiratory depression:*
    - Increased $PaCO_2$
    - Increased cerebral blood flow (CBF) and ICP
- *Hypoxemia:* Increased brain edema.

PLAN FOR CRANIOTOMY PAIN RELIEF

- *Preempt analgesia:*
  - Acetaminophen
  - Local anesthetic infiltration—bupivacaine with epinephrine
  - Dexamethasone
  - Gabapentin.
- *Intraoperative management:*
  - Narcotics
  - Infusion of lidocaine
  - Infusion of magnesium
  - IV acetaminophen
- *Post-surgery management (Table 3):*
  - *Codeine:*
    - Pro-drug converted to morphine
    - Genetic variability in acetylation rates may affect the therapeutic response.
    - Avoided in pediatric patients
  - *Other narcotics:* Hydromorphone, morphine, pethidine, methadone
  - Acetaminophen oral/intravenous
  - Patient-controlled analgesia (PCA) with fentanyl/morphine
    - Narcotic PCA better than PRN doses
  - Dexamethasone
  - Ketamine
  - Regional: Scalp block
  - *Adjuvants:*
    - Gabapentin
    - Antiemetics
    - COX-2 selective inhibitors: e.g., Parecoxib, Celebrex, and Vioxx

CASE REPORTS FOR FURTHER DISCUSSION

Case 1: A 36-year-old female underwent an uneventful left frontal craniotomy for a metastatic brain tumor. She was interviewed for pain assessment as a part of an ongoing research project on the fifth postoperative day. She has had several past surgeries, but she considered this to be the

Table 3: Pharmacological interventions for craniotomy.

Class type: Example	Mechanism of action	Side effects	Effectiveness as analgesic
Anticonvulsants: Gabapentin	Block voltage-gated Ca^{++} channels, Na^+ channels, NMDA receptors, and via the opioid pathway	Peripheral edema, dizziness, fatigue, and ataxia	Minimal benefit
Steroids: Dexamethasone	Anti-inflammatory decreases vasogenic edema, antiemetic and euphoric effects	Impaired glucose homeostasis and hyperglycemia	Decreases narcotic side effects
Narcotics: Codeine, fentanyl, morphine, hydromorphone	μ receptor-mediated analgesia, euphoria, and sedation	Sedation, respiratory depression with hypoxia and hypercapnia, and miosis	Excellent in appropriate doses
COX-2 selective inhibitors: Parecoxib	NSAIDs without platelet function inhibition	Potential thrombotic complications, limited use	Mild benefit
NSAIDs: Acetaminophen	Inhibits central COX-3, activates serotonergic pathway, substance P, and NMDA antagonism	Well-tolerated, no platelet inhibition	Routinely used with narcotics
NMDA antagonists: Ketamine	Decreases opioid tolerance and central hypersensitivity to pain	Low-dose ketamine may have psychogenic side effects	CNS side effects and limited use
Methadone	Narcotic μ receptor agonist, σ and K antagonist; NMDA antagonist	Dependence possible; prolongation of QTc; torsades de pointes	For multi-modality and chronic pain management
Tramadol	Mild μ agonist, serotonergic effects and inhibits norepinephrine uptake	More effective with narcotics but increases the risk of vomiting	Benefits vary across studies
Dexmedetomidine	α-2 agonist	Sedation	Can decrease opioid requirements
Preoperative regional scalp block	Decreases post-trauma pain sensitization	Limited by the duration of action of the local anesthetic drug	Decreases postoperative narcotic requirements
Post-surgery regional block	Block pain transmission	Low bupivacaine concentrations of 0.25% and less effective than 0.5%	Decreases pain and narcotic requirements

(CNS: central nervous system; COX: cyclooxygenase; MOA: mechanism of action; NMDA: N-methyl-D-aspartate; NSAIDs: nonsteroidal anti-inflammatory drugs)

CHAPTER 60 Post-craniotomy Pain Management

worst pain. She described several types of pain: (1) Pain related to arm or leg movements, sitting up, and coughing. It had very severe intensity; (2) Throbbing pain with each heartbeat; (3) Vibrating pain that went up the spine as she walked. She was prescribed: Hydromorphone, oxycodone, morphine, fentanyl, and oxycodone/acetaminophen. Records revealed that she was taking pain medications every 2 hours. The researcher described the pain trajectory as declining over time, with the greatest severity on the day of surgery. *Based on the description, what are the most likely causes of pain in this case? Are you satisfied with the selection of treatment drugs? What else could have been used to treat this pain?*

Case 2: A 62-year-old woman presented with a history of adenocarcinoma of the lungs. She underwent resection of occipital metastases around seven years earlier. Subsequently, she presented with a new-onset headache and gait disturbances. MRI revealed tumor recurrence in the right occipital lobe. An uneventful craniotomy was undertaken in the prone position. The patient recovered uneventfully from anesthesia. Three hours after surgery, the patient developed a severe headache. Her consciousness rapidly deteriorated. A repeat CT scan revealed a large contralateral frontal hematoma. Immediate decompressive surgery was done. A case review revealed no contributing hemodynamic, coagulation issue, or evidence of venous obstruction. *What is the etiology of postoperative hemorrhage after a craniotomy? Are there known risk factors that could be influenced by anesthesia? Is headache a reliable presentation of such bleeding?*

Case 3: A 52-year-old woman underwent craniotomy for a right frontal meningioma. The patient recovered from surgery but complained of right supraorbital pain extending into the forehead on the third postoperative day. On examination, there was tenderness in the supraorbital notch. The patient was treated with ibuprofen, oxycodone, and carbamazepine. Despite the treatment, the pain progressively worsened and was rated 9/10 on the visual analog scale (VAS). On the 12th postoperative day, a supraorbital nerve block with local anesthetic completely resolved the pain (0/10 VAS). The benefit lasted over two days when the pain score was 6/10 on the VAS. Based on the positive results of the regional block, radiofrequency ablation of the supraorbital nerve was undertaken. Post-treatment, VAS was 3/10, which decreased to 0/10 on day 3. There was no loss of sensation in the nerve distribution. *What are the other causes of chronic headaches after a craniotomy?*

Case 4: A 40-year-old woman was diagnosed with Arnold–Chiari malformation. MR imaging revealed inferiorly displaced optic chiasma, flattening of the pons, and a tonsillar herniation. She underwent suboccipital decompressive craniotomy. The onset of a severe postural headache complicated the postoperative course. A hypotensive headache was suspected and confirmed by CT myelography that revealed a spontaneous CSF leak at the C7 nerve roots. *What is the presentation of postoperative CSF leak? What are the potential complications of such a leak? What are the other causes of headaches in such patients?*

CASE REPORT REFERENCES

Case 1: Foust RE. The experience of post-craniotomy pain among patients with brain tumors. Ph.D. dissertation, Indiana University; 2018.

Case 2: Nagasaki H, et al. Remote supratentorial hemorrhage following supratentorial craniotomy: a case report. NMC Case Rep J. 2016;3(1):13-6.

Case 3: Xiao X et al. Treatment of post-craniotomy acute severe supraorbital neuralgia using ultrasound-guided pulsed radiofrequency: a case report. J Pain Res. 2018;11:1497-501.

Case 4: Schievink WI. Misdiagnosis of spontaneous intracranial hypotension. Arch Neurol. 2003;60(12):1713-8.

FURTHER READING

1. Guenther F et al. Pre- and postoperative headache in patients with meningioma. Cephalalgia. 2019;39(4):533-43.
2. Manohar N et al. Scalp Block: Tool for Diagnosis in Postoperative Headache of Unknown Origin. J Neurosurg Anesthesiol. 2018;30(4):381-2.
3. Matsota PK et al. Factors associated with the presence of postoperative headache in elective surgery patients: a prospective single center cohort study. J Anesth. 2017;31(2):225-36.
4. Ravn Munkvold BK et al. Preoperative and Postoperative Headache in Patients with Intracranial Tumors. World Neurosurg. 2018;115:e322-e330.
5. Sabab A et al. Postoperative headache following treatment of vestibular schwannoma: A literature review. J Clin Neurosci. 2018;52:26-31.

Vignette: Hickman's "Anesthesia" was no Humbug!

Henry Hill Hickman was a Scottish physician born in 1800. He was 20 years old when he became a member of the Royal College of Surgeons. In early 1823, he anesthetized animals by administering carbon dioxide to perform painless amputations. Hickman first used the term "Anesthesia" to describe the state of suspended animation that permitted surgery perceiving pain. He wrote about his experiments to Sir Humphry Davy, who had experimented with gases two decades earlier. It seems that Hickman's letter never reached Sir Davy. Hickman submitted his results to the Lancet. The journal rejected his findings, belittled him, and called him a "Surgical humbug". Hickman wrote to Napoleon, but despite the encouragement of Napoleon's physician, Boron Dominique-Jean Larrey, his findings were dismissed in France as well. Boron Larrey had witnessed the painless amputation of frozen limbs when Napoleon's army retreated from Russia in the winter of 1812. Hickman died in 1830 at the age of 30 years, and his achievements went unrecognized. However, on October 16, 1846, after Morton's successful ether demonstration, Dr John Collins Warren, then the Dean of Harvard Medical School, who had arranged for Morton's demonstration, announced, "Gentlemen, this is no humbug!" How ironic!

Chapter 61: Massive Blood Transfusion

INTRODUCTION

Massive hemorrhage is defined as losing total blood volume in 24 hours, half blood volume in 3 hours, or bleeding at >150 mL/min. A massive blood transfusion involves the transfusion of 10 units of blood in 24 hours. However, such a definition does not capture the intensity of blood loss. Alternately, massive transfusion involves the transfusion of three or more packed cells in an hour or 1L crystalloid + 0.5 L of colloid + 1 unit of any blood product in 30 min. This chapter describes fluid replacements in the setting of massive blood loss.

NEUROANESTHETIC CONCERNS

- *Fluid resuscitation:*
  - *Volume replacement:*
    - Colloids versus crystalloids
    - Packed cell transfusion
  - *Coagulation correction:*
    - Assessment of coagulation
    - Oral anticoagulants, e.g., warfarin:
      - *Urgent correction:* Fresh frozen plasma (FFP)
      - *Time permits:* Vitamin K
    - *Heparin and low molecular heparin:* Protamine
    - *Aspirin and Antiplatelet drugs:* Platelet transfusions
  - Management of dilutional coagulopathy
    - Fresh frozen plasma (FFP)
    - Cryoprecipitate (Factor VIII)
    - Recombinant Factor VII
- Risk of blood transfusion
- MBT management.

Fluid Replacement: Crystalloids vs. Colloids

- Euvolemic anemia [hematocrit (Hct) of 20%] is tolerated by healthy subjects.
- Crystalloids have a short circulating half-life (30 minutes) **(Table 1)**.

SECTION 3 Neuroanesthesia Case Management

Table 1: Common clinically used crystalloids and colloids.

	Ringer lactate	0.9% normal saline	25% albumin	5% albumin	3% saline	20% mannitol
Type and composition						
Type	Crystalloid	Crystalloid	Colloid	Colloid	Crystalloid	Crystalloid
Colloid	None	None	Albumin	Albumin	None	None
Molecular weight	–	–	69 kDa	69 kDa	–	182 Da
Composition (unless stated the concentration is in mEq/L)	pH: 6.5 Na: 130 Cl: 100 K: 4.0 Ca: 3.0 Lactate: 28	pH: 5.5 Na: 154 Cl: 154	pH: 7.0 albumin 25 g/dL	pH: 7.0 albumin 5 g/dL Na: 150	pH: 5.0 Na: 513 Cl: 513	pH: 5.0 Mannitol: 20 g/dL
Functional characteristics						
Tonicity	Hypotonic#	Isotonic	Isotonic	Isotonic	Hypertonic	Hypertonic
Osmolality (mOsm/L)	280	300	310	290	1,020	1,200
COP (mm Hg)	–	–	100	25	–	–
Plasma half-life	30 minutes	30 minutes	24 hours	24 hours	20–40 min	90 minutes
Volume limit	As per clinical needs	As per clinical needs	2 g/kg/day Albumin dose	2 g/kg/day Albumin dose	As per clinical needs	As per clinical needs
Maximum expansion volume*	25%	25%	400%	80%	200%	120%
Duration of volume expansion	2 hours	2 hours	24 hours	24 hours	2 hours	90 minutes
Clinical use						
Indications	Routine Intraoperative maintenance fluid	Preferred IV fluid in a neuro ICU	Hypoproteinemia Neonates Burns Renal failure	Colloid Resuscitation with major blood loss or burns	Inc. ICP, Trauma resuscitation	Inc. ICP, Inc. IOP, Forced diuresis, Oliguric renal failure, IA for BBBD
Side effects incidence	Very rare	Rare	Rare	Rare	Likely with 7.5% and 23.4%	Likely with rapid infusions
Side effects	Can increase brain edema.	Hyperchloremic metabolic acidosis	Allergic reaction Potential viral infection	Allergic reaction Potential viral Infection	Hyperchloremic metabolic acidosis	Rapid infusion hazardous with CHF, acidosis, hyperkalemia

(COP: colloid osmotic pressure; ICP: intracranial pressure; ICU: intensive care unit; IOP: intraocular pressure; IV: intravenous; IA for BBBD: intraarterial injection for blood-brain barrier disruption. Inc.: Increased)
#Marginally hypotonic; *Expressed as a % of administered fluid volume.

CHAPTER 61 Massive Blood Transfusion

- *Synthetic colloids (dextran, hetastarch, haemaccel, gelofusine):* Effective but can cause allergic reactions, coagulopathy, and renal failure.
- Balanced crystalloids are ideal for resuscitating healthy individuals with a large protein pool.
- Colloids are probably more beneficial in patients with a depleted interstitial protein pool, such as renal failure, burn, or sepsis.

Blood Transfusion: Packed Cell Transfusion

- Packed Cell preservation at 1–6°C lasts 21 days with Acid Citrate Dextrose (ACD) or Citrate Phosphate Dextrose (CPD). 35 days with CPD-Adenosine. 42 days with Saline Adenosine Dextrose (SAD) with mannitol. Less than 1% of RBCs should hemolyze with such storage. Other preservatives include Adsol® (AS) variants AS-1, AS-3, and AS-5.
- Leukocyte-depleted blood has fewer transfusion reactions.
- Expected to increase hemoglobin by 1gm/dL with each unit of transfusion.
- Biconcave discoid shape augments gas exchange.
- *Change with storage:*
  - The normal RBC life span is 120 days; aging continues during storage.
  - Change in shape from biconcave to oval increases RBC clearance after transfusion.
  - Time-dependent increase in K^+.
  - Decrease in 2-3 di-phosphoglyceraldehyde (2,3-DPG).
  - More significant is the scavenging of nitric oxide that cause vasoconstriction on transfusion and can injure organs such as the kidneys.

Hemoglobin

- In mature RBCs, hemoglobin (Hb) accounts for 95% of all proteins.
- Hb molecule has four structural protein chains, a pair of α and β chains.
- Hb variants have different oxygen affinities.
- It has four oxygen-binding sites with Fe^{++} at the center of the molecule.
- Besides O_2 and CO_2 Hb also binds to NO, a potent vasodilator.
- Carbon monoxide (CO) has a 200–300–fold greater affinity for Hb than O_2. CO decreases the oxygen binding capacity and shifts the O_2-hemoglobin dissociation curve to the left.

Oxygen–hemoglobin Dissociation Curve

- The binding of O_2 to hemoglobin shows a characteristic sigmoid curve due to the cooperative nature of the binding, i.e., the binding of an O_2 molecule increases the affinity for the second one. The cooperative nature of O_2-hemoglobin binding is described by Hill's equation:

$$\theta = \frac{[L]^n}{K_d + [L]^n} = \frac{[L]^n}{(K_a)^n + [L]^n} = \frac{1}{1 + (K_a/[L])^n}$$

θ = Fraction of receptor protein bound to ligand
[L] = Free ligand concentration
K_d = Apparent dissociation constant
K_a = Ligand concentration at 50% receptor saturation
n = Hill coefficient

2,3-DPG

- The most important allosteric modulator of oxygen binding
- A glycolytic pathway intermediate
- Concentration in RBCs (5 mmol/L), equimolar to Hb
- Increases during adaptation to anemia, congestive heart failure, chronic lung disease, and hypoxia.
- Decreases in acidosis and during storage of blood.
- Depletion of 2,3-DPG during blood storage can impair tissue oxygenation.

The Shift of Oxygen–hemoglobin Dissociation Curve (Fig. 1)

- *Shift to the right (decreased affinity, lower P50):* ↓pH, ↑PCO_2, ↑Temperature, ↑2,3-DPG with pregnancy, anemia, and hypoxemia.
- *Shift to the left (increased affinity higher P50):* ↑pH, ↓PCO_2, ↓Temperature, ↓2,3-DPG, abnormal Hb, carbon monoxide poisoning, and hypophosphatemia.

Indications for Packed Cell Transfusion

- Hb of 10 g/dL and Hct of 30% optimum for micro-circulation O_2 delivery, with sufficient O_2 carrying capacity and optimum blood viscosity to perfuse tissues.

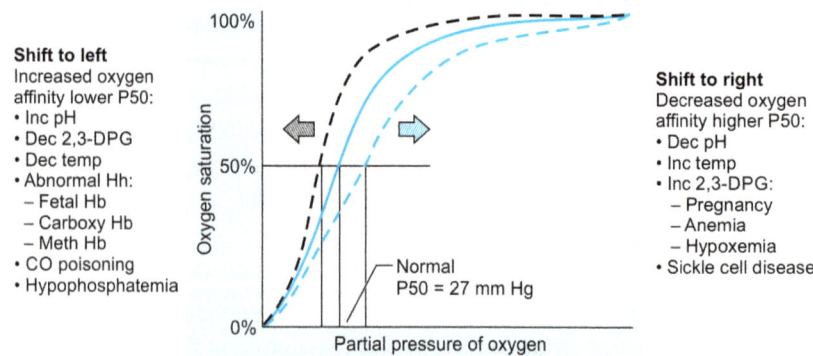

Fig. 1: Oxyhemoglobin dissociation curve. (Dec: decreased; Hb: hemoglobin; Inc: increased; P50: partial pressure of oxygen with 50% saturation)

CHAPTER 61 Massive Blood Transfusion

- Packed cell transfusion is indicated for a healthy individual with an acute decrease in Hb concentrations to 7 g/dL or a Hct <20%.
- Transfusion is indicated with a Hct of 30% in patients with unstable angina or recent myocardial infarction (MI).
- In chronically anemic patients, such as those with chronic renal insufficiency, a lower Hct of 20–25% may be acceptable.
- Higher Hb concentration might be needed in patients with intrapulmonary shunts to maintain O_2 delivery.

Coagulation and Fibrinolysis

Clotting and fibrinolysis represent the sequential activation of proteins **(Table 2)** that result in clot formation and dissolution, respectively **(Figs. 2 and 3)**.

Table 3 summarizes the various clinically used coagulation tests.

Table 2 : Coagulation and fibrinolytic factors.

	Clotting factors		
Designation	Name	Half-life (hours)	Concentration (mg/L)
I	Fibrinogen	90	3,000
II	Prothrombin	60	100
III	Tissue factor	–	–
IV	Calcium	–	–
V	Labile factor and proaccelerin	15	10
VII	Stable factor	5	0.5
VIII	Antihemophilic factor A	10	0.1
IX	Christmas/antihemophilic factor B	25	5
X	Stuart–Prower factor	40	10
XI	Plasma thromboplastin antecedent	40	5
XII	Hageman factor	–	–

Aid to remembering: **F**iendish **P**oliticians **T**rumpet **C**oncocted **L**egends **S**adly **A**bout **C**ovid-vaccines **S**upremely **P**osing **H**ealth-hazards.

	Fibrinolytic factors		
XIII	Fibrin stabilizing factor	200	300
XIV	Prekallikrein (Fletcher)	25	–
XV	HMWK (Fitzgerald)	150	–
XVI	von Willebrand factor	15	10
XVII	Antithrombin III	75	200
XVIII	Heparin cofactor II	60	–
XIX	Protein C	0.5	–
XX	Protein S	–	–

Table 3: Coagulation tests.			
Test	Principle	Value	Significance of increase
Tests for abnormal bleeding			
Bleeding time	Ivy method: 10 mm × 1 mm incision on the upper arm; replaced largely by in-vitro tests	3–10 minutes	Thrombocytopenia, vWD, platelet disorders, and abnormal vascular reactivity; correlates poorly with bleeding
Capillary fragility test	Cuff at the average of systolic and diastolic pressures, 1-inch diameter 4 cm below the elbow for 15 min	>20 petechial spots <10 petechial spot normal	• Idiopathic thrombo-cytopenic purpura • Increased capillary fragility
Platelet count	Microcytometer	• 100,000/μL: Normal • 20–50,000/μL: Bleeding after trauma • <20,000/μL: Spontaneous bleeding • <5,000/μL: Life-threatening major bleeding	
Platelet function analyzer	Assess platelet by in-vitro platelet plug formation and to assess vWF functions	Normal <3 minutes	• Thrombocytopenia • von Willebrand disease • Abnormal platelets
Tests for abnormal coagulation			
Mixing test	Mix test and normal plasma and assess clotting	Clot formation yes/no	Need for further testing: If a clot is seen: It indicates factor deficiency; if the clot is absent: A clotting inhibitor
Prothrombin time*: Tests extrinsic pathway— More sensitive to V, VII, X Less to I and II	Platelet poor plasma + thromboplastin + calcium	10–12 seconds (human thromboplastin)	Liver failure, vitamin K deficiency, oral anticoagulants, and DIC
Activated thromboplastin time: Tests intrinsic pathway— Sensitive to VIII, IX, XI, XII, heparin	Activates contact factors (kaolin, silica, ellagic acid) + CaCl2 + phospholipids	25–40 seconds	Hemophilia A and B, liver failure, DIC, massive blood transfusion, and heparin, for Vit K deficiency less than PT
Thrombin time Downstream of both intrinsic and extrinsic pathways	Clotting with added thrombin	>20 seconds	• Hypofibrinogenemia • Dysfibrinogenemia • Liver disease, multiple myeloma, DIC
Fibrinogen assay: High levels of FDP can interfere with the result	Diluted plasma clotting time with thrombin	2.5–4 g/L; A 50% reduction is clinically significant	• Increase in pregnancy. • Dysfibrinogenemia • Hypofibrinogenemia • Liver disease
Factor VII assay/activity	Congenital or acquired deficiency of Factor VII such as, due to liver disease, Vit K deficiency	• Normal range: 65–140% • Clinical symptoms may occur below 30%	Vit K-resistant coagulopathy
Factor VIII assay/activity	Congenital or acquired deficiency of Factor VIII. Latter due to antibodies to factor VIII	• Normal range: 50-200% • Deficiency: <15 Severe 1-5%: Moderate >5%: Mild	• Decreased: Detection and Rx of hemophilia A • Increased: Stress, liver disease, obesity, age, pregnancy, malignancy
Factor IX assay/activity	Congenital or acquired deficiency of Factor IX.	• Normal range: 50–200% • Deficiency: <15 severe 1–5%: Moderate >5%: Mild	Decreased: Detection and Rx of hemophilia B, Vit K deficiency, liver disease, DIC, anticoagulants, fat malabsorption

Contd...

Contd...

Test	Principle	Value	Significance of increase
Test for abnormal fibrinolysis			
Clot solubility test	Lack of factor XIII dissolves the clot	Clot stable for 24 hours	Screening test for Factor XIII
Fibrin degradation products Includes fibrinopeptides A, B and C and D dimers	Agglutination of latex particles coated with FDP antibodies	<10 µg/mL	10–40 µg/mL: MI, pneumonia, thromboembolism, >40 µg/mL DIC, and thrombolytic drugs
D-dimer assay (D-D fragment)	Agglutination of latex coated with antibodies to D-dimer (automated testing improved results)	Normally undetected Abnormal if >500 ng/ml D-Dimer Units or >250 Fibrin equivalent units	DIC, or increased clotting such as, during DVT or PE
Fibrin monomer assay	Proteolysis of fibrinogen and release fibrin free of peptides A/B	Hemagglutination assay	Increased DIC with increased thrombin activity

*INR or International Normalized Ratio: Prothrombin time (PT) assay may vary between laboratories therefore PT values for a given patient are compared to a control sample and expressed as a the normalized value. INR assesses the extrinsic and the common pathways. For patients on anticoagulant treatment for DVT or Atrial fibrillation, the therapeutic value is 2–3, peripheral nerve and spinal block can be undertaken with INR values </=1.5.
(APTT: activated partial thromboplastin time; DIC: disseminated intravascular coagulation; DVT: deep vein thrombosis; FDP: fibrin degradation product; PE: pulmonary embolism; PT: prothrombin time; vWD: von Willebrand disease; vWF: von Willebrand factor).

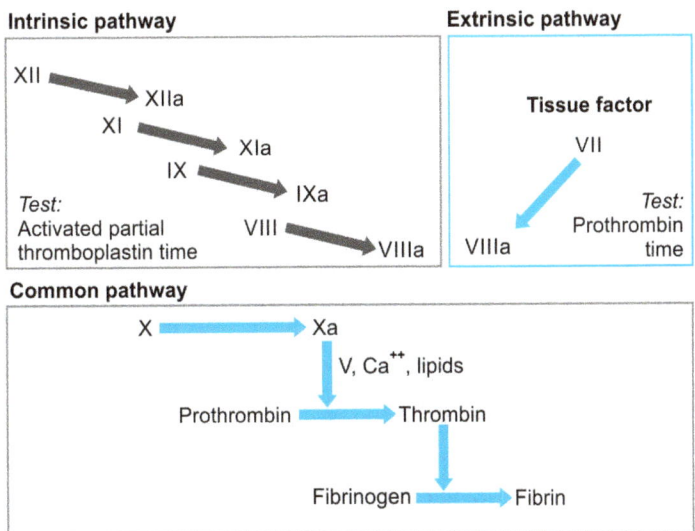

Fig. 2: Coagulation cascade.

Point of Care Testing for Clotting and Fibrinolysis

Viscoelastic properties of blood clots can be mechanically tested to assess coagulation and fibrinolysis. Rotational thromboelastogram (ROTEM) measures the stress on a rotating wire by the clot. In thromboelastography

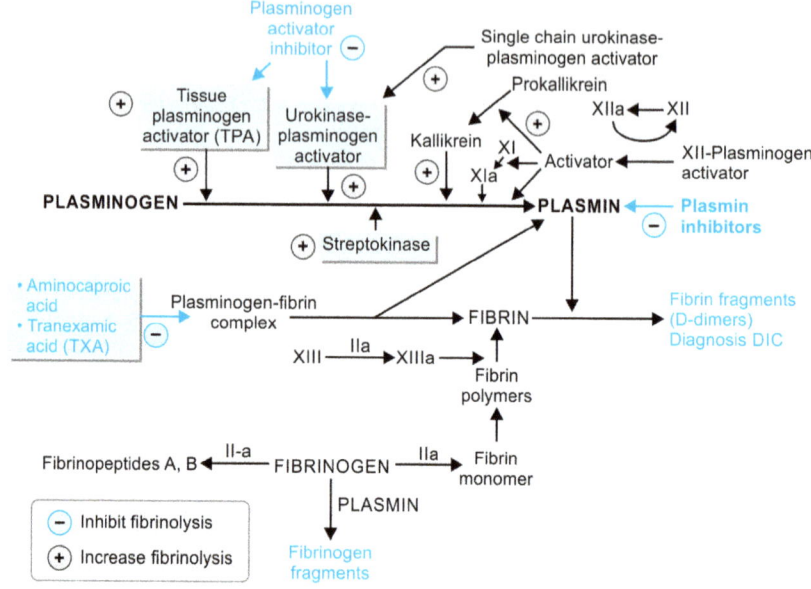

Fig. 3: Activation and inhibition of fibrinolysis and effect of drugs.

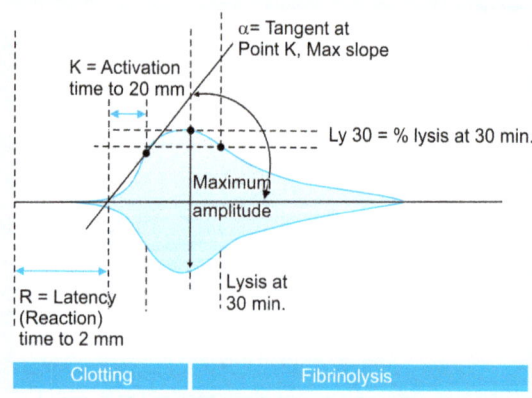

Fig. 4: Key thromboelastographic parameters. (MA: maximum amplitude)

(TEG), the clot forms in an oscillating cup, and the torsion wire suspended generate the displayed waveform **(Figs. 4 and 5)**. **Table 4** describes how pathological processes affect the key TEG parameters.

TEG and ROTEM **(Figs. 4 to 6)** are rapid coagulation tests based on viscoelastic clot properties. These tests are particularly useful in the settings of coagulopathy. The benefits of the techniques are as follows:
- A quick assessment of intraoperative coagulopathy
- Identify and correct specific corrective measures, for example, with TEG:
  - *Prolonged R:* Fresh Frozen Plasma
  - *Prolonged K:* Cryoprecipitate

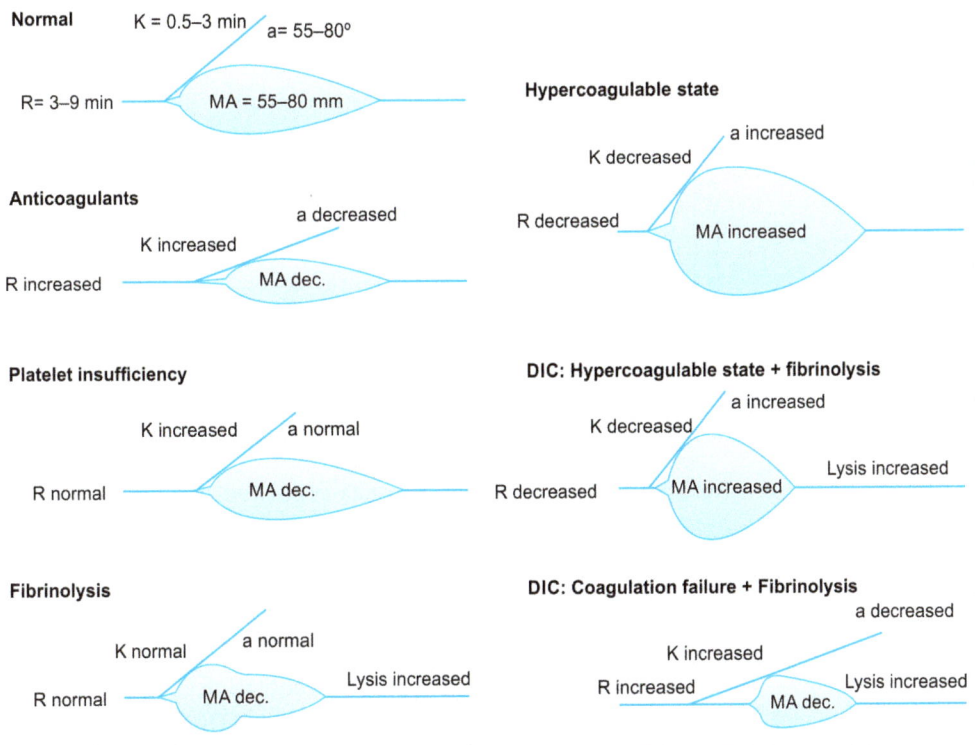

Fig. 5: TEG parameters in pathological conditions.

Table 4: TEG parameters.

Pathological process	TEG finding
Tissue factor activation	• Rapid (<10 minutes) to maximum amplitude (MA) • Shortening of reaction time (R value)
Heparin/heparinase	• R value of TEG is sensitive heparin • Adding heparinase can reverse heparin effect
Fibrinogen and platelet function	MA directly correlated with log platelet count
Fibrinolysis	Elastic modulus (amplitude)
Hypercoagulability	Shorter R value, accelerated clot propagation

  - *Decreased MA:* Platelet correction/DDVAP
  - *Increased Lysis 30:* Antifibrinolytics
- Further, identify specific coagulation defects by repeating ROTEM with correction factors.
- Rapidly assess treatment response
- Decrease blood loss and blood transfusion by rapidly correcting deficiencies in coagulation and fibrinolytic pathways.

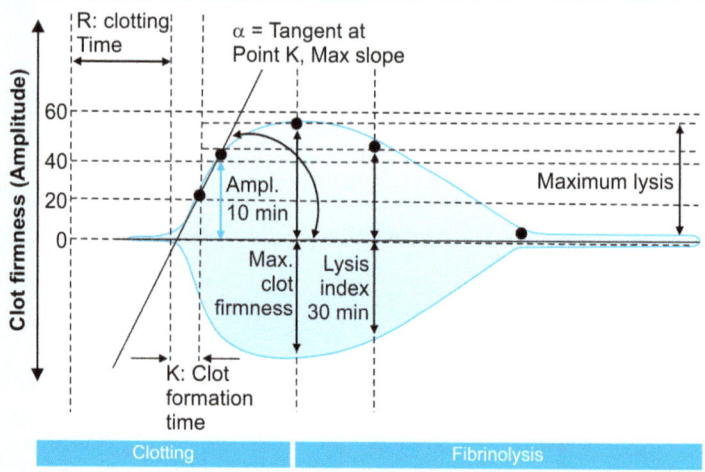

Fig. 6: ROTEM parameters, some amplitude at specified times, are not shown.

- *The overall impact of TEG and ROTEM:*
  - It decreases blood loss.
  - It decreases transfusion needs.
  - It decreases the duration of post-op ventilation.
  - It decreases the length of intensive care unit (ICU) stay.
  - It decreases 6-month mortality in high blood loss surgeries.

Platelet Function Tests
- The bleeding time test
- Platelet size, number, and morphology
- *Light transmission aggregometry:* Adenosine diphosphate (ADP; 0.5–20 µM), collagen (1–5 µg/mL), and epinephrine (0.5–10 µM) are used to test platelet aggregation. If abnormal, higher concentrations and other agents are subsequently used for testing.
- *Nucleotides release testing:* ADP to adenosine triphosphate (ATP) values and ratios.
- TEG and ROTEM.

Blood Product Transfusion

Platelet Transfusion
- The normal platelet count is 150,000–450,000 platelets/µL
- 1 unit of platelets transfusion increases the platelets count by 5,000–10,000/µL
- ABO compatibility is not essential.
- Stored at 22°C for 5–7 days.

- *Indications:*
  - Transfusion threshold at 50,000/µL with bleeding.
  - Prophylactic transfusion at <20,000/µL without bleeding.
  - A higher platelet count, of 80,000/ µL is preferred during neurosurgery.
- *Risks:* Infection, febrile reaction, hypotension, and allergic reactions. Nonspecific replacement of specific factor deficiency.

Fresh Frozen Plasma (FFP)

- FFP is group specific, except for AB plasma.
- *Indications:*
  - MBT
  - Liver failure
  - Disseminated intravascular coagulation (DIC)
  - Reversal of warfarin
  - Reversing increased international normalized ratio (INR), prothrombin time (PT), and activated partial thromboplastin time (APTT)
  - Nonspecific replacement in the absence of a specific factor deficiency

Cryoprecipitate

- *Normal fibrinogen levels:* 200–400 mg/dL
- ABO compatibility is not essential
- 1 unit/kg infusion increases fibrinogen by 5 mg/dL
- *Indications:*
  - Bleeding likely at fibrinogen levels ≤ 80 mg/dL
  - Bleeding after MBT, awaiting coagulation testing
  - Congenital fibrinogen deficiency
  - Nonspecific treatment of hemophilia A and von Willebrand disease.

Factor VII Replacement

- The normal concentration of factor VII
- Only 10–15% of factor VII is adequate for coagulation.
- Target level ≥ 20 U/dL
- Dose 15–20 mL/kg
- Indication for off-label use of factor VII includes intracranial hemorrhage.
- Empirical use does not seem to improve survival and could increase the chances of thromboembolism.

Antifibrinolytic Drugs

- *Protease inhibitor (nonspecific):* Aprotinin inhibits trypsin
- *Plasminogen inhibitor and lysine analogs:* E-Aminocaproic acid and tranexamic acid (TXA)

Risks and Benefits of Antifibrinolytic Drugs

- They are widely used in spine surgery and cranial reconstructive surgery.
- The role of antifibrinolytic drugs in intracranial neurosurgery is unclear.
- *Side-effects:* Seizures (4–8 × greater than in untreated patients); thrombosis, bradycardia, hypotension, renal impairment, injection site reactions.
- *Seizures due to TXA:*
  - *Etiology:*
    - Inhibition of GABA
    - Inhibition of glycine receptors.
    - Micro emboli
    - Altered blood-brain barrier.
- TXA is better tolerated than E-Aminocaproic acid.
- Several studies describe the use of antifibrinolytic in subarachnoid hemorrhage (SAH), where early treatment decreases the risk of rebleeding, but ischemic complications are increased.
- The availability of bedside monitoring of fibrinolysis may help in case selection and dose optimization.

Benefits

- Decrease blood loss.
- Decrease transfusion requirements.
- Decrease postoperative anemia.
- Decrease the risk of bleeding and hematoma formation.

Risks

- Thromboembolic risks
- Seizures due to the inhibition of glycine and gamma-aminobutyric acid (GABA) receptors

Indications for Anti-Fibrinolytic Therapy in Neurosurgery

- Spine surgery with significant blood loss
- Aneurysmal subarachnoid hemorrhage
- Vascular tumors

Hazards of Blood Transfusion

- Acute transfusion reaction and ABO incompatibility
  - A high level of vigilance is needed at all times but particularly during massive blood transfusions
  - *Acute intravascular hemolysis*
    - *Under anesthesia:* Bronchospasm, tachycardia, hypotension, decreased urine output, fever, rash, and DIC.

CHAPTER 61 Massive Blood Transfusion

- *Awake patient:* Complaints of anxiety, chest pain, breathlessness, sweating, fever with chills, and flushing with signs listed above
- *Investigations:*
  - *Confirmation:* Direct Coomb's test
  - *Serum:* ↑ hemoglobin, ↓ haptoglobin, ↑ bilirubin
  - *Urine:* ↑ hemoglobin
  - *Coagulation:* ↓ platelets, ↑ PT, PTT, and INR; ↓ fibrinogen and ↑ fibrin degradation products (FDPs)
- *Delayed hemolytic reactions:*
  - Due to the incompatibility of minor antigens (such as, Kelly, Duff, or Lewis)
  - Extravascular hemolysis
  - Occurs 2–21 days after transfusion.
  - Malaise, jaundice, and fever
- *Allergic reactions:* Serum platelet or RBC induced—Steroid useful.
- *Febrile reaction:* Mild, usually due to leukocyte antigens
- *Urticarial reaction:* Erythema, hives, and itching without fever
- *Post-transfusion purpura:* Due to platelet antibodies
- *Graft versus host reaction:* Transfused lymphocytes cause an immune response; presents as pancytopenia due to donor lymphocytes and may be prevented by irradiation of blood.
- Infections after blood transfusion:
  - HIV and Hepatitis C: 1:1,000,000
  - Hepatitis B: 1:200,000
  - Others: Cytomegalovirus, West Nile, Creutzfeldt–Jakob disease
- Transfusion-induced acute lung injury (TRALI):
  - Incidence 1/500,000 RBC and 1/500 platelet unit transfusions
  - The overall risk to transfused patients is 1:1,000 to 1:50,000.
  - Deposition of white cells in the pulmonary bed
  - Mimics acute respiratory distress syndrome (ARDS)
  - Presents lung injury after 6 hours with acute respiratory distress and failure
  - Resolves in 96 hours with supportive treatment.
  - Steroids and diuretics are ineffective.
  - Fatal in 5–10% of cases
- Transfusion-associated circulatory overload (TACO)
- Immunosuppression leads to cancer recurrence or activation of latent viral infections. Therefore, limit the transfusions to <5 units or use irradiated blood.

Massive Blood Transfusion

Criteria based on the replacement of large volume of blood:
- 100% blood volume/24 hours
- 50% blood volume/3 hours

Table 5: Infusion rates through commonly used peripheral venous cannulae.

Manufacturer	Size	Internal diameter	Internal area	Length	Flow rate
Braun	24G	0.7 mm	0.38 mm^2	19 mm	22 mL/min
	22G	0.9 mm	0.64 mm^2	25 mm	35 mL/min
	22G	0.9 mm	0.64 mm^2	64 mm	24 mL/min
	20G	1.1 mm	0.95 mm^2	32 mm	60 mL/min
	22G	1.1 mm	0.95 mm^2	64 mm	51 mL/min
	18G	1.3 mm	1.32 mm^2	32 mm	105 mL/min
	16G	1.7 mm	2.27 mm^2	32 mm	215 mL/min
	14G	2.2 mm	3.46 mm^2	50 mm	345 mL/min
Angio catheter	20G	1.1 mm	0.95 mm^2	48 mm	42 mL/min

- Three units/h
- 1 L crystalloid + 500 mL colloid + 1 unit blood product in 30 min
- 150 mL/min.

Basic Setup

- Central venous catheters, large (>18-16 G) peripheral lines, or intraosseous access is required. The narrow lumen peripherally inserted central catheter (PICC) is inadequate. Flow rates through different IV cannulae are shown in **Table 5**.
- The blood set has a 170–200-micron filter. Filter sequesters platelets yet are used for platelet transfusion.
- Any infusion >500 mL should be warmed. The Target transfusion temperature is 37°C and should not exceed 43°C.
- Blood should be isolated from other infusions and drugs: a separate catheter or a separate channel of a multi-lumen catheter.
- *Avoid contact with Calcium containing fluids:* Lactated Ringer, synthetic colloids (Haemaccel or Gelofusine). Also, hypotonic 5% dextrose can cause hemolysis.

Hazards of Massive Blood Transfusion

- MBT is needed to prevent and treat hemorrhagic shock.
- Clinical features of hemorrhagic shock severity are listed in **Table 6**.
- Erroneous assessment of circulating volume can lead to TACO
- MBT increases the risk of ABO incompatibility.
- *Lead to electrolyte imbalances:* Hypocalcemia (citrate toxicity), hyperkalemia (increased hemolysis during storage), and acidosis due to the decrease in pH during storage
- Hypothermia
- Dilutional coagulopathy

Table 6: Grades of hemorrhagic shock.

	Grade I	Grade II	Grade III	Grade IV
Stage	Initial	Compensatory	Progressive	Refractory
Blood loss % TBV	15%	30%	30–40%	>40%
Blood loss	750 mL	1500 mL	2000 mL	>2000 mL
Heart rate (beats/min)	100-120	120–140	120–140	>140
Blood pressure	Normal	Normal	Decreased	Decreased
Respiratory rate (breaths/min)	12–15	15–30	30–40	>35
Capillary refill	Normal	Sluggish	Absent	Absent
Urine output (mL/hr)	30+	15–30	5–15	Negligible
Cognition	Normal	Anxious	Confused	Obtunded
Resuscitation strategy	Crystalloids	Crystalloids, colloid (±)	Crystalloid, colloid (±), blood	Crystalloid, colloid (±), blood, products

(TBV: total blood volume)

- Left shift of oxygen-hemoglobin dissociation curve, decreased concentrations of 2,3-DPG, and poor tissue O_2 release.
- Increased risks of all complications of blood transfusion, such as TRALI, infection, sepsis, and allergic and immune reactions
- Possibility of air embolism with rapid infuser malfunction.

Management

- Anticipate and ensure that adequate IV access is available.
- Monitor volume response during infusion on critical vital signs:
  - Arterial blood pressure
  - Pulse pressure variation
  - Central venous pressure (CVP) and/or pulmonary capillary wedge pressure (PCWP)
  - Urine output
  - Hct. and base deficit
- Tabulate hourly blood loss, urine output, blood, fluid replacement, and Hct. and base deficits.
- Preserve bags of used blood and blood products.
- Establish the baseline coagulation profile.
- Inform the blood bank as per evolving needs for blood and blood products.
- *Aggressively treat hypothermia:* Blankets, fluid warmers, and consider low gas flows.
- Watch for and treat hypocalcemia (<1.1mEq/L).

- Correct acidosis (pH <7.2) and hyperkalemia (>6.5 mEq/L, with 20 U insulin in 50 mL 50% dextrose).
- Replace coagulation factors.
- Plan for postoperative ICU care and ventilation.

Hypotension with Adequate Volume Replacement
Consider:
- Hypocalcemia
- Acidosis
- Persistent low Hct
- Anesthetic overdose
- Sepsis
- Cardiogenic shock
- Thrombus or air embolism.

High Flow Rapid Infusion Technology
- It can provide steady basal infusion.
- Can replace fluid at a rate of 100–1000 mL/min in bolus mode.
- Requires large-bore catheters, connectors, and unrestricted fluid flow from the fluid bags.
- In high-flow situations, an optional reservoir is recommended to minimize changing bags.
- Monitors infusion temperature, air emboli, and infusion pressure.
- It does not require pre-warmed fluids that can lead to an over-temperature alarm.
- *Fluids not to be delivered through rapid infuser:*
  - Platelets and granulocytes
  - Cryoprecipitate
  - *Avoid mixing blood with:*
    - *Ringer's lactate:* due to Ca^{++} that can negate anticoagulation.
    - *Hypotonic solutions:* Dextrose and hypotonic sodium chloride
    - Calcium that would negate anticoagulation.

Major Causes of Mortality after Transfusion
- TRALI
- Sepsis
- ABO incompatibility.

CASE REPORTS FOR FURTHER DISCUSSION

Case 1: A 72-year-old obese patient weighing 122 kg underwent resection of a sphenoid wing meningioma. The patient had a solitary kidney, and serum creatinine was 1.5 mg/dL. During surgery, he received TXA (loading dose 8 mg/kg and infusion 4 mg/kg/h) in anticipation of significant bleeding. The surgery lasted 9 hours with an estimated blood loss of 1,000 mL. Five minutes after arrival in the recovery room, the patient lost consciousness and had a grand mal seizure with asystolic arrest. He was resuscitated and reintubated. Seizures were treated with propofol infusion and phenytoin. Postoperative laboratory reports were significant for lactic acidosis and increased creatinine of 2 mg/dL. His CT scan was negative, and EEG on the second postoperative day revealed no epileptic activity. He was weaned off propofol on the third postoperative day. *What are the possible risk factors for seizures with TXA in this case?*

Case 2: A 69-year-old patient with ankylosing spondylitis sustained a fall three weeks earlier. The initial scan at another hospital was said to be "normal". He developed progressively increasing back pain and lower limb weakness due to cord compression and L2 and L3 nerve roots. Repeat scans revealed a complex fracture of the lumbar spine with epidural hematoma. His history was significant for hypertension, coronary artery disease (CAD; treated with hydrochlorothiazide and captopril), and colonic resection with an ileostomy. He had fallen in the past and sustained a cervical fracture treated with traction. The preoperative workup revealed a Hb level of 13.8 g/dL; an echocardiogram revealed an ejection fraction of 55% and a negative stress test. Planned surgery would involve the monitoring of somatosensory evoked potential (SSEP). During surgery, massive blood loss was anticipated. Around 17 L of blood was lost during surgery. *What are the factors that contributed to this massive bleeding? How would you have planned for such a case?*

Case 3: A 57-year-old, 167 kg male with chronic back pain due to spinal stenosis for several years was scheduled for decompressive lumbar surgery. The surgery included bone grafting and spinal instrumentation from L3 to S1. In preparation for surgery, autologous blood was harvested for intraoperative use. During the 9-hour surgery, the patient lost 16 L of blood. He was resuscitated with 20 L of crystalloid, 5.2 L of cell-saver blood, nine units of blood (5 autologous units), ten units of FFP, and 6 U of platelets. The systolic blood pressure was maintained at 90 mm Hg. The lowest Hct was 24% transiently. On the fifth day, the patient's vision was noted to be markedly decreased in both eyes, with no reaction to light in the left eye and minimal response in the right eye. The ophthalmological exam of the fundus was negative. There was no loss of corneal sensation or ocular movements. The CT scan of the orbit and the brain was negative. *Can you explain the loss of vision in this case? Do you agree with the management? What additional precautions can you take to prevent this outcome?*

Case 4: A 25-year-old male with a history of a fall one year earlier that required surgical treatment. He presented with worsening back pain and weakness in the lower limbs. MRI revealed an aggressive spinal T12 tumor extending from T11 to L1. There was no evidence of metastasis to the lungs. He underwent total vertebrectomy from T11 to L1 with en-block tumor resection with extended posterior fusion from T8 to L4. Three spinal arteries were ligated during the process to insert a metal cage. The total blood loss during the procedure was 7.7 L. A dural tear complicated the postoperative course. There was no hemopneumothorax, but despite ventilation, the oxygenation remained poor. *What steps can you take to minimize blood loss in the case of a spinal tumor? How can you decrease the chances of postoperative respiratory failure?*

CASE REPORT REFERENCES

Case 1: Merriman B et al. Postoperative seizure in a neurosurgical patient: should tranexamic acid be on the differential? Can J Anaesth. 2013;60(5):506-7.

Case 2: Tetzlaff JE et al. Massive bleeding during spine surgery in a patient with ankylosing spondylitis. Can J Anaesth. 1998;45(9):903-6.

Case 3: Katzman SS et al. Amaurosis secondary to massive blood loss after lumbar spine surgery. Spine. 1994;19(4):468-9.

Case 4: Faruk NA et al. Three level thoracolumbar spondylectomy for recurrent giant cell tumor of the spine: a case report. Malays Orthop J. 2018;12(3):50-2.

FURTHER READING

1. Black JA et al. Complications of hemorrhagic shock and massive transfusion-a comparison before and after the damage control Resuscitation Era. Shock. 2021;56(1):42-51.
2. Blaine KP et al. Viscoelastic monitoring to guide the correction of perioperative coagulopathy and massive transfusion in patients with life-threatening hemorrhage. Anesthesiol Clin. 2019;37(1):51-66.
3. Hu P et al. A new definition for massive transfusion in the modern era of whole blood resuscitation. Transfusion. 2021;61(Suppl 1):S252-263.
4. Meneses E et al. Massive transfusion protocol in adult trauma population. Am J Emerg Med. 2020;38(12):2661-6.
5. Rankin D et al. Massive blood loss in elective spinal and orthopedic surgery: Retrospective review of intraoperative transfusion strategy. J Clin Anesth. 2017;37:69-73.

CHAPTER 61 Massive Blood Transfusion

Vignette: A Brief History of Intravenous Fluid Therapy

1492   The record of the first blood transfusion to Pope Innocent VIII is a matter of dispute. The comatose Pope was transfused blood after a stroke.
1628   William Harvey published "De Motu Cordis", describing blood circulation.
1656   Robert Boyle and Christopher Wren injected a tincture of opium intravenously, using a pig bladder and a quill, in a dog successfully.
1662   The first intravenous infusion and blood transfusion by Johann Major had fatal results.
1667   Richard Lower and Edmond King did the first blood transfusion from sheep to humans. Subsequent efforts were fatal, and research in blood transfusion was banned.
1829   The first human-to-human blood transfusion by James Brundell
1832   Thomas Latta used saline transfusion to treat cholera.
1844   First hypodermic needle by Francis Rynd
1853   Alexander Wood developed a syringe with a hypodermic needle for human use.
1880   Sidney Ringer introduced the mixed electrolyte "Ringer's" solution
1888   Hartog Jakob Hamburger described normal saline: A 0.92% solution did not cause hemolysis.
1900   Karl Landsteiner identified the main blood groups.
1914   Citrate was first used as an anticoagulant for blood storage.
1930   Alexis Frank Hartman added lactate to formulate Ringer's lactate solution.

Chapter 62

Brain Death and Organ Harvest

INTRODUCTION

An estimated 100,000 Americans were awaiting transplants in 2020, and some 40,000 transplant surgeries were performed that year. These figures reveal the shortage of donor organs. Optimum preharvest donor care is needed to maximize the benefits of the donated organs. Most of the transplant organs were obtained from cadaveric sources after the diagnosis of brain death. Brain death describes the complete cessation of neurological functions characterized by coma, absence of brainstem reflexes, and apnea. Before such a determination is made, the confounding effects of hypothermia, hypotension, metabolic abnormality, and drugs must be ruled out. In children, brain death determination may require repeat testing. After determining brain death, supportive care can be provided as needed to enable organ harvest. Donor care requires optimum electrolyte and fluid balance, hemodynamic support to ensure organ perfusion and viability, inflammation mitigation, and infection prevention. Vasopressin, corticosteroids, and thyroid hormones may be needed. Many anesthesiologists continue to provide anesthetic care once the diagnosis of brain death is confirmed until the terminal cessation of circulation during the harvesting procedure. Anesthesiologists need to coordinate with the organ harvest team to ensure that organs are harvested in the most pristine condition.

NEUROANESTHETIC CONCERNS

- Definition of brain death
- Determination of brain death
- Physiological changes after death
- Surgical approaches to organ harvest
- Anesthesia for organ harvest
- Organ preservation
- Warm perfusion
- Cold preservation time limits.

Definition of Brain Death

Brain death is the irreversible loss of brain function, including the brain stem. Brain death is diagnosed in the settings of significant brain injury by coma, brainstem areflexia, and apnea, without a confounding effect of hypothermia, hypotension, metabolic abnormalities, or drugs.

Clinical Determination of Brain Death

- *Prerequisites:* The cause of loss of brain function should be known and demonstrably irreversible:
  - A clinical exam, or neuroimaging, should demonstrate catastrophic neurological injury consistent with brain death.
  - No confounding medical condition, such as severe electrolyte imbalance, acid-base imbalance, or endocrine disturbance
  - No hypotension, a mean blood pressure of 70–90 mm Hg
  - No drug intoxication or overdose.
  - *No hypothermia:* The temperature should be >36.5°C or 97.7°C. For apnea testing, the core temperature should be ≥36.5°C. A core temperature <32°C or 90°F can lead to coma without brain injury.
- *Clinical exam:*
  - Absence of response to pain.
  - *Absence of brainstem reflexes:*
  - *No pupillary response:*
    - Pupils fixed (4–9 mm).
    - Unresponsive to light.
  - *No ocular response:*
    - *No oculocephalic reflex:* The eyes rotate opposite to the direction of movement to the head.
    - *No oculovestibular reflex:* Cold saline irrigation of the ear causes fast nystagmus away and slow return towards the irrigated side.
  - *No facial response:*
    - No corneal reflex
    - No jaw reflex.
    - No grimace in response to pain.
  - No pharyngeal gag response.
  - No tracheal cough response.
- *Clinical observations consistent with brain death:*
  - Isolated spontaneous limb movements.
  - Atypical respiratory-like movements but no measurable tidal volumes.
  - *Autonomic changes:* Flushing, sweating, tachycardia, and hypertension.
  - Certain reflexes may be present, such as deep tendon, Babinski, or superficial abdominal reflexes.

Pitfalls in the Clinical Diagnosis of Brain Death
- Facial trauma may limit the examination of cranial nerves.
- Pupillary abnormalities may be difficult to assess due to injuries.
- *Drug overdose:* Sedatives, antipsychotics, anticonvulsants, muscle relaxants, aminoglycosides, and others.
- Sleep apnea or severe chronic obstructive pulmonary disease (COPD)

Differential Diagnosis
- Hypothermia
- Locked-in syndrome
- Guillain–Barre syndrome
- Sedative drug overdose.
- Residual neuromuscular blockade

Apnea Testing
- *Prerequisites:*
  - Core temperature ≥36.5°C or 97.7°F
  - Systolic blood pressure (SBP) ≥100 mm Hg, mean BP 70–90 mm Hg
  - Euvolemia or positive fluid balance over the last 6 hours
  - Normal $PaCO_2$ or $PaCO_2$ ≥40 mm Hg.
  - Normal PaO_2 or PaO_2 >200 on 100% inspired oxygen concentration.
  - No central nervous system (CNS) depression due to sedative drugs.
  - Ensure reversal of paralysis by neuromuscular monitoring.
- *Test:*
  - Connect the pulse oximeter and obtain a baseline arterial blood sample.
  - Disconnect the ventilator and insert a cannula for O_2 delivery into the trachea.
  - Ensure O_2 of 6 L/min into the trachea at the level of the carina.
  - Watch out for any abdominal or chest excursions.
  - Terminate at 8 minutes after obtaining an arterial blood sample.
- *Abort the test if:*
  - Respiratory movements are observed, then obtain an arterial sample and abort the test.
  - The patient becomes hypotensive (SBP <90 mm Hg).
  - SaO_2 <90%
  - The onset of arrhythmias.
- *Test results:*
  - *Positive:* No respiratory effort is seen in 8 minutes with a $PaCO_2$ >60 mm Hg or a 20-mm increase from baseline $PaCO_2$.
  - *Negative:* Respiratory effort is evident within 8 minutes.
  - *Indeterminate:* Test aborted.

CONFIRMATORY TESTS

- Brain death diagnosis is based on clinical examination.
- Confirmatory tests are used when some clinical assessment is ambiguous.
- Confirmatory tests could be positive in a patient who has not met the clinical criteria of brain death.
- *Confirmatory tests in order of sensitivity are:*
  - *Angiography:* No intracranial perfusion as evidenced by external carotid artery (ECA) but not internal carotid artery (ICA) perfusion on common carotid injection of contrast.
  - *Electroencephalography (EEG):* 16-channel EEG reveals no electrical activity for 30 minutes per the American Encephalographic Society (AES) specification.
  - *Transcranial Doppler (TCD):*
    - TCD can be unreliable; 10% of the patients do not have a suitable TCD window.
    - Small systolic peaks with either no diastolic flow or a diastolic flow reversal suggest a grossly increased ICP.
- *Technetium-99m* brain scan demonstrates a "hollow skull", with no intracranial isotope uptake.
- *Other tests:*
  - Magnetic resonance angiography
  - Computed tomographic angiography
- *Ancillary electrophysiologic tests in order of sensitivity are:*
  - Nasopharyngeal SSEP electrode recording
  - Somatosensory evoked potential (SSEP): Bilateral absence of N22–P22 response to median nerve stimulation as per the AES criteria.
  - Bispectral index (unreliable).

Physiological Changes after Brain Death

- *Diabetes insipidus:*
  - Loss of antidiuretic hormone (ADH)
  - Hypo-osmotic urine (<300 mOsm/kg) and diuresis (5–10 mL/kg/h)
  - *Results in:*
    - Contraction of blood volume.
    - Increased serum osmolality >295 mOsm/kg
    - *Electrolyte imbalance:*
      - Increased serum Na >150 mEq/L
      - Hypokalemia
      - Hypocalcemia
      - Hypophosphatemia
  - *Treatment:*
    - Sodium-free fluids

- Desmopressin
- IV vasopressin
  - Both desmopressin and vasopressin cause splanchnic constriction and could decrease blood flow to visceral organs.
- Concurrent with sodium-free fluids, diuretics, e.g., furosemide, may be used.
- *Hypothermia:* Loss of central hypothalamic control
- *Autonomic storm:*
  - Is a massive surge of catecholamine release with resulting hypertension and inflammation.
  - Requires aggressive antihypertensive treatment.
  - Steroids
- *Hypotension due to:*
  - Contraction of blood volume
  - Decreased vasomotor responses
  - Stunned myocardium
  - *Treatment:*
    - Fluids
    - Triple hormone therapy;
      - Methylprednisolone
      - L-thyroxine
      - Vasopressin
    - Dopamine before adrenergic drugs
- *Arrhythmias due to:*
  - Electrolyte imbalances
  - Pressor therapy
  - Metabolic abnormalities
- *Pulmonary complications due to:*
  - CPR
  - Fluid overload
  - Aspiration
  - Ventilator-associated pneumonia
- *Organ failure due to:*
  - Hypotension
  - Contracted blood volume
  - Pressor treatment.

Surgical Approaches

Organ harvest requires clear communication with the transplant team as institution protocols may vary. The surgeons may need an extra sterile A-line. The goals are to ensure organ perfusion, minimize stress and prevent infection.

CHAPTER 62 Brain Death and Organ Harvest

- *Midline incision:* Provides the usual access for organ harvest in sequence:
  - Kidneys and pancreas
  - Heart and lungs
  - Skin, corneas, and bone
- *Organ preservation:* Typical time limits with cold preservation:
  - *Heart and lungs:* <6 hours
  - *Liver:* 18 hours
  - *Pancreas:* 24 hours
  - *Kidneys:* 72 hours

  Warm perfusion can increase the duration and quality of organ preservation.

Anesthesia for Organ Harvest

- Institution-specific policies and protocols determine organ harvest.
- Discuss protocol and harvest sequence with the transplant team.
- No anesthesia is necessary; however, after the diagnosis of brain death, anesthesia is sometimes continued until terminal circulatory arrest.
- Anesthetics may cause hemodynamic instability.
- The donor is hemodynamically optimized before transfer for harvest.
- Thyroxin drip increases metabolism and blood pressure without concomitant vasoconstriction seen with pressor drugs.

Physiological Targets

- Systolic arterial pressure (SAP) >100 mm Hg
- Central venous pressure (CVP) >5 mm Hg
- Urine output (UO) >100 mL/h
- Temperature >35°C
- Oxygen saturation >90%, room air

Usual Interventions

- *At the start of harvest:*
  - Blood (100 mL) drawn for type matching
  - Antibiotics (Cefazolin 1 g)
  - Hydrocortisone 1 g.
- *15 minutes before cross clamp:*
  - Mannitol 0.5 g/kg
  - Lasix 0.5 mg/kg
- *5 minutes before cross clamp:*
  - 30,000 units of heparin

For Heart Harvest

- Withdraw the pulmonary artery catheter.
- Drop the lungs during sternotomy.

CASE REPORTS FOR FURTHER DISCUSSION

Case 1: A 62-year-old female patient was found unresponsive and pulseless at home by the paramedics. Basic and advanced cardiac life support was instituted, and the pulse returned after 35 minutes. On arrival in the ER, laboratory reports revealed a white cell count of 16, hematocrit of 25, blood urea nitrogen (BUN) of 41 mg/dL, and glucose of 584 mg/dL. She had a history of hypothyroidism, hypertension, coronary artery disease, chronic renal disease, and noninsulin-dependent diabetes mellitus. On clinical examination, she was unresponsive to noxious stimuli, and the core temperature was 33.1°C. *What problems do you see in assessing unresponsiveness in this patient? Would you wait to correct hyperglycemia before declaring brain death? What about normalizing thyroid functions before announcing brain death?*

Case 2: A 13-year-old otherwise healthy patient had anaphylaxis and cardiac arrest after peanut exposure. She received multiple doses of epinephrine, and the cardiopulmonary resuscitation lasted 45 minutes. She was severely acidotic and hypothermic. In the ICU, the patient was hypothermic for the next 24 hours and then gradually rewarmed over the next 14 hours. After rewarming, the core temperature was 35.9°C.

No pain response, no gag or cough response, and no brainstem response could be elicited. There was no respiratory effort even when the $PaCO_2$ doubled from 35 to 72 mm Hg. However, it was noted that there was a shoulder shrug when the CO_2 was increased. Similarly, when the clavicles were pinched, there was bilateral lower limb withdrawal. *Can you consider the lower limb response to upper body stimulation a spinal reflex? What are the prerequisites for doing apnea testing? What further investigations will you request?*

Case 3: A 68-year-old obese patient with chronic hydrocephalus was unresponsive to verbal and pain stimulation. CT scan showed signs of uncal herniation. Sixteen hours after admission to the ICU, her consciousness had not improved. Her brainstem tests were negative. The apnea test revealed no ventilatory effort despite a significant increase in $PaCO_2$. Having met the American Academy of Neurology (AAN 2010) criteria for brain death, her family consented to an organ harvest. In preparation for the procedure, she was given 1 g of methylprednisolone. After that, spontaneous breathing returned for the next 2 hours, and the patient breathed spontaneously using a T piece. With the return of spontaneous breathing, the organ harvest was aborted. Over the next 20 hours, breathing effort waned and eventually ceased. The repeat brainstem testing led to a second brain death declaration. *What are the possible causes for the breathing to return after negative brainstem tests? Could high-dose steroids affect brain death diagnosis?*

Case 4: A 49-year-old man failed to regain consciousness after a 5-minute cardiac arrest following an epileptic seizure. MR imaging on the second day showed significant hypoxic-ischemic injury. EEG showed low-amplitude delta activity. Five days after the arrest, his pupils were nonreactive, and brainstem reflexes and apnea tests were negative. No pain response was elicited. It was concluded that the criteria for brain death had been met. However, a few hours later, it was reported that there was a movement of arms, neck, and back on sternal rubbing. At the request of the organ donation team, a cerebral perfusion single-photon emission computerized tomography (SPECT) scan was undertaken. The scan revealed prominent hemispheric perfusion. On the sixth day, while there were no brainstem reflexes, the gross motor response to sternal rub could still be elicited. On that day, the patient suffered another cardiac arrest from which he could not be resuscitated. *What are the limitations of perfusion scans in diagnosing brain death?*

Case 5: A 61-year-old patient sustained a transient cardiac arrest of uncertain duration. Upon arrival at the ICU, he was unresponsive. EEG showed slow persistent activity, while the initial CT scan was negative for raised ICP. Over time, his neurological condition worsened. On the fourth post-arrest day, there were no brainstem reflexes, no respiratory effort was seen in response to a rise in CO_2, and the EEG revealed no significant activity. Yet the TCD revealed good blood flow in both middle cerebral arteries with flow velocities around 40 cm/s in diastole and a pulsatility index of 1.4. The condition did not change over until the sixth day. The EEG and toxicological screens were negative. CT revealed loss of gray and white matter differentiation but with a normal volume of lateral ventricles. Under the country's laws, he was declared brain-dead on the sixth day. *Can neuronal death be associated with a relatively intact cerebral blood flow?*

CASE REPORT REFERENCES

Case 1: Burns JM et al. Confounding factors in diagnosing brain death: a case report. BMC Neurol. 2002;2:5.

Case 2: Joffe AR et al. Some questions about brain death: a case report. Pediatr Neurol. 2007;37(4):289-91.

Case 3: Glass D et al. A patient declared brain dead who subsequently breathed spontaneously. Crit Care Med. 2016;44(12):528.

Case 4: Ala TA et al. A case meeting clinical brain death criteria with residual cerebral perfusion. Am J Neuroradiol. 2006; 27(9):1805-6.

Case 5: Nguyen M et al. Rapid brain death following cardiac arrest without intracranial pressure rise and cerebral circulation arrest. Case Rep Crit Care. 2018;2018:2709174.

FURTHER READING

1. Busl KM et al. Apnea testing for the determination of brain death: a systematic scoping review. Neurocrit Care. 2021;34(2):608-20.
2. Greer DM et al. Determination of Brain Death/Death by Neurologic Criteria: The World Brain Death Project. JAMA. 2020;324(11):1078-97.
3. Meneses E et al. Massive transfusion protocol in adult trauma population. Am J Emerg Med. 2020;38(12):2661-6.
4. Murphy L et al. Toxicologic confounders of brain death determination: a narrative review. Neurocrit Care. 2021;34(3):1072-89.
5. Rabinstein AA. Coma and brain death. Continuum (Minneap Minn), 2018; 24(6):1708-31.

Vignette: Determining Death

Dick Teresi 2012 book titled "The Undead." describes how death was determined over time and across cultures. The Romans did so by cutting the finger. Others rubbed warm water or waited for putrefaction. Still, others used smelling salts, sharp pain, skin blistering by caustic compound, and recently electric shocks to determine death. The classical criteria of cessation of breathing or stoppage of the heart were unreliable but became more redundant as cardiovascular and respiratory support technologies improved. In 1968, Harvard criteria were introduced to diagnose brain death that could be used to determine the cessation of life support or candidacy for organ harvest.

Section 4

Appendices

Appendix 1

COMMON INFUSION RATES OF DRUGS IN NEUROANESTHESIA

Class	Drug	Infusion rate
Sedatives		
	Propofol	25–200 µg/kg/min
	Dexmedetomidine	0.2–0.7 µg/kg/h
	Ketamine	0.2–1.2 mg/kg/h
	Etomidate	0.02–0.1 mg/kg/h
	Methohexital	0.05–0.2 mg/kg/min
Narcotics		
	Remifentanil	0.03–0.5 µg/kg/min
	Sufentanil	0.1–1 µg/kg/h
	Alfentanil	0.5–3 µg/kg/min
Muscle relaxants		
	Vecuronium	1–2 µg/kg/min
	Rocuronium	10–12 µg/kg/min
Pressors		
	Phenylephrine	10–200 µg/min
	Norepinephrine	0.5–20 µg/min
	Vasopressin	0.2–2.4 U/h
	Dopamine	2.5–20 µg/kg/min
	Epinephrine	0.05–20 µg/min
	Amrinone	5–15 µg/kg/min
	Milrinone	0.4–0.8 µg/kg/min
Hypotensive agents		
	Esmolol	25–300 µg/kg/min
	Nicardipine	1–3 µg/kg/min
	Nitroglycerin	0.25–10 µg/kg/min
	Nitroprusside	0.25–5 µg/kg/min
Antiarrhythmic		
	Lidocaine	20–50 µg/kg/min
	Amiodarone	1,000 mg/24 h not exceeding 30 mg/min
	Flecainide	50 mg q 12 h
	Procainamide	20 mg/min total 17 mg/kg
	Tocainide	400–600 mg q 8 h
Antifibrinolytics		
	Tranexamic acid	10 mg/kg over 15 minutes with 1 mg/kg/h
	Aminocaproic acid	100 mg/kg in 1 h, followed by 33 mg/kg/h; to a maximum of 25 g/24 h

Appendix 2

KEY PROPERTIES OF VOLATILE ANESTHETICS

	Sevoflurane	Desflurane	Isoflurane	Nitrous
Minimum alveolar concentration (adults, %)	1.8	6.6	1.2	104
Other relevant characteristics				
Class	Halogenated ether	Halogenated ether	Halogenated ether	Inorganic
Molecular weight	200	168	184	44
Boiling point (°C)	60	25	50	−90
Vapor pressure at 20°C (mm Hg)	165	670	250	39,000
Stability with moist soda lime	No	Yes	Yes	Yes
% Metabolized	2–5%	0.02%	0.2%	None
Solubility				
Olive Oil/gas partition coefficient	50	20	100	1.5
Blood/gas partition coefficient	0.7	0.4	1.5	0.5
Brain/blood solubility	1.7	1.3	1.6	1.1
Fat/blood solubility	55	30	50	2
Muscle/fat solubility	2.6	1.7	2.5	1.2

Sevoflurane: Introduced in 1990. Non-inflammable, sweet-smelling, nonirritating volatile fluorinated methyl isopropyl ether. It has a low blood-gas partition coefficient compared to isoflurane but has similar fat and muscle solubilities. Compared to isoflurane, the benefit of quick emergence is attenuated with prolonged anesthesia. The liver metabolizes about 2% of sevoflurane. The kidneys excrete metabolite hexafluoro- isopropanol. Sevoflurane decreases cerebral metabolism, causes vasodilation, increases ICP, impairs flow-metabolism coupling, and impairs electro-physiological monitoring.

Desflurane: Introduced in 1993. Irritant, low-potency, a highly volatile racemic mixture of two enantiomers of a fluorinated methyl-ethyl-ether. Cerebrovascular effects are like sevoflurane but at higher MAC values. About 0.002% of the administered dose is metabolized. Any hepatic or renal toxicity is exceedingly unlikely.

Nitrous oxide: It was introduced in 1844. It is a sweet-smelling, non-irritant, low-potency, analgesic inorganic gas. Nitrous oxide is often used with other volatile agents, complicating clinical assessment. When used in isolation, traditionally reported adverse effects such as increased cerebral metabolism, blood flow, and intracranial pressure might be less significant.

Appendix 3

INDUCTION AGENTS

	Propofol	Etomidate	Ketamine	Methohexital	Thiopental
Class	Alcohol	Imidazole	Phencyclidine	Oxybarbiturate	Thiobarbiturate
Typical neurosurgical doses					
Induction dose (mg/kg)	2–3	0.3	2	1.5–2	5–7
Infusion dose (µg/kg/min)	25–200 µg/kg/min	10–25 µg/kg/min	0.2–1.2 mg/kg/hr	0.5 µg/kg/min	3–5 mg/kg/hr
Key pharmacokinetic parameters					
Early $T_{1/2}$ (min)	2	3–5	8	6	10
$T_{1/2}\beta$ (hours)	4	4	3	4	10
Vd SS (L)	300	300	200	120	300
Clearance (mL/kg/min)	30	15	15	10	3.0
Induction features					
Injection pain	+	++	0	++	0
Movements	++	+++	+	+	0
Hiccups	+	++	+	+++	0
Apnea	+++	++	0	++	+
Hypotension	++	0	0	+	+
Tachycardia	+	+	+++	++	++
Post-operative nausea and vomiting (PONV)	0: anti-emetic	++	+++	+	+

Caution with propofol: Serum concentration of about 4 µg/mL is associated with anesthesia. Propofol decreases cerebral oxygen requirements and cerebral blood flow by about 20% and 30%, respectively, while lactate and glucose metabolism is unaffected. There is a linear correlation between the decrease in cerebral oxygen consumption and blood flow. In healthy subjects, propofol, unlike volatile anesthetics, has favorable effects on cerebral hemodynamics. However, in patients with brain tumors, despite a decrease in ICP, cerebral perfusion pressure might decrease with propofol induction due to systemic hypotension. Similarly, in head-injured patients with impaired autoregulation despite preserved flow metabolism coupling, cerebral blood flow may decrease. Thus, avoiding systemic hypotension during propofol induction is necessary for such patients.

Propofol infusion syndrome (PRIS) was first reported in 1990 in pediatric cases. PRIS is seen with high-dose propofol infusion. Risk factors include prolonged infusion, usually lasting >48 hours in doses >4mg/kg/hr., carbohydrate depletion, increased severity of illness, sepsis, inborn errors of fatty acid metabolism, catecholamine, and steroid use. Dose-dependent incidence: 20% with 5 mg/kg/hr and 30% with 6 mg/kg/hr. A leading cause of PRIS is the inhibition of mitochondrial oxidative metabolism. Propofol increases free fatty acid concentrations. Clinically, it results in increased metabolic acidosis with an increased anionic gap. Organ failures of the kidney, heart, and liver. Rhabdomyolysis and hyperkalemia. Treatment includes immediate propofol discontinuation and supportive care.

Appendix 4

NARCOTIC USE IN NEUROSURGICAL CASES

	Fentanyl	Sufentanil	Remifentanil	Methadone	Hydro-morphone	Morphine
Bolus dose	0.5–2 µg/kg	0.2 µg/kg	0.05–1 µg/kg	0.1–0.3 mg/kg	0.4–2 mg	0.02–0.2 mg/kg
Infusion rate	0.2–0.4 µg/kg/h	0.1–0.1 µg/kg/h	0.05–0.3 µg/kg/min	–	0.2 mg/h	0.02–0.03 mg/kg/h
T1/2γ (hours)	8	10	0.5	35	5	3
Vd steady state (L)	350	550	22	400	325	150
Cl (L/min)	0.6	1	3	0.2	2	2
Active metabolites (AM)	No	No	No	No	Yes	Yes
Renal elimination	10%	0%	0%	20%	0%	10%
Liver failure	Single dose NC MD: reduction advised	Single dose NC MD: reduction advised	No change	Avoided Unless part of detoxification Rx	50% reduction	50% reduction
Renal failure	Generally safe	Generally safe	Ideal	Generally safe	Caution AM acc	Caution AM acc.

(AM: active metabolite; Cl: clearance; MD: maintenance dose; Vd: Volume of distribution)

Context-sensitive half-time: Describes that the target site concentrations/effects of narcotics depend on the dose and duration of infusion. Context sensitivity ranges from very significant for fentanyl to minimal for sufentanil, propofol, remifentanil and alfentanil. Although even with the latter drugs, their half-life increases with the duration of their infusion. Context-sensitive half-time is due to the saturation of various body compartments, such that when the infusion stops, the drugs are offloaded at different rates. Context-sensitive half-life provides a better measure of clearance of drugs compared to a simple elimination half-life. However, active metabolites of drugs can also accumulate and prolong the effects.

Appendix 5

ALTERNATIVES TO OPIOID ANALGESIA

	Route	LD	MD/Frequency
Gabapentin	Oral	300 mg	Daily
Pregabalin	Oral	150 mg	Daily
Acetaminophen	IV	15 mg/kg	6 hourly
Dexmedetomidine	IV	0.3 to 0.7 µg/kg bolus	0.5 µg/kg/hr
Lidocaine	IV	1 mg/kg bolus	1–2 mg/kg/hr
Ketorolac	IV	30 mg	6 hourly
Ketamine	IV	0.25 mg/kg bolus	0.1 mg/kg/hr
Magnesium	IV	30 mg/kg	10 mg/kg/hr

(LD: loading dose; MD: maintenance dose)

Narcotic independent total intravenous anesthesia (TIVA): Infusion with propofol, dexmedetomidine, and lidocaine or propofol-ketamine can be used when narcotics cannot be used for TIVA.

Appendix 6

KEY PROPERTIES OF MUSCLE RELAXANTS

	Rocuronium	*Vecuronium*	*Cisatracurium*
Class	Aminosteroid	Aminosteroid	Benzylisoquinoline
Duration of action	Intermediate	Intermediate	Short
ED95 (mg/kg)	0.3	0.05	0.05
Priming dose (mg/kg)	0.3	0.01	0.01
Intubating dose (mg/kg)	1	0.25	0.3
Onset (min)	2	2.5	5
Recovery index (min)	15	20	15
Complete recovery (min)	105	150	90

Rocuronium: Introduced in 1994. Non-depolarizing, rapid-onset, intermediate-duration muscle relaxant. It is an amino steroid and a desacetoxy analog or vecuronium. ED 95 of 0.3 mg/kg. In a dose range of 0.6–1.2 mg/kg, intubation is possible in a minute, and the effects last 20–35 min. Hemodynamically stable. It has fewer hemodynamic side effects compared to atracurium and mivacurium. Allergic reactions are possible with hypotension and rash, with immunological response reported in 1/2500 patients.

Sugammadex: Introduced in Europe in 2008 and in the US in 2015. "Su"= sugar; "gammadex" = gamma-cyclodextrin. The compound (ORG 25969) was developed to improve rocuronium formulation. Sugammadex has a high affinity for amino-steroid muscle relaxants. At a molar ratio of 1:1, the affinity is rocuronium> vecuronium>>pancuronium. The free-to-bound rocuronium to sugammadex ratio is estimated at 1:25 million. The sugammadex distribution volume is about 20 L, and clearance is about 100 mL/min. Excretion via urine in 24 hours. No dose adjustments are needed with mild to moderate renal failure. It is not recommended in severe renal failure or patients on dialysis.

Dose: Intravenous injections are recommended over ten sec. The dose recommended is 2 mg/kg with moderate (two twitches) neuromuscular bloc and 4 mg/kg with a significant residual block (1–2 post-tetanic twitches). A higher dose is recommended if no reversal is seen at 3 minutes.

Side effects: Adverse reactions (nausea, vomiting, pain, headache, rash, and itching) are dose-dependent (5–10%). Anaphylaxis and bradycardia are possible.

Redosing with rocuronium after sugammadex: The waiting time for redosing rocuronium when usual doses are used is 25 minutes. Although, Rocuronium (1.2 mg/kg) can provide neuromuscular blockade within five minutes after sugammadex reversal.

Drug interactions: Interactions with toremifene (anti-estrogen used for breast cancer treatment) and oral contraceptives (OCP). An additional contraceptive method for patients on OCPs is needed for seven days. Sugammadex can interfere with serum progesterone assay.

Appendix 7

VASOPRESSORS

	Adrenergic receptors or MOA	Dose	Indications	Side effects
Dopamine	D1: ++++++ β1: +++ β2: ++ α1: +	D1: 0.5–3 µg/kg/min β1: 3–10 µg/kg/min α1: 10–20 µg/kg/min Max: 50 µg/kg/min	• Hypotension • Bradycardia	• Tachyarrhythmia • Hypertension • Cardiac ischemia • Tissue ischemia
Epinephrine	α1: +++++ β1: ++++ β2: +++	0.01–0.1 µg/kg/min CPR/anaphylaxis: 1 mg 3 q min	• Hypotension • Bronchospasm • Bradycardia • Anaphylaxis	• Hypertension • Arrhythmias • Cardiac ischemia • Tissue ischemia
Nor-epi-nephrine	α1: +++++ β1: +++ β2: ++	• 0.01–2 µg/kg/min • Max: 5 µg/kg/min	Hypotension	• Bradycardia • Hypertension • Cardiac ischemia • Tissue ischemia
Ephedrine	α1: ++ β1: ++ β2: ++ PS NE release	5–10 mg q 5 min	• Hypotension • Bradycardia	Tachyarrhythmia
Dobutamine	β1: ++++++ β2: ++ α1: +	• 2–20 µg/kg/min • Max: 40 µg/kg/min	• Hypotension • Bradycardia	• Tachyarrhythmia • Ventricular arrhythmias • Hypertension • Cardiac ischemia • Hypotension
Isoproterenol	β1: +++++	2–10 µg/min^{-1}	• Bradycardia • Torsade des pointes/Brugada syndrome	• Ventricular arrhythmias • Hypertension • Cardiac ischemia • Hypotension
Phenylephrine	α1: +++++	0.1–0.5 mg bolus 0.1–10 µg/kg^{-1}/min^{-1}	Hypotension	• Bradycardia • Hypertension • Tissue ischemia
Milrinone	PDEI	Bolus: 50 µg/kg^{-1} over 20 minutes; infusion: 0.4–0.8 µg/kg^{-1}/min^{-1}	Refractory CHF	• Ventricular arrhythmias • Cardiac ischemia • Hypotension

Contd...

Contd...

	Adrenergic receptors or MOA	Dose	Indications	Side effects
Amrinone	PDEI	Bolus: 1 mg/kg^{-1} over 3 minutes; infusion: 5–10 µg/kg^{-1}/min^{-1}	Refractory CHF	• Ventricular arrhythmias • Cardiac ischemia • Hypotension • Thrombocytopenia • Hepatotoxicity
Vasopressin	V1: +++++	Bolus: 0.5 U/kg^{-1} Infusion: 50 U/kg^{-1}/min^{-1}	Shock Hypotension due to ACE inhibitors	• Ventricular arrhythmias • Hypertension • Cardiac, peripheral, and mesenteric ischemia • Hypotension
Methylene blue	GC inhibitor NOS inhibitor	LD: 2 mg/kg over 30 minutes; infusion: 0.25–2 mg/kg/h	Shock: CPB-septic methemoglobinemia	• Hypersensitivity • Hemolytic anemia
Levosimendan	ATP-dependent Ca^{++} channel opener; Ca^{++} sensitizer	LD: 5–10 µg/kg in 10 min. Infusion: 0.05–0.2 µg/kg/min	Refractory CHF	• Tachycardia • Hypotension
Steroids	Inhibits phospholipases and vasodilator synthesis	Hydrocortisone: 50 mg q 6 hourly	• Septic shock • Steroid withdrawal • Anaphylaxis	Immunesuppression

(ACE: angiotensin-converting enzyme; CHF: congestive heart failure; CPB: cardiopulmonary bypass; CPR: cardiopulmonary resuscitation; GC: guanylyl cyclase; MOA: mechanism of action; NOS: nitric oxide synthase; PDEI: phosphodiesterase inhibitor; PS: presynaptic)

INOTROPE AND VASOPRESSORS

Catecholamines

Factors Modulating Response
- Receptor-type sensitivity
- Reflex response
- Up- or downregulation
- *Modulators:* Acidosis or hypoxia.

SPECIFIC FEATURES

Dopamine
- Increases regional blood flow
- *D1 (postsynaptic):* Coronary, mesenteric, renal, and cerebral vascular beds
- *D2 (presynaptic):* Systemic vasculature and renal beds
- *β1:* Weak while α1 effect at higher infusion rates
- The renal protective role of low-dose dopamine infusions is unclear.

Dobutamine
- β1:β2 effect: 3:1
- Inotropic effect > chronotropic effect
- Lower doses (≤5 µg/kg/min) decrease systemic vascular resistance (SVR)
- Intermediate doses (5–15 µg/kg/min) increase cardiac contractility
- Higher doses (≥15 µg/kg/min) increase SVR
- It increases myocardial oxygen consumption
- Used for stress testing

Norepinephrine
- Predominantly α1 effect increases SVR and has minimal impact on cardiac output.
- It increases systolic and diastolic blood pressure, and the latter can improve coronary perfusion.
- Prolonged infusions have a direct toxic effect on the heart.

Epinephrine
- Acts via β1, β2, and α1 adrenergic receptors in cardiac, pulmonary, and systemic blood vessels
- β effects at a low dose and α effects a higher infusion rates
- Increases heart rate (HR), BP, and CO
- It increases coronary blood flow, but higher doses can lead to myocardial injury.

Isoproterenol
- Nonselective β agonist
- Increases HR and myocardial contractility
- Decreases pulmonary and systemic vascular resistance
- Decreases in SVR can cause hypotension.

Vasopressin
- *Receptors:* V1a: Vascular smooth muscles; V1b: Hypothalamus; V2: Renal collecting ducts.

- Increases sensitivity to norepinephrine.
- Increases SVR reflexes, decreases HR, and causes coronary and cerebral vasoconstriction.
- Effects preserved in acidosis and hypoxia.

Levosimendan
- Calcium-sensitizing drugs
- *In chronic heart failure:*
  - Increase Ca^{++} binding to tropomyosin to improve myocardial contractility
  - Activates ATP-dependent K^+ channels and causes vasodilation
  - Hence improves cardiac output.

Phosphodiesterase 3 Inhibitors
- *Decreases the breakdown of cyclic adenosine monophosphate (cAMP):*
  - Increases myocardial contractility
  - Decreases systemic vascular resistance
  - Improves diastolic relaxation
- *Milrinone:*
  - Half-life 2–4 hours
  - Useful in chronic congestive heart failure (CHF) when there is downregulation of receptors
- *Amrinone:*
  - Dose-dependent thrombocytopenia.

Type of shock	Common etiology	CO	HR	CVP	PCWP	SVR	SvO_2
Distributive	Septic shock Hyperdy	Inc	Inc	Dec	Dec	Dec	Inc
	Septic shock Hypody	Dec	Inc	Dec	Dec	Inc	Dec
	Anaphylactic	Dec	Inc	Dec	Dec	Dec	Dec
	Neurogenic	Dec	Inc	Var	Dec	Var	Dec
	Endocrine	Dec	Inc	Var	Var	Dec	Dec
Hypovolemic	Hemorrhage	Dec	Inc	Dec	Dec	Inc	Dec
	Fluid GI/Skin	Dec	Inc	Dec	Dec	Inc	Dec
	Third space	Dec	Inc	Dec	Dec	Inc	Dec
Cardiogenic	Myopathies	Dec	Inc	Inc	Inc	Inc	Dec
	Arrhythmias	Dec	Inc/Dec	Inc	Var	Inc	Dec
	Mechanical, e.g., valves	Dec	Var	Inc	Var	Inc	Dec
Obstructive	Right heart inflow	Dec	Inc	Inc	Dec	Inc	Dec
	Pulmonary outflow	Dec	Inc	Inc	Inc	Inc	Dec

(Dec: decrease; Hyperdy: hyperdynamic; Hypody: hypodynamic; Inc: increase; Var: variable)

Appendix 8

HYPOTENSIVE AGENTS

Drug	Adrenergic receptors or MOA	Pharmacokinetics	Dose	Indications	Contraindications/ side effects
Labetalol	α1 and nonselective β antagonist 1:7	Onset: <1 minute Peak: 5 minutes DOE: 4 hours Half-life: 6 hours	20–80 mg IV bolus; infusion 0.5–2 mg/min	Hypertensive emergencies; pheochromo-cytomas	Allergic reactions; bronchospasm; congestive heart failure; heart block
Esmolol	β1 selective antagonist	Onset: <1 minute Peak: 10 minutes DOE: 30 minutes Half-life: 9 minutes	0.2–1 mg/kg bolus; infusion 0.15 mg/kg/min	Supraventricular arrhythmias; tachycardia/ hypertension/acute MI	Sinus bradycardia/ heart block/ CHF/diabetes/ bronchospasm
Metoprolol	β1 selective antagonist	Onset: Immediate Peak: 20 minutes DOE: 5–8 hours Half-life: 3–7 hours	0.01–2 µg/kg/min Max: 5 µg/kg/min	Hypertension/ acute MI/angina/ cardiomyopathy	Sinus bradycardia/ heart block/ CHF/diabetes/ bronchospasm
Hydralazine	Directly acting vasodilator	Onset: 5 minutes Peak: 10 minutes DOE: 2–6 hours Half-life: 2–8 hours	5–10 mg q 5 min	Hypertension/severe CHF	Drug-induced SLE, allergic reactions, polyneuritis, rash, orthostatic hypotension
Nicardipine	CCB	Onset: Immediate Peak: Immediate DOE: 10–15 min Half-life: 45 minutes	2–20 µg/kg/min Max: 40 µg/kg/min	Hypertension	Tachyarrhythmia Ventricular arrhythmias Hypertension Cardiac ischemia Hypotension
Clevidipine	CCB	Onset: Immediate Peak: 1-2 min DOE: 5-10 minutes Half-life: 15 min	1–2 mg/h to a max of 16 mg/h	Hypertensive crisis	CI to patients with egg allergy, lipid sensitivity
Phentolamine	α Adrenergic antagonist	Onset: Immediate Peak: 10-15 min DOE: 30 min Half-life: 30 min	2–10 µg/min	Pheochromocytoma, dermal necrosis due to norepinephrine, LVF	Ventricular arrhythmias Hypertension Cardiac ischemia Hypotension
Phenoxybezamine	α Adrenergic antagonist	Slow onset Sustained duration of effect	Oral dose 10 mg BD	Pheochromocytoma Preparation for surgery	Potential carcinogenic compound and potential teratogenicity
Fenoldopam	Dopamine D1 receptor agonist	Onset: <5 minutes Peak: 20 min DOE: 30–60 min Half-life: 5 minutes	Infusion: 0.025–0.25 µg/kg/min	Hypertensive crisis, Promotes diuresis natriuresis. Decreases PVR	Allergic reaction to metabisulfite, hypotension, and increased IOP

Contd...

Contd...

Drug	Adrenergic receptors or MOA	Pharmacokinetics	Dose	Indications	Contraindications/ side effects
Nitro glycerine	Nitric oxide donor	Onset: Immediate Peak: Immediate DOE: 5 minutes Half-life: 2 minutes	Bolus: 12.5–25 µg; infusion: 5–200 µg/min	Angina Refractory CHF Acute MI Hypertensive crisis	Increases ICP and IOP, met-hemoglobinemia and tolerance
Nitroprusside	Nitric oxide donor	Onset: Immediate Peak: Immediate DOE: 1–2 minutes Half-life: 90 seconds	0.3–10 µg/kg/min	Severe hypertension, CHF	Cyanide toxicity >10 µg/kg/min, severe hypotension possible, increased ICP, decreased CPP

(CCB: calcium channel blockers; CHF: congestive heart failure; CPP: cerebral perfusion pressure; DOE: duration of effect; ICP: intracranial pressure; IOP: intraocular pressure; PVR: Peripheral vascular resistance; LVF: left ventricular failure; MI: myocardial infarction; MOA: mechanism of action; SLE: systemic lupus erythematosus)

HYPERTENSION IN NEUROANESTHESIA

- *Underlying hypertensive disease*
  - Inadequate perioperative management
  - Drug withdrawal: Clonidine, beta-blockers
  - Steroid-induced hypertension
- *Intubation and extubation response*
- *Neurological conditions:*
  - *Cushing's reflex:* Increased ICP results in increased pulse pressure, bradycardia, irregular respirations
  - Autonomic hyper-reflexia
  - *Neuroendocrine syndromes:* Cushing's syndrome, acromegaly
- *Neurosurgical events:*
  - *Surgical pain:*
    - Pinning
    - Incision
    - *Tissue retraction:* Especially in CN-V distribution
    - Craniotomy
  - Cranial nerve traction
  - Brainstem manipulation

Induced Hypertension

- Carotid surgery
- Temporary intracranial vascular occlusion
- Ischemic stroke
- Vasospasm
- Improve spinal cord perfusion
- Testing homeostasis after tumor or AVM resection

Induced Hypotension
- Decrease blood loss during surgery
  - Spine surgery
  - Tumors
  - AVM surgery
- *Endovascular:*
  - AVM embolization
  - For testing cerebrovascular reserve during carotid occlusion.

Appendix 9

ANTIBIOTIC PROPHYLAXIS

Antibiotic	Dose	Interval	Spectrum	Side effects
Cefazolin	1 g IV <80 kg 2 g IV >80 kg 30 mg/kg	4 hours	• Gm +ve: *Staphylococcus aureus* and streptococci • Gm −ve: *Moraxella*; *Escherichia coli*, *Klebsiella* and *Proteus*	• Allergic reactions • Anaphylaxis • Skin reaction • Marrow suppression • Liver dysfunction
Cefuroxime (crosses BBB)	1.5 g IV 50 mg/kg	6 hours	• Gm +ve: *S. aureus*; streptococci • Gm −ve: *Moraxella, E. coli, Hemophilus influenzae* and *Neisseria*	• Allergic reactions • Anaphylaxis • Skin reaction • Marrow suppression • Eosinophilia
Cefamandole	1 g IV 40 mg/kg	6 hours	• Gm +ve: *S. aureus* and streptococci • Gm −ve: *Moraxella, E. coli, H. influenzae,* and *Neisseria*	• Allergic reactions • Anaphylaxis • Skin reaction • Marrow suppression • Interstitial nephritis
Cefotetan	1–2 g 40 mg/kg	4 hours	• Gm +ve: *S. aureus* and streptococci • Gm −ve: *Moraxella, E. coli, H. influenzae, Neisseria,* and *Bacteroides* species	• Allergic reactions • Anaphylaxis • Skin reaction • Marrow suppression • Interstitial nephritis
Clindamycin	600–900 mg IV 3–6 mg/kg	6 hours	• Gm +ve: *S. aureus* Streptococci • Gm −ve: *Moraxella, E. coli, H. influenzae, Neisseria,* and *Bacteroides* species	• Allergic reactions • Anaphylaxis • Stevens-Johnson syndrome • *Clostridium difficile* diarrhea • Skin reactions
Gentamycin	80–120 mg 1.5 mg/kg IV	8 hours	• GM −ve: *Pseudomonas, E. coli, Proetus, Klebsiella, Enterobacter, Serratia, Providencia, Acinetobacter, Citrobacter, Morganella, Enterococcus* • *Mycobacterium* spp. • Gm +: *Staphylococcus* species, *Viridans streptococci*	• Ototoxicity • Nephrotoxicity • Neuromuscular blockade
Metronidazole	0.8–1 g IV 15 mg/kg initially 7.5 mg/kg afterward	8 hours	• Anaerobic Gm −ve: *Bacteroides, Fusobacterium, Porphyromonas, Prevotella* Anaerobic • Gm +ve: *Clostridium*; Anaerobic cocci: Peptostreptococci Protozoa: *Blastocystis hominis, Entamoeba histolytica, Giardia lamblia, Trichomonas vaginalis*	Gastrointestinal disturbances, metallic taste, neurological symptoms, leukopenia, thrombocytopenia, hypersensitivity reaction, and alcohol intolerance
Vancomycin	1 g IV 10–15 mg/kg	8 hours	Gm +ve: *S. aureus*; streptococci; Gm −ve: Enterococci; *Clostridium*; *Listeria*; *Actinomyces*	Redman syndrome with rapid infusion, nephrotoxicity, neutropenia, and drug fever

(Gm: gram; +ve: positive; −ve: negative; IV: intravenous)

Appendix 10

ANTICONVULSANTS

Drug	Average Half-life	Indications/ Typical daily dose	Side-effects Relevant comment
Commonly used anticonvulsant drugs			
Lamotrigine (Lamictal)	15–60 hours	• CPS/GTC >2 years • 50–100 mg 12 hourly • Requires gradual discontinuation	• Allergic reactions • Drug interactions • Dizziness, diplopia, ataxia; skin rash; teratogenic; nephrotoxic
Gabapentin (Neurontin)	6 hours	CPS usually >12 years 300 mg increasing to 1,800 mg in three doses	Sedation, dizziness, ataxia, nystagmus, and eosinophilia systemic reaction; allergic reactions
Levetiracetam (Keppra)	8 hours	GTC; Myotonic; CPS >6 years. 500 mg increasing to 1500 mg 12 hourly, as tolerated.	Somnolence, fatigue, impaired coordination, behavioral change, and can impair renal functions
Phenytoin (Dilantin)	20 hours	GTC/CPS/SE 100 mg to 300 mg 8 hourly	IV doses cause bradycardia, heart blocks, and hypotension; infuse slowly
Zonisamide (Zonegran)	60 hours	CPS >16 years 100 mg increasing to 200 mg OD	Rash, cognitive dysfunction; tremors, kidney stones, aplastic anemia; sudden death. Caution with driving.
Carbamazepine (Tegretol)	35 hours	CPS/mixed seizures and GTC seizures 200 mg bid gradually increased to max of 1000 mg/day	Sedation; cognitive side effects; rash; dry mouth; Steven Johnson syndrome, bone marrow depression, SIADH and hyponatremia (2-40%), and drug interactions
Oxacarbazine (Trileptal)	• 3 hours • Long half-life of an active	CPS typically >4 years 150 mg increasing to 1,200 mg OD	SIADH, hyponatremia, skin rash, cognitive dysfunction, ataxia, blurred vision, and tinnitus; Steven Johnson syndrome
Valproic acid (Depakene)	10–20 hours	Absence seizures; Mixed seizures;CPS 750 mg/day, to max 2000 mg/day	GI side effects, cognitive dysfunction, blurred vision tinnitus, weight gain, Hepatotoxicity, pancreatitis, neural tube defects, and suicidal ideation
Topiramate (Topamax)	20 hours	CPS and GTC seizures 25 mg increased to 50 mg q 6 hourly, extended-release formulations given OD	Cognitive side effects, weight loss, metabolic acidosis, hyperammonemia, decreased sweating, and teratogenicity

Contd...

Contd...

Drug	Average Half-life	Indications/ Typical daily dose	Side-effects Relevant comment
Other anticonvulsant drugs			
Phenobarbital (Luminal)	100 hours	GTC; SE; Myotonic seizures; inc. ICP, neuroprotection. 4–6 mg/kg/day	Sedation, ataxia, confusion, psychosis, dependence, developmental defects, and carcinogenicity
Primidone (Mysoline)	10 hours	• GTC, CPS, and mixed seizures • 100 mg po, gradually increased, maximum 2 g/day BID	Ataxia, vertigo, psychosis, sedation, nausea and vomiting, anemia, suicidal ideation, and sudden withdrawal may cause convulsions
Ethosuximide (Zarontin)	48 hours	Absence seizures, 250 mg/day gradually to 1500 mg/day	GI symptoms, cognitive S/E, cramps, Blood dyscrasia, hepatic or renal toxicity, facial growth, macroglossia, suicidal ideation
Divalproex (Depakote: Combination valproic acid and sod valproate)	6 hours	Absence seizures; Mixed seizures; CPS 10 mg/kg/day, increasing to 20 mg/kg/day	GI side effects, Hepatotoxicity, pancreatitis, cognitive dysfunction, blurred vision tinnitus, tremors, weight gain, and suicidal ideation
Clonazepam (Klonopin)	40 hours	Absence seizures, focal seizures, non-convulsive SE. 0.25 – 1 mg BID	Drowsiness, ataxia, cognitive changes, excessive salivation, and withdrawal risk
Felbamate (Felbatol)	20 hours	CPS refractory to Rx 1.2 g/day increased to 3.6 g/day in divided 3 or 4 doses	Vison disturbances, weight loss, anorexia, aplastic anemia and acute hepatic failure
Tiagabine (Gabitril)	8 hours	CPS >12 years 4 mg increases substantially if with a hepatic enzyme inducer.	GI side effects, seizures initially, with dose escalation and on withdrawal, cognitive and behavioral changes, suicidal ideation, and teratogenesis

(GTC: generalized tonic clonic seizures; CPS: complex partial seizures; SE: Status epilepticus, GI: gastrointestinal side-effects, LD: loading dose; SIADH: syndrome of inappropriate antidiuretic hormone)

Appendix 11

RAPID NEURO EXAM

- *Higher functions:*
  - *Consciousness:* Awake, verbal command, pain, and none
  - *Orientation:* Time/Place
  - Mood and affect
  - Attention
  - *Language:* Fluency, reading, writing, comprehension, naming, and repetition
  - *Memory:* Immediate, recent, and remote
  - *Higher functions:* Abstraction, judgment, insight, reasoning, and general knowledge
- *Cranial nerves:*
  - *Cranial nerve (CN) I:* Olfactory: R/O local pathology. Test one nostril with a nonirritating odorant: Soap, lemon, vanilla, or coffee.
  - *CN II:* Optic: Acuity, field, and fundus
  - *CN II and III:* Optic and oculomotor: Pupillary reaction and accommodation
  - *CN III, IV, and VI:* Oculomotor, trochlear, and abducens:
    - Ocular alignment, smooth movements, and nystagmus
    - III vertical, IV medial, and VI lateral
  - *CN V:* Trigeminal three divisions: Ophthalmic; maxillary, and mandibular
    - Masseter muscle strength, corneal reflex, and jaw jerk
  - *CN VII:* Facial nerve: Forehead bilateral supranuclear
    - *Rest of face:* Smile, close eyelids, and blow your cheek infra-nuclear
  - *CN VIII:* Cochlear: Hearing finger rubbing at arm length
  - *CN IX and X:* Swallowing, gagging, coughing, and voice
  - *CN XI:* Spinal accessory: Shrug shoulder
  - *CN XII:* Hypoglossal: Deviation of the protruded tongue
- *Muscle strength, tone, and bulk:*
  - Motor exam
    - *Muscle exam:* BESST: *B*ulk, *E*ndurance, *S*peed, *S*trength, *T*one
    - *Muscle strength scale:*
      - 0: No movement
      - 1: Visible contraction without movement
      - 2: Movement seen
      - 3: Antigravity
      - 4: Against some resistance
      - 5: Against normal resistance
  - Muscles tested **(Table 1)**

Table 1: Upper extremity and lower extremity muscles tested.

Upper extremity	Lower extremity
Deltoid	Iliopsoas
Biceps	Quadriceps
Triceps	Hamstrings
Extensor carpi radialis	Tibialis anterior
Abductor pollicis brevis	Gastrocnemius/soleus
Interossei	

- *Reflexes:*
  - *Tested reflexes:* Biceps (C5-6), triceps (C6-7), patellar (L2-4), and ankle (S1-2)
  - *Grading scale:*
    - 0: Absent
    - 1: Sluggish
    - 2: Normal
    - 3: Brisk
    - 4: Clonus
  - *Reinforcement:* Contraction of another group, pulling apart the arms, and increases reflex response
  - *Babinski reflex (L4-S2):*
    - *Normal:* Toes flex
    - *Abnormal:* Toes extended
    - *Positive:* Corticospinal dysfunction
- *Coordination:*
  - *Tests:*
    - Finger nose test
    - Finger tapping
    - Heel shin test
    - Rapid alternate movements
  - *Evaluate:* Control, precision, and smoothness
- *Sensory function:*
  - Tests and key dermatomes are listed in **Table 2**.
  - Explain the test, with the eyes closed, compare the left and right sides, and ask, "About the same?"
    - Light touch/pressure
    - Pain/temperature
    - Proprioception
    - Vibration (128 Hz)
  - *Grades:* Absent, reduced, normal, exaggerated, and abnormal (perverted)
  - *Stereognosis:* Object recognition with eyes closed
  - *Graphesthesia:* Recognizing shapes drawn on hand with eyes closed
  - *Romberg sign:* Swaying or falling with the eyes closed

Table 2: Key dermatomes.

Site	Dermatome
Neck	C4
Lateral elbow	C5
Thumb	C6
Middle finger	C7
Little finger	C8
Medial elbow	T1
Axilla	T2
Nipple	T4
Umbilicus	T10
Inguinal region	T12
Anterior thigh	L2
Medial femoral condyle	L3
Medial malleolus	L4
Dorsum of foot	L5
Lateral heel	S1
Popliteal fossa midline	S2
Ischial tuberosity	S3
Perineum	S4–S5

- *Gait:*
    - *Posture:* Body and limbs
    - *Walk on a line:* Normal, on toes, on the heel, and tandem
    - Stride length, speed, and rhythm
    - *Walking pattern:* Base, steadiness, arm swing, and symmetry
    - *Control:* Start, stop and turn on the cue
- *Meningeal signs and symptoms:*
    - *Symptoms:*
        - Headache
        - Photophobia
        - Neck stiffness
        - Seizures with meningitis
    - *Signs:*
        - *Nuchal rigidity:* Resists neck flexion
        - *Kernig's sign:* Pain on the extension of the knee with a flexed hip.
        - *Brudzenski's sign:* Flexion of the hip and knees on flexing the neck
- *Assessment of coma patients*
    - Posture **(Fig. 1 and Table 3)**

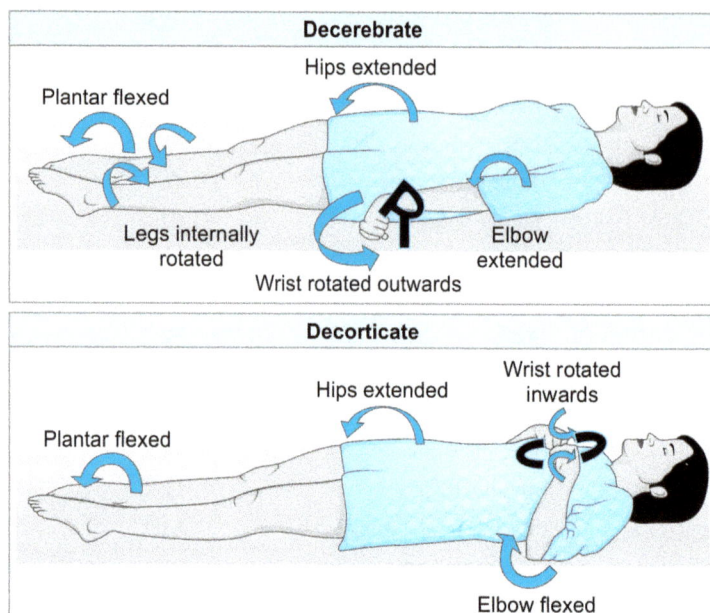

Fig. 1: Mnemonic for Dece"R"ebrate and dec"O"rticate posture.

Table 3: Decerebrate and decorticate postures and the sites affected.

	Decorticate	Decerebrate
Injury site	• Upper midbrain • Above the red nucleus • Upper limb flexors dominate	• Upper pons • Below the red nucleus • Upper limb extensors dominate
Shoulder	Adducted	Adducted
Elbow	Flexed	Extended
Forearm	Supinated	Pronated
Wrist	Flexed inward	Flexed outward
Hip	Internally rotated	Normal
Knees	Extended	Extended
Ankle	Plantar flexed	Plantar flexed
Summary	"Mummy" like	

- Abnormal breathing patterns **(Table 4)**
- Localizing signs
- Neck rigidity
- *Coma broad etiologies:*
  - *Coma without focal signs or neck stiffness:*
    - Ischemia, hypoxia, toxemia, trauma, inflammation, post-seizure

Table 4: Pathological breathing patterns.

Breathing	Pattern	Waveform	Injury site
Central neurogenic hyperventilation	Increased tidal volume and respiratory rate of at least 25 bpm		Upper pons and midbrain tumor or trauma
Cheyne-Stokes breathing	Periods of apnea and hyperventilation of 45 to 90 seconds in duration		Congestive heart failure, loss of cortical control
Apneustic breathing	Prolonged inspiration and expiration		Lower midbrain and upper pons
Cluster breathing	A cluster of breath with intervening apnea		Lower pons, higher medulla
Ataxic breathing	Completely irregular, with pauses in between		Medulla and reticular activating system
Biot's breathing	Hyperventilation with regular apneic pauses		Uncal or tentorial herniation
Kussmaul breathing	Persistent hyperventilation		Metabolic acidosis of acidosis from other causes

- *Coma with focal signs:*
    - Tumor, vascular (stroke, hemorrhage, thrombosis), abscess, trauma
- *Coma with neck stiffness:*
    - Subarachnoid hemorrhage, meningitis, meningoencephalitis.

Appendix 12

GENERAL PEDIATRIC CONCERNS

NEURAL DEVELOPMENT IN INFANCY

- *Neural development activity:*
  - Apoptosis and developmental changes occur throughout early childhood
  - Myelination of the peripheral nervous system affects the local anesthetic response and the latency of evoked potentials
  - Pain pathways are immature. Sensitization is possible with chronic pain.
- The spine and skull are cartilaginous.
- The posterior fontanelle closes by 3 months and the anterior by 18 months.
- The spinal cord extends to L3/4 at birth and L1 vertebrae by 1 year.
- The dural sac extends to S3/4 at S2 by 1 year.
- *Cerebral blood flow (CBF)* is lower in neonates (40 mL/100 g/min) but higher in young children (100 mL/100 g/min) compared to adults (50 mL/100 g/min).
- Autoregulation and metabolic regulation are operational.
- Sutures are not closed. An increase in intracranial pressure (ICP), such as with hydrocephalus in infancy, increases head circumference without a concomitant increase in the pressure until the late stages.

Pharmacological Factors

- *The total body water content of 75% is higher in neonates as compared to 55% in adults* resulting in an increased volume of distribution of water-soluble drugs
- Muscle compartment small (20%) as compared to adults (50%)
- The fat compartment is also smaller than adults
- The brain/body weight ratio is higher in children compared to adults
- Hepatic and renal functions immature
- Total serum protein (albumin and alpha-1-glycoproteins) low
- Drug half-life prolonged due to slower metabolism and elimination
- *Minimum alveolar concentration (MAC):*
  - MAC is higher in children than in adults
  - For isoflurane and desflurane, it peaks at 3-months
  - With sevoflurane, it linearly decreases with age
- Despite higher MAC values, induction is faster in neonates due to a smaller functional residual capacity (FRC), increased cerebral blood flow, lower tissue/blood solubility, and lower blood/gas solubility.

Pediatric Airway (Fig. 1)

- An airway exam may not be possible
- Cephalad larynx
- Prominent occiput
- Large tongue
- Large floppy epiglottis
- Narrow laryngeal inlet
- Large tonsils
- Low FRC, high closing volumes, and high metabolic rate result in rapid desaturation
- *The formula for determining tube sizes in children:*
  - Uncuffed endotracheal tube (ETT) size for children 1–10 years of age, internal diameter (mm) = age/4 + 4 mm
  - *Nasogastric/orogastric or Foley catheter size:* 2× the ETT size in mm = Catheter size in French gauge
  - *ETT depth of placement:* 3 × numeral value of ETT tube size in cm
  - *Chest tube maximum:* Not exceeding 4 × ETT size
  - *ETT sizes for neonates:* <1 kg, 2.5 mm; <2 kg, 3 mm; <3 kg, 3.5 mm; >3 kg, 4 mm.

Fasting Status

- *Minimum fasting time:*
  - *Clear fluid:* 2 hours
  - *Breast milk:* 4 hours

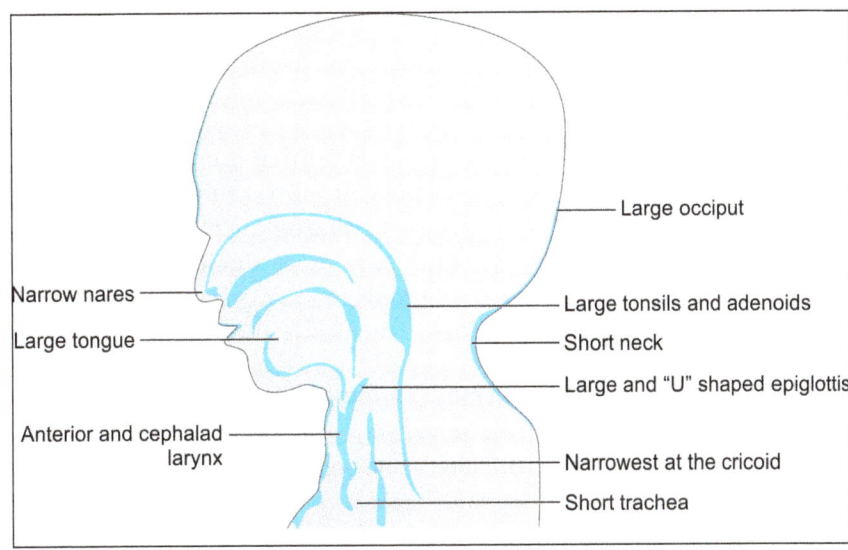

Fig 1: Anatomical features of pediatric airway.

- *Light meal with minimal fat:* 6 hours
- *Solid food:* 8 hours.

Premedication
- Rarely used for neurosurgery due to the risk of respiratory depression and raised ICP
- *Nonpharmacological anxiolysis:*
  - *Audiovisual distraction:* Video games, movies, child-life specialists
  - Role in cognitively impaired cases debatable
- The participation of parents is debated and has to be individually assessed
- Oral midazolam if needed; Fentanyl lollipops
- Intranasal midazolam, dexmedetomidine, and ketamine
- Rectal delivery possible for benzodiazepine and ketamine
- IV sedation if there is pre-existing access.

Vascular Access: Indication of Central Venous Pressure in Pediatric Neurosurgery
- Significant blood loss
- Poor IV access
- Monitoring central venous line (CVL)
- Repeated blood sample
- Hypertonic fluid use anticipated
- Venous air embolism.

Thermoregulation in Children
- *Hypothermia:* A core temperature <36°C if >5 years or 36.5°C if <5 years
- Larger surface area to body weight ratio
- Lacks subcutaneous fat
- Lacks muscle mass to generate heat
- It relies on non-shivering thermogenesis through brown fat
- Radiative heat loss is the most significant. Minimizing it by keeping OR at 80°F or cautiously using infrared heaters helps.
- Radiative heat loss is more significant than convective (airflow), evaporative (humidification of gases), and conductive (contact with table) heat loss.

Fluid Replacement Formula in Children

The total body water content decreases with age; hence, fluid requirements decrease with increasing body weight **(Table 1)**:
- *01–10 kg:* 4 mL/kg/h
- *10–20 kg:* 40 mL/h + 2 mL/kg/h for weight between 10 and 20 kg
- *>20 kg:* 60 mL/h + 1 mL/kg/h for body weight exceeding 20 kg.

Table 1: Assessment of hydration.

Dehydration	Weight loss % body weight	Clinical features	Replacement volume/10 kg weight
Mild	5%	Dry tongue, loss of skin turgor	50 mL
Moderate	10%	Increased HR, decreased UO, and sunken fontanelles	100 mL
Severe	15%	Absent tears, hypotension (late sign), and anuria	150 mL

(HR: heart rate; UO: urine output)

Recommended fluids in neuroanesthesia: Normal saline/Plasmalyte; Ringer's lactate is considered hypotonic.

Anesthetic Neurotoxicity: Children
- There is no scientific basis for delaying necessary surgery.
- Hazards of anesthetic exposure remain unproven.
- The risk of minimizing anesthesia exposure must be balanced against inadequate pain relief during surgery, which can cause long-term harm.

Appendix 13

ANTIEMETIC DRUGS

Class	Drug	Dose	Notable Side effects
Central sedatives			
Anxiolytics	Lorazepam	2–4 mg	May enhance sedative effects of concurrent sedatives
Steroids	Dexamethasone	4 mg	Via NK1 receptors; S/E: Immunosuppression
Anesthetics	Propofol		Via 5HT3 receptors; S/E: Sedation
Chemoreceptor trigger zone			
D2 receptor blockers	Metoclopramide (oral or IV)	10 mg Max: 60 mg/day	Drowsiness, restlessness, fatigue; Tardive dyskinesia, C/I: children, gastrointestinal obstruction, epilepsy, and allergy to a drug
5HT3	Ondansetron	4–8 mg	QT prolongation, serotonergic syndrome, and allergic reactions are possible
	Dolansetron	100–200 mg	Highly selective serotonin (HT3) blocker; HT3 receptors are on the vagal nerve; prolonged QTc, IV injections, hypotension, bradycardia, syncope; and allergic reactions possible
	Palonosetron	0.25 mg	0.075–0.25 mg in 6 mL over 30 seconds; serotonergic syndrome; and allergic reactions are possible
NK1	Aprepitant	40–120 mg PO	Hepatic enzyme inducer, hence interaction with cytochrome P3A4 inhibitors and inducers, bone marrow depression, and allergic reactions
	Netupitant	300 mg capsule	Capsule 300 mg with palonosetron 0.5 mg; allergic reactions, serotonin syndrome, hepatic enzyme inducer, and hence interaction with cytochrome P3A4 inhibitors and inducers
H2 blockers	Ranitidine (Zantac)	150 mg	**Recalled due to possible carcinogenic contaminant. N-nitrosodimethylamine whose concentrations increase time and temperature**
	Famotidine (Pepcid)	20–40 mg OD	Headache, dizziness, bowel disturbances: Constipation, diarrhea, and allergic reactions
	Cimetidine (Tagamet)	200–400 mg	Doses 2–3× per day, max dose 2,400 mg; headache, dizziness, and diarrhea; allergic reactions; and drug interactions
H1 generation 1	Promethazine (Phenergan)	12.5–25 mg	Drowsiness, difficulty in sleeping, dry mouth, blurred vision, urinary retention, and vomiting
	Diphenhydramine (Benadryl)	25–50 mg	Sedation, tiredness, sleepiness, dizziness, constipation, disturbed coordination, urinary retention, hypotension, tachycardia, palpitations, and confusion
	Prochlorperazine Compazine)	5–10 mg	Dizziness, blurred vision, dry mouth, stuffed nose, headache, nausea, constipation, and difficulty in urinating
	Meclizine (Antivert)	25–100 mg	Drowsiness, tiredness, headache, blurred vision, and dry mouth
	Doxylamine	25 mg	Dry mouth, dizziness, constipation, decreased sweating, and decreased urinating
H1 generation 2	Loratadine (Claritin)	10 mg	Headache, dry mouth, sore throat, mouth sore, and allergic reactions

ONDANSETRON DOSES

- *Mild risk of nausea and vomiting:* 8 mg IV 30 minutes before a trigger event
- *Moderate risk of severe nausea and vomiting:* 8 mg IV 30 minutes before trigger and 8 mg every 8–12 hours
- *Severe risk of significant nausea and vomiting:* Rx limited to 8 mg single dose 30-60 minutes before trigger event; a higher dose (32 mg) was previously used but was withdrawn due to cardiac concerns.

Serotonin syndrome: Features: agitation, hallucination, delirium, coma, fever, autonomic hyperreflexia/tremors/seizures/diarrhea. Etiology: Antiemetics and antidepressants. Possible drug interactions, antidepressants, narcotics, and side effects of several drugs, above.

Etiology of serotonergic syndrome	
Mechanism	Drugs
Increased substrate	Tryptophan, lithium
Increased release	CNS stimulants: Cocaine and amphetamines
Decreased reuptake	Antidepressants, opioids, antiemetics, and antiepileptics
Decreased breakdown	Monoamine oxidase inhibitors, oxazolidinone antibiotics, methylene blue, procarbazine
Decreased metabolism	Hepatic micro enzyme inhibitors: anti-fungal agents, anti-viral and antibiotics

Appendix 14

ANTIPLATELET DRUGS

Drug	Daily dose	Route	Half-life	Desired withdrawal	Neuro-applications	Common side-effects
Cox 2 inhibitors						
Aspirin	Fever dose> anti-coagulant dose (81mg/day)	PO	20 minutes	7 days	TIA and stroke Rx	• Allergic reaction • Hemorrhagic complications
ADP receptor blockers						
Clopidogrel (Plavix)	75 mg OD	PO	6 hours	5 days	TIA stroke, stent	• Allergic reaction • Serious hemorrhagic complications
Prasugrel (Effient)	5–10 mg OD	PO	7 hours	7 days	3.75 mg OD effective in stroke prevention	• Allergic reaction • Serious hemorrhagic complications
Ticagrelor (Brilinta)	60–90 mg BD	PO	7 hours	5 days	• Acute ischemic stroke • High risk TIA	• Dyspnea • Serious hemorrhagic complications
Ticlopidine (Ticlid)	250 mg BD	PO	12 hours	14 days	• Second-line • Rx for stroke prevention	• Neutropenia • Thrombotic thrombocyto-penic purpura
Phosphodiesterase inhibitors						
Dipyridamole (Persantin)	PO: 75–10 µg 6–8 h 0.14 mg/kg/min IV Dose: Max 60 mg	PO/IV	α:40 minutes β:10 hours	2 days	Prevention of stroke	• Allergic reactions • Serious S/E possible • GI, CVS, CNS, and ocular side-effects
Cilostazol (Pletal)	100 mg BD	PO	10 hours	5 days	Possible stroke prevention	Headache, GI S/E and palpitations. C/I with CHF
GP IIb/IIIa inhibitors						
Abciximab (ReoPro)	LD: 0.25 µg/kg MD: 0.1 µg/kg/min Dose: Max 10 µg/min	IV	α:10 minutes β:40 minutes	2–3 days platelet recovery 48 hours	• Possible stroke thrombolysis • Use in INR	GI symptoms; Allergic reaction Hemorrhagic complications
Epitifibatide (Integrilin)	LD: 180 µg/kg MD: 2 µg/kg/min	IV	2.5 hours	8 hours	Possible stroke thrombolysis	Hemorrhagic complications
Tirofiban (Aggrastat)	LD: 25 µg/kg MD: 0.1 µg/kg/min	IV	2 hours	4 hours	After mechanical thrombectomy for stroke	Hemorrhagic complications; allergic reaction; thrombocytopenia

(ACS: acute coronary syndrome; ADP: adenosine diphosphate; CHF: congestive heart failure; CVA: cerebrovascular accident; GI: gastrointestinal; ICH: intracranial hemorrhage; LD: loading dose; MD: maintenance dose; PAD: peripheral arterial disease; PCI: percutaneous coronary intervention; TIA: transient ischemic attack)

Appendix 15

IV FLUID MANAGEMENT

- *Osmolarity:* Osm/L while osmolality: Osm/kg
- *Calculated plasma osmolality:* 2 × (Na⁺ mEq/L) + [BUN (mg/dL)/2.8] + [Glucose (mg/dL)/18]
- However, even when raised, BUN remains inconsequential. BUN is lipid-soluble and diffuses across the capillary membrane. Therefore, A simpler formula for plasma osmolarity is:
  - *Calculated plasma osmolality:* 2 × (Na⁺ mEq/L) + + [Glucose (mg/dL)/18]
- *Free water deficit:* [(serum Na – 140)/140] × total body water.

Characteristics of intravenous fluids.

Fluid	pH	mOsm/L	Na	Cl	K	Ca	Mg	Dextrose	Lactate
5% Dextrose	4.3	278	–	–	–	–	–	50	–
5% Dextrose +0.45 saline	4.3	405	77	77	–	–	–	50	–
0.9 NaCl	5.5	308	154	154	–	–	–	–	–
Ringer lactate	6.5	274	130	109	4	3	–	–	28
3% Saline	7.4	1,026	513	513	–	–	–	–	–
20% Mannitol	6.3	1,098	–	–	–	–	–	–	–
5% Albumin	6.9	290	145	130	1–2	–	–	–	–

Clinical features and management of electrolyte imbalances.

Condition	Symptoms	Treatment concerns
Hyponatremia <130	Cognitive changes, seizures, focal symptoms, headache, and brain edema	Rapid correction of Na (>2 mEq/h) central pontine myelinolysis
Hypernatremia >160	Cognitive changes, seizures, rigidity, tremors, and myoclonus	Rapid correction with hypotonic solutions can cause brain edema
Hypokalemia <2.5	Cardiac arrhythmias, muscle weakness, and tetany	Cardiac monitoring essential
Hyperkalemia >7.0	Cardiac toxicity, tall peaked T waves, and muscle weakness (±)	Urgent treatment is often required with glucose/insulin or calcium
Hypocalcemia	Acute decrease requires immediate IV replacement Chronic: Cognitive changes, seizures, tetany, and pseudotumor cerebri	Long-term complications with Ca⁺⁺ replacement and vitamin D can be due to nephrocalcinosis, renal impairment, soft tissue calcium deposits

Contd...

Contd...

Condition	Symptoms	Treatment concerns
Hypercalcemia	Headache, cognitive changes, increased reflexes, increased urination, and thirst	Serum Ca^{++} of >14 mg/dL or with CNS symptoms need treatment; normal saline infusion; calcitonin is helpful, but tachyphylaxis may occur
Hypomagnesemia	Cognitive changes increased reflexes, tetany, tremors, and myoclonus	IV magnesium replacement needs careful monitoring in renal failure
Hypermagnesemia	Cognitive changes decreased reflexes and muscle weakness	Rx affected by renal functions, if impaired; Rx with IV saline, $CaCl_2$, furosemide, and hemodialysis
Hypophosphatemia	Cognitive changes, decreased reflexes, muscle weakness, and focal signs	Normal saline, diuretics, phosphate binders orally, and hemodialysis
Hyperphosphatemia	Muscle weakness	Oral or IV phosphate replacement

Pseudohyponatremia is seen with hyperglycemia, hyperlipidemia, hyperproteinemia, or mannitol administration. Usually seen in diabetes, multiple myeloma, liver, and kidney diseases that increase nonsodium solutes in the blood.

Appendix 16

NEUROLOGICAL CONDITIONS WITH ELECTROLYTE IMBALANCES

Diabetes insipidus (DI): Major causes are idiopathic, pituitary tumors, postoperative, and head injury. Nephrogenic DI is the failure of kidneys to respond to antidiuretic hormone (ADH). The latter can be due to drugs such as lithium.

	Diabetes insipidus	Syndrome of inappropriate ADH	Central salt wasting syndrome
Pathogenesis			
Mechanism	Central: Dec. ADH Or, Nephrogenic: Decreased renal ADH response	Increased and inappropriate ADH release	Renal Na^+ loss: Inc. BNP Neurogenic
Etiology	*Shock; pain; anxiety; surgery; Trauma, trauma, infections*	*Trauma, trauma, infections, drugs*	*Trauma, trauma, infections, drugs*
Drugs	Lithium, Propofol	Opiates, NSAIDs, anesthetics, Oral hypoglycemic agents	
General features			
Urine Output	>250 mL/hr	Decreased	Increased
ECF Volume	Decreased	Increased	Decreased
Serum Osmolarity (mOsm/kg)	Increased >295	Decreased <285	Decreased <285
Urine Osmolarity (mOsm/kg)	Decreased <200	Increased >200	Decreased <200
Body weight Cognition	Decreased	Increased	Decreased
Cognition	Normal, impaired	• Confusion/lethargy • Nausea/vomiting • Tremors/cramps	Impaired, agitation, coma
Serum parameters			
Serum Na^+ (mEq/L)	>145	<135	<135
Serum K^+ (mEq/L)	Decreased	Normal	Normal/increased
Serum Albumin	Increased	Normal	Increased
BUN	Decreased	Decreased	Increased
Hct	Increased	Normal	Increased
Urine parameters			
Urine Sp. gravity	<1.005	>1.010	>1.010
Urine Na^+ mEq/L	Dec	>40	>40
Treatment	• Water Replacement • Vasopressin or Desmopressin • Hydrochlorothiazide • Chlorpropamide	• Fluid restriction • Hypertonic saline • Furosemide • ADH receptor antagonists • Demeclocycline	• Fluid and Na replacement • Fludrocortisone

ADH receptor antagonists:
- Arginine vasopressin or ADH receptor antagonists.
- V2 receptor antagonists increased Na and promoted free water clearance.
- They help treat the syndrome of inappropriate antidiuretic hormone (SIADH) and euvolemic or hypovolemic hyponatremia.
- *Examples:* Conivaptan and tolvaptan.

Propofol-induced diabetes insipidus (DI): Propofol infusions have resulted in DI with hypotonic urine (sp. gravity <1.005), increased urine output (<->400 mL/hr.), and increased serum sodium. It is responsive to desmopressin treatment. Treatment includes discontinuation of propofol, and treatment with desmopressin may be required.

Sodium and water content	
Water balance	
Total body water (% weight)	• Males: 60%; Females 50% • Less on obese more in lean habitus
Water distribution (% Total)	Intracellular 70%; Interstitial 20%; Intracellular 10%
Daily water intake	*Average:* 2.5L; Recommended minimum 1.5 L; Short term: 200 mL
Obligatory water loss	0.5 mL/kg/hr
Sodium balance	
Total body sodium	Average males 85 g
Na distribution	40 g extracellular; 10 g intracellular; 35 g in bones
Extracellular Na	140 mEq/L (contrast from K 4 mEq/L)
Intracellular Na	4 mEq/L (contrast from K 140 mEq/L)
Plasma osmolality	
Total mOsm/Kg	2X (Na mEq/L) + (glucose mg/dL)/18 + Urea (mg/dL)/2.8
Range	275–290 mOsm/kg
Osmolar gap	• Measured Osmolarity - calculated osmolality >10 mOsm/L • Decreased water content: Increased serum lipids and proteins • Increased Alcohols, mannitol, ethylene glycol, glycine

Appendix 17

CARDIAC IMPLANTABLE ELECTRONIC DEVICES (CIEDS): PACEMAKERS AND INTERNAL CARDIAC DEFIBRILLATORS

Pacemakers and internal cardiac defibrillators:
- An estimated 250,000 patients are implanted in the US annually.
- It consists of a sensor, amplifiers, microprocessor, output circuitry, and battery.
- At rest, a pacemaker uses around 7-microampere current, with a battery life of about seven years.
- Typical generates pulse: 3.5 V for 0.4 ms in duration.
- *Usual indication:* High degree AV block and sick sinus syndrome.

Examples
- *VVI:* Ventricle paced, ventricle sensed, pacing inhibited by spontaneous ventricular beats
- *DDD:* Ventricle and atrium sensed; Ventricle and atrium paced; each chamber is paced if the beat is not sensed. Common programming combinations:
    - Dual chambers sensed, both chambers inhibited by spontaneous depolarization at a set rate. It enables cardiac pacing at a desired rate.
    - Atrial pacing with ventricular sensing as for sick sinus syndrome with normal AV conduction. Spontaneous ventricular depolarization inhibits atrial pacing.
    - Atrial sensed and ventricle pacing for normal SA node with AV block. Spontaneous atrial depolarization leads to ventricular stimulation.
    - Atrial and ventricular are sensed and paced when the electrical activity is undetected within a specified time window.

Designation of pacemakers: The pacemaker code				
1st letter	2nd letter	3rd letter	4th letter	5th letter
Chamber paced	Chamber sensed	Response to sensed	Programmability	Arrhythmia control
A = Atrium	A = Atrium	I = Pacing inhibited	P = Rate + Output	P = Pacing
V = Ventricle	V = Ventricle	T = Pacing triggered	M = Multiprogrammable	S = Shock
D = Dual (V+A)	D = Dual (V+A)	D = Dual (I+T)	C = Communicating	
	O = None	O = None	R = Rate adaptive	
			O = None	

- *VVIR:* Ventricle paced, ventricle sensed, Rate adaptive ventricular pacing in response to exercise as sensed by an internal accelerometer.
- *DDDR:* Dual chambers sensed and paced at a rate adaptive to exercise
- *Asynchronous pacing modes:*
  - For atrial pacing (AOO), ventricular pacing (VOO), dual chamber pacing (DOO)
  - An asynchronous mode can be achieved by placing a magnet though it may not always be reliable
  - In the asynchronous mode, the pacemaker at 60–70 bpm
  - The asynchronous discharge rate decreased with lower battery life
  - May not meet the physiological needs during surgery
  - ICD with pacemaker function – magnet prevents defibrillation but does not affect the pacemaker function.

Chamber paced:
- *Single chamber:* Right atrium (RA) or right ventricle (RV) is paced, usually by a single lead.
- *Dual chamber:* RA ad RV are both paced by two separate leads.
- *Biventricular pacing:* Programmed RA, RV, and left ventricle pacing to enable optimal ventricular performance using three leads.

Synchronous/asynchronous:
- *Synchronous pacing:* Inhibits discharge during a regular beat.
- *Asynchronous activity:* Independent of muscle depolarization, discharge at a fixed rate, such as by application of a magnet.

Leadless pacemakers:
- Used in patients with a limited life expectancy
- For right ventricular pacing for bradyarrhythmia
- Implanted in the ventricle along the outflow tract
- Avoid complications associated with pacemaker leads.

Complications of pacemaker:
- Trauma at placement
- *Infection:*
  - Endocarditis
  - Pacemaker pocket infection
- *Thrombosis and pulmonary embolism*
- *Trigger arrhythmias:* Asynchronous pacing can cause R on T, leading to reentrant arrhythmias that can be minimized by VOO pacing.
  - Sensing problems failure to detect depolarization
  - *Output problems:* Failure to stimulate effectively
  - Pacemaker-induced tachycardia.
- *Lead-related complications:*
  - Trauma at placement

- Displacement and fracture of leads
- Valvular regurgitation
- Infection
- Perforation
- Venous obstruction
- *Magnet-related problems:*
  - Failure to convert to the asynchronous rhythm.
  - Accidental reprogramming with a longer duration of magnet application
  - Trigger pacemaker-induced tachycardia.
- *Unipolar/Bipolar leads:*
  - *Unipolar:* Cathode at the tip of the lead anode being the pacemaker shell
  - *Bipolar:* The more frequent type. Cathode at the end of the lead with anode just proximal to it.

LOOP RECORDERS

- Small, sub-cutaneous, sometimes injectable, leadless monitoring devices
- Record arrhythmias either spontaneously, during an event, or when interrogated.
- *Indications:* Diagnosis of unexplained syncope, palpitations, or monitoring atrial fibrillation.
- Do not require resetting before diathermy use.

IMPLANTABLE CARDIAC DEFIBRILLATORS

- Components are similar to pacemakers but with a capacitor capable of delivering the much higher voltage needed for defibrillation. The shock is about 750 V and 30–50 J of power.
- Like the pacemaker can be inactivated by a magnet.
- *Indications:*
  - Inpatients with poor heart functions, significant structural heart damage, low ejection fraction (<35%)
  - *Useful for:*
    - Anti-tachyarrhythmia pacing
    - Cardioversion
    - Defibrillation
    - Bradyarrhythmia pacing
- *Types:* Defibrillators like the pacemakers can be:
  - Single chamber
  - Dual chamber
  - Biventricular.

PREOPERATIVE PACEMAKER ASSESSMENT

- *Clinical review:*
  - Review pacemaker identification card/MRI compatibility.
  - Indication for pacemaker placement.
  - Underlying cardiac disease and cardiac function.
  - Type of device, placement date, last interrogation.
  - Functional status of the patient and comorbidities.
  - *Nature of surgery:*
    - Site of surgery
    - Location of pads
    - Use of cautery, bipolar diathermy
- *Bedside assessment:*
  - Vital signs blood pressure/heart rate
  - Rhythm on ECG monitor
  - Observing pulse pleth with a pulse oximeter or pressure variations of an arterial line might help to assess the effect of the paced versus non-paced rhythm
  - Valsalva maneuver or carotid massage can decrease spontaneous heart rate to test the pacemaker.
- *Investigations:*
  - *Chest X-ray:* Pacemaker type, lead location, and integrity
  - *EKG:* Type and extent of pacing
  - *Laboratory:* Electrolytes, including magnesium and blood gases, in critically ill
  - Underlying cardiac status by echocardiography or stress tests should be reviewed based on case needs.
- *Interrogation of the pacemaker:* It is required to assess the risk of electromagnetic interference, appropriate corrective strategies, and the consequences of discontinuing the pacemaker.
  - Type of device
  - *ICD functions:* Yes/No
  - The extent of pacemaker dependency: Insignificant/frequent/dependent
    - Dependent implies 40% paced beats
  - *Frequency of ICD use:* Never/rare/frequent
  - *Lead integrity and function:* Normal/impaired/malfunction
  - *Sensing amplitude:* Normal: Yes/No
  - *Pacing threshold:* Normal/excessive
- Place pacing pads for external defibrillation/pacing before deactivating an ICD.

FAILURE TO CAPTURE THE PACING PULSE

- *Device failure:*
  - Programming errors

- Lead malfunction and displacement
  - CVP or PAC placement
  - VA shunt placement
- Battery drainage
- Post-ICD discharge pacemaker failure
- Positive pressure ventilation may displace leads
- *Cardiac:*
  - Progressive cardiomyopathy
  - Inflammation and fibrosis
- *Non-cardiac:*
  - *Electrolyte imbalance:* Hyperkalemia, hypermagnesemia
  - Acidosis
  - Hypoxia
  - Hypercarbia
  - Hypothermia
  - *Drugs:*
    - Anti-arrhythmic drugs, e.g., amiodarone, flecainide
    - Hyperkalemia due to succinylcholine
    - Movements such as fasciculation with succinylcholine or excitatory movements with etomidate may impair pacemaker function
  - Electrical interference
- *Management:*
  - Identification and correction of the underlying cause
  - *Pharmacological:* Atropine, isoproterenol, or epinephrine to enhance capture
  - External pacing and defibrillation as needed
  - Temporary transvenous pacing.

PACEMAKER AND SPECIAL ENVIRONMENTS

Interference	Effect	Corrective strategy
Electromagnetic interference	Inhibit pacemaker/ activate ICD	• Avoid using electrical diathermy • Interrogate CIED and program to asynchronous mode • Use magnets with caution • Use bipolar, avoid unipolar • *Grounding pads are placed to ensure the current path away from CIED* • Use in short bursts (1–2 s) with pauses (10s) • Coagulation mode is worse than cutting
Radiofrequency ablation	Inhibit pacemaker/ activate ICD	• Reprogram pacemaker • Minimize RF use
Peripheral stimulators: vagus nerve, phrenic nerve, and TENS	Inhibit pacemaker	• Assess individual safety of device and placement location • TENS contraindicated with a pacemaker

Contd...

Contd...

Interference	Effect	Corrective strategy
Magnetic resonance imaging	• None: MRI-safe pacemakers • Static field: displace CIED • Modulated field: sensing errors; heat lead tips • Gradient field: sensing errors	• CIED-specific injury possible • Requires device interrogation and reprogramming to asynchronous mode • Resuscitation is available if needed • Assessment after imaging completed
Electroconvulsive therapy	• Usually safe • Seizure may affect sensing • Adverse cardiac effects of ECT may affect the device	• Need EP assessment • Conversion to fixed-mode pacing • Reassessment after the procedure ICD disabled
Radiation treatment	• >1000 rads run away pacemaker • >5000 rads pacemaker malfunction; X-rays and CT safe	Keep CIED outside the radiation field
Extracorporeal shock wave lithotripsy	Suppress pacemaker	Keep CIED 6 inches away from the lithotripsy focus

DEEP BRAIN STIMULATORS AND CIEDS

- Deep brain stimulators (DBS) are used to treat Parkinson's disease, essential tremors, and dystonia but are also helpful in treating epilepsy, severe depression, and behavioral disorders.
- DBS and CIEDs can interfere with each other.
- While inhibiting DBS by CIED has a minimal effect, the inhibition of CIED conversely can be fatal.
- DBS pulse typically is 1–4V, 100–200 Hz for 50–500 μs.
- *To minimize DBS and CIED interference:*
    - Both the DBS and CIED sensing leads should be in bipolar mode.
    - The risk of sensing DBS stimuli by CIEDs decreases with the CIED using bipolar leads.
    - Set the DBS at a minimum stimulating frequency of >60 Hz.
    - However, optimal functioning of the DBS typically requires unipolar configuration. The electrodes are at the catheter tip and the body of the device.
    - When DBS and CIEDs generators are implanted, they should be at least 20 cm apart.

- A joint team of cardiac and neuro-electrophysiologists should assess the risk.
- Use leadless cardiac pacemakers if possible.

MAGNETS AND CIEDS

- Pacemakers and AICD have magnet-sensitive Reed or Hall switches in the sensing circuit:
  - A Reed switch is a glass tube with magnet-sensitive material. However, the extent of the magnetic field and orientation can affect the functioning of the Reed switch. Reed switch can be affected by MRI's magnetic field. It can malfunction if its glass capsule is damaged.
  - While the Hall switch is a solid-state sensor that is immune to MRI's magnetic field yet can be reliably triggered by the application of a magnet.
  - In most devices, the application of a magnet inactivates the sensing circuit.
  - It converts the pacemaker output into an asynchronous pacing mode.
  - The pacing rate is slightly higher than the resting rate.
  - In the case of an AICD, the application of a magnet inhibits cardioversion, but the pacing mode is unaffected.
  - Modern pacemakers can be programmed to be immune to the magnet.

MAGNET USE DURING NEUROSURGERY

- *Magnet application in neurosurgical patients is challenging for several reasons:*
  - Placement may not be possible in prone, lateral, or sitting positions.
  - Surgical procedures requiring access to the chest and neck may prevent the positioning of the magnet.
  - CIEDs are often inaccessible and at a distant location under drapes.
  - Neurosurgical procedures tend to be extended:
    - Magnets can be dislodged from their placement site.
    - A prolonged magnet application might reset the pacemakers.
  - Should a CIED malfunction occur, the chances of instituting CPR can be challenging.
  - It is best left to an electrophysiologist to assess the device unless the effect of magnet application is known or can be determined beforehand.

Appendix 18

APPROACH TO FAST TRACK WAKE-UP AFTER CRANIOTOMY AND ITS ASSESSMENT

Appendix 18A: Author's wake-up score

Score	Features
1	• Extubation is achieved within 5 minutes of the end of surgery. • No coughing or bucking; permissible hemodynamic response. • Fully cooperative with neuro exam.
2	• Extubation is achieved within 5 minutes of the end of surgery. • Transient coughing bucking, easily treatable hemodynamic response, no restraining required. • Adequate neuro exam before extubation. • Or, Grade 1 extubation that is delayed for 15 minutes.
3	• Extubation with coughing and bucking, no restraints needed. • Response to simple verbal command before extubation. • Aggressive but adequate hemodynamic treatment is needed before extubation. • Or, Grade 1/2 extubation that is delayed for 30 min.
4	• Coughing and bucking occur with agitation requiring restraints. • Neuroexam not possible prior to extubation • Aggressive hemodynamic treatment • Or, wake is delayed for more than 30 minutes but imaging is not needed.
5	• Significant coughing bucking, neuro exam not possible, restrained by OR staff. • Additional sedation reinstituted • Aggressive hemodynamic management • Or, delayed wake up which needed imaging with negative findings. • Or, the patient needed reintubation.

Appendix 18B: Preparation for fast track wake up after craniotomy

Preoperative risk factors

Patient factors	Large tumors, surgery in eloquent areas of the brain, elderly, impaired cognition, significant seizure history
Prolonged surgery	Long duration, prolonged TIVA infusions, long-acting drugs

Early in surgery

Intraoperative events	Excessive CSF drainage, pneumocephalus, prolonged retraction, prolonged surgery, surgical complication, drug interactions
Lidocaine 5% ointment on the distal 7.5 cm, including the cuff	To prevent coughing at extubation. Supplement with intratracheal lido 2% 3–5 mL for more lengthy procedures.
Bupivacaine/lido/epi scalp block	Decrease incision site pain and pressure may permit lighter anesthesia at wake up.

During surgery

Selection of short-acting drugs	Propofol, fentanyl, remifentanil, sevoflurane, desflurane
Burst analgesia (tunnel and pins)	Remifentanil, propofol bolus, of burst of nitrous inhalation
Avoid hydromorphone	Use small doses if necessary; neuro-patients may be abnormally sensitive to sedation by narcotics.
Avoid hypothermia (aneurysm surgery, target temp 34°C)	Water blanket rewarming takes time, set to 35°C when the core temperature is 34.5°C; the rewarming rate is about 0.1°C/10 min.
	Air warmer activated after aneurysm exposure; Target temp at the end of surgery >36°C.

T-30 minutes, towards the end of surgery

Hypocapnia correction	Establish A-a (CO_2) gradient to guide ventilation; Restore normocapnia after surgical resection is complete.
Reduce/shut off sevoflurane	Plan to achieve complete sevoflurane washout by the end of the case; switch to propofol or desflurane. Use processed EEG to guide propofol infusions.
Tylenol	15 mg/kg IV; An order often needed; onset 15 min; peak 1 hour, duration 6 hours.
Steroids repeat dose of dexamethasone	Decrease neuroinflammation, airway irritability, antiemetic, and analgesic effect
Antiemetics	Odansetron 4 mg

Just before extubation

I/T lidocaine	Delivered with a 26G needle as a fine particle size spray, give small 0.5 mL volumes 2% slowly with 2–3 in between breaths. Give 2.5 to 5 mL. It decreases coughing and bucking and probably attenuates hypertensive response.
Antihypertensive drugs	Nicardipine/hydralazine if HR <70 bpm, Labetalol if HR >70 bpm

Appendix 18C: Fast-track wake-up after craniotomy

Three things to avoid: Hypothermia, hypocapnia, excessive drugs

T + 30 min

1. Titrate anesthesia requirements to neurological status
2. Optimize temperature management
3. Judicious use of long-acting drugs (e.g., avoid hydromorphone)
4. Curtail sufentanil infusion switch to remifentanil

T- 30 min

1. Restore normocapnia with dura closure
2. Stop sevoflurane, change to desflurane 2–3%, FGF at 3L to not more than 0.5 MAC combined sevoflurane residue + desflurane
3. Propofol infusion 20–40 mcg/kg/min (Processed EEG at 25–50% power)
4. Decrease remifentanil infusion to 0.05 mcg/kg/min
5. Tylenol 15 mg/kg IV
6. Dexamethasone 4 mg if <6 hr; or 10 mg if >6 hr
7. Odansetron 4 mg
8. Check temperature
9. Avoid muscle relaxants

T- 15 min

1. Adjust desflurane 2–4% to 0.5 total MAC (sevoflurane residue+ desflurane)
2. Increase FGF to 4L
3. Decrease Remifentanil (0.03 mcg/kg/min)
4. Keep IV propofol ready for a premature wake-up
5. Propofol infusion around 40–60 mcg/kg/min (Processed EEG 40–60% power), desflurane wake up preferred.

T- 2 min

1. Intratracheal (I/T) lidocaine (2%) spray 26 needle
2. Antihypertensive treatment
3. Shut desflurane
4. FGF to 8 to 10 L for rapid washout of desflurane
5. Shift to pressure support with a respiratory rate of 8

T- 0

1. Complete 4–5 mL total lidocaine (2%) I/T spray injection
2. Removal from pins, dressing
3. Oral suction
4. Sugammadex, confirm sustained tetanus
5. Stop propofol
6. Stop remifentanil after oral suction
7. Antihypertensive treatment as needed
8. Pressure support with a respiratory rate of 4

Appendix 19

ALLERGIC REACTIONS TO DRUGS

Allergic reactions to drugs: Common allergens: Antibiotics and anticonvulsants.

Types of adverse drug reactions:

Immunological:
- *Type I:* IgE mediated: Anaphylaxis: Rash, hypotension, and bronchospasm.
- *Type II:* Cytotoxic: Hemolytic anemia, neutropenia, thrombocytopenia
- *Type III:* Immune-complex disease: Serum sickness with fever, rash, arthralgia, vasculitis, glomerulonephritis, e.g., with immunoglobulins
- *Type IV:* Delayed cell-mediated, e.g., contact dermatitis with a rash
- *Others:* T cell activation (rash with sulfonamides); Fas/Fas ligand-induced apoptosis: Stevens-Johnson syndrome/toxic epidermolysis; drug-induced systemic lupus erythematous (anticonvulsants).

Anaphylaxis
- IgE mediated
- Acute reaction characterized by the classic triad of prophylactic shock: hypotension, bronchospasm, and urticaria
- *Other symptoms:* itching, vomiting, diarrhea, and angioedema.

Diagnosis:
- History, presentation, symptoms, and time course of events
- Detect circulating IgE by standardized skin tests.
- Detect mast cell activation (histamine, tryptase, β-tryptase) in < 4 hours.

Management:
- *Acute reaction:*
  - Identification and discontinuation of the drug,
  - Epinephrine (150–300 μg),
  - Antihistamines (diphenhydramine 50 mg),
  - Corticosteroids and
  - *Supportive treatment:* IV fluids, oxygen, intubation, and ventilation.
- *Preventive protocol, e.g., contrast allergy:*
  - Prednisolone 50 mg at 12.6 and 1 hour before contrast exposure
  - Diphenhydramine 50 mg 1-hour pre-exposure.

Non-immunological side-effects of drugs
- *Anaphylactoid:* Dose-dependent histamine release, e.g., muscle relaxants

- *Idiosyncratic:* G6PD deficiency-associated drug reactions
- *Drug intolerance:* Unusual side effects in a given patient.
- *Side effects of drugs:*
  - *Known side effects:* Such as, respiratory depression and constipation with narcotics.
  - *Known drug toxicities:* Such as, cardiotoxicity with daunorubicin.
  - *Indirect side effects:* Such as, oral fungal infections with antibiotics.
  - Side effects due to drug interactions.

Appendix 20

ADVANCED CARDIAC LIFE SUPPORT DRUGS AND DOSES

Drug	Indication	Dose	Side effects
Epinephrine	Cardiac arrest Bradycardia Hypotension	1 mg q 3–5 min ETT: 2 × IV for arrest but lower doses for bradycardia and hypotension	Increase in myocardial oxygen consumption, ischemia
Atropine	Bradycardia	0.5–1 mg q 3–5 min Max dose: 3 mg	Increase in myocardial oxygen consumption, ischemia
Lidocaine	Stable monomorphic VT	1–1.5 mg/kg bolus Max: 3 mg/kg ETT: 2–4 mg/kg	CNS side effects: Slurred speech
Adenosine (Avoid with 2° or 3° heart block)	PSVT	6 mg, repeat 12 mg	Asystole, flushing, and bronchospasm
Amiodarone	Irregular, narrow, complex, and tachycardia. Stable, regular, complex, and tachycardia	300 mg IV bolus, followed by 150 mg IV bolus; LD 150 mg of over 10 min and then 1 mg/min over 6 hours and 0.5 mg/min in the next 18 hours	CNS side effects: Increased liver and enzymes
Procainamide (avoid with CHF or QT prolongation)	Stable monomorphic VT	20–50 mg/min until suppressed stop with hypotension; QRS increased by 50%; dose limit of 17 mg/kg	Bone marrow depression
Vasopressin	• Cardiac arrest • Severe hypotension	40 U IV	Severe vasoconstriction
Sotalol (avoid with CHF or QTc prolongation)	Stable monomorphic VT	1.5 mg/kg over 5 minutes	Hypotension and bradycardia

(CHF: congestive heart failure; ETT: endotracheal tube; LD: loading dose; PSVT: paroxysmal supraventricular tachycardia; VT: ventricular tachycardia)

Refractory arrest: 7 Hs and 4 Ts:
- Hypoxia, Hypovolemia, Hypothermia, Hypoglycemia, Hyper or hypokalemia, Hydrogen ions. (*To remember the 7 Hs: "During Hypoxia. Small-Volumes of Cold Glucose Increase not decrease Potassium due to Acidosis"*)
- Trauma, Tamponade, Thrombus (heart or lungs), and Toxins

In Memoriam

Dr Nielamber Chintamani Joshi, FACS
(1888–1947)

Nielamber Chintamani Joshi was born on August 2, 1888. He was the only child of Kaushaliya and Chintamani Joshi. He was orphaned early on and brought up by his extended family. He graduated in medicine from the King George Medical College in Lahore, now in Pakistan. In 1917 he joined the Mayo Clinic as the first minority surgical trainee. His training paved the way for other minority students to be trained at the Clinic two years later. On completion of his training, he returned to India in 1921.

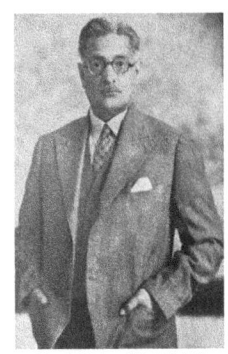

Dr NC Joshi, FACS
(1888–1947)

Instead of working in an urban center, he went to Deoria, a village in an impoverished part of the country. In a short time, he turned Deoria into a medical "oasis." He pioneered surgery for goiter and elephantiasis, which was endemic in the region. Later, he became the Chief Medical Officer for the erstwhile State of Bharatpur.

In 1930, he resigned from the state service and started his surgical practice in Delhi. It began in a small office with one assistant. His practice rapidly grew, and his clinic developed into a 100-bed hospital with advanced treatment facilities and several doctors on the roll. The hospital still functions some ninety years later. The nearby road bears his name. Dr Joshi was a founder-member and later presided over the Association of Surgeons of India. For many years he was the President of the Delhi Medical Association. The Association holds an oration in his name that honors some of the country's leading surgeons. Dr Joshi remained in touch with the Mayo Clinic throughout his life. He wanted to build a similar clinic in India and had even brought the land to do so.

Dr Joshi was widely known for his charitable care of his poor and downtrodden countrymen. He helped many freedom fighters who took shelter in his clinic. He was a close friend of Mahatma Gandhi, the Father of the Nation, who often visited his hospital. On September 9th, 1947, amid the communal violence of the time, Dr Joshi was fatally shot while trying to calm a frenzied mob. Yet even after his death, he continued to save lives. In a prisoner swap that followed, the alleged assassin was exchanged for safe passage for 900 Indians. Although the bullet had closed a fascinating page in India's medical history, Dr Joshi's life and creed, *"To leave the world a little better than you found it",* remains an eternal inspiration.

On Teaching and Learning

"Information is not knowledge"
Albert Einstein (1879–1955)
Theoretical physicist

"The noblest pleasure is the joy of understanding"
Leonardo Da Vinci (1452–1519)
Painter, scientist, architect-engineer

*"Reserve your right to think,
for even to think wrongly is better than not to think at all"*
Hypatia (350–415)
Mathematician astronomer philosopher

"Simplify, simplify"
Henry David Thoreau (1817–1862)
Naturalist writer philosopher

"A wealth of information creates a poverty of attention"
Lucius Annaeus Seneca (4 BC–65 AD)
Roman philosopher

"A short saying oft contains much wisdom"
Sophocles (496–406 BC)
Greek playwright

"The fewer words, the better the prayer"
Martin Luther (1483–1546)
Priest theologian

"Self-education is the only kind of education there is"
Isaac Asimov (1920–1992)
Science fiction writer

*"Live as if you will die tomorrow.
Learn as if you will live forever"*
Mohandas Karamchand Gandhi (1869–1948)
Lawyer nationalist philosopher

Index

Page numbers followed by *f* refer to figure, *fc* refer to flowchart, and *t* refer to table.

A

Abdominal compression 124
Ablative procedures 198
Abscess 118
Accessory monitors 349
Acetaminophen 200, 546
Acetazolamide 416, 515
  perfusion scan 117
Acetylcholine 7
Achondroplastic dwarf 268
Acid citrate dextrose 551
Acid-base imbalances 251
Acoustic neuromas 448
Acquired hydrocephalus 146
Acromegaly 88, 460, 461
Activated clotting time 265
Acute coronary syndrome 608
Acute lung injury
  transfusion-induced 561
  transfusion-related 183, 184
Acute respiratory distress
  syndrome 183
Acute spinal injury 428
  clinical evaluation 430
  radiology 432
  surgical management 433
Adam's test 205
Adamkiewicz, artery of 25
Addisonian crisis 460
Adenohypophysis, cells of 85*t*
Adenomas 87
Adenosine 372, 625
  arrest, clinical use of 373
  diphosphate 608
  doses 372*t*
  high-dose 372
    complications of 372
Adrenal insufficiency,
  secondary 89
Adrenocorticotropic hormone
  85, 460
  secreting tumors 87
Adrenocorticotropin hormone,
  lack of 89

Adult human neuron types 4*f*
Advanced cardiac life support
  drugs 625
Adverse drug reactions, types
  of 623
Aggressive hemodynamic
  management 357
Agraphesthesia 31
Air
  aspiration 230
  embolism, clinical severity
    of 231*t*
  entrainment, sites of 226
  leak 298
  slow entrainment of 227
Airway 206, 274, 453
  assessment 420, 462
  difficult 501
  equipment 275, 497
  examination 263
  management devices 383
  obstruction 211, 297
Akinetic mutism 507
Allergic reactions 274, 561, 623
  management of 321
Allergy 274
Alpha-amino propionic acid 7
Alpha-amino-3-hydroxy-5-methyl-
  4-isoxazolepropionic
  acid 154
Alveolar concentration, minimum
  351, 602
Alzheimer's disease 14
  cognition of 6
  treatment drugs 265
Amantadine 218
Amaurosis fugax 151
Ambulatory neurosurgery 291,
  294, 297
Amiodarone 247, 617
Amitriptyline 200
Amnesia, post-traumatic 379
Amrinone 588, 590
Amygdala 18
Amyotrophic lateral sclerosis 34

Analgesia, preempt 545
Analgesics 79
Anaphylactoid 623
Anaphylaxis 623
Ancillary electrophysiologic
  tests 571
Anemia 294
  correction of 206
  euvolemic 549
  potential hazards of 384
Anesthesia 94, 165, 273, 280, 308,
    336*t*, 350, 477, 501, 536
  care, monitored 317, 326, 535
  effects of 104
  general 132, 248, 272, 297, 301,
    302, 308, 309*t*, 325*f*, 326,
    342, 535
  induction of 520, 527
  machine 498, 526
  maintenance of 279, 279*t*,
    351, 384
  management 472
  monitors, routine 421, 462
  reversal of 473
  techniques 534
  without coughing and bucking
    312
Anesthetic choice 162
Anesthetic concerns 148, 161
Anesthetic drugs 60*t*, 334
  effects of 99
  short-acting 477
Anesthetic implications 160,
  188, 248
Anesthetic management 323, 325,
  362, 407, 461
Anesthetic neuroprotection 127
Anesthetic neurotoxicity 127,
  131, 605
Anesthetic pharmacology 67
Anesthetic techniques 296, 451
Aneurysm 176, 177, 188, 189*t*, 336*t*,
  344, 347, 448
  bleeding accounts 343
  clipping of 93, 346, 352

Index

coiling of 346
formation, risk factors for 174*fc*
protected 281
unruptured 175, 281, 344
Aneurysm rupture 542
biomechanics of 345
risk treatment 346*t*
Angiographic procedures 319*t*
Angiographic spasm 181
Angiographic suzuki grades 190
Angiographic vasospasm 360
Angiography 571
Angioplasty 317, 360
Angiotensin-converting enzyme inhibitors 265, 488, 588
Animal prion diseases 506
Anisocoria 169
Anterior cord syndrome 210, 430
Anterior spinal
artery 25
injury syndrome 37, 37*f*
Antiarrhythmic drug 372, 617
Antibiotics 274, 278, 607
prophylaxis 594
Anticoagulation 305, 537
management of 537
Anticonvulsant drugs 219, 258, 595, 596, 607
serum concentrations of 294
Antidepressants, tricyclic 244
Antidiuretic hormone 460
loss of 571
receptor
antagonists 612
blockers 608
Antiemetic drugs 606
Antiepileptic drugs 265, 278
side-effects 225
Antifibrinolytic drugs 207, 559
risks and benefits of 560
use of 560
Antifibrinolytic therapy 560
Anti-fungal agents 607
Anti-hypertensive 265
drugs 308, 621
Anti-intercellular adhesion molecule antibody 131
Antiplatelet drugs 311, 325*t*, 549, 608
Antishock trousers, use of 230
Anti-vascular endothelial growth factor treatment 161
Anton syndrome 17
Anxiety, perioperative 259
Anxiolytics 265, 606
Aortic surgery 92
Aortocaval compression 491

Apert's syndrome 496
Aphasia 155
Apnea test 252, 570
primary 252
Apneustic breathing 395, 601
Apoplexy 177, 185
Apoptotic cell death 154, 155
Aprepitant 162, 606
Aprotinin inhibits trypsin 559
Aqueductal stenosis 146
Arachnoid cysts 146
Arachnoid villi 412
Arnold Chiari malformation 146, 202, 203, 547, 448
Arrhythmias 183, 242, 572
surgery-triggered 454
treatment of 537
Arterial access
advantages of 319*t*
disadvantages of 319*t*
Arterial blood flow, complex biomechanics of 56
Arterial blood gas 359, 381
monitoring 499
Arterial blood pressure 350*f*
recording 56*f*
Arterial cannulation 349
Arterial line 276, 370, 384
placement 311
Arterial occlusion 319
Arterial pressure
upstroke 56*f*
value 57*f*
Arterial wall, biomechanics of 56*f*
Arteriotomy 305
Arteriovenous fistulae 53
Arteriovenous malformation 186, 187*f*, 189, 372, 486, 542
clinical presentation 187
hemorrhages 81
investigations 188
pathophysiology of 186
resection 58, 281
Artery forming, variations in 51
Aryl-hydrocarbon interacting gene 87
Aseptic meningitis 80
Asleep-awake-asleep technique 296
Aspiration 297
pneumonia 184
Aspirin 200, 325, 549, 608
clopidogrel 265
Astereognosis 31
Astrocytes 4, 13
Asymmetric pupils 169
Asymmetric shoulders 204

Asynchronous pacing modes 614
Ataxia 20
Ataxic breathing 395, 601
Ataxic dysarthria 20
Atheromatous plaques 151
Atherosclerotic cerebrovascular disease 151
differential diagnosis 152
investigations 152
pathology 151
Atherosclerotic disease, risk factors for 151
Atomic nuclei 117
Atonic seizures 222, 292
Atrial ectopy 183
Atrial fibrillation 538
Atropine 6, 308, 482, 617, 625
Audiometry 46
Audiovisual distraction 604
Auditory pathway 44, 45, 47*f*, 48
Auditory system 44
functions of 44
organization of 44
Augmented hyperventilation 141
Autoimmune diseases 80
Autonomic disturbances 244
Autonomic hyper-reflexia 210, 211, 435
Autonomic nervous system 7
Autonomic regulation 60
Autonomic response assessment 248
Autonomic storm 572
Autoregulation, loss of 26
Autosomal dominant disease 86
Awake craniotomy 291, 294, 295
complications of 297
scalp block for 295
Awake fiberoptic intubation 421, 431
Axial flow device 533

B

Babinski's reflex 598
Babinski's sign 34
Back pain, chronic 565
Backup intubation technique 462
Bacterial meningitis 80
Bacterial pathogens 80
Bacterial vaginosis 487
Baer technique 99
Balint's syndrome 17
Balloon test occlusion 51
Barbiturates 68, 95, 212
coma 405
Basal ganglia 18, 32

Index

Baseline neurological examination 308
Battle sign 235, 378
Bed rest, supine 415
Benserazide 217
Benzodiazepines 68, 212, 219, 224, 245, 285, 311
Best eye opening 236, 379
Beta-blockers 219t, 265
Bevacizumab 161
Biperiden 218
Biot's breathing 601
Bipolar disorders 478
Bipolar leads 615
Bispectral analysis 94
Bispectral index 93, 287, 370, 423, 434
Biventricular pacing 614
Bladder dysfunction 78, 202
Bleeding 187, 337, 537
  causes of 537
  greater, risk of 462
  potential risk for major 259
  tests for abnormal 554
Blindness, transient unilateral 151
Blood
  conservation 206
  direct effects of 181
  features of 180t
  glucose 264
  indirect effects of 181
  oxygen level 64
  product transfusion 558
  volume 139f, 140, 487
Blood flow 316
  velocity, measurement of 108f
Blood loss 164, 207, 407, 419, 500, 563
  excessive 500, 512
  monitor 279
Blood pressure 274, 361, 563
  changes 169
  management 281
    principles of 310
  support 232
  systolic 350f, 372
  targets 182
Blood transfusion 266, 267, 551
  hazards of 560
  risk of 549
Blood-brain barrier 11, 403
  components of 11f
  disruption 550
  functions
    loss of 14
    pathologies of 14
  iatrogenic disruption of 15

physiological functions of 14
transport across 13
Body mass index 261, 517
Body metabolism 487
Bone
  characteristics 432
  marrow suppression 161
Botox injections 219
Bougie-assisted intubation 275
Bowel dysfunction 78
Brachial plexus 199
  injury 125
Brachiocephalic trunk 50f
Bradycardia 211, 274, 297, 381, 398, 435, 500
Bradykinin 15
Brain 198
  arteriovenous malformation 192
  capillary endothelium 12
  deep venous drainage of 53f
  development 104
  disease, progressive 221
  edema 166
  function, loss of 569
  herniating 258
  imaging 116
  injury 170
  management of tight 171
  parenchymal 61
  swelling 297
  temperature 240
  venous drainage of 52f
  watershed regions of 391
Brain aneurysms 177, 181, 345
  location of 173f
  risk of developing 343
Brain death 250, 568, 569, 575
  clinical determination of 569
  clinical diagnosis of 570
  diagnosis of 250-252, 568
Brain herniation 166, 169, 389
  consequences of 392t
  differential diagnosis of 170
  intraoperative 171
  mechanism of 392t
  pathology of 389, 390
  treatment of 389
  types of 170f
Brain metabolism 64, 65
  imaging 66
  overview 64
Brain tissue 11, 107
  oxygen monitoring 106
Brain tumor 117, 137, 159, 160, 163, 258
  distribution of primary 159f

false 79
imaging, intraoperative 164
metastatic 524
pathology 159
primary 159, 524
secondary 160
Brainstem 19, 53, 198
  anatomy of 20t
  auditory evoked responses 47f, 93, 99, 100f, 100t, 440
  decompression 448
  pathology, levels of 20
  reflexes, absence of 569
  tumor surgery 440
Branch retinal artery occlusion 515
Breathing 601
  circuits 498
  patterns, pathological 601
Broca's injuries 16
Brodmann's areas injuries 16
Bromocriptine 217, 461
Brown–Sequard syndrome 36, 36f, 210
Brudzenski's sign 179, 599
Bullard's laryngoscope 433
Bypass
  institution of 371
  surgical exposure of 371

C

Cabergoline 461
Caffeine 79
Calcium
  antagonists 131
  channel blockers 131, 361, 592
  chelators 131
  metabolism, autosomal dominant disorder of 243
Caloric test 252
Capillary fragility test 554
Capillary refill 563
Carbamazepine 200, 201, 243, 595
Carbidopa 217
Carbon dioxide 59
Carbon monoxide 551
Carbonic anhydrase inhibitor 515
Carcinomas 160
Cardiac arrest 371, 539
Cardiac arrhythmias 273, 453
Cardiac disease, significant 324
Cardiac implantable electronic devices 613
Cardiac injury 183
Cardiac output, pulse contour analysis for 349

Index

Cardiac rhythm 532
Cardiogenic pulmonary
    edema 184
Cardiomyopathy, progressive 617
Cardiopulmonary bypass 370f,
    513, 588
    machine 369
Cardiopulmonary resuscitation
    239, 267, 588
Cardiorespiratory arrest 112
Cardiovascular assessment 258,
    449, 477
Cardiovascular collapse 228
Cardiovascular complications, risk
    factors for 260
Cardiovascular effects 121, 205,
    248, 479
Cardiovascular status 347
Cardiovascular system 273
Carotid arterial disease
    pathology of 301, 302
    treatment of 301, 303, 303t
Carotid artery 327f
    external 305
    ipsilateral
        external 327
        internal 182
    origins of 50
    stenting 317
    stenting
        contraindications 318
        indications 318
Carotid bulb manipulation 305
Carotid disease 309t
    regional anesthesia for 309t
    significant 324
Carotid endarterectomy 281, 301,
    317, 440
    general anesthesia for 309
    regional anesthesia for 309
Carotid sheath 305
Carotid stenosis 152t
    assessment of 304
Carotid stenting 301, 325t
Carotid surgery 92, 93, 592
Carpal tunnel syndrome 197, 199
Carpenter's syndrome 497
Catatonia, acute 478
Catecholamine 588
    methyl transferase 216f, 218
Catheter, placement of
    long-arm 230
Cauda equina syndrome 35, 36f,
    211, 431
Cavernous malformation 486
Cavernous sinus 52, 53
Cefamandole 594

Cefazolin 594
Cefotetan 594
Cefuroxime 594
Celebrex 545
Cell
    abnormal growth of 159
    cluster level resolution 94
    types 16, 85
Cellular infiltration 14
Central cholinergic syndrome 283
Central cord syndrome 35, 35f,
    210, 430
Central fever 243
Central herniation 393
Central nervous system 7, 8, 13, 16,
    202, 546
    applied anatomy of 16
    effects 479
    mass 22
    tumors 162
Central neurogenic
    hyperventilation 601
Central respiratory
    dysregulation 258
Central retinal artery
    occlusion 515, 516
Central venous catheters 562
    placement 450f
Central venous line 403
Central venous pressure 231, 349,
    370, 434
    indication of 604
    monitoring 450
Cephalad larynx 603
Cephalosporin 274
Cerebellar artery injury, posterior
    inferior 203
Cerebellar damage affects 33
Cerebellar hemispheres, lateral 20
Cerebellar herniation, signs of 447
Cerebellar injury 20
Cerebellar lesions 447
Cerebellar nerves 448
Cerebellar symptoms 448, 507
Cerebellar tonsillar herniation 394
Cerebellar vermis 448
Cerebellopontine
    angle lesions 448
Cerebellum 20, 32
Cerebral air embolism 233
Cerebral aneurysms 173, 342
    clinical presentation 175
    clipping of 342
    pathology 173
Cerebral angiography 188, 320f
Cerebral arteriovenous
    malformation 336t
    resection 331

Cerebral artery
    anterior 42f, 171, 346
    infarct, right anterior 365
    middle 191
    posterior 171, 175, 346, 394, 42f
Cerebral autoregulation 58f, 60,
    149
Cerebral blood flow 26, 50, 58, 60,
    61, 61t, 67, 68, 68t, 148,
    191, 405, 453
    regulation 55
        cellular mechanisms of 60
    siphon augment 54
Cerebral blood volume 61
Cerebral circulation 49, 392f
Cerebral cortex, layers of 16t
Cerebral edema 166, 167, 389, 390
    high altitude 168
    management of 169
    prevention of 169
    treatment of 169
    types of 166, 390
Cerebral elastance curves 138
Cerebral herniation, types of 171t
Cerebral hyperperfusion
    syndrome 62, 313
Cerebral hypoperfusion, detection
    of 307
Cerebral hypotension 78
Cerebral injury, traumatic 382
Cerebral lesions 448
Cerebral metabolic rate 65, 148
Cerebral metabolism 60, 65, 65t
Cerebral microdialysis 363
Cerebral oxygen monitoring 382
Cerebral palsy 204
Cerebral perfusion
    monitoring 382
    pressure 57, 67, 170, 381,
        402, 592
    measure of 306
Cerebral sinuses 53
Cerebral spinal fluid circulation,
    abnormalities of 77
Cerebral steal 163, 339
Cerebral vasospasm 178, 181,
    357, 363
    management of 182
    treatment of 357, 361t
    ultrasonic diagnosis of 182
Cerebral veins 52
Cerebral venous drainage 51
Cerebrocerebellums 20
Cerebrospinal fluid 72, 74, 76f, 124,
    248, 394, 412
    characteristics 73
    circulation 72, 74, 412

Index

collecting system 143*f*
drain 371
    attenuates 26
    complications of 143
drainage procedures 137
dynamics 411
excessive 146
formation of 72, 74, 76*f*
functions 72
leak 411, 542
    characteristics of 413
    pathophysiology 413
obstruct flow of 159
reabsorption, routes of 77
rhinorrhea 378
viscosity of 73
Cerebrovascular accident 261, 608
Cerebrovascular effects 186, 453
Cerebrovascular surgery 92
Cervical
  collar limits access 422
  decompression 419
  deformities, extreme 422
  disc herniation,
    symptoms of 420*t*
  laminectomies 226
  lesion 433
  nerves 544
  sympathetic nerves 544
Cervical plexus block 310
  superficial 302, 309
  ultrasound-guided 310
Cervicomedullary syndrome 210
Cervicothoracic spine 439
Charcot Marie-Tooth disease 246
Chemoreceptor trigger zone 606
Chemotherapy 160, 162
  side effects of 161
Cheyne-Stokes breathing 601
Chiari malformation 202
Cholecystokinin 198*f*
Choroid plexectomy 148
Choroid plexus
  ablation 469, 472
  cells 72
  tumors 160
Chronic obstructive pulmonary
    disease 295
  severe 570
Chronic pain
  pathogenesis of 194*f*
  pathology of 193
  surgica
    interventions for 197
    treatment of 193
  syndromes 199
Cilostazol 361, 608

Cimetidine 162, 322
Circle of Duret 49
Circle of Willis 51, 51*f*, 190
Cisplatin 161, 247
Cisterna
  ambiens 75
  chiasmaticus 74
  magna 74
  pontis 75
Citrate phosphate dextrose 551
Clarke's column 28
Clarke's, dorsal nucleus of 23
Classic cerebellar signs 448
Clazosentan 361
Clevidipine 591
Clindamycin 594
Clinical blood pressure
    manipulation 58
Clinical congestive heart
    failure 348
Clinical syndrome 180, 244, 302
Clipping, potential complications
    of 347
Clomethiazole 131
Clonazepam 219
Clonic seizures 222, 292
Clonidine 265
Clopidogrel 608
Clot aspiration 157
Clotting, point of care
    testing for 555
Cluster breathing 395, 601
Coagulation 206, 553
  assessment of 499, 549
  correction 549
  defects 81
  tests 554, 554*t*
Coagulopathy 384
  risk factors for 384
Cobb's angle 204
  determination of 204*f*
  significance of 205
Cochlear implants 48
Cochlear nerve 100
Cochlear nucleus 100
Cochlear pathway 45
Codeine 545, 546
Cognition, impaired 169, 282
Cognitive impairment 78, 90
Cognitive status 274
Coiling, potential complications
    of 347
Collagen disorders 247
Colliculus, inferior 100
Colloid osmotic pressure 550
Coma 600
  scales 237

Comatose 258
Common carotid artery 152
Common cortical sensory
    disorders 31
Communicating
    hydrocephalus 78, 146
Communication 259
Complete blood
    count 294, 347, 359
Computed tomography 180, 188,
    358, 359, 432
  perfusion scan 117
Congenital hydrocephalus 146
Conscious sedation 535
Consciousness,
    loss of 179, 379, 482
Contralateral neglect 17
Contrast allergy, history of 321
Conus medullaris
    syndrome 37, 37*f*, 211
Cooling devices, surface 398
Cord
  complete transection of 430
  hemisection 430
  partial transection of 430
Core temperature
    management 273
Cornea 40
Corneal abrasion 517
Corneal reflex 252
Corneal sensation, loss of 565
Coronary artery
    disease 261, 301, 480
Coronavirus disease-2019, testing
    of 263*fc*
Cortex 16
  transmits, transcranial
    electrical stimulation
    of 441
Cortical blindness 17, 512, 516
Cortical stimulating electrode 102
Corticobulbar tract 33
Corticospinal tract 33
  anterior 33
  injuries, lateral 33, 34
Corticosteroids 568
Corticotropes 85
Corticotropin-releasing
    hormone 84
Cough reflex 252
Coughing, complications of 281
Cranial cisterns 74
Cranial defects 201
Cranial nerve 27, 84*f*, 171, 197,
    313, 597
  compression 141
  examination 378, 380*t*

injuries 313
  microvascular decompression of 448
  monitoring 450
  paralysis 448
  tests for 46
  tumors 448
Cranial trephination 172
Craniocaudal sequence 74
Craniofrontal-nasal syndrome 497
Craniopharyngiomas 89, 90
Craniosynostosis 495
  management of 495
Craniotomy 542
  pain
    mechanism of 543
    relief 545
  pharmacological interventions for 546*t*
  routine 272
Creutzfeldt-Jakob disease 505, 507*t*
  anesthetic management 508
  clinical features 507
  infection risk 507
  pathogenesis of 505, 506*f*
  surgical management 509
  variant 507
Crouzon's syndrome 497
Cryoprecipitate 549, 559
Crystalloids 549
Cubital tunnel syndrome 199
Cushing's disease 88, 460, 461
Cushing's reflex 592
Cushing's signs 140
Cushing's triad 112, 381, 395, 470
Cushing's ulcers 386
Cutaneous nerve, lateral 199
Cyclic adenosine monophosphate 590
Cyclooxygenase 546
Cyproheptadine 461
Cysticercosis 293
Cytotoxic
  brain edema 390
  edema 167

D

Dandy's point 142
Dandy-Walker syndrome 146
Dantrolene 244
Deafness 47, 161
Death 208
Declamping carotid artery 312
Decompressive craniectomy 169, 398, 401, 406
  rationale of 406

Decompressive procedures 197
Deep brain
  stimulation 218, 219, 618
  structures 16, 18
Deep cerebral veins 52
Deep cervical plexus block 302, 309, 310
Deep hypothermic circulatory arrest 372
  technique 368, 369
Deep vein thrombosis 241, 243, 267, 274, 353, 453, 487
  prophylaxis 382
Defibrillators 615
Degenerative diseases 204
Degenerative plaques 302
Dehydration 605
Deliberate hypotension 348, 515
Delirium tremens 245
Density spectral array 94
Depression 478
Depth electrodes, removal of 520
Dermatome 22, 599
Desamino-8-D-arginine vasopressin 465
Desflurane 68, 580
Desipramine 200
Desloratadine 162
Device
  failure 616
  loss 539
  types of 532
Dexamethasone 162, 278, 545, 546, 606
  steroid repeat dose of 621
Dexmedetomidine 95, 99, 212, 335, 423, 546
  low-dose 522
Dextran 551
Dextrose 73
Diabetes 247
  worsening 161
Diabetes insipidus 246, 261, 460, 571, 611
  postoperative 464
  propofol-induced 612
  treatment of 465*t*
Diadochokinesia 21
Diastematomyelia 202
Diazepam 224
Diffuse injury 237
Diffusion-weighted imaging 117
Digital nerve compression 199
Digital subtraction
  angiography 332
  imaging system 320*f*

Dilutional coagulopathy, management of 549
Diphenhydramine 321, 606
Diplopia 79
Dipyridamole 608
Disc herniation 29
Disinhibition 297
Disseminated intravascular coagulation 261, 385
Distal emboli entrapment devices 317
Divalproex 596
Dobutamine 587, 589
Dolasetron 162, 286
Doll's eyes 251
Donepezil 265
  binds 6
Dopamine 6, 7, 218, 587, 589
  antagonist 461
  receptor agonist 461
Dorsal column
  ascends 27
  sensation 38
Dorsal group 23
Dorsal horn 22
Dorsal root ganglion 195
Double-ring sign 235
Doxorubicin 247
Doxylamine 162, 606
Driveline infections 538
Droperidol 244, 286
Drug 258, 482
  antiemetic 606
  antiepileptic 265, 278
  antifibrinolytic 207, 559
  anti-hypertensive 308, 621
  antiplatelet 311, 325*t*, 549, 608
  pressor 308
  refractory disease 218
  resistant rigidity 217
  selection 536
  sulfa 243
  third-line 224
  transfers across placenta 491
  withdrawal 283
Dual chamber 614
Dural venous sinuses 52
Durant's maneuver 232
Dynamic visual acuity testing 47
Dysdiadochokinesia 448
Dyslipidemias 151
Dysmetria 21, 448
Dysphagia 217, 288
Dysphoric reactions 297
Dysplastic vessels, region of 186
Dyspnea 183
Dyssynergia 21

Index

E

E-aminocaproic acid 559
Ear, anatomy of 45*f*
Eclampsia triad 489
Edaravone 131
Edema, mixed 390
Ehlers-Danlos syndrome 174, 343
Ejection fraction 261
Elbow 441
Electrical failure 539
Electrical stimulation parameters 102
Electrocardiogram 229
Electroconvulsive therapy 477, 482, 482*t*, 618
   anesthesia for 481
   bilateral 478
   modified 477
   procedures, types of 477
   steps for 481
   ultra-brief 478
   unilateral 477
Electrode
   implantation 448
      technique of 520
   monitoring of depth 520
Electroencephalogram 252
Electroencephalography 65, 92, 93, 238, 571
Electrolyte 294
   imbalances 242, 258, 347, 611, 617
      clinical features of 609
      management of 609
Electromagnetic interference 617
Electromyograph
   indications 95
   technique 95
Electrophysiological monitoring 92, 93*t*, 419
   intraoperative 439
Eliciting pain response, typical sites for 251
Emboli 178
Embolic prevention device 323
Embolism 151
Emergence hypertension 281, 282
Emergence hypotension 282
Emergency surgery 497
Emissary veins 447
Encephalo-duro-arterio-synangiosis 191
   procedure, left 327
Encephalo-myo-synangiosis 191
End-diastolic velocity 152
End-expiratory pressure, positive 184, 230

Endocrine 386
   abnormalities 251
   anatomy 459*f*
   functions 83
   organs 83
   syndromes 459
Endocrinopathies 90
Endoscopic surgery 462
Endoscopic third ventriculostomy 469, 470
Endothelial cells 4, 11-13
Endothelin 361
Endothelin antagonist 361
Endotracheal intubation 287
Endotracheal tube 422, 423, 497, 625
   lumen 523
Endovascular embolization 331, 333
   anesthesia for 334
Endovascular resection 331
Endovascular surgery 257
End-stage renal disease 261
Enflurane 95
Entacapone 218
Enzymatic barrier 12
Ependymal cells 4
Ephedrine 277, 482, 538, 587
Epicritic touch 28
Epidermoid cysts 448
Epidural bolt 111
Epidural hematoma 382
Epilepsy 221, 225, 257, 521, 523
   clinical features of 223*t*
   preoperative assessment of 521
   surgery 294, 565
Epileptic seizure 291
Epinephrine 7, 321, 587, 589, 625
Erythropoietin 361
Escherichia coli 80
Esmolol 277, 482, 591
Esophageal temperature probe 276
Essential tremors 215, 217
   etiology 217
   pathology 217
   treatment of 219*t*
Estrogen 361
Ethosuximide 596
Ethylcysteinate dimer 61
Etomidate 68, 95, 212, 382, 482
Evoked potentials 238, 439
   deteriorates 443
   monitoring 203
Evoked response monitoring 441
Excessive volume resuscitation 207

Extracorporeal shock wave lithotripsy 618
Extra-pyramidal symptoms 507

F

Face, edema of 207
Facial asymmetry 313
Facial trauma 570
Familial cluster 175
Famotidine 162
Fasudil 361
Fatal familial insomnia 506
Febrile reaction 561
Felbamate 294, 596
Femoral
   artery 318, 371
   nerve 246
   vein 327*f*
Fenoldopam 591
Fentanyl 277, 337, 382, 546
Ferromagnetic implants 118
Fetal concerns 490
Fetal monitoring 490, 491
Fever 244
Fiberoptic devices 433
Fibers usually transmit pain, types of 194
Fibrinogen 557
Fibrinolysis 553, 557
   activation of 556*f*
   inhibition of 556*f*
   point of care testing for 555
   test for abnormal 555
Fibromuscular dysplasia 343
Fibrosis 617
Fisher's grade, modified 180
Flecainide 617
Flocculonodular lobe 20
Floppy epiglottis, large 603
Flow metabolism coupling 60, 71
Fluid 79, 232, 383, 564, 605
   associated inversion recovery imaging 507
   attenuated inversion recovery 117
   imbalances 242
   management 499, 609
   overload 532
   replacement formula 604
   resuscitation 549
   selection 384
Flumazenil 483
Fluorescein 415
Fluorodeoxyglucose-PET imaging 292
Focal seizures 223

Follicle-stimulating hormone 85
Foramen of Monro 76, 470
Forbes-Albright syndrome 460
Fornix 18
Fracture, depressed 382
Frazier's point 142
Free radical scavengers 131
Fresh frozen plasma 434, 549, 559
Frontal lobe syndrome 16
Functional residual capacity 487
Fungi 80, 538
Funiculus injury
    lateral 29
    posterior 29
Furosemide 416
    actions of 416
Fusiform aneurysms 174

G

Gabapentin 200, 219, 290, 545, 546, 595
Gag reflex 252, 378
Gait 599
    wide-based 268, 448
Gamma-aminobutyric acid 7, 154, 216f
    antagonists 131
Ganglionectomy 198
Gap junctions 6
Gastric decompression 162
Gastrointestinal system 211
Gateway control theory 195, 196f
Gelfoam 338
Gelofusine 551
Genitourinary system 211
Gentamycin 594
Gerstmann syndrome 17
Gerstmann-Straussler-Scheinker syndrome 506
Gigantism 88, 460
Giraffe, cerebral blood flow of 63
Girard's scale 228
Glasgow coma scale 185, 235, 236t, 379f, 386, 395t
    modified 237
    pitfalls of 236
Glasgow coma score 181
Glasgow outcome scale 238
Glaucoma 516
    acute 512
Glial cells 4
Glial fibrillary protein 238
Glide scope 275, 462
Glioblastoma multiforme 159
    treat 288
Gliomas 159, 447

Globus pallidus 18
Glossopharyngeal nerve block 421
Glucose 65
Glutamate 7
    antagonists 131
    receptors, excitatory 8
Glycine 7
    receptors, inhibition of 560
Glycopyrrolate 308, 482
Gonadotropin 85
    releasing hormone 87
Graft vs. host reaction 561
Graphesthesia 598
Gray commissure injury 29
Gray matter organization 22
Growth hormone 461
    releasing hormone 84, 87
    treatment 79
Guanylyl cyclase 588
Guillain-Barré syndrome 247, 570

H

H_1 blockers, second-generation 162
Haemophilus influenzae 80
Hagen-Poiseuille formula 55
Harner scale 543
Hazards, positioning 453
Head
    fixation, type of 120
    trauma 343
Head injury
    clinical features of 379t
    signs of direct 378
    symptoms of direct 378
Headache 140, 266, 331, 332, 542
    chronic 543
    clinical features of 542
    postural 79
    sudden severe 81
    worsening 269
Hearing, mechanism of 46f
Heart
    disease, congenital 496
    harvest 573
    rate 169, 372, 423, 563
    strain, right 228
Heart failure, chronic 403, 532
    congestive 273, 301, 361, 478, 588, 592, 608, 625
    correction of right 206
Helium release 526
HELLP syndrome 489
Hemangioblastoma 447
Hematoma 282
    decompression of 191

Hemihypesthesia 31
Hemiplegia 155
Hemispheric electroencephalogram, bilateral 370
Hemodilution 360
Hemodynamic 499
    changes 325, 454
    instability 124, 454
    lability, excessive 500
    management 307
    monitoring 307, 317, 348, 419
    status 532
Hemoglobin 551, 552f
Hemolytic reactions, delayed 561
Hemorrhage 144
    intracerebral 189, 282
    intracranial 183, 187, 313, 340, 368, 486, 538, 608
    intraventricular 146, 180, 243
    retinal 179
    sentinel 175, 178, 343
    subdural 282
Hemorrhagic shock 56f
    grades of 563t
Hemorrhagic strokes 153t
Heparin 361, 549
Hepatic micro enzyme inhibitors 607
Hereditary hemorrhagic telangiectasia 331
Herniation syndromes 389, 391
Herniation, impending 381
Hexamethylpropyleneamine oxime 61
High-resolution fluoroscopy 319
Hippocampus 18
Histamine 7
Hoarseness 313
Hoffman's sign 34
Homonymous hemianopsia 528
Horn injury, anterior 33
Horner's syndrome 313
Human growth hormone 85
Human prion diseases 506
Hunt and Hess grade 180, 344
Huntington's chorea 215, 220
Hydralazine 247, 591
Hydration, assessment of 605
Hydrocephalus 77, 78, 146, 257, 288, 469
    acute 170
    classification of 146, 469
    clinical features of 147f
    early 448
    treatment of 150
Hydrocortisone 321
Hydrogen clearance 61

Index

Hydromorphone 546
Hydrostatic brain edema 391
Hyperactive tendon reflexes 29
Hyper-angulated
    videolaryngoscopic
    blades 422
Hyperbaric oxygenation 232
Hypercapnia 58*f*
Hypercoagulability 557
Hyperglycemia 239
Hyperkalemia 617
Hyperlipidemia 288, 301
Hyperosmolar agents 384, 402
Hyperprolactinemia 90
Hyperpyrexia 244, 283
Hypertension 151, 273, 297, 360, 489, 523, 532, 592
  induced 58, 592
  treatment 363
Hypertensive
  bleed 542
  crisis 486
  disease 592
Hyperthermia 239, 243
  malignant 243
Hypertonic agents 169
Hypertonic saline 141, 384, 403*t*, 404
Hyperventilation 60, 95, 139*f*, 141, 169, 395, 396, 402
  aggressive 141
  effects of 59
  levels of 141
  pros and cons of 59
Hypervolemia 360
Hypocapnia 163, 622
  correction 621
Hypoglossal nerve 313
Hyponatremia 299, 435
Hypo-osmolal edema 391
Hypophyseal portal system 86*f*
Hypotension 239, 297, 435, 532, 538, 564, 572
  at induction, treatment of 421
  induced 59, 593
  postural 217
  transient 373
Hypotensive agents 591
Hypothalamic boundaries 83
Hypothalamic hormones 84
Hypothalamic insufficiency 169
Hypothalamic ischemia 348
Hypothalamic sulcus separates 83
Hypothalamic-hypophyseal portal system 84, 85
Hypothalamic-pituitary
  gonadotropic axes 83

hormones 87*t*
  thyroid 83
Hypothalamus 19, 83
  functions 83
Hypothermia 26, 64, 127, 128, 203, 241, 397, 405, 500, 569, 572, 604, 622
  benefits of 127
  clinical status of 127
  induce 241*t*
  intraoperative 352
  mild 241
  treatment 128
Hypotonia 21
Hypovolemia 230, 258
Hypoxemia 297, 545
Hypoxia 239, 391, 526, 625
Hypoxic injuries 293

I

Ibuprofen 200
Idiopathic cardiomyopathy 532
Idiopathic intracranial
  hypertension 140
Immune disorders 293
Immunosuppression leads 561
Immunotherapy 161
Implantable cardiac defibrillators 615
Induction 383, 434, 462
  agents 581
  technique 498
Infection 14, 207, 257, 343, 472
  control strategies 508
  prevention 415
Infective mass lesions 293
Inferolateral injuries 19
Inflammation 617
Inflammatory mediator release 543
Infusion pumps 434
  external 527
Inhaled nitric oxide 537
Injury
  below, side of 36
  consequences of 23*f*
  levels of 36, 430
  manifestations of 29
  mechanism of 125*f*
  posterior 19
  prevention of secondary 434
  primary 209, 377, 391
  secondary 209, 377, 391
  severity score 385
  site 600
  types of primary 209

Inotrope 588
Inotropic receptors 8
Instantaneous blood flow velocity 57*f*
Intensive care unit 353, 370*f*, 550
  postoperative care in 353
  transfer from 406
Internal cardiac defibrillators 613
Internal carotid artery 42*f*, 152, 175, 346
International normalized ratio 265, 399
International Study of Unruptured Intracranial Aneurysms 346
Interstitial cerebral edema 168
Interstitial edema 390
Interventional neuroradiology 336
Interventional radiology suite, setup of 317
Intra-arterial
  blood pressure 535
  vasodilator treatment 360
Intracranial aneurysms, types of 174*f*
Intracranial arteries 50*f*
Intracranial bleed 269, 339
Intracranial compartmental sizes 139*f*
Intracranial compliance curve 113
Intracranial hemorrhage 183, 187, 313, 340, 368, 486, 538, 608
  risk of 181, 275
  significant 337
Intracranial hypotension syndrome 414
Intracranial pressure 67, 68, 137, 163, 169, 171, 181, 241, 258, 394, 550, 592
  dynamic assessment of 112
  monitoring 110
    methods 111*t*
  values 112
  volume 138*f*
Intractable seizures, anesthetic doses for 224
Intraocular pressure 515, 550, 592
Intraparenchymal probe 111
Intrathecal chemotherapy 80
Intratracheal lidocaine 424, 523
Intravascular hemolysis, acute 560
Intravenous anesthetics, effects of 68
Intravenous fluids, characteristics of 609
Intraventricular catheter 111

Intubation 206, 434, 462
  response 349
In-utero surgery 202
Invasive arterial blood
    pressure 536
Invasive neurosurgical
    procedures 201
Iodinated contrast
  allergy 321
  nephropathy, prevention of 322
Ionic edema 167
Ionic homeostasis, disruption
    of 14
Ionotropic receptors 8
Ipsilateral stroke 151
Ipsilateral transient ischemic
    attack 151
Ischemia 391
Ischemic brain
  injury 391
    pathways of 130*f*
    multiple pathways of 154*fc*
Ischemic cardiomyopathy 269, 532
Ischemic lesions 246
Ischemic neurological deficit,
    delayed 181
Ischemic optic neuropathy
    512, 515
  anterior 515, 516
  posterior 515, 516
Ischemic stroke 153*t*, 281, 592
Isoflurane 68
Isonicotinic acid hydrazide 247
Isoproterenol 587, 589, 617

J

J point, elevation of 398*f*
Jackson frame 121
Jaw protraction 420
Jerky movements 293
Judicious narcotic analgesia 502
Jugular bulb 52, 109*f*
Jugular compression, effects
    of 113*f*
Jugular vein compression 112
Jugular venous oximetry 61, 65,
    66, 108
Juvenile myoclonic epilepsy
    223, 293

K

Kainate receptors 9
Keen's point 142
Kernig's sign 179, 599
Ketamine 60, 68, 95, 131, 212, 482,
    502, 545, 546

Ketoconazole 461
Ketorolac 483
Kety-Schmidt method 61
Kinesthesia 28
Kocher's point 142
Kussmaul breathing 601

L

Labetalol 277, 482, 591
Labor, preventing premature 488
Lacosamide 224
Lactate 65
Lactotropes 85
Lamictal 595
Lamotrigine 200
Laryngeal mask airway 431
Laryngeal nerve
  block, superior 421
  inferior 421
Laryngoscopes 275, 497
Laryngoscopy
  direct 275, 431
  test 351
Laser ablation, complications
    of 528
Laser Doppler 61
Laser interstitial thermal therapy
    15, 520, 523
  anesthesia for 527
  indication of 523
  technique of 523
Laser probe, stereotactic
    placement of 527
Leak test 207
Left ventricular
  assist devices 531
  failure 592
  functions 532
Lemniscal pathway 45
Lemniscus, lateral 100
Lennox-Gastaut syndrome 223
Lens 40
  dislocation 512, 515, 517
Leukocyte
  adhesion inhibitors 131
  depleted blood 551
Levetiracetam 224, 595
Levodopa 6, 217
Levosimendan 588, 590
Lidocaine 277, 279, 353, 482, 625
  bolus 337, 523
  effects of 67
Light reflex 251
Limbic system 18
Lindegaard's ratio 182
Listeria monocytogenes 80

Lithium 607
Liver
  dysfunction 539
  function test 294
Local anesthesia 421
Local anesthetic agents 9
Locked-in syndrome 250, 570
Lomustine 160
Loop diuretics 397
Loop recorders 615
Loratadine 162
Lorazepam 162, 219, 224, 285, 606
Low molecular heparin 549
Lower extremity muscles 598
Lower motor neuron lesion 34
Low-pressure ventilation 163, 537
Lubeluzole 131
Lumbar cerebrospinal fluid
    drain 144
Lumbar cistern 75
Lumbar drain
  complications of 144
  management 415
Lumbar puncture 78, 111, 180, 213,
    344, 370*f*
Lumbar symptoms 35
Luminal surfaces 12
Lung
  adenocarcinoma of 547
  maturation 491
Luteinizing hormone 85
Lysine analogs 559

M

MacEwen's crackpot sign 147
Macromolecules, limits influx
    of 14
Magnesium 131, 361
Magnetic resonance imaging
    188, 333
  facility, transport to 527
  functional 64
  perfusion-weighted 61
  scans, types of 117
Magnetic resonance
    spectroscopy 117
Malignancy 80
Mallampati
  classification 264*f*
  grade 420
Mammillary bodies 18
Mania disorders 478
Mannitol 278, 384, 403, 551
  typical dose of 403
Marfan's syndrome 174, 343
Marvelous brains 316

Index

Mass effects 178
Massive bleeding 565
Massive blood transfusion 549, 561
  hazards of 562
Massive catecholamine surge 183
Massive resuscitation 499
Maternal concerns 490
Mean arterial pressure 229, 231,
  306, 487
Mechanical thrombectomy 536
Mechanical ventilation 296
Mechanoreceptors 28
Meclizine 162, 606
Medial geniculate nucleus 100
Medial pathway 33
Median nerve 441
Medulla oblongata 20
Meissner's corpuscles 195
Memory, impaired 17
Meningeal signs 179
Meningioma 160, 448
  right frontal 547
Meningitis 80, 170, 542
Meningocele 201
Mental status 244
Meralgia paresthetica 199
Mesial temporal sclerosis 292
Metabolic abnormalities 251
Metabolic dysfunction 184
Metabolic glutamate receptors 154
Metabolic panel, basic 264
Metabolic receptors 8
Metabolic regulation 60
Metabolic testing 252
Metabotropic receptors 9
Metastasis, detection of 118
Methadone 546
Methohexital 212, 483
  infusions 95
Methylated O6-methylguanine-
  DNA-methyltransferase
  promoter gene 159
Methylene blue 588, 607
Metoclopramide 162, 244, 286, 606
Metoprolol 219, 591
Metronidazole 594
Microcatheters 365
Microdialysis 65
Microglial cells 4
Microsurgical resection 335
Midazolam 224, 277, 335
Mid-brain, anatomy of 20t
Middle cerebral artery 42f, 175f,
  182, 190, 306, 346
Milrinone 184, 361, 587, 590
Minimal sedation technique 296
Minocycline 79

Mitigates hyperthermic injury 241
Mitotane 461
Mixing test 554
Modulation, abnormal 195
Molecular weight 550
Monoamine oxidase inhibitors
  218, 244, 607
Monro-Kellie doctrine 137,
  389, 390
Morbid obesity 295
Morphine 546
Morton's neuroma 199
Motor cortex 31
  primary 31
Motor evoked
  potential 419, 441
  response 101
    monitoring, complications
    of 104
Motor pathway injuries 33
Motor power, clinical assessment
  of 247
Motor system, organization of 31
Motor tracts, organization of 32f
Movement disorders 215, 219, 220
  cluster of 219
Moyamoya disease 189, 343, 486
Muenke syndrome 496
Multimodal analgesia 502
Multiple endocrine neoplasia 459
  syndrome 86
Multipolar neurons 4
Mural cells 12
Muscarinic acetylcholine 6
Muscle
  paralysis 499
  relaxants 382, 498
    properties of 585
  relaxation 206, 383
  rigidity 243
  strength scale 597
  tone, loss of 112
  weakness 29
Muscular dystrophy 204
Muscular hypertrophy 151
Mycotic aneurysms 174
Myelocele 202
Myelomeningocele 202
Myocardial contractility 276
Myocardial dysfunction 348
Myocardial infarction 267, 478, 532
Myocardial injuries 183
Myocardium, neurogenic stunning
  of 348
Myoclonic seizures 222, 292
Myoclonus 507
Myopia 40

N

Naloxone 131
Narcotics 212, 311, 382
  effects of 67
  pharmacokinetics of 336t
  receptors 544t
  supplements 278, 473
Narrow laryngeal inlet 603
Nasal fiberoptic might 420
Nasal speculum 417
Nasogastric tube 383
National Institute of Health Stroke
  Scale 155, 156t
Nausea 161, 162, 266, 297, 501, 607
  prevent postoperative 473
Near-infrared
  light, ability of 116
  spectroscopy 65, 66, 93, 306
Near-sightedness 40
Neck
  flexion 124, 125
  hematoma 313
  movements, range of 420
  rigidity 81, 179
  stiffness 79, 600
Necrotic death 154
Neisseria meningitides 80
Nerve
  conduction studies 247
  decompression 197
  injuries 121, 199, 312
  sheath tumors 160
Nerve fibers
  characteristics of 9t
  classification of 9t
  differential sensitivity of 10
  types of 9
Nerve root 103
  injury, posterior 29
Nerve-muscle biopsy 248
Nervous system 21
  cell 3
    biology of 3
    diversity of 3f
Neural circuits 41
Neural hypothalamic-hypophyseal
  tract 84
Neural stem cells 5
Neural tube defects 146, 257
Neuraxial anesthesia 535
Neuroanesthesia 59, 255, 579,
  592, 605
Neuroanesthetic concerns 272,
  291, 301, 317, 331, 342,
  357, 368, 376, 389, 401,
  411, 419, 428, 439, 446,
  458, 469, 477, 486,
  495, 549

Index

Neurofibromatosis 293
Neurogenic pulmonary edema
    183, 258
Neurogenic shock 210, 432*t*, 435
Neurohypophysis 86
Neuroleptic malignant
    syndrome 244
Neurologic syndromes 210
Neurological assessment 347, 448
Neurological deficits 161, 201,
    206, 528
    postoperative 208
    unmasking of 283
Neurological deterioration 282
Neurological diseases 258
    systemic manifestations of 257
Neurological dysfunction,
    management of
    postoperative 282
Neurological injury 203, 348, 458
    protect against 127
Neurological monitoring 106,
    305, 310
Neurological symptoms 266, 459
Neuromuscular block
    minimal potentiation of 225
    resistance to 225
Neuromuscular junction 7
Neuromuscular monitoring 277
Neuronal death 14
Neuronal functions 240
Neuronal nitric oxide
    synthetase 154
Neurons 3
    first-order 45
    fourth-order 46
    loose cluster of 285
    second-order 28, 45
    third-order 28, 45
Neuro-ocular syndrome 145
Neuropathic pain 193*t*
    syndromes 199
Neuroprotection, cellular
    mechanism of 128
Neurosurgery 486, 560
    positioning during 120
    pregnant patient for 486
Neurosurgical case, preoperative
    assessment of 257
Neurosurgical diseases 181
Neurosurgical interventions 64
Neurosurgical monitoring 492
Neurotransmitters 6
Newtonian fluid 55
Nicardipine 277, 361, 482, 591
Nidus 186
Nimodipine 131, 361

Nitric oxide 361
    antagonists 131
    donor 592
    synthase 361, 588
Nitroglycerine 592
Nitroprusside 592
Nitrous oxide 68, 99, 212, 580
    pros and cons of 69
N-methyl-D-aspartate 7, 154, 198*f*,
    216*f*, 546
Nociceptive receptors 194
Nocturia 217
Noise 525
Non-anesthetic neuroprotective
    agents 129
Non-communicating
    hydrocephalus 78, 146
Nonepileptic seizures 223, 293
Nonfunctioning adenomas 87
Noninvasive blood pressure
    276, 370
    monitoring 538
Nonlemniscal pathway 46
Nonophthalmic surgery 512
Nonsteroidal anti-inflammatory
    drugs 80, 198*f*, 546
Non-thermal interstitial
    electroporation 15
Norepinephrine 7, 196*f*, 587, 589
    doses of 232
Normocapnia 141
Normothermia 241
Nuchal rigidity 599
Nucleus 18, 23
    proprius 23
    tractus solitarius 286
Nystagmus 21, 448

O

Obesity 79, 151
Obstructive sleep apnea 258,
    261, 295
Occipital lobe syndromes 17
Occlusion sequence 305
Octreotide 461
Ocular abnormalities 144
Ocular injuries 121
Ocular movements 565
Ocular signs 112, 448
Oligodendrocytes 4
Olivary complex, superior 100
Omental graft 191
Oncolytic viruses 161
Ondansetron 162, 286, 287,
    483, 606
    doses 607

Operating room, setup of 275
Ophthalmic injuries, site of
    perioperative 514*f*
Opiate antagonists 131
Opioid 68
    analgesia 584
Optic chiasma 42
Optic nerve 42
    blood supply of 514*f*
Optic radiations 42
Optic tracts 42
Optical pathway 42*f*
Optical spectroscopy, diffuse 116
Optimum preharvest donor 568
Oral airways 497
Oral contraceptives 586
Organ failure 572
Organ harvest 568
    anesthesia for 573
Osborn wave 398, 398*f*
Osler Rendu Weber disease 331
Osmolarity 609
Osmotic diuretics 163
Oxacarbazine 595
Oxazolidinone antibiotics 607
Oximetry catheter, placement
    of 109*f*
Oxygen 60, 65
    cascade 106
    consumption 118
    demand 377
    hemoglobin dissociation curve,
        shift of 552
    partial pressure of 107, 552*f*
    supplementation 378
Oxyhemoglobin dissociation curve
    551, 552*f*

P

Pacemaker 613, 617
    assessment, preoperative 616
    complications of 614
    designation of 613
    interrogation of 616
    leadless 614
Pacinian corpuscles 195
Packed cell
    preservation 551
    transfusion 549, 551, 552
Pain 27
    chronic 198*f*
        treatment 197*f*
    hypersensitivity 193
    medications 265
    nociceptive 193*t*
    pathways 544

Index

personification of 200
postoperative 543
post-surgery 207
precordial 228
pretreatment strategy 206
receptors
  modulation of 195
  sensitization of 543
  scale 543
  scores 543*t*
  syndrome 542
  throbbing 547
  vibrating 547
Paine's point 142
Palonosetron 162, 606
Panhypopituitarism 460
Papaverine 361
Papilledema 179, 448
  bilateral 268
Papillomas 160
Paradoxical air embolism 232
Parahippocampal gyrus 18
Paramedian injuries 19
Paraplegia 430
Parasites 80
Parecoxib 545
Parenchymal basement membrane 13
Parietal association cortex 31
Parietal lobe injury
  left 17
  right 17
Parietal lobe syndrome 17
Parietal-temporal lesions 17
Parkinson's disease 215
  clinical features 216
  etiology 215
  idiopathic 215
  pathology 215
  treatment 216*f*, 217, 217*t*
    drugs 265
Paroxysmal supraventricular tachycardia 625
Partial seizure 222, 292
Partial thromboplastin time 265
Patent foramen ovale 369
Pathogenic prion protein 506*f*
Pathological prion proteins 506
Pathological vasoconstriction 62
Pathological waves 114
Peak systolic velocity 152
Pediatric airway 603
  anatomical features of 603*f*
Pediatric anesthesia
    neurodevelopment trial 133
Pediatric coma scale 237

Pediatric neurosurgery 495, 604
Pediatric spine surgery 202
Pediatrics evoked potential monitoring 104
Pegvisomant 461
Penicillin 243
Pentobarbiturate 60
Percent alpha variability 238
Percussion wave 56
Perfusion-weighted scans 117
Pericallosal cistern 74
Peri-cranial tissues 543
Pericytes 4, 13
Peripheral arterial disease 608
Peripheral nerve 197, 198
  injury 29
Peripheral nervous system 7
Peripheral neuropathy 246
  clinical features 247
  etiology 246
Peripheral steroid conversion, block 461
Peripheral vascular
  disease 151, 301
  resistance 592
Peritoneum 471
Persistent hemodynamic instability 501
Persistent vegetative state 250
Pfeiffer's syndrome 497
Pharmacologic neuroprotection 127
Pharmacological burst suppression 397
Pharmacological modulation 60
Phenergan 606
Phenobarbital 224, 596
Phenothiazine 244
Phenoxy bezamine 591
Phentol amine 591
Phenylephrine 277, 279, 423, 482, 538, 587
  pumps for 308
Phenytoin 243, 247, 595
Phosphatidylcholine precursor 131
Phosphodiesterase inhibitor 361, 588, 590, 608
Phospholipases 588
Photophobia 81
Pial arterial plexus 26
Piezoelectric sensors 229
Pin fixation 122
  cons 122
  precautions 122
  pros 122
Piracetam 131

Pituitary adenoma, familial isolated 87
Pituitary anatomy 84*f*
Pituitary apoplexy 89, 460
Pituitary dysfunction 184
Pituitary gland 85
Pituitary hormones 459*f*
  anterior 87
Pituitary insufficiency 459
Pituitary surgery 458
Pituitary syndromes 86
Pituitary tumors 160, 459
  medical management of 461*t*
Plaque
  maturation of 302
  removal 305
Plasma osmolality 609, 612
Plasminogen inhibitor 559
Platelet
  count 554
  function 557
    analyzer 554
    tests 558
  transfusion 549, 558
Pneumocephalus 282
  causes of 289
Pneumonia 258
Pneumonitis 184
Poliomyelitis 33
Polyarteritis nodosa 246, 247
Polycystic kidney disease 343
Polycystic ovary syndrome 79
Polydipsia 460
Polyuria 460
Positron emission tomography 61, 118
Positron imaging technology 66
Postcardiotomy 532
Postclamping 308
Post-craniotomy pain
  inadequate treatment of 544
  management 542, 543
Posterior cord syndrome 210
Posterior fossa 226
  anatomy 446
  surgery 382, 446, 448, 449, 452*t*
  venous system 53
Posterior pituitary 86
  hormones 87
Posterior spinal injury syndrome 38
Postintubation management 423
Postoperative blindness, incidence of 512
Postoperative delirium 284
  management 284
  risk factors 284

Post-surgery management 545
Postsynaptic
  receptors 8
  response 7
Postural tilt 204
Potency *vs.* fentanyl 336
Potential complications 121, 408, 454
Potential interventions 131
Potential neuroprotection targets 131
Pramipexole 217
Prasugrel 608
Preanesthesia evaluation 461
Pre-anesthetic concerns 342
Precordial Doppler 229, 499
Predominant afferent 16
Pre-eclampsia 489
Pregnancy
  physiological changes in 487
  physiological effects of 487*t*
  surgery during 490
Premedication 324
Premotor complex 31
Premotor cortex injury produces 16
Pressure 28
  autoregulation 58
  sores 121
  zero flow 57
Primidone 219, 596
Primitive neuroectodermal tumors 160
Procainamide 625
Procarbazine 161, 607
Prochlorperazine 162, 244
  compazine 606
Prodromal symptoms 178
Prolactin 85
Prolactinomas 87, 88, 461
Promethazine 162, 606
Pronator drift 34
Propofol 60, 68, 95, 212, 224, 277, 279, 287, 308, 335, 337, 382, 383, 405, 423, 482, 483, 581, 606
  induction 225
  infusion of 288
    syndrome 582
  pros and cons of 70
Propranolol 219
Protamine 549
Protease inhibitor 559
Proteins 73
  abnormal 506
Proteinuria 489
Protopathic touch 29

Pseudohyponatremia 610
Pseudotumor cerebri 79
Psychotropic drugs,
  pharmacological
    interaction of 480*t*
Pulmonary artery 229
  catheter 370
  hypertension 232
Pulmonary edema 183
Pulmonary embolism 267, 614
Pulmonary functions 205, 206
  impaired 205
Pulmonary hypertension,
  treatment of 537
Pulmonary injury 183
  etiology 183
Pulmonary vascular resistance 487
Pulsatility index 534
Pulse pressure 350*f*
  analysis 349
Pump
  controls 533
  flow 533
  power 534
  speed 534
  thrombosis 538
Pupil 40
Pupillary abnormalities 570
Pupillary dilation 169
Pupillary response 386
Purpura, post-transfusion 561

Q

Quadrantanopia 528
Quadrigeminal cistern 74
Quality of life 259
Quenching 526

R

Raccoon's eyes 235, 378
Radial nerve 246, 441
Radiation 160, 193
  necrosis 524
  safety 317, 320
  treatment 618
Radicular artery 25*f*, 26
Radiofrequency
  ablation 617
  coils 524
Radionucleotide scan 252
Raised intracranial pressure 78, 137, 272
  clinical signs of 112
  management of 141
  pathology of 137
Ramsay sedation score 334*t*

Ranitidine 162, 606
Rankin's scale, modified 157*t*
Rankin's score, pre-stroke modified 156
Rapid air entrainment 227
Rapid coagulation tests 556
Rapid infusion technology, high flow 564
Rapid-sequence intubation 380
Rasagiline 218
Rathke's pouch 89
Reabsorption 412
Rebleeding, risk of 181
Reconstructive surgery 202
Rectus abdominis 103
Recumbency related 144
Reflexes 598
  tested 598
Reflow phenomenon 57
Refractory arrest 625
Regional anesthesia 248, 302, 308, 310, 491, 535
  conduct of 310
Regional block, post-surgery 546
Regional cooling 128
Regional injuries, effects of 17*f*
Regional scalp block, preoperative 546
Regional techniques 302
Remacemide 131
Remifentanil 279, 288, 423
  low-dose 522
Renal dysfunction 539
Renal failure 347
  acute 403
Reperfusion injury, multiple pathways of 154*fc*
Residual anesthetics 282
Residual cardiac function 534
Residual neck pain 203
Residual neuromuscular blockade 570
Residual paralysis 283
Residual volatile agents 283
Respiratory complications 211
  risk factors for 261
Respiratory concerns 258, 496
Respiratory cycle 350*f*
Respiratory depression 545
Respiratory effects 121
Respiratory failure, postoperative 566
Respiratory function, impaired 258
Respiratory insufficiency 430, 431, 435
Respiratory irregularities 169
Respiratory mechanics 487

Index

Respiratory monitoring 277
Respiratory rate 563
Respiratory volumes 487
Restless leg syndrome 215, 219
Resuscitation 431
    strategy 563
Retching 285
Rete mirabile 49, 190
Reticulospinal tract 33
Retina 41, 42
Retinal signals 41
Rexed laminae 24
Rheumatoid arthritis 247
Rho kinase inhibitor 361
Right atrial junction 450
Right ventricle 231
Right ventricular
    failure 537
    functions 532
    outflow obstruction 228
    outflow tract volume 228
Road mapping function enables 320
Robot-assisted
    electrode implantation, technique of 521
    stereotactic lead implantation, anesthesia for 520
    surgery 520
Rocuronium 277, 279, 382, 423, 482, 585
Romberg's sign, positive 29
Romberg's test 21, 598
    positive 29
Ropinirole 217
Rotational chair 47
Rubrospinal tract 33
Rule out rare causes 172
Ruptured aneurysms 175, 343, 344
Ruptured intracranial aneurysm, complete coil embolization of 365

S

Saccular aneurysms 174
Safe tissue exposure limits 320
Safety precautions 321
Safinamide 218
Saline adenosine dextrose 551
Sampling errors 115
SARS-CoV-2, testing of 263*fc*
Schizophrenia 478
Sciatic nerve 199
Sclerosis, multiple 14, 118
Scoliosis 93, 203, 205
    correction 439

developmental abnormalities of 201
    etiology of 203
    severity of 205
Scopolamine 287
Sedation 310, 544
    doses 336
    score 334
Sedative drug overdose 570
Sedative hypnotics 265
    pharmacokinetics of 335*t*
Saethre-Chotzen syndrome 497
Seizure 161, 169, 170, 222, 297, 331, 332, 489, 560
    absence 222, 223, 292
    activity 95
    classification of 222*t*
    clinical features of 222*t*
    complex partial 222, 596
    disorders 291
    electroencephalographic features of 222*t*
    generalized 222, 223
    mixed 293
    persist 225
    post-traumatic 381
    types and treatment 221
        pathology 221
    unclassified 293
Selegiline 218
Sella turcica permits 458
Sensory
    disassociation 29
    function 598
    system, organization of 27
Sensory cortex 30, 30*f*
    primary 30
    secondary 30
Sensory pathways 27, 29
    organization of 27*f*
Sepsis 538
Septal nuclei 18
Serotonergic syndrome, etiology of 607
Serotonin 7
    antagonist 461
    reuptake inhibitor, selective 244, 480
    syndrome 244, 607
Sevoflurane 68, 95, 580
Shivering 242, 283
    scale 242
Shock
    syndrome, hemodynamic features of 590
    types of 590
Short tau inversion recovery 117

Shunt 312, 471
    centriculoperitoneal 148, 268, 416
    placement 268
    procedures 148
    right-to-left 124, 449
    surgery 149
    ventriculoarterial 148
    ventriculoatrial 124
Sialorrhea 217
Sigmoid sinus 52
Silvius, aqueduct of 77, 470
Single chamber 614
Single-photon emission computed tomography 61, 119
Sinoatrial node 450*f*
Sinus
    inferior petrosal 52
    inferior sagittal 52
    superior 52
Sitting surgery 451
Skin changes 193
Skull deformity 140, 496
Skull-base tumors 160
Sleep apnea 570
Small mouth opening 422
Smooth extubation strategies 424
Smooth wakeup, strategies for 473
Sodium
    balance 612
    bicarbonate 322
    valproate 224
Soft plaque, formation of 302
Solitary intraparenchymal lesions 447
Somatolactotropinomas 87
Somatosensory
    baseline-evoked 421
    evoked potential 93, 97, 98*f*, 212, 307, 382, 419, 440, 441, 571
    monitoring 441*t*
    monitoring, part of 93
Somatostatin 461
Somatotropes 85
Somatotropinomas 87
Sore throat 259, 266
Sotalol 625
Spasticity 29
Specific herniation syndrome 169
Spectral edge frequency 94
Speech function location 297
Spetzler–Martin arteriovenous malformation grading 333
    scale 333*t*
Spheno-parietal sinus 52

Index

Spina bifida occulta 201
Spinal arteries, posterior 24, 26
Spinal canal, surgical enlargement of 419
Spinal cord 16, 25f, 198
  anatomy 22
  blood, segmental 24f
  dorsal root ganglia of 4
  functional anatomy of 22
  hemi-section of 36
  ischemia, preventing 26
  protection 213
  stabilization 213
  syndromes 35
Spinal cord blood flow 24
  organization of 24
  regulation of 26
Spinal cord injury 34
  complete 34
  delayed complications of 213
  levels of 430t
  pathology of 209
  pathophysiology of 209
Spinal deformities 201
Spinal gray matter, organization of 23f
Spinal headache 144
Spinal injuries, shock after 431
Spinal malformations 202
Spinal muscular atrophy 204
Spinal nerve 27
  roots 22
Spinal pain modulation 195
Spinal reflexes 251
Spinal shock 432t, 435
Spinal stenosis 93, 419
Spinal subarachnoid granulations 77
Spinal tracts 23f
Spinal trauma 429
  etiology 429
  pathophysiology 429
Spinal tumor surgery 440
Spine
  developmental abnormalities of 201
  lateral bending of 203
  stability of 433
  trauma 93
  tumor 93, 257
Spine surgery 207, 257
  complex 439
  complications of 207
  intradural 439
  risk factors during 512
Spinocerebellar tract
  anterior 28
  posterior 28

Spinocerebellum, mid-line 20
Splenic infarctions 298
Staphylococci 538
Statins 361
Status epilepticus 223, 596
  absence 221
  management of 223
  treatment of 224t
Stenosis 151
  assessment of 301
  severity of 152
Stent
  contraindication 317
  indications 317
  placement
    anesthesia for 317
    complications of 326
  retriever 157
Stereognosis 598
Steroid 278, 397, 405, 588, 606
  induced diabetes 258
  perioperative 161
  psychosis 283
  replacement 278
  withdrawal 79
Steroidal anti-inflammatory drugs 162
Stiffness 203
Stiles–Crawford effect 40
Stimulation
  artifacts 103
  method 102
  threshold, selection of 483
Stimulatory procedures 198
Stoke 312
Streptococcus pneumonia 80
Stress 243
Striatum 18
Stroke 127, 130, 154, 157, 257, 258, 298, 329, 536, 538
  assessment 155
  etiology of 152
  investigations 156
  precipitating factors 302
  suspected 155
  treatment 155
Stump pressure 306
Subarachnoid hemorrhage 58, 80, 142, 178, 184, 243, 258, 282, 357, 358, 560
  complications of 181
  incidence of 343
  pathology 178
  presentation 178
Subarachnoid space 74, 357
Subclavian artery, right 50f
Subconscious proprioception 28

Subcortical structures 32
Subdural bolt 111
Subdural catheter 111
Subdural hematoma 258, 382
Subhuman primates 131
Sublabial transsphenoid 458
Substantia
  gelatinosa 23
  nigra 18
Subthalamic nuclei 18
Succinylcholine 243, 277, 382, 473, 483, 617
Suction tube 383
Sufentanil 279, 423
Sugammadex 277, 482, 585, 586
Sulfa drugs 243
Sunset sign 147
Supplemental propofol bolus 351
Supplementary motor complex 31
Supraglottic anesthesia 421
Suprascapular nerve 199
Supraspinal pain modulation 196
Surgery
  preparation for 495, 497
  prolonged 207
Surgical complications 331
Surgical management 333
Surgical positionings 121
Surgical resection 331
Sympathectomy 198
Symptomatic vasospasm 181
Synaptic transmission 6
Syndrome of antidiuretic hormone 258
Syndrome of inappropriate antidiuretic hormone 596
  secretion 378, 480
Syndromic craniosynostosis 496
Synostosis 496
Synthetic colloids 551
Syringomyelia 29, 201, 448
Systemic emboli 538
Systemic lupus erythematosus 246
Systemic malignancy 162

T

Tachycardia 243, 297
Takotsubo syndrome 183, 348
Tandem gait, impaired 268
Technetium-99m brain scan 571
Tectospinal tract 33
Temozolomide 160
Temperature 27
Temporal artery, superior 191
Temporal lobe syndrome 17

Index

Tension pneumocephalus 170, 282
   development of 289
Teratogenicity 488, 491
Tethered cord 202
Tetracyclines 79
Tetralogy of Fallot 423
Tetraplegia 430
Thalamic injury 19*t*
Thalamic nuclei 19
Thalamic pain syndrome 19
Thalamocortical projections 100
Thalamotomy, unilateral 219
Thalamus 18, 19, 32
Thermal diffusion 61
Thermoreceptors 9
Thermoregulation, impaired 211
Third ventricle 76
   floor of 471*f*
Thoracolumbar lesion 433
Thrombocytopenia 294
Thromboelastographic parameters 556*f*
Thrombogenesi 155, 211
Thrombosis embolism 614
Thunderclap headache 175, 179, 343
Thyroid hormones 568
Thyroid-stimulating hormone 85
Thyrotoxicosis 460
Thyrotropes 85
Thyrotropin-releasing hormone 84, 87
Tiagabine 596
Tibial nerve, stimulating posterior 98*f*
Ticagrelor 608
Ticlopidine 608
Tidal wave 56
Tinnitus 332
Tissue
   factor activation 557
   injury 378
   oximetry 65, 66
   perfusion 138*f*
      failure of 139*f*
   retraction 592
   trauma 543
   water content, regulation of 13
Tobacco smoke, puff of 189
Tocolytics 488
Todd's paralysis 223
Tolcapone 218
Tongue
   deviation of 313
   injury 207
   large 603
   swelling 207

Tonic seizures 222
Tonic-clonic
   seizures 222
   status epilepticus, generalized 221
Tonsillar herniation during placement 144
Topiramate 219, 595
Total blood volume 563
Total intravenous anesthesia 70, 132, 163, 277, 338, 352, 423*t*, 434, 441
   setup 206
Touch 28
   and vibration 20
Tourette's syndrome 220
Toxins 247
Toxoplasmosis 293
Trachea, angulation of 423
Tramadol 546
Tranexamic acid 559
Tranquilizers 219
Transalar herniation 394
Transcarotid artery revascularization procedures 317, 326, 327*f*
Transcranial Doppler 61, 93, 107, 252, 571
   ultrasound 107
Transcranial magnetic stimulation 478
Transcranial motor evoked potentials 102*f*, 440
Transduction, abnormal 193, 194
Transesophageal Doppler 228
Transesophageal echocardiogram 229, 231, 535
Transesophageal echocardiography, role of 349
Transforms
   associated circulatory overload 561
   endogenous cellular prion proteins 506*f*
   reaction 243
Transient cerebral ischemia 66
Transient circulatory arrest 352, 372
   methods 368
Transient ischemic attacks 298
Transmural pressure 345
Transplant organs 568
Transsphenoid hypophysectomy 458
   clinical presentation 459

   investigations 461
   treatment 461
Transsphenoid surgery 458
Transtentorial herniation 392, 393
   upward 394
Trauma 515
Traumatic brain injury 127, 169, 181, 234, 236, 257, 293, 386
   assessment of 236
   clinical features 235
   high-risk 238
   magnetic resonance imaging assessment of 238
   management of 376
   pathophysiology of 376
   serum markers of 237
Tremors 20
   causes of 219
Trendelenburg position 311
Trigeminal neuralgia 199
Trigger arrhythmias 614
Triggering agents 243
Trihexyphenidyl 218
Triphasic response 479
Trismus 243
Truncal ataxia 448
Tryptophan 607
Tubb's point 142
Tube selection 463
Tuber cinereum 83
Tuberous sclerosis 293
Tumor 448, 486
   blood flow 163
      autoregulation 163
   excisions 294
   fourth ventricle 448
   resection 164
   treatment modalities 160
Tylenol 621
Tympanic membrane displacement 111
Tyrosine kinase inhibitors 161

U

Ulnar nerve 441
Ultrasonic guidance 535
Uncinate seizure 223
Unipolar leads 615
Unstable angina 478
Upper extremity 598
Upper motor neuron lesion 34
Upper respiratory infection
   diagnosis of 262
   differential diagnosis of 262*t*
Urinary catheter 381

Index

Urinary output 276
Urinary tract infection 267, 435
Urinary urgency 217
Urine
  osmolality 460
  output 563
  parameters 611
Urticarial reaction 561
Uterine blood flow 488

V

Valproic acid 201, 224, 294, 595
Valsalva maneuver 415
Valvular heart disease 369
Vancomycin 594
Vascular access 161, 206, 317, 318, 499, 604
  assessment of 347
Vascular clamps, guarded release of 305
Vascular complications 203
Vascular lumen 151
Vascular malformation 257
Vascular pedicle 191
Vascular resistance 55
Vascular sacrifice 345
Vascular territories 42*f*
Vasculitis 246
Vasodilator synthesis 588
Vasogenic brain edema 390
Vasogenic edema 166
Vasopressin 588, 589, 625
Vasopressors 587, 588
Vasospasm 282
  differential diagnosis of 358
  incidence of 357
  pathology of 358
  systolic blood pressure, settings of 281
Vena cava
  inferior 450*f*
  superior 450, 450*f*
Venous air embolism 226, 500
  detection of 229
  during neurosurgery, risk of 226
  hemodynamic effects of 227
  pathology 226
  prevention of 230
Venous sinus injury, superficial 53

Venous system, arrangement of 52
Ventilation 380, 499
  difficult 498
Ventral group 24
Ventricular assist device 531
Ventricular drain 81
  external 243, 364
  placement 536
Ventricular ectopy 183
Ventricular pacing 614
Ventricular tachycardia 372, 625
Ventriculostomy 142
  indications 142
  landmarks 142*t*
  third 148
Verapamil 361, 365
  blocks voltage-gated calcium channels 360
Vertebral artery injury 203
Vertebrates 4
Vestibular pathway 45
Vestibular schwannomas 448
Vestibulocochlear dysfunction 144
Vestibulospinal tracts 33
Vibratory sense, loss of 29
Vincristine 161
Viral myocarditis 532
Viscoelastic clot properties 556
Viscosity, reduction of 56
Vision loss 79
  causes of postoperative 512
  incidence postoperative 513
  management of postoperative 514
  postoperative 512
  prevention of postoperative 514
  risk factors postoperative 513
Vision painless
  impairment of 516
  loss of 517
Visual changes 179
Visual cortex 42
Visual disturbances 90, 414
Visual evoked responses 100, 101*f*, 440
  indications 100
  technique 100
Visual field
  anomaly 42

  cuts 79
  defects 42*f*, 528
Visual loss 79
Visual pathway 40, 42*t*
Visual signs 140
Visual symptoms 140, 507
Visual system
  functions of 40
  organization of 40
Vital brain region 159
Vital signs 112, 274, 283, 398
Vitamin
  A overdose 79
  B_{12} deficiency 246
Volatile 68
  agents 60, 68, 212, 243, 473
    pros and cons of 69
    suppress evoked responses 99
  anesthetics 132, 580
    vasodilate cortical vessels 339
Volume replacement 549
Volume resuscitation 276
Vomiting 140, 161, 162, 266, 297, 501, 607
  prevent postoperative 473
von Willebrand's disease, acquired 537

W

Wada test 292, 333
Warfarin 265
Water balance 612
Waves, plateau of 169
Weight gain 161
Werner syndrome 86
Wernicke aphasia 17
West syndrome 223
Whiplash injury 429
Willis–Ekbom disease 219
Wilson's disease 220
Winston Churchill's strokes 330
Wound closure, start of 424
Wrist 441
  abnormal 496

Z

Zonisamide 219, 595

EU GSPR Authorised Reprsentative
Logos Europe, 9 rue Nicolas Poussin
1700, La Rochelle, France
Phone: +33 (0) 6 67 93 73 78
E-mail: contact@logoseurope.eu

www.ingramcontent.com/pod-product-compliance
Ingram Content Group UK Ltd.
Pitfield, Milton Keynes, MK11 3LW, UK
UKHW051846210426
5322IPUK00019B/282